Cancer Epidemiology

METHODS IN MOLECULAR BIOLOGY™

John M. Walker, SERIES EDITOR

METHODS IN MOLECULAR BIOLOGY™

Cancer Epidemiology

Volume II
Modifiable Factors

Edited by

Mukesh Verma, PhD

Division of Cancer Control and Population Sciences, National Cancer Institute, Bethesda, Maryland

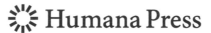 Humana Press

Editor
Mukesh Verma
Division of Cancer Control and Population Sciences
Bethesda, Maryland 20892
USA

Series Editor
John M. Walker
School of Life Sciences
University of Hertfordshire
Hatfield, Hertfordshire, AL10 9AB, UK

ISBN: 978-1-60327-491-3   e-ISSN: 1940-6029
ISSN: 1064-3745   e-ISBN: 978-1-60327-492-0
DOI: 10.1007/978-1-60327-492-0

Library of Congress Control Number: 2008938206

Printed on acid-free paper

9 8 7 6 5 4 3 2 1

springer.com

Preface

Population studies facilitate the discovery of genetic and environmental determinants of cancer and the development of new approaches to cancer control and prevention. Furthermore, epidemiology studies play a central role in making health policies. Cancer epidemiology may address a number of research areas such as:

- familial predispositions to colon cancer and breast cancer study to determine whether families who carry a genetic predisposition to breast cancer may also be at risk of colon cancer, and vice versa;

- prospective examination of whether baseline dietary intakes and serum levels of carotenoids and vitamin A are associated with subsequent risk of lung cancer;

- analysis of the relationship between serum levels of sex-steroid hormones and genetic polymorphisms in biosynthesis enzymes in a prospective cohort of pre-menopausal women;

- analysis of the role of HLA-Class II similarity/dissimilarity between sexual partners and the role in HIV transmission, using the multicenter hemophilia cohort study population for the data set;

- multiple comparisons and the effect of stratifying data on study power.

This two-volume set compiles areas of research that cover etiological factors or determinants that contribute in the development of cancer as well as describe the latest technologies in cancer epidemiology. Emphasis is placed on translating clinical observations into interdisciplinary approaches involving clinical, genetic, epidemiologic, statistical, and laboratory methods to define the role of susceptibility genes in cancer etiology; translating molecular genetics advances into evidence-based management strategies (including screening and chemoprevention) for persons at increased genetic risk of cancer; identifying and characterizing phenotypic manifestations of genetic and familial cancer syndromes; counseling individuals at high risk of cancer; investigating genetic polymorphisms as determinants of treatment-related second cancers; and pursuing astute clinical observations of unusual cancer occurrences that might provide new clues to cancer etiology. All the chapters in these two books are divided into three categories:

Volume 1:

> Cancer Incidence, Prevalence, Mortality, and Surveillance
>
> Methods, Technologies, and Study Design in Cancer Epidemiology
>
> Host Susceptibility Factors in Cancer Epidemiology

Volume 2:

> Modifiable Factors in Cancer Epidemiology
>
> Epidemiology of Organ-Specific Cancer

These chapters have been written in a way that allows readers to get the maximum advantage of the methods involved in cancer epidemiology. Several examples of specific organ sites would be helpful in understanding cancer etiology.

Mukesh Verma, Ph.D.

Contents

Contributors

VOLKER ARNDT, M.D., M.P.H. • *Division of Clinical Epidemiology and Aging Research, German Cancer Research Center, Heidelberg, Germany*

MARC BISSONNETTE, M.D. • *Department of Medicine, University of Chicago, Chicago, IL, USA*

EVE BOURGKARD, Ph.D. • *Department of Occupational Epidemiology, INRS, Vandoeuvre, France*

NORMAN F. BOYD, M.D., D.Sc. • *The Campbell Family Institute for Breast Cancer Research, Ontario Cancer Institute, Toronto, Canada*

HERMANN BRENNER, M.D., M.P.H. • *Division of Clinical Epidemiology and Aging Research, German Cancer Research Center, Heidelberg, Germany*

MAI BROOKS, M.D., F.A.C.S. • *Division of Surgical Oncology, School of Medicine, University of California, Los Angeles, CA, USA*

IRENE BRÜSKE-HOHLFELD, M.D. • *Institute of Epidemiology, Helmholtz Zentrum München, German Research Center for Environmental Health (GmbH), Neuherberg, Germany*

ROBERT G. CARLILE, M.D. • *Department of Surgery and Pathology, University of Hawaii School of Medicine, Honolulu, HI, USA*

ROBERT CARROLL, M.D. • *Department of Medicine, University of Illinois Chicago, IL, USA*

JEFFREY S. CHANG, M.D., Ph.D., M.P.H. • *Department of Epidemiology and Biostatistics, University of California, San Francisco, CA, USA*

KAMRAN CHAUDHARY, M.D. • *Department of Medicine, University of Illinois, Chicago, IL, USA*

CHIN HIN CHO, Ph.D. • *Department of Pharmacology, Faculty of Medicine, The Chinese University of Hong Kong, Shatin, N.T., Hong Kong, China*

YVONNE M. COYLE, M.D. • *Department of Internal Medicine, UT Southwestern Medical Center, Dallas, TX, USA*

MARIE DESMEULES, M.Sc. • *Centre for Chronic Disease Prevention and Control, Public Health Agency of Canada, Ottawa, Ontario, Canada*

ALECIA MALIN FAIR, Dr.PH. • *Department of Surgery, Meharry Medical College, Nashville, TN, USA*

TAKASHI FUKAGAI, M.D. • *Department of Surgery and Pathology, University of Hawaii School of Medicine, Honolulu, HI, USA*

JOHN L. HOPPER, Ph.D. • *Centre for Molecular, Environmental, Genetic and Analytic Epidemiology, University of Melbourne, Australia*

SHARAD KHARE, Ph.D. • *Department of Medicine, Loyola University, Maywood, IL, USA*

ANNE E. KILTIE, M.A., D. M. MRCP(UK), F.R.C.R. • *Molecular Radiobiology Group, Cancer Research UK Clinical Centre, St James's University Hospital, Leeds, West Yorkshire, UK*

ARTO LEMINEN, M.D., Ph.D. • *Department of Obstetrics and Gynecology. HUCH Hospital Area, Hospital District of Helsinki and Uusimaa, Helsinki, Finland*

OTTO S. LIN, M.D., M.Sc. • *Digestive Diseases Institute, Virginia Mason Medical Center, Seattle, WA, USA*

JAN LUBINSKI, M.D. • *International Hereditary Cancer Center, Pomeranian Medical University, Szczecin, Poland*

LISA J. MARTIN, Ph.D. • *The Campbell Family Institute for Breast Cancer Research, Ontario Cancer Institute, Toronto, Canada*

MICHAEL MICHAEL, B.Sc. (Hons), M.B.B.S (Hons), FRACP. • *GI Clinical Service, Division of Haematology and Medical Oncology, Peter MacCallum Cancer Centre, Victoria, Australia*

SALOMON MINKIN, Ph.D. • *The Campbell Family Institute for Breast Cancer Research, Ontario Cancer Institute, Toronto, Canada*

KARA MONTGOMERY, Dr.PH. • *Department of Health Promotion, Education, and Behavior, University of South Carolina, Columbia, SC, USA*

MIKIO NAMIKI, M.D. • *Department of Urology, Kanazawa University School of Medicine, Kanazawa, Japan*

THOMAS NAMIKI, M.D. • *Department of Surgery and Pathology, University of Hawaii School of Medicine, Honolulu, HI, USA*

HIROKO OHGAKI, Ph.D. • *Pathology Group, International Agency for Research on Cancer, Lyon, France*

SAI YI PAN, M.D. • *Centre for Chronic Disease Prevention and Control, Public Health Agency of Canada, Ottawa, Ontario, Canada*

CHRISTOPHE PARIS, M.D., Ph.D. • *Department of Occupational Health and Epidemiology, Medical School, Vandoeuvre, France*

ANDREW D. PATERSON, M.B., B.Ch. • *Department of Public Health Sciences, University of Toronto, Toronto, Canada*

JENNIFER PERMUTH-WEY, M.S. • *Division of Cancer Prevention and Control, H. Lee Moffitt Cancer Center and Research Institute, Tampa, FL, USA*

ISAAC J. POWELL, M.D. • *Department of Urology, Wayne State University Detroit, MI, USA*

BEVERLY S. REIGLE, Ph.D., R.N. • *College of Nursing, University of Cincinnati, Cincinnati, OH, USA*

ANNIKA RISKA, M.D. • *Department of Obstetrics and Gynecology, Hospital District of Helsinki and Uusimaa, Helsinki, Finland*

JOHANNA M. ROMMENS, Ph.D. • *Program in Genetics and Genomic Biology, The Hospital for Sick Children, Toronto, Canada*

DIETRICH ROTHENBACHER, M.D., M.P.H. • *Division of Clinical Epidemiology and Aging Research, German Cancer Research Center, Heidelberg, Germany*

RODNEY J. SCOTT, Ph.D., FRCPath. • *Discipline of Medical Genetics, School of Biomedical Sciences, Faculty of Health, University of Newcastle and the Hunter Medical Research Institute, Newcastle New South Wales, Australia*

HELMUT K. SEITZ, M.D. • *Department of Medicine, and Center of Alcohol Research, Liver Disease and Nutrition, Salem Medical Center, University of Heidelberg, Heidelberg, Germany*

THOMAS A. SELLERS, Ph.D. • *Division of Cancer Prevention and Control, H. Lee Moffitt Cancer Center and Research Institute, Tampa, FL, USA*

MAHDU S. SINGH, M.B.B.S. • *Division of Haematology and Medical Oncology, Peter MacCallum Cancer Centre, Victoria, Australia*

JENNIFER STONE, Ph.D. • *Centre for Molecular, Environmental, Genetic and Analytic Epidemiology, University of Melbourne, Australia*

CHEE-KEONG TOH, M.B.B.S, MRCP. • *Department of Medical Oncology, National Cancer Centre, Singapore*

PASCAL WILD, Ph.D. • *Department of Occupational Epidemiology, INRS, Vandoeuvre, France*

HEINRIC WILLIAMS, M.D. • *Department of Urology, Wayne State University Detroit, MI, USA*

KAREN WONDERS, Ph.D. • *Department of Health, Physical Education and Recreation, Wright State University, Dayton, OH, USA*

MARTIN J. YAFFE, Ph.D. • *Imaging Research, Sunnybrook and Women's Health Sciences Centre, and Department of Public Health Sciences, University of Toronto, Toronto, Canada*

WEI ZHENG, M.D., Ph.D. • *Vanderbilt Epidemiology Center and Vanderbilt-Ingram Cancer Center, Vanderbilt University School of Medicine, Nashville, TN, USA*

Contents of Volume I

Part I

Modifiable Factors in Cancer Epidemiology

Chapter 1

Environmental and Occupational Risk Factors for Lung Cancer

Irene Brüske-Hohlfeld

Abstract

Lung cancer is the world's leading cause of cancer death. It is primarily due to the inhalation of carcinogens and highly accessible to prevention by diminishing exposures to lung carcinogens. Most important will be the complete cessation of exposure to cigarette smoke (first and second hand) and to asbestos. Two environmental exposures—radon in homes and arsenic in drinking water—cannot be totally avoided, but people in certain geographical regions would greatly benefit from a reduction in exposure magnitude. And last but not least, workers all over the world deserve that preventive measures at the workplace are observed with regard to exposures, such as arsenic, beryllium, bis-chloromethyl ether (BCME), cadmium, chromium, polycyclic aromatic hydrocarbons (PAHs), and nickel.

Key words: Lung cancer, cigarette smoke, asbestos, radon in homes, arsenic in drinking water, beryllium, bis-chloromethyl ether (BCME), cadmium, chromium, nickel, polycyclic aromatic hydrocarbon (PAH).

1. Introduction

1.1. Short Descriptive Epidemiology

Incidence and mortality rates for lung cancer have risen dramatically since the turn of the last century. In 1878, malignant lung tumors represented only 1% of all cancers seen at autopsy in the Institute of Pathology of the University of Dresden in Germany *(1)*. By 1918, the percentage had risen to almost 10%, and, in 2004, lung cancer was the most common cause of cancer death (27% of all cancer deaths) in men in the European community, resulting in a lifetime risk of dying from lung cancer of 5.5% *(2)*. In the USA, 215,020 new cases and 161,840 deaths from lung

M. Verma (ed.), *Methods of Molecular Biology, Cancer Epidemiology, vol. 472*
© 2009 Humana Press, a part of Springer Science+Business Media, Totowa, NJ
Book doi: 10.1007/978-1-60327-492-0

cancer are predicted for 2008[1]. Worldwide lung cancer causes the largest disease burden of all cancers, accounting for more than 1.2 million new cases annually, a figure that is still increasing.

The likelihood of getting lung cancer increases with age. Only one in ten patients diagnosed with this disease will survive the following 5 years. While smoking prevalence has declined in many developed countries, it is increasing in developing countries and also among women. Throughout the world the incidence of lung cancer among men exceeds, usually by twofold or more, that among women. This sex difference is shrinking, however, as gender differences in smoking have become less pronounced. Although the causes of lung cancer are almost exclusively environmental, it is likely that there is a substantial individual variation in the susceptibility to respiratory carcinogens. The risk of the disease can be conceptualized as reflecting the joint consequences of the interrelationship between exposure to etiologic/protective agents and the individual susceptibility to these agents. A familial aggregation of lung cancer has been described in numerous studies, including segregation analyses *(3)*, and a higher concordance for monozygotic than for dizygotic twins has been noted *(4)*. However, it is still open to what degree the familial aggregation of lung cancer can be explained by heritability of cancer susceptibility compared with 'inheritance' of smoking behaviour and other factors, such as passive smoking and eating habits.

1.2. The Lung as a Main Entry Portal to the Organism

The lung consists of two different parts, the airways transporting the air in and out of the lung and the alveoli, which consist of specialized cells that form millions of tiny, exceptionally thin-walled air sacs (~200 nm) for gas exchange. Whereas the airways have a relatively robust barrier of ciliated epithelium and viscous mucus—the so-called mucociliary escalator—the gas exchange region is only protected by alveolar macrophages. During a typical day, the average adult inhales about 10,000 L air. All inhaled gases diffuse from the alveolar air to the blood in the pulmonary capillaries, as carbon dioxide diffuses in the opposite direction, from capillary blood to alveolar air. The large surface of the alveoli and the intense air blood contact is often illustrated by the metaphor of one wineglass of blood spread over the surface of a tennis court. As permeability is the main function of the alveoli, there are structural and functional limits to act at the same time as a barrier against inhaled gases and particles, including bacteria and viruses. The phagocytosis of particles and fibres from the

---

[1]http://www.cancer.gov/cancertopics/types/lung

inhaled gas induces macrophages to release chemokines, cytokines, reactive oxygen species, and other mediators that can lead to a sustained inflammation and eventually to fibrotic changes.

Lung cancer develops through a series of progressive pathological changes occurring in the respiratory epithelium. According to the histological appearance of the malignant cells, lung cancer can be classified into small cell lung cancer and non-small cell lung cancer. Although this classification based on simple pathomorphological criteria has very important implications for clinical management and prognosis of the disease, it generally cannot be used to distinguish between the potential exposures that might have caused it.

1.3. Risk Factors of Lung Cancer

What is accepted as a "known" risk factor of lung cancer is judged differently all over the world, and is heavily influenced by political, financial, and industrial interests. Trying to find an objective point of view, the International Agency for Research on Cancer (IARC) is considered as an organization adopting such a neutral scientific position. The IARC is an arm of the World Health Organisation (WHO). It conducts and promotes epidemiological and laboratory-based research and training, and is most famous for its series 'Monographs on the Evaluation of Carcinogenic Risks to Humans'[2]. Based on animal and human data, interdisciplinary working groups of expert scientists—selected on the basis of competence and the absence of conflicts of interest— review published studies and evaluate the weight of the evidence that an agent can increase the risk of cancer. They assign an agent, mixture, or exposure circumstance to one of five categories:

- Group 1 (agent is carcinogenic to humans)
- Group 2a (agent is probably carcinogenic to humans)
- Group 2b (agent is possibly carcinogenic to humans)
- Group 3 (agent is not classifiable regarding its carcinogenicity)
- Group 4 (agent is agent is probably not carcinogenic to humans).

The principles, procedures, and scientific criteria that guide the evaluations are described in the Preamble to the IARC Monographs[3]. Group 1 pulmonary carcinogens, which will be covered in this chapter, include arsenic *(5, 6)*, asbestos *(7)*, beryllium *(8)*, bis-chloromethyl ether (BCME) *(8)*, cadmium *(8)*, chromium (VI) *(9)*, nickel *(9)*, radon *(10)*, silica *(11)*, as well as active *(12)* and passive smoking *(13)*.

---

[2]http://monographs.iarc.fr/
[3]http://monographs.iarc.fr/ENG/Preamble/index.php

2. Environmental and Occupational Exposures

2.1. Arsenic

Arsenic is widely distributed throughout the earth's crust and is introduced into the groundwater by dissolution of minerals and ores. Arsenic contamination of groundwater has occurred in various parts of the world, most notably the Ganges Delta of Bangladesh and West Bengal, India, but parts of Thailand, Taiwan, Argentina, Chile, and China have also been affected.

Inorganic arsenic can occur in the environment in several forms but in natural waters, and thus in drinking water, it is mostly found as trivalent arsenite, As(III), or pentavalent arsenate, As (V). Drinking water poses the greatest threat to public health from arsenic. Absorption of arsenic through the skin is minimal and thus hand-washing, bathing, laundry, etc. with water containing arsenic do not pose a human health risk. Organic arsenic species, abundant in seafood, are very much less harmful to health, and are readily eliminated by the body.

In Bangladesh, West Bengal (India), and some other areas, it was common practice to collect drinking water from open dug wells and ponds. This water was often contaminated with micro-organisms contributing to transmitting diseases, such as diarrhea, dysentery, typhoid, cholera, and hepatitis. To prevent morbidity and mortality from gastrointestinal disease in children, the United Nations Children's Fund (UNICEF) started a program to install tube-wells to provide what was then thought to be a safe source of drinking water *(14)*. However, in 1993 it was discovered that about half of these wells contained arsenic levels of greater than the maximum level of 50 µg/L permitted in Bangladesh. The WHO recommendations on the acceptability and safety of levels of arsenic in drinking water are even lower, having dropped 20-fold, from a concentration of 200 µg/L in 1958 to 10 µg/L in the 1993 WHO Drinking Water Guidelines[4]. The latest statistics indicate that 80% of Bangladesh and an estimated 40 million people are at risk of arsenic poisoning-related diseases, including lung cancer, because the ground water in these wells is contaminated with arsenic *(15)*.

Long-term exposure to arsenic via drinking water causes skin changes such as pigmentation changes and thickening (hyper-keratosis), and, after a latency period, various cancers of the skin, lungs, urinary bladder, and kidney, liver, and colon. An increased risk of lung, probably from inhalation of water vapor, has been

---

[4]http://www.who.int/mediacentre/factsheets/fs210/en/index.html

observed at drinking water arsenic concentrations of 350–1140 μg/L[5]. According to some estimates, arsenic in drinking water will cause 200,000–270,000 deaths from all cancers in Bangladesh *(14)*.

Arsenic is used in wood preservatives and pesticides, and industrial emissions may also be significant locally. Occupational exposure to inorganic arsenic, especially in mining and copper smelting, has very consistently been associated with an increased risk of cancer. An almost tenfold increase in the incidence of lung cancer was found in workers most heavily exposed to arsenic, and relatively clear dose—response relationships have been obtained with regard to cumulative exposure *(16)*. Other US smelter worker populations have been shown to have consistent increases in lung cancer incidence *(17)*. A dose—response analysis indicated that the roasters and arsenic departments were risk places for the development of cancer, especially lung cancer, among Swedish smelter workers *(18)*.

2.2. Asbestos

The term asbestos refers to a family of naturally occurring, flexible, fibrous hydrous silicate minerals. Although many minerals can crystallize in fibrous, asbestiform habit, only a few have been of industrial use, like chrysotile, anthophyllite, crocidolite, amosite, and tremolite. The crystal structure of chrysotile, which represents 94% of world asbestos consumption, is snakelike (hence also named "serpentine"); the others are called amphibole minerals. Asbestos is of commercial interest because of properties such as resistance to heat and traction, flexibility and ease of spinning for textile products, chemical resistance to alkalines, all giving rise to a startling range of uses *(19)*. From the beginning of the 20th century, world production of asbestos grew steadily escalating after World War II in a rush for asbestos cement and textile products, vinyl asbestos floor tile, friction materials, and spray products to name just a few. In Western Europe, Scandinavia, North America, and Australia, the manufacture and use of asbestos products peaked around 1970 with about 5 million tons/year.

Deposition of inhaled asbestos fibers is diffuse through the lung and extends to the subpleural lung tissue. Clearance of asbestos fibers occurs by a variety of pathways, including the mucociliary escalator, the translocation into the interstitium to the lymphatic system and the dissolution, degradation and breakdown of the original material. Fibers <3 μm are phagocytosed and eliminated via the lymphatics. But, if fibers are longer than 5 μm, phagocytosis will be incomplete and they will stay in the tissue longer. This will initiate and sustain a cascade of events leading

---

[5]http://www.who.int/water_sanitation_health/dwq/arsenic2/en/

first to local and later to more diffuse fibrosis, named asbestosis of the lungs. The relative toxicity of different forms and structures of asbestos minerals can be linked to their morphology—long, thin amphibole fibers are more pathogenic. Asbestos is not a classic gene mutagen in bacterial systems, but it does have the capacity to induce chromosomal aberrations and transformation in mammalian cells.

Problems stemming from the inhalation of asbestos in milling and manufacturing plants had been observed since the turn of the century. Early reports *(20–22)* linking asbestos and cancer of the lung in the 1950–1960s laid the foundation for the definitive investigations of insulation workers in the USA by Irving Selikoff and his colleagues *(23)*. A very good historical overview of the growing evidence of adverse health effects related to asbestos exposure is given in the article by the European Environmental Agency (EEA) "Late Lessons from Early Warnings: The Precautionary Principle 1896–2000"[6].

Asbestos-induced lung cancer is generally characterized by a latency period of 20 years or longer between start of exposure and onset of the disease. In a mortality follow-up of 17,800 US and Canadian asbestos insulation workers *(24)*, there was a twofold increase of lung cancer during the period 10–14 years after initial employment, reaching nearly sixfold 30–34 years after employment, and declining at longer intervals. Because of the long latency period, the peak level of lung cancer and mesothelioma—a form of cancer that is extremely rare in the general population and much more specific to asbestos exposure than lung cancer, as it is not associated with smoking—has not been reached yet. Peto et al. *(25)* predicted that deaths from mesothelioma among men in Western Europe would increase from just over 5,000 deaths per year in 1998 to about 9,000 per year in 2018. In Western Europe alone, past asbestos exposure will give rise to a quarter of a million deaths from mesothelioma over the next 35 years. The number of lung cancer deaths caused by asbestos is at least equal to the number of deaths from mesothelioma, but the ratio may be higher.

Worldwide many million of workers have been exposed to asbestos at the workplace. About 20–40% of adult men report some past occupations and jobs that may have entailed asbestos exposure at work *(26, 27)*. A number of studies have projected the number of premature deaths that will result from the asbestos cancer epidemic *(27–29)*. When the various estimates from these and other studies are extrapolated to include the world popula-

---

[6]http://reports.eea.europa.eu/environmental_issue_report_2001_22/en/issue-22-part-05.pdf

tion, they project that at least 100,000 workers die each year from asbestos exposure resulting in cancer *(29)*. In this conservative estimate, it is assumed that asbestos exposures are going to cease and that the epidemic will run itself out. But the world's production of asbestos, which went down by half in 1990s due to the asbestos ban in many developed countries, seems to have stabilized now at around 2 million tons/year *(30, 31)*.

By the beginning of 2006, 39 countries in Europe, the Americas, the Middle East, and Australia had imposed national bans. With dwindling markets in developed countries, the global asbestos industry is focusing on emerging markets in developing countries. Asbestos use in developing countries is increasing at an annual rate of 7%. Asia has emerged as one of the largest markets for asbestos consumption, with China, India, Japan, Indonesia, and South Korea among the world's top ten consumers in the year 2000 *(31)*. Asian countries accounted for about 60% of the global asbestos consumption in the year 2000 *(32)*. Only Singapore and recently Japan have adopted a total ban on asbestos. The only way to assure an end to the asbestos cancer epidemic is to ban all asbestos mining and manufacture, which will be even more necessary in developing countries, where enforcement of health and safety regulations is not a viable alternative. But, even if exposure to asbestos were to stop soon, somewhere between 5 and 10 million people would ultimately die from asbestos related diseases [7] .

How much the ubiquitous low-dose exposure to asbestos fibres in the environment contributes to the burden of lung cancer in the general population is not known. Camus and co-workers found no measurable excess of death due to lung cancer among women in two chrysotile asbestos-mining areas in the province of Quebec *(33)*. However, there is some evidence that family members and others living with asbestos workers have an increased risk of developing mesothelioma. For example, Schneider and co-workers *(34)* described six fatal diseases of pleural mesothelioma: five wives and one son of asbestos industry workers. The wives had been exposed to asbestos fibres while cleaning the contaminated work clothes and shoes of their husbands at home, and the son used to visit his father throughout his childhood at the workplace. Even pet dogs may develop mesothelioma if their owners are exposed to asbestos *(35)*.

2.3. Beryllium

Beryllium is most commonly used in high-tech devices where it is bound into electronic components. Although only a relatively small number of workers worldwide are potentially exposed to high levels of beryllium, mainly in the refining and machining of

---

[7]http://www.bwint.org/pdfs/chrysotileasbestos.pdf

the metal and in production of beryllium-containing products, a growing number of workers are potentially exposed to lower levels of beryllium in the aircraft, aerospace, electronics, and nuclear industries.

Ward et al. *(36)* reported the results of a cohort mortality study of 9,225 workers at seven beryllium plants in the USA, where a small but significant excess in mortality from lung cancer was found in the total cohort. The risk of lung cancer was consistently higher in those plants in which there was also excess mortality from non-malignant respiratory disease. Also, the risk for lung cancer increased with time since first exposure and was greater in workers first hired in the period when exposures to beryllium in the work place were relatively uncontrolled.

The IARC *(8)*, the National Toxicology Program, and the American Conference of Governmental Industrial Hygienists (ACGIH) have classified beryllium as a human carcinogen, but only at airborne exposure levels well in excess of the current occupational exposure limits. The US Environmental Protection Agency (EPA) classifies beryllium as a probable human carcinogen and the European Union states that beryllium may cause cancer by inhalation.

However, a reanalysis of the original data from the 1992 publication *(36)* of a cohort mortality study conducted by the National Institute of Occupational Safety and Health (NIOSH) of workers employed in seven plants producing beryllium in the USA found lower and generally not statistically significant standard mortality ratios that are not compatible with the interpretation of a likely causal association *(37)*.

2.4. Bis-Chloromethyl Ether and Chloromethyl Methyl Ether

In the past, bis-chloromethyl ether (BCME) was used to make several types of polymers, resins, and textiles. In 1962, suspicion arose that an excess of lung cancers was developing in a chemical plant. A prospective cohort study of 125 male workers was begun, and the group was followed from January 1963 to the end of 1979. A small epidemic of respiratory cancer evolved, including 14 cases of lung cancer and 2 cases of laryngeal cancer among 91 men exposed to chloromethyl ethers (CMEs) in the 17-year period, as compared with 2 cases of lung cancer among 34 unexposed men. The lung cancer epidemic peaked 15–19 years after onset of exposure and began to subside thereafter *(38)*. Numerous epidemiological studies have demonstrated that workers exposed to chloromethyl methyl ether and/or BCME have an increased risk for lung cancer *(39–41)*. Among heavily exposed workers, the relative risks (RRs) are tenfold or more. Risks increase with duration and cumulative exposure and latency is shortened among workers with heavier exposure. Histological evaluation indicates that exposure results primarily in lung cancer of the small cell type.

The small quantities that are produced nowadays are only used in enclosed systems to make other chemicals. Strict controls have been established to minimize exposure to this chemical [8] in the USA and worldwide.

2.5. Cadmium

Cadmium is used in electroplating for the manufacture of automotive, aircraft, and electronic parts, and marine equipment and industrial machinery. Cadmium compounds serve as stabilizers for plastics and as pigments. Cadmium is also widely used in nickel—cadmium storage batteries and is combined with other metals in alloys. Most exposure to cadmium and its compounds occurs in the working environment via inhalation.

Experimentally, cadmium induces lung tumors in rats, but various epidemiological studies of cadmium-exposed workers did not show any clear results due to concomitant exposures to other occupational carcinogens, mainly nickel and arsenic. In a cohort mortality study conducted at a US plant where cadmium metals and compounds were processed since 1925, Stayner et al. *(42)* observed an excess in mortality from lung cancer for the entire cohort. Mortality from lung cancer was greatest among workers in the highest cadmium exposure group, and among workers with 20 or more years since the first exposure. A statistically significant dose—response relationship was evident in nearly all of the regression models evaluated.

2.6. Chromium (VI)

Chromium occurs primarily in the trivalent state, in which it is unable to enter cells and has a low toxicity. However, hexavalent chromium, Cr (VI), enters the cell through membrane anionic transporters. It is a strong oxidizing agent, as well as a skin and mucous membrane irritant. At the cellular level, Cr exposure may lead to cell cycle arrest, apoptosis, premature terminal growth arrest, or neoplastic transformation. Cr-induced DNA—DNA interstrand crosslinks (DDC), the tumor suppressor gene p53, and oxidative processes are some of the major factors that might play a significant role in determining the cellular outcome in response to Cr exposure *(43)*. The increased risk of lung cancer occurs primarily in workers exposed to hexavalent chromium dust during the refining of chromite ore and the production of chromate pigments *(44, 45)*. Chromium is a human carcinogen primarily by inhalation exposure in occupational settings *(46)*; little is known about the health risks of environmental exposures to chromium.

---

[8]http://www.atsdr.cdc.gov/tfacts128.html

2.7. Nickel

Nickel is used in many industrial and consumer products, including stainless steel, magnets, coinage, and special alloys. It is also used for plating and as a green tint in glass. Nickel is preeminently an alloy metal, and its chief use is in the nickel steels and nickel cast irons.

A large epidemiologic report on cancer mortality in 10 cohorts of occupationally exposed workers showed *(47)* that the mortality from cancers of the lung was associated with exposure to high levels of oxidic nickel compounds, exposure to sulfidic nickel in combination with oxidic nickel, and exposure to water-soluble nickel, alone or together with less soluble compounds.

Grimsrud and co-workers demonstrated a dose-related association between lung cancer and cumulative exposure to water-soluble nickel compounds *(48)*. In a case—control study of Norwegian nickel refinery workers, the authors examined dose-related associations between lung cancer and cumulative exposure to four forms of nickel: water soluble, sulfidic, oxidic, and metallic. A job-exposure matrix was based on personal measurements of total nickel in air and the quantification of the four forms of nickel in dusts and aerosols. The nickel exposures were moderately to highly correlated. A clear dose-related effect was seen for water-soluble nickel (odds ratio, 1.7; 95% confidence interval (CI], 1.3–2.2). A general rise in risk from other types of nickel could not be excluded, but no further dose-dependent increase was seen.

2.8. Particulate Air Pollution

Particulate matter (PM) is a complex mixture of airborne solid and liquid particles including soot, organic material, sulfates, nitrates, other salts, metals, and biologic material. Many carcinogens, including a multitude of polycyclic aromatic hydrocarbons (PAHs), adsorb to particles and can be deposited throughout the respiratory tract. Also, combustion of fossil fuels is a source of arsenic in the environment through disperse atmospheric deposition.

Air pollution may increase lung cancer risk in a number of ways. Inhalation of fine particles can lead to production of radical oxygen species that cause DNA damage, which can lead to cancer. Some of the metals that are found in fine PM are carcinogenic. Several studies found an association between external measures of exposure to air pollution and increased levels of DNA adducts, with an apparent levelling-off of the dose—response relationship. The experimental work, combined with the data on frequent oxidative DNA damage in lymphocytes in people exposed to urban air pollution, suggests 8-oxo-dG as one of the important promutagenic lesions *(49)*.

In general, ambient levels of PM are characterized as total suspended matter (TSP), or PM with an effective aerodynamic diameter of less than 10 μm (PM_{10}) or 2.5 μm ($PM_{2.5}$). Particles in the sub micrometer ranges, particularly in the size range

<100 nm, are labelled as ultrafine particles in epidemiology. The number concentration of these small particles exceeds by far that of larger ones in the urban area, but their contribution to the total mass concentration, which is measured on a routinely basis nowadays in the USA and Europe, is relatively low. Typically, the biological activity of particles increases as the particle size decreases and surface area becomes larger. Alveolar deposition is highest for inhaled ultrafine particles of about 20 nm diameter, higher than for any other particle size (50). Thus, although inhaled mass concentration of ultrafine particles in urban areas may be low, numbers of ultrafine particles in the alveolar region of the lung may be very high. Studies on rodents demonstrate that ultrafine particles administered to the lung cause greater inflammatory response than do larger particles per given mass (51).

Air pollution has always been an attractive explanation for the 10–40% increase in lung cancer mortality observed in urban versus rural areas, but confounding from smoking and other factors has been a great limitation in interpreting geographical comparisons (52). Two large American cohort studies showed a link between air pollution and lung cancer: in the Harvard Six Cities Study—a prospective cohort study—exposure was estimated on the basis of average levels of pollution over the risk period from 1974 through 1989, assuming residential stability. For 8,111 residents of six US cities, individual-level information was available for age, gender, smoking habits, body mass index, and education, all confounders or potential effect modifiers. In the cohort, 1,429 deaths occurred, 120 due to lung cancer. The difference in the long-term average PM concentrations between the most and least polluted cities was approximately 20 µg/m³ and the RR of lung cancer was increased (RR 1.37). Assuming a linear relationship between exposure and lung cancer, the RR increased by approximately 19% per 10 µg/m³ increase of PM (53).

The second study was the American Cancer Society study that followed the mortality of approximately 500,000 adult men and women from 1982 to 1998. Participants were assigned to metropolitan areas of residence, and mean PM 2.5 concentrations were compiled for each metropolitan area from several data sources. Personal information on risk factors (confounders or effect modifiers) was collected by questionnaire at enrolment. The last follow-up in 2002 (54) indicated a significantly increased mortality risk ratio for lung cancer (RR 1.14; 95% CI, 1.04–1.23) for a difference of 10 µg/m³ of PM 2.5. These results were controlled for age, gender, race, smoking, education, marital status, body mass, alcohol consumption, occupational exposure, and diet.

Several recent studies have addressed whether socioeconomic position modifies the health effects of particulate air pollution (55). The majority of studies evaluating individual-level characteristics showed higher effects (in general) among those of lower socioeconomic position. Low educational attainment seems to be a particularly consistent indicator of vulnerability in these studies. Groups with lower socioeconomic position may receive higher exposure to air pollution at work and at home, living closer to major roads, and they may experience compromised health status due to material deprivation, psychosocial stress, and personal behaviour. International organizations have identified both air pollution and poverty as priority areas for public health intervention, as approximately 1 billion people live in poverty (World Bank 2002; http://www.worldbank.org/) and an estimated 1.5 billion people currently live in polluted urban areas (WHO, 2000).

When interpreting the findings regarding the impact of air pollution on the general population, it should not be forgotten that one main component of urban air pollution will always be diesel motor emissions (DME) coming from a wide variety of sources, including large trucks, earth-moving equipment, farm machinery, and diesel-powered cars. Most epidemiological studies show an association between exposure to DME and lung cancer risk *(56)*. In the light of biological plausibility, making a causal inference seems to be justified, as DME contain both highly mutagenic substances *(57)* and recognized human carcinogens *(58)*. Increased levels of human peripheral blood DNA adducts are associated with occupational exposure to DME *(59)*. Furthermore, DME have been shown to induce lung cancer in laboratory animals *(60, 61)*.

2.9. Radon

Radon, as well as polonium-218 and polonium-214, are characterized by alpha radiation, a type of radioactive decay in which an atom emits an alpha particle (two neutrons and two electrons) and transforms into an atom with a mass number 4 less and atomic number 2 less. The range of alpha radiation in the body is limited to less than 100 μm, which implies that the skin is a sufficient barrier against alpha radiation, but the alveolar epithelium is not. When radon gas itself is inhaled, most is exhaled before it decays. But, if solid decay products are deposited in the lung, they undergo further radioactive decay, releasing energy in the form of alpha particles that can either cause double-stranded DNA breaks or create free radicals that can also damage the DNA and thereby cause lung cancer. A small part of the inhaled radon and its progeny may be transferred from the lungs to the blood and finally to other organs, but the corresponding doses and associated cancer risk are negligible compared with the lung cancer risk.

Originating from the decay of uranium and thorium contained in the crust of the earth, radon gas and its solid decay products occur naturally in the air worldwide. Its concentration depends on the highly variable uranium content of the soil. Due to dilution in the air, outdoor levels of radon are generally low in comparison with what can be found indoors. Radon gas enters houses through openings such as cracks at concrete floor—wall junctions, gaps in the floor, small pores in hollow-block walls, and through sumps and drains. Exchange of indoor air with the outside exerts a strong influence on indoor air concentration of radon and depends on the construction of the house, the sealing of windows, and the ventilation habits of the inhabitants. Consequently, radon levels are usually higher in basements, cellars, or other structural areas in contact with soil. Even higher radon concentrations can be found in places such as mines, caves, and water treatment facilities.

For a century, it has been known that some underground miners suffered from higher rates of lung cancer than the general population. During the past three decades, several epidemiological studies (for example, refs. (62–72)) on uranium miners have been conducted, all showing an increased risk of lung cancer. The connection between radon and lung cancer in miners has raised concern that radon in homes might be causing lung cancer in the general population. Studies in Europe, North America, and China have confirmed that radon in homes contributes substantially to the occurrence of lung cancers worldwide. A recent pooled analysis of European studies estimated the risk of lung cancer increased by 8.4% (95% CI, 3.0–15.8%) per 100 Bq/m^3 increase in measured radon (p=0.0007). This corresponds to an increase of 16% (5–31%) per 100 Bq/m^3 increase in usual radon—that is, after correction for the dilution caused by random uncertainties in measuring radon concentrations (73). The dose—response relation seems to be linear without evidence of a threshold.

In 1999, the National Research Council published the BEIR VI report, which confirms that radon is the second leading cause of lung cancer in the USA, accounting for 15,000 to 22,000 lung cancer deaths per year in the USA. One of the most comprehensive case—control epidemiologic radon studies, performed by Field and colleagues (74), demonstrated a 50% increased lung cancer risk with prolonged radon exposure at the EPA's action level of 4 pCi/L. A systematic analysis of pooled data from seven large-scale case—control studies of residential radon studies was undertaken to provide a more direct characterization of the public health risk posed by prolonged radon exposure. The combined data set included a total of 4,081 cases and 5,281 controls. Residential radon concentrations were determined primarily by α-track detectors placed in the living areas of homes of the study subjects in order to obtain an integrated 1-year average radon concentration in indoor air. Conditional likelihood regression was used to estimate the excess risk of lung cancer due to residential radon exposure, with adjustment for attained age, sex, study, smoking factors, residential mobility, and completeness of radon measurements. For subjects who had resided in only one or two houses in the 5–30 exposure time window and who had α-track radon measurements for at least 20 years of this 25-year period, the excess odds ratio was 0.18 (0.02, 0.43) per 100 Bq/m³. Recent pooled epidemiologic radon studies by Dan Krewski et al. *(75, 76)* have also shown an increased lung cancer risk from radon below the US EPA's action level of 4 pCi/L.

2.10. Silica

The chemical compound silicon dioxide (SiO_2), also known as silica, is one of the most common minerals in the continental crust. Sand mostly consists of silica, usually in the form of quartz, but there are many other crystalline forms—like, for example, cristobalite and tridymite. Whereas silica in the environment do not present a public health problem, in occupational settings, such as mines, stone quarries and granite production, ceramic and pottery industries, steel production, and sandblasting, silica can provoke fibrotic changes and cancer of the lung, especially if inhaled as freshly ground crystalline silica dust.

Several studies have been published on the relation between occupational silica exposure and lung cancer. In a review of epidemiological studies between 1996 and 2005 *(77)*, the pooled RR of lung cancer, calculated using random effects models, from all cohort studies was 1.34. The RR was higher, 1.69, in cohort studies of silicotics only. The pooled RR was 1.41 for all case—control studies. And, again, the RR was 3.27 in case—control studies of silicotics only. In summary, in this re-analysis, the association with lung cancer was consistent for silicotics, but less clear for non-silicotics. This leaves open the question whether silicosis is a surrogate for a more pronounced exposure relating to higher cancer risk or whether is in itself a prerequisite in the development of lung cancer.

In a pooled data set of 10 cohort studies, Steenland and co-workers *(78)* examined a total of 65,980 subjects, two thirds of them miners. There were 1,072 deaths from lung cancer. The authors found an increasing trend in risk of lung cancer with cumulative silica exposure: RR 1.0 (95% CI, 0.85–1.3); RR 1.3 (95% CI, 1.1–1.7); RR 1.5 (95% CI, 1.2–1.9); and RR 1.6 (95% CI, 1.3–2.1) compared with the lowest quintile. This dose—risk relation supports the conclusion of a causal relationship.

2.11. Smoking

Current research indicates that the factor with the greatest impact on risk of lung cancer is long-term exposure to inhaled tobacco smoke from cigarettes. But other forms of tobacco smoking, such as cigars and pipes, also increase risks for cancer of the lung, cancer of the head and neck, and other cancers. The particulate phase of the smoke contains most of the 55 carcinogens identified by the IARC *(12)*. Of these, polycyclic aromatic hydrocarbons and the tobacco-specific nitrosamine 4-(methylnitrosamino)-1-(3-pyridyl)-1-butanone are likely to play major roles *(79)*. Also, the alpha-emitting radioisotope polonium-210 has been identified by the US EPA as a cause of lung cancer in humans when inhaled. Nicotine itself is not considered to be carcinogenic. Smoking produces gene mutations and chromosomal abnormalities. Urine from smokers is mutagenic and tobacco smoke is assessed as geno-toxic in humans and experimental animals by the IARC.

The US Centers for Disease Control and Prevention describes tobacco use as "the single most important preventable risk to human health in developed countries and an important cause of premature death worldwide". On average, cigarette smokers die about 10 years younger than nonsmokers, and stopping at age 60 years, 50 years, 40 years, or 30 years gains, respectively 3, 6, 9, or 10 years of life expectancy (80).

Although tobacco smoking accounts for the majority of lung cancer, approximately 10% of patients with lung cancer in the USA are lifelong never smokers, women disproportionately more often than men (81).

2.12. Second-Hand Tobacco Smoke

Second-hand tobacco smoke, also known as environmental tobacco smoke (ETS), is a mixture of the smoke given off by the burning end of tobacco products (side stream smoke) and the mainstream smoke exhaled by smokers. Because side stream smoke is generated at lower temperatures and under different conditions than mainstream smoke, it contains higher concentrations of many of the toxins found in cigarette smoke, such as formaldehyde, lead, arsenic, benzene, and radioactive polonium-210.

Second-hand smoke was first considered as a possible risk factor for lung cancer in 1981 when two studies were published that described increased lung cancer risk among never-smoking women who were married to smokers. In a case—control study from Athens, the odds ratio of lung cancer associated with having a husband who smokes was 3.4 for nonsmoking women whose husbands smoked more than one pack of cigarettes per day (82). In a study from Japan 91,540 non-smoking wives aged 40 years and older were followed up for 14 years (1966–1979), and standardized mortality rates for lung cancer were assessed according to the smoking habits of their husbands. Wives of heavy smokers were found to have a higher risk of developing lung cancer and a dose—response relation was observed (83).

More than 50 studies of involuntary smoking and lung cancer risk in never smokers, especially spouses of smokers, have been published during the last 25 years. Meta-analyses of those studies show that there is a statistically significant and consistent association between lung cancer risk in spouses of smokers and exposure to second-hand tobacco smoke from the spouse who smokes. Furthermore, meta-analyses of lung cancer in never smokers exposed to second-hand tobacco smoke at the workplace have found a statistically significant increased risk of lung cancer[9].

---

[9]http://www.cdc.gov/tobacco/data_statistics/Factsheets/LungCancer.htm

The National Research Council *(84)* estimated in 1986 that almost one fourth of lung cancer cases among non-smokers could be attributed to passive smoking. In May 2006, the US government's Centers for Disease Control issued its first new study on second-hand smoke in 20 years. Surgeon General Richard Carmona summarized, "The health effects of second hand smoke exposure are more pervasive than we previously thought. The scientific evidence is indisputable: second hand smoke is not a mere annoyance. It is a serious health hazard that can lead to disease and premature death in children and non-smoking adults." The study estimated that living or working in a place where smoking is permitted increases the non-smokers' risk of developing lung cancer by 20–30%.

The US EPA, the National Institutes of Health National Toxicology Program, and the IARC have concluded that second-hand smoke is a known human carcinogen. If it occurs at the workplace, it is considered to be an occupational carcinogen (NIOSH).

3. Outlook

Although lung cancer is the world's leading cause of cancer death, it is also highly accessible to prevention by diminishing exposure to known lung carcinogens. So, looking on the bright side, these are the options for prevention:

Number one on the list is tobacco *smoking*. As a response to the global tobacco epidemic "The Tobacco-Free Initiative" was established by the WHO in 1998[10]. The WHO Framework Convention on Tobacco Control (FCTC) was the first public health treaty negotiated under the auspices of the WHO[11]. It was unanimously adopted by the WHO's 192 Member States in May 2003. It officially entered into force in 2005 and, by the end of 2006, the total number of contracting parties had reached 142, covering more than three quarters of the world's population. In the end, the prevention of smoking seems to be on the way.

Less successful has been the call for a global ban on *asbestos* sales, though national bans on asbestos exist in most industrialized countries. If a substance such as chrysotile is too hazardous

[10]http://www.who.int/tobacco/resources/publications/TFI%20primer-English.pdf
[11]http://www.who.int/tobacco/framework/download/en/index.html

to be used in industrialized countries, it should not be exported; if it is exported, then full disclosure of the hazards should be made mandatory. But, the Rotterdam Convention, an international treaty governing trade in toxic substances, which creates legally binding obligations for the implementation of the Prior Informed Consent (PIC) procedure, failed to agree to add chrysotile to a list of more than 30 substances about which exporting countries must inform importers before shipping[12]. While the inclusion of chrysotile asbestos on the PIC list of the Rotterdam Convention does not constitute a ban on global sales, it would at least have enabled developing economies to make informed decisions on whether they wish to import a chemical that has been found to be carcinogenic by the International Labor Organization, the WHO, the IARC, the International Program on Chemical Safety, the Collegium Ramazzini, and the World Trade Organization.

Current levels of radon in dwellings and other buildings are of public health concern. The US EPA recommends fixing the home if radon levels exceed 4 pCi/L[13]. Radon levels less than 4 pCi/L still pose a risk, and in many cases may be reduced. A person living in an average European house with a *radon* concentration of 50 Bq/m^3 has a lifetime excess lung cancer risk of $1.5-3\times10^{-3}$. A lifetime lung cancer risk below about 1×10^{-4} cannot be expected to be achievable because the natural concentration of radon in ambient outdoor air is about 10 Bq/m^3. Nevertheless, the risk can be reduced effectively based on procedures that include optimization and evaluation of available control techniques. In general, simple remedial measures should be considered for buildings with radon progeny concentrations of more than 100 Bq/m^3 or 2.7 pCi/L equilibrium equivalent radon as an annual average, with a view to reducing such concentrations wherever possible[14].

The scale of the contamination of drinking water by *arsenic* in Bangladesh has rightly been called a mass poisoning, with millions of people exposed. A United Nations Foundation grant was approved in 2000 to enable UNICEF and the WHO to support a project to provide clean drinking water alternatives to 1.1 million people in three of the worst-affected sub-districts in Bangladesh[15]. The project utilizes an integrated approach involving communication, capacity building for arsenic mitigation of all stakeholders at subdistrict level and

---

[12]http://www.lkaz.demon.co.uk/chrys_hazard_rott_conv_06.pdf
[13]1 pCi/L equals 37 Bq/m^3
[14]http://www.euro.who.int/document/e71922.pdf
[15]http://www.who.int/mediacentre/factsheets/fs210/en/

below, tube-well testing, patient management, and provision of alternative water supply options. Urgent requirements include a large-scale support to the most severely affected populations, with a simple, reliable, and low-cost equipment for field measurement of arsenic levels in drinking water as well as robust and affordable technologies for arsenic removal at wells and in households.

References

1. Witschi H., (2001) A short history of lung cancer, *Toxicol. Sci.* **64** pp 4–6.
2. Boyle P., and Ferlay J., (2005) Cancer incidence and mortality in Europe, 2004, *Ann. Oncol.* **16** pp 481–488.
3. Sellers T. A., Chen P. L., Potter J. D., Bailey-Wilson J. E., Rothschild H., Elston R. C., (1994) Segregation analysis of smoking-associated malignancies: evidence for Mendelian inheritance, *Am. J. Med Genet.* **52** pp 308–314.
4. Braun M. M., Caporaso N. E., Page W. F., Hoover R. N., (1995) A cohort study of twins and cancer, *Cancer Epidemiol. Biomarkers Prev.* **4** pp 469–473.
5. International Agency for Research on Cancer, (1980) IARC Monographs Volume 23: Some Metals and Metallic Compounds, IARC, Lyon.
6. International Agency for Research on Cancer, (1987) IARC Monographs on the Evaluation of the Carcinogenic Risk of Chemicals to Humans. Supplement 7 Overall evaluations of carcinogenicity: An updating of IARC Monographs Volumes 1 to 42, **IARC**, Lyon.
7. International Agency for Research on Cancer, (1977) IARC Monographs Volume 14: Asbestos, **IARC**, Lyon.
8. International Agency for Research on Cancer, (1993) IARC Monographs Volume 58: Beryllium, Cadmium, Mercury, and Exposures in the Glass Manufacturing Industry, **IARC**, Lyon.
9. International Agency for Research on Cancer, (1990) IARC Monographs Volume 49: Chromium, Nickel and Welding, **IARC**, Lyon.
10. International Agency for Research on Cancer, (1988) IARC Monographs Volume 43: Man-Made Mineral Fibres and Radon, **IARC**, Lyon.
11. International Agency for Research on Cancer, (1997) IARC Monographs Volume 68: Silica, Some Silicates, Coal Dust and para-Aramid Fibrils, **IARC**, Lyon.
12. International Agency for Research on Cancer, (1986) IARC Monographs Volume 38: Tobacco, **IARC**, Lyon.
13. International Agency for Research on Cancer, (2004) IARC Monographs Volume 83: Tobacco Smoke and Involuntary Smoking 2004, **IARC**, Lyon.
14. Smith A. H., Lingas E. O., Rahman M., (2000) Contamination of drinking-water by arsenic in Bangladesh: a public health emergency, *Bull. World Health Organ.* **78** pp 1093–1103.
15. Alam M. G., Allinson G., Stagnitti F., Tanaka A., Westbrooke M., (2002) Arsenic contamination in Bangladesh groundwater: a major environmental and social disaster, *Int. J. Environ. Environ Health Res.* **12** pp 235–253.
16. Lee Feldstein A., (1989) A comparison of several measures of exposure to arsenic. Matched case-control study of copper smelter employees, *Am. J. Epidemiol.* **129** pp 112–124.
17. Enterline P. E., Henderson V. L., Marsh G. M., (1987) Exposure to arsenic and respiratory cancer. A reanalysis, *Am. J. Epidemiol.* **125** pp 929–938.
18. Wall S., (1980) Survival and mortality pattern among Swedish smelter workers, *Int. J. Epidemiol.* **9** pp 73–87.
19. Alleman J. E., and Mossman B. T., (1997) Asbestos revisited., *Sci. Am.* **July** pp 54–57.
20. Doll R., (1955) Mortality from lung cancer in asbestos workers, *Br. J. Ind. Med.* **12** pp 81–86.
21. Wagner J. C., Sleggs C. A., Marchand P., (1960) Diffuse pleural mesothelioma and asbestos exposure in the North Western Cape Province, *Br. J. Ind. Med.* **17** pp 260–271.
22. Tweedale G., (2000) Science or public relations? The inside story of the asbestosis research council, 1957–1990, *Am. J. Ind. Med.* **38** pp 723–734.
23. Selikoff I. J., Churg J., Hammond E. C., (1964) Asbestos exposure and neoplasia, *JAMA.* **188** pp 22–26.

24. Selikoff I. J., Hammond E. C., Seidman H., (1979) Mortality experience of insulation workers in the United States and Canada, 1943–1976, *Ann N Y. Acad. Sci.* **330** pp 91–116.

25. Peto J., Decarli A., La Vecchia C., Levi F., Negri E., (1999) The European mesothelioma epidemic, *Br. J. Cancer* **79** pp 666–672.

26. Brüske-Hohlfeld I., Mohner M., Pohlabeln H., Ahrens W., Bolm-Audorff U., Kreienbrock L., Kreuzer M., Jahn I., Wichmann H. E., Jockel K. H., (2000) Occupational lung cancer risk for men in Germany: results from a pooled case-control study, *Am. J. Epidemiol.* **151** pp 384–395.

27. Goldberg M., Banaei A., Goldberg S., Auvert B., Luce D., Gueguen A., (2000) Past occupational exposure to asbestos among men in France, *Scand. J. Work Environ. Health.* **26** pp 52–61.

28. Howie R. M., (2001) Asbestos and cancer risk, *Ann Occup. Hyg.* **45** pp 335–336.

29. Tossavainen A., (2004) Global use of asbestos and the incidence of mesothelioma, *Int. J. Occup. Environ. Environ Health.* **10** pp 22–25.

30. LaDou J., (2003) International occupational health, *Int. J. Hyg. Environ. Environ Health.* **206** pp 303–313.

31. LaDou J., (2004) The asbestos cancer epidemic, *Environ. Environ Health Perspect.* **112** pp 285–290.

32. Takahashi K., and Karjalainen A., (2003) A cross-country comparative overview of the asbestos situation in ten Asian countries, *Int. J. Occup. Environ. Health.* **9** pp 244–248.

33. Camus M., Siemiatycki J., Meek B., (1998) Nonoccupational exposure to chrysotile asbestos and the risk of lung cancer [see comments], *N. Engl J. Med.* **338** pp 1565–1571.

34. Schneider J., Straif K., Woitowitz H.-J., (1996) Pleural mesothelioma and household asbestos exposure, *Rev. Environ. Health.* **11** pp 65–70.

35. Glickman L. T., Domanski L. M., Maguire T. G., Dubielzig R. R., Curg A., (1983) Mesothelioma in pet dogs associated with exposure of the owners to asbestos, *Environ. Res.* **32** pp 305–313.

36. Ward E., Okun A., Ruder A., Fingerhut M., Steenland K., (1992) A mortality study of workers at seven beryllium processing plants, *Am. J. Ind. Med.* **22** pp 885–904.

37. Levy P. S., Roth H. D., Hwang P. M., Powers T. E., (2002) Beryllium and lung cancer: a reanalysis of a NIOSH cohort mortality study, *Inhal. Toxicol.* **14** pp 1003–1015.

38. Weiss W., (1982) Epidemic curve of respiratory cancer due to chloromethyl ethers, *J. Natl. Cancer Inst.* **69** pp 1265–1270.

39. Figueroa W. G., Raszkowski R., Weiss W., (1973) Lung cancer in chloromethyl methyl ether workers, *New. Engl. J. Med.* **288** pp 1096–1097.

40. Albert R. E., Pasternack B. S., Shore R. E., Lippmann M., Nelson N., Ferris B., (1975) Mortality patterns among workers exposed to chloromethyl ethers—a preliminary report, *Environ. Health Perspect.* **11** pp 209–214.

41. Pasternack B. S., Shore R. E., Albert R. E., (1977) Occupational exposure to chloromethyl ethers. A retrospective cohort mortality study (1948–1972), *J. Occup. Med.* **19** pp 741–746.

42. Stayner L., Smith R., Thun M., Schnorr T., Lemen R., (1992) A dose-response analysis and quantitative assessment of lung cancer risk and occupational cadmium exposure [see comments], *Ann. Epidemiol.* **2** pp 177–194.

43. Singh J., Carlisle D. L., Pritchard D. E., Patierno S. R., (1998) Chromium-induced genotoxicity and apoptosis: relationship to chromium carcinogenesis (review), *Oncol. Rep.* **5** pp 1307–1318.

44. Barceloux D. G., (1999) Chromium, *J. Toxicol. Clin. Toxicol.* **37** pp 173–194.

45. Birk T., Mundt K. A., Dell L. D., Luippold R. S., Miksche L., Steinmann-Steiner-Haldenstaett W., Mundt D. J., (2006) Lung cancer mortality in the German chromate industry, 1958 to 1998, *J. Occup. Environ. Environ Med.* **48** pp 426–433.

46. Luippold R. S., Mundt K. A., Austin R. P., Liebig E., Panko J., Crump C., Crump K., Proctor D., (2003) Lung cancer mortality among chromate production workers, *Occup. Environ. Med.* **60** pp 451–457.

47. Report of the International Committee on Nickel Carcinogenesis in Man, (1990) *Scand. J. Work Environ. Environ Health.* **16** pp 1–82.

48. Grimsrud T. K., Berge S. R., Haldorsen T., Andersen A., (2002) Exposure to different forms of nickel and risk of lung cancer, *Am. J. Epidemiol.* **156** pp 1123–1132.

49. Vineis P., and Husgafvel-Pursiainen K., (2005) Air pollution and cancer: biomarker studies in human populations, *Carcinogenesis.* **26** pp 1846–1855.

50. International CommissonCommission on Radiological Protection, (1994) ICRP publication 66: Human respiratory tract model for radiological protection, Pergamon Press, 1994.

51. Oberdörster G., (2001) Pulmonary effects of inhaled ultrafine particles, *Int. Arch. Occup. Environ. Health.* **74** pp 1–8.

52. Forastiere F., (2004) Fine particles and lung cancer, *Occup. Environ. Environ Med.* **61** pp 797–798.

53. Dockery D. W., Pope C. A., Xu X., Spengler J. D., Ware J. H., Fay M. E., Ferris B. G., Speizer F. E., (1993) An association between air pollution and mortality in six U.S. cities, *N. Engl. J. Med.* **329** pp 1753–1759.

54. Pope C. A., Burnett R. T., Thun M. J., Calle E. E., Krewski D., Ito K., Thurston G. D., (2002) Lung cancer, cardiopulmonary mortality, and long-term exposure to fine particulate air pollution, *JAMA.* **287** pp 1132–1141.

55. O'Neill M. S., Jerrett M., Kawachi I., Levy J. I., Cohen A. J., Gouveia N., Wilkinson P., Fletcher T., Cifuentes L., Schwartz J., (2003) Health, wealth, and air pollution: advancing theory and methods, *Environ. Health Perspect.* **111** pp 1861–1870.

56. Bhatia R., Lopipero P., Smith A. H., (1998) Diesel exhaust exposure and lung cancer, *Epidemiology.* **9** pp 84–91.

57. Claxton L. D., (1983) Characterization of automotive emissions by bacterial mutagenesis bioassay: a review., *Environ. Mutagen.* **5** pp 609–631.

58. International Agency for Research on Cancer, (1989) IARC Monographs Volume 46: Diesel and gasoline engine exhaust and some nitroarenes, **IARC**, Lyon.

59. Nielsen P. S., Andreassen A., Farmer P. B., Ovrebo S., Autrup H., (1996) Biomonitoring of diesel exhaust-exposed workers. DNA and hemoglobin adducts and urinary 1-hydroxypyrene as markers of exposure, *Toxicol. Lett.* **86** pp 27–37.

60. Mauderly J. L., (1994) Toxicological and epidemiological evidence for health risks from inhaled engine emissions, *Environ. Environ Health Perspect.* **102** Suppl 4 pp 165–171.

61. Vainio H., Sorsa M., and Hemminki K., (1983). Biological monitoring in surveillance of exposure to genotoxicants. *Am. J. Ind. Med.* **4** (1–2):87–103.

62. Hornung R. W., and Meinhardt T. J., (1987) Quantitative risk assessment of lung cancer in U.S. uranium miners, *Health Phys.* **52** pp 417–430.

63. Howe G., and Stager R., (1996) Risk of lung cancer mortality after exposure to radon decay products in the beaverlodge cohort based on revised exposure estimates, *Radiat. Res.* **146** pp 37–42.

64. Kunz E., Sevc J., Placek V., Haracek J., (1979) Lung cancer mortality in uranium miners, *Health Phys.* **35** pp 579–580.

65. Kunz E., Sevc J., Placek V., Horacek J., (1979) Lung cancer in man in relation to different time distribution of radiation exposure, *Health Phys.* **36** pp 699–706.

66. L'Abbe K. A., Howe G. R., Burch J. D., Miller A. B., Abbatt J. D., Band P., Choi W., Du J., Feather J., Gallagher R., et al, (1991) Radon exposure, cigarette smoking, and other mining experience in the beaverlodge uranium miners cohort, *Health Phys.* **60** pp 489–495.

67. Morgan M. V., and Samet J. M., (1986) Radon daughter exposures of New Mexico U miners, 1967–1982, *Health Phys.* **50** pp 656–662.

68. Samet J. M., Pathak D. R., Morgan M. V., Marbury M. C., Key C. R., Valdivia A. A., (1989) Radon progeny exposure and lung cancer risk in New Mexico uranium miners: a case-control study, *Health Phys.* **56** pp 415–421.

69. Samet J. M., Pathak D. R., Moran M. V., Key C. R., Valdivia A. A., (1991) Lung cancer mortality and exposure to radon progeny in a cohort of New Mexico underground uranium miners, *Health Phys.* **61** pp 745–752.

70. Sevc J., Kunz E., Placek V., (1976) Lung cancer in uranium miners and long-term exposure to radon daughter products, *Health Phys.* **30** pp 433–437.

71. Tirmarche M., Raphalen A., Allin F., Chameaud J., Bredon P., (1993) Mortality of a cohort of French uranium miners exposed to relatively low radon concentrations, *Br. J. Cancer.* **67** pp 1090–1097.

72. Woodward A., Roder D., McMichael A. J., Crouch P., Mylvaganam A., (1991) Radon daughter exposures at the Radium Hill uranium mine and lung cancer rates among former workers, 1952–87, *Cancer Causes Control.* **2** pp 213–220.

73. Darby S., Hill D., Auvinen A., Barros-Dios J. M., Baysson H., Bochicchio F., Deo H., Falk R., Forastiere F., Hakama M., Heid I., Kreienbrock L., Kreuzer M., Lagarde F., Makelainen I., Muirhead C., Oberaigner W., Pershagen G., Ruano-Ravina A., Ruosteenoja E., Rosario A. S., Tirmarche M., Tomasek L., Whitley E., Wichmann H. E.,

Doll R., (2005) Radon in homes and risk of lung cancer: collaborative analysis of individual data from 13 European case-control studies, *Br. Med. J.* **330** pp 223.

74. Field R. W., Steck D. J., Smith B. J., Brus C. P., Fisher E. L., Neuberger J. S., Platz C. E., Robinson R. A., Woolson R. F., Lynch C. F., (2000) Residential radon gas exposure and lung cancer: the Iowa Radon Lung Cancer Study, *Am. J. Epidemiol.* **151** pp 1091–1102.

75. Krewski D., Lubin J. H., Zielinski J. M., Alavanja M., Catalan V. S., Field R. W., Klotz J. B., Letourneau E. G., Lynch C. F., Lyon J. I., Sandler D. P., Schoenberg J. B., Steck D. J., Stolwijk J. A., Weinberg C., Wilcox H. B., (2005) Residential radon and risk of lung cancer: a combined analysis of 7 North American case-control studies, *Epidemiology.* **16** pp 137–145.

76. Krewski D., Lubin J. H., Zielinski J. M., Alavanja M., Catalan V. S., Field R. W., Klotz J. B., Letourneau E. G., Lynch C. F., Lyon J. L., Sandler D. P., Schoenberg J. B., Steck D. J., Stolwijk J. A., Weinberg C., Wilcox H. B., (2006) A combined analysis of North American case-control studies of residential radon and lung cancer, *J. Toxicol. Environ. Environ Health A.* **69** pp 533–597.

77. Pelucchi C., Pira E., Piolatto G., Coggiola M., Carta P., La Vecchia C., (2006) Occupational silica exposure and lung cancer risk: a review of epidemiological studies 1996–2005, *Ann. Oncol.* **17** pp 1039–1050.

78. Steenland K., Mannetje A., Boffetta P., Stayner L., Attfield M., Chen J., Dosemeci M., DeKlerk N., Hnizdo E., Koskela R., Checkoway H., (2001) Pooled exposure-response analyses and risk assessment for lung cancer in 10 cohorts of silica-exposed workers: an IARC multicentre study, *Cancer Causes Control.* **12** pp 773–784.

79. Hecht S. S., (1999) Tobacco smoke carcinogens and lung cancer, *J. Natl. Cancer Inst.* **91** pp 1194–1210.

80. Doll R., Peto R., Boreham J., Sutherland I., (2004) Mortality in relation to smoking: 50 years' observations on male British doctors, *Br. Med. J.* **328** pp 1519.

81. Subramanian J., and Govindan R., (2007) Lung cancer in never smokers: a review, *J. Clin. Oncol.* **25** pp 561–570.

82. Trichopoulos D., Kalandidi A., Sparros L., MacMahon B., (1981) Lung cancer and passive smoking, *Int. J. Cancer.* **27** pp 1–4.

83. Hirayama T., (1981) Non-smoking wives of heavy smokers have a higher risk of lung cancer: a study from Japan, *Br. Med. J. Clin. Res. Ed.* **282** pp 183–185.

84. National Research Council (USA) and Committee on Passive Smoking, (1986) Environmental tobacco smoke: measuring exposures and assessing health effects, National Academy Press, Whashington, DC, 1986.

Chapter 2

Lifestyle, Genes, and Cancer

Yvonne M. Coyle

Abstract

It is estimated that almost 1.5 million people in the USA are diagnosed with cancer every year. However, due to the substantial effect of modifiable lifestyle factors on the most prevalent cancers, it has been estimated that 50% of cancer is preventable.

Physical activity, weight loss, and a reduction in alcohol use can strongly be recommended for the reduction of breast cancer risk. Similarly, weight loss, physical activity, and cessation of tobacco use are important behavior changes to reduce colorectal cancer risk, along with the potential benefit for the reduction of red meat consumption and the increase in folic acid intake. Smoking cessation is still the most important prevention intervention for reducing lung cancer risk, but recent evidence indicates that increasing physical activity may also be an important prevention intervention for this disease. The potential benefit of lifestyle change to reduce prostate cancer risk is growing, with recent evidence indicating the importance of a diet rich in tomato-based foods and weight loss. Also, in the cancers for which there are established lifestyle risk factors, such as physical inactivity for breast cancer and obesity for colorectal cancer, there is emerging information on the role that genetics plays in interacting with these factors, as well as the interaction of combinations of lifestyle factors. Integration of genetic information into lifestyle factors can help to clarify the causal relationships between lifestyle and genetic factors and assist in better identifying cancer risk, ultimately leading to better-informed choices about effective methods to enhance health and prevent cancer.

Key words: Cancer prevention, diet, lifestyle, obesity and overweight, physical activity, smoking, tobacco.

1. Introduction

It is estimated that almost 1.5 million people in the USA are diagnosed with cancer every year (*1*). There is also evidence that lifestyle factors increase cancer risk and, if modified, could significantly reduce the cancer burden (*2*). This chapter reviews

M. Verma (ed.), *Methods of Molecular Biology, Cancer Epidemiology, vol. 472*
© 2009 Humana Press, a part of Springer Science+Business Media, Totowa, NJ
Book doi: 10.1007/978-1-60327-492-0

the current epidemiological evidence on the contributions of the major modifiable risk factors to cancer incidence and mortality for the most common cancers diagnosed in the USA and developed world—breast, colorectal, lung, and prostate cancer (3). Due to the substantial effect of modifiable lifestyle factors on the most prevalent cancers, it has been estimated that 50% of cancer is preventable (4). Current recommendations for the major risk factors that can be modified to decrease risk for these cancers include reducing tobacco use, increasing physical activity, controlling weight, improving diet, and limiting alcohol consumption (5). When defining the cancer prevention strategies used to modify these risk factors, it is also important to integrate genetic information that may play a role in determining the effectiveness for modifying these factors.

2. Breast Cancer

Breast cancer is the most common cancer in women, with nearly 180,000 women diagnosed with breast cancer in the USA annually (1). The fact that lifestyle changes can decrease the risk for developing breast cancer is supported by several lines of evidence. First, studies indicate that as populations migrate from the low- to the high-risk geographical areas for breast cancer, the incidence of breast cancer approaches that of the host country in one to two generations (6–8). Second, only a small part of breast cancer risk is linked to genetic inheritance and environmental exposures from chemicals or physical agents. Third, modification in lifestyle due to behavior change has been shown to be associated with a lower breast cancer risk in population studies. Last, experimental animal and human models provide confirmation that several lifestyle behaviors have a positive effect on breast biology. The major modifiable risk factors for breast cancer are physical inactivity, obesity and the overweight condition, alcohol use, and possibly diet (9).

2.1. Physical Activity

A recent systemic review that included all cohort and case-control studies that assessed total and leisure time activities in relation to the occurrence or mortality of breast cancer indicated that there was strong evidence for an inverse association between physical activity and breast cancer risk (10). The risk reduction for the cohort studies with a higher quality score ranged from 21% to 39%. Evidence for an inverse dose-response relationship was seen in all but one of the cohort studies. The risk reduction for the case-control studies ranged from 23% to 65%, and evidence for a dose-response was noted in most of the case-control studies.

A lower risk breast cancer was also noted for both premenopausal and postmenopausal breast cancer in nearly all of the studies in which this relationship was assessed. Several of these studies quantified the level of physical activity required to reduce breast cancer risk, finding that this risk reduction was on the average about 30% lower for women who exercised for 3–4 hours per week at moderate and vigorous levels. In addition, most studies have been conducted in non-Hispanic white women, although data from some studies suggest that physical activity is associated with a lower risk for breast cancer in women of diverse races and ethnicities (11–15). Physical activity at adolescence has also been observed to be associated with a delayed age at breast cancer onset among women with mutations in the tumor suppressor genes (TSGs), *BRCA1* and *BRCA2*, which substantially increase the risk for breast cancer (16). Likewise, the benefit of physical activity has been apparent among breast cancer survivors in recent studies (17, 18). In one study that involved 2,987 women diagnosed with stage I, II, and II breast cancer, the age-adjusted risk of death from breast cancer was inversely associated with physical activity after the diagnosis of breast cancer (17). In this study, the greatest benefit was noted in women who performed the equivalent of walking 3–5 hours per week at an average pace. In another study, among 1,264 women ages 20 to 54 years, it was found that recreational physical activity undertaken in the year before a diagnosis of breast cancer was associated with a lower all-cause mortality at the 8–10 year follow-up (18). Thus, it appears that physical activity may play an important role in preventing breast cancer in women with and without a personal history of breast cancer, as well as delaying the onset of breast cancer in women with genetic susceptibility.

It is thought that the relationship between physical activity and breast cancer risk may have a hormonal mechanism. Increased physical activity measured through self-report has been found to be associated with lower estrogen levels in premenopausal and postmenopausal women (19, 20). Exercise interventions have also been shown to decrease estrogen levels and increase sex hormone-binding globulin (SHBG) levels in postmenopausal women (21, 22). A recent pooled analysis of nine cohort studies showed that the risk for breast cancer in postmenopausal women increased significantly with increasing concentrations of total estradiol, free estradiol, and estrone (23). In addition, lower concentrations of SHBG, which binds to estradiol, is associated with a higher risk for breast cancer (23). Other findings from epidemiological studies further support the etiologic role of estrogen in breast cancer, showing that breast cancer risk is associated with early menarche, late menopause, low parity, and the use of exogenous estrogens, all of which are linked to prolonged or extensive exposure of breast tissue to estrogen stimulation (*24*). High endogenous estrogen levels have also been shown to be associated with shortening of the disease-free interval in postmenopausal women with breast cancer recurrence (*25*). Finally, a number of clinical trials have shown that estrogen ablation increases survival after a diagnosis of breast cancer (*26*). In addition, estrogens can increase the production of insulin-like growth factor (IGF)-I (*27*), and higher estrogen and IGF-I levels have both been shown to be associated with increased mammographic density (*28*). Mammographic density is a strong risk factor for breast cancer, and reflects proliferation of the breast epithelium and stroma (*29*). Several epidemiological studies have shown that IGF-I is positively associated with breast cancer risk, especially in premenopausal women (*30–33*). Thus, several randomized studies with exercise interventions have been performed to identify the potential benefit of aerobic exercise or strength training for reducing IGF-I levels. These studies have shown that aerobic training produces a decrease in mean serum IGF-I levels in prepubertal girls (*34*), adolescent female subjects (*35*), and postmenopausal breast cancer survivors (*36*). However, most of the weight training intervention studies that involved premenopausal postmenopausal women or premenopausal and postmenopausal breast cancer survivors reported no change in IGF-I levels (*37–39*).

There is also growing evidence that estrogens play a dual role in the etiology of breast cancer by not only stimulating cell proliferation (*40*), but by silencing genes implicated in breast carcinogenesis (*41–43*). For breast cancer, as well as many other cancers, promoter region hypermethylation of TSGs is an early and frequent event in carcinogenesis and occurs in conjunction with transcriptional silencing of these genes. The mechanism driving promoter hypermethylation is unknown, however, it has been noted in tissues where there is chronic exposure to carcinogens that a continuum of increasing gene promoter hypermethylation occurs from hyperplasia through invasive carcinoma (*44*). The process of promoter hypermethylation has been referred to as "epigenetic" and is potentially reversible (*45*). DNA methylation of promoter CpG islands of genes prevents them from being transcribed for apoptosis, senescence, and other important physiological processes in cells, which makes cells that have accumulated DNA methylation prone to becoming tumor cells (*45*). Although the relationship between estrogen, which has been shown to have carcinogenic effects in human breast epithelial cells (*46*), and the methylation of genes is unknown, there is some evidence that estrogen alters the methylation patterns of genes. Studies in mice have shown that diethylstilbestrol (DES) (*47*) and estradiol (*48*) elicit genetic methylation changes that result in heavier uteri (*47*) and uterine tumors (*48*). Recently, it was demonstrated that estradiol and DES induced promoter hypermethylation of the putative TSGs, *E-cadherin* and *p*16, in human breast epithelial cells (*42*).

There is direct evidence that promoter hypermethylation of several putative TSGs, including *APC*, *RASSF1A*, and *RARβ2*, are associated with breast carcinogenesis (*45, 49–56*). In a recent study that included women with and without a personal history of breast cancer, it was shown that promoter hypermethylation of *APC*, *RASSF1A*, and *RARβ2* in nonmalignant breast tissue was associated with epidemiological markers of breast cancer risk (*56*). More specifically, *APC* and *RASSF1A* were positively associated with breast cancer risk, as defined by the Gail mathematical risk model (*57*); whereas promoter hypermethylation of *RARβ2* was positively associated with a personal history of breast cancer (*57*). Several studies (*51, 52, 58–60*) have shown that treatment of breast cancer cells with promoter hypermethylation of the putative TSGs, *RASSF1A* and *RARβ2*, with the DNA methyltransferase inhibitor 5-Aza-2′-deoxycytidine has led to their demethylation and re-expression. Thus, promoter hypermethylation of TSGs can be reversed by small molecules, making them promising targets for cancer prevention interventions. Alternatively, it is thought that lifestyle changes, such as physical activity, may reverse promoter methylation of TSGs. A recent cross-sectional study was conducted to determine the association of lifetime physical activity with promoter hypermethylation of *APC* and *RASSF1A* in nonmalignant breast tissue, among premenopausal and postmenopausal women without breast cancer (*61*). This study provided evidence to support the hypothesis that physical activity is inversely associated with promoter hypermethylation of TSGs, such as *APC*, in nonmalignant breast tissue (*61*).

In summary, observational studies have shown that there is a strong inverse association between moderate or vigorous physical activity and breast cancer risk, in which there may be a hormonal mechanism, particularly involving estrogen and its related effect on IGF-I.

2.2. Obesity and Overweight

The association of the overweight condition and obesity with breast cancer risk has been well studied. Extensive data from cohort and case-control studies provide convincing evidence that there is a 30–50% greater risk of postmenopausal breast cancer from the overweight condition and obesity, and a larger twofold increase in risk for adult weight gain (*62, 63*). Estimates from a meta-analysis of cohort studies found gradual increases in risk of postmenopausal breast cancer up to a body mass index (BMI) of 28, after which the risk did not increase further, with the relative risk (RR) of 1.26 for a BMI of 28 compared with a BMI of less than 21 (*64*). However, risk estimates vary by age at diagnosis, history of hormone-replacement therapy (HRT), and estrogen receptor (ER) status of the tumor. Another meta-analysis, involving prospective cohort and population-based case-control studies, found that this increased risk for postmenopausal breast cancer corresponded to a 12% increase for overweight women and a 25% increase for obese women (65). In fact, in a prospective cohort study among premenopausal and postmenopausal women, there was an even stronger association for adult weight gain, with a doubling of risk among women who have never used HRT and who gained over 20 kg from age 18 years (66). A meta-analysis of cohort studies found an inverse association between BMI and premenopausal breast cancer, with a RR reduction of 46% for women with a BMI greater than 31 compared with a BMI of less than 21 (64).

There are several plausible mechanisms linking adiposity to breast cancer risk. These mechanisms have evolved from a focus on estrogen excess, to the combined effect of estrogen and progesterone, and most recently, to attempts to understand the factors defining the bioavailability and effects of estrogens and androgens and their metabolites on specific end organs. Increases in obesity have been associated with increases in androgens, triglycerides, and insulin; and decreases in SHBG. These hormonal changes increase the bioavailability of estradiol and its metabolites and may also directly promote tumor growth (67–73). The bioavailability of estradiol is dependent on the degree and strength of binding to several protein carriers. SHBG is the predominant protein carrier of estradiol and the percentage of free estradiol is inversely related to the level of SHBG (23). Increases in free fatty acids, such as triglycerides, has been reported to increase the level of free estradiol by displacing estradiol from SHBG (23). Therefore, both decreases in SHBG and increases in triglycerides may result in increases in free estradiol. Key and Pike (74, 75) first hypothesized that the effect of adiposity on the estrogen bioavailability was modulated by menopausal changes in estrogen and progesterone production, and as a result explained the contradictory findings for premenopausal and postmenopausal breast cancer. Before menopause, ovarian production of estrogen overwhelms changes in estrogen metabolism related to the overall level of adiposity. As a result, estradiol in ovulatory cycles does not differ significantly in obese compared with lean women. However, estradiol levels are reduced in anovulatory cycles that are more frequent in obese than lean premenopausal women. In addition, obese premenopausal women have been found to have markedly reduced progesterone levels, both due to anovulation and decreased production during the luteal phase of the menstrual cycle. After menopause, the lower risk associated with premenopausal obesity diminishes over time. In addition, in postmenopausal women, the overall level of adiposity results in increased estrogenic activity due to an increase in estrogen production from the aromatization of higher levels of androgens in adipose tissue (*76*), decreased estrogen binding (*77*) due to decreases in SHBG (*70, 72, 78*), and increases in triglycerides (*72*). Furthermore, insulin and insulin-like growth factors have been found to promote cancer cell growth, and their production can be increased by estrogen (*79*). However, although five studies have shown that higher IGF-I levels are associated with a higher risk for breast cancer (*80–84*), only one of these studies found this association to be statistically significant (*81*). In addition, published studies, thus far, have not found an association between IGF-I and postmenopausal breast cancer (*81, 83, 85*). Similarly, one of two published studies found C-peptide, a marker of hyperinsulinemia, to be associated with breast cancer risk (*85, 86*). Data on the association between IGF-I and BMI or fat mass in men and women are also mixed (*87*), with some studies showing no association and others an inverse association. Therefore, it has been hypothesized that IGF-I is positively associated with muscle mass, which may explain the increased premenopausal breast cancer risk among tall and lean women. Another hormonal hypothesis is that leptin, a hormone that reflects total fat mass, may be positively related to breast cancer risk. Leptin has been characterized as a growth factor for breast cancer (*88–91*). Thus far, one study has been published that has examined this relationship among premenopausal women finding nonsignificant lower levels of leptin in breast cancer cases compared with controls (*92*), which is consistent with an inverse association between BMI and premenopausal breast cancer. No published studies have examined the relationship of leptin to breast cancer risk in postmenopausal women. Thus, current studies do not provide convincing data to support a link between insulin, IGF-I, or leptin with breast cancer risk. However, one study found that there was a multiplicative interaction between adult exercise and sports activity and BMI, with inactive women in the upper BMI quartile being at increased risk compared with their lean and active counterparts (*93*).

2.3. Alcohol

The literature over the last 2½ decades provides convincing evidence that alcohol consumption has a modest impact on breast cancer risk (*94*). That is, the RR associated with alcohol consumption is not great, since it has been found to be associated with an approximately 10% increase in risk for an increase in average consumption of one drink per day (*95*). However, because of the high prevalence of alcohol consumption, the attributable risk is likely to exceed 10% in those who consume alcohol regularly (*96*). The dose-response relationship between alcohol and breast cancer risk is well demonstrated in the results of a meta-analysis by Smith-Warner and colleagues (*95*), where breast cancer risk rose by 7% for every 10-g increase in daily alcohol consumption. However, there is also some evidence that this risk does not substantially increase until a threshold of 15 g/day of alcohol is reached. Furthermore, there is little evidence that this risk is modified by menopausal status (97, 98).

One plausible explanation for an etiologic association between alcohol and breast cancer carcinogenesis is that it increases circulating estrogen levels. Circulating estrogens originate from ovarian synthesis or from peripheral conversion (aromatization) pathways involving androgens, such as testosterone. For premenopausal women, alcohol intake has been associated with higher concentrations of estrogens and androgens, as well as decreases in follicle-stimulating hormone levels (99–106). It has also been found that in postmenopausal women not using HRT, moderate alcohol intake can lead to increased estrogen and androgen levels, although the findings have been variable (107–109). Studies have shown that alcohol is associated with mammographically dense breast tissue (110–115), which is also positively associated with levels of estrogen and IGF-I (27, 116). As previously mentioned, estrogen can increase the production of IGF-I (27). The dense patterns seen on mammography are associated with atypical hyperplasia and/or carcinoma in situ (117) and with cytological atypia in nipple aspirates (118), which may be a result of mitogenesis or mutagenesis in the breast (119).

In addition, whether dietary and genetic factors modify the effect of alcohol use in breast cancer risk has been of interest. Zhang and colleagues reported that women consuming more than 15 g of alcohol per day and whose intake of folate was less than 300 μg/day had a higher risk for breast cancer, compared with women who had the same level of alcohol consumption, along with folate levels greater than 300 μg/day (120). Other reports (121–123) confirm this relationship. It is important to note, however, that low-to-moderate alcohol consumption, in contrast to heavy drinking, may not result in folate depletion (124–127). Thus, it is thought that in combination with low folate intake, ethanol and/or its primary metabolite acetaldehyde may alter folate or methionine metabolism so that an imbalance in DNA methylation or in DNA repair processes results; leading to DNA instability or aberrant gene expression (128–132). Alcohol consumption also has been associated with decreased blood levels of β-carotene, lutein/zeaxanthin, and vitamin C, which are thought to be cancer protective (133, 134). Thus, these studies collectively suggest that alcohol consumption, particularly at higher levels, may be associated with increased breast cancer risk, in part because of the negative impact of alcohol intake on the dietary factors that are thought to be cancer protective. There is also some evidence that the relationship between alcohol and breast cancer risk could differ according to the gentotype of several metabolizing enzymes. Park and colleagues have found that premenopausal women that consume alcohol and lack the glutathione-*S*-transferase genes (*GSTM1* and *GSTT1*) were at 5.3-fold greater risk for developing breast cancer compared with women with these genes, suggesting that the lack of these genes potentiates the adverse effects of alcohol on the breast due to the decreased capacity to detoxify alcohol (*135*).

2.4. Diet

Fat is the dietary component that has most often been found to relate to the risk of cancer in general (*136*). In a pooled analysis of case-control studies, a highly significant and positive association was seen between dietary fat and breast cancer risk (*137*). However, prospective studies have consistently shown no association (*138*). In a pooled analysis of large prospective studies, breast cancer risk for a higher total fat intake was minimal (RR = 1.03) (*139*). Similarly, the largest randomized controlled dietary cancer prevention intervention study to date, which involved 48,800 postmenopausal women, found only a modest statistically nonsignificant 9% decrease in invasive breast cancer in those who consumed a low-fat diet (*140*).

Early epidemiological studies suggested that vegetables and fruits may lower breast cancer risk (*141*). However, a pooled analysis of eight prospective cohort studies involving 351,825 women found no association between the intake of vegetables and fruits and breast cancer risk (*142*). A recent prospective study in which 285,526 women participated, ages 25–70 years, found no significant association between vegetable and fruit intake and breast cancer risk, adjusting for potentially important confounders, such as menopausal status (*143*). Although these studies collectively indicate that vegetables and fruits may not modify breast cancer risk, it is possible that specific genotypes may interact with vegetable and fruit intake to lower breast cancer risk. A recent large case-control study was performed to assess the effect of different variants of myeloperoxidase (MPO), an antimicrobial enzyme in the breast that generates reactive oxygen species, on breast cancer risk. This study showed that specific variants of MPO were associated with a lower breast cancer risk among premenopausal and postmenopausal women who consumed higher amounts of vegetables and fruits that was not noted among the lower consumption group (*144*).

Soy products contain phytoestrogens, which can act as weak estrogens and as estrogen antagonists, depending on the hormonal milieu of the host. Epidemiological data suggest that the consumption of soy products may reduce breast cancer risk (*145, 146*). However, recent evidence suggests that a component of soy, genistein, may promote the growth of some estrogen-sensitive tumors and reduce the efficacy of tamoxifen, emphasizing the need to perform additional studies to determine whether soy products are safe for women with breast cancer or at high risk for breast cancer (*147, 148*).

Several epidemiological studies have investigated the association between dietary and supplement intakes of various vitamins and minerals and the risk of breast cancer. Those micronutrients that have been found to be potentially associated with a lower risk for breast cancer include the carotenoids, folate (particularly in association with alcohol intake), calcium, vitamin D, and vitamin C (*141, 149–151*).

3. Colorectal Cancer

Colorectal cancer is the second most commonly occurring cancer in the USA and was estimated and to affect over 150,000 men and women in 2005 (*1*). Based on epidemiological studies, there is convincing data that obesity is an important risk factor for colorectal cancer (*152*), and that a high level of physical activity is a strong protective factor for colorectal cancer, which may reduce its risk by 50% (*153, 154*). Convincing data from epidemiological studies also support tobacco use as significant risk factor for colorectal cancer. Another potential risk factor for colorectal cancer is the consumption of red meat. However, the numerous studies with both cohort and case-control designs have not consistently supported a positive association between the consumption of red meat and colorectal cancer. On the other hand, a dietary factor that may be related to colorectal cancer risk is the micronutrient, folate, which has an inverse association.

3.1. Physical Activity

Colorectal cancer is one of the most commonly studied cancers with respect to physical activity. Numerous case-control and cohort studies have found an inverse association between physical activity and colon cancer risk (*152, 155–159*). This relationship has been observed in men and women of all age groups, in various racial and ethnic groups, and in diverse geographic areas around the world. In some of these studies, the effect of physical activity on colon cancer risk is attenuated in women compared with men, the reason for which is unknown. In most of the cohort studies described in a past review (*152*), as well as several more recent cohort studies (*155–159*), the risk of colon cancer was decreased in the highest physical activity compared with the lowest category, with risk reductions ranging from 10% to 60%. In addition, adjustment for potential confounding factors, such as age, diet, and obesity, did not reduce the strength of the associations between physical activity and colon cancer risk (*152, 155–159*). However, with regard to rectal cancer, these studies as a whole did not support an inverse association between physical activity and rectal cancer risk (*152, 155–159*). There is also some evidence that physical activity reduces neoplastic growth in the colon and rectum. In a recent prospective cohort study among African-American women, higher levels of physical activity were inversely associated with risk for the development of colorectal adenomas (160), which are thought to be precursors to most colon and rectal cancers (161). In another recent study, a 12-month moderate-to-vigorous intensity aerobic exercise intervention resulted in a significant decrease in colon crypt cell proliferation indices in men who exercised ≥250 min/week or whose cardiopulmonary fitness, as measured by VO_2 max, increased by ≥5% (162). In this study, patients with colon cancer and persons with an elevated risk for colon cancer (history of sporadic adenoma, ulcerative colitis, familial polyposis, family history of colon cancer, age, etc.) exhibited in macroscopically normal colon mucosa both an increased epithelial cell proliferation rate and an extension of the normal zone of epithelial cell proliferation extending from the base to the luminal portion of the colonic crypt (163).

Biological mechanisms for the effect of physical activity on colon and perhaps rectal cancer risk are unknown. However, several biologically plausible mechanisms have been proposed, including alterations in the immune system, reduced bowel transit time (increasing exposure to fecal carcinogens), higher prostaglandin levels, and bile acid secretion, as well as higher levels of insulin and insulin-like growth factors (164). Although studies are limited in number, there is convincing data to support the latter of these mechanisms, in that both insulin and IGF-I are potent mitogens of colonic carcinoma cells. Several studies have now shown that high levels of IGF-I increase the risk for colorectal cancer, whereas high levels of insulin-like growth factor binding protein (IGFBP)-3, which can reduce IGF-I levels, are associated with a reduced risk for colorectal cancer (165, 166). Likewise, the interaction of physical activity with inherited genetic polymorphisms or mutations in colorectal tumors is limited. Although the interaction of gene polymorphisms and physical activity are unavailable, there is evidence that mutations in the genes APC, p53, and Ki-ras may be inversely associated with physical activity. These genes are thought to regulate cell growth and apoptosis, with mutations in these genes resulting in tumor growth (155). APC mutations are thought to be an early event in the carcinogenic process, with other gene mutations occurring afterward (155). Studies have not been done to determine the association of physical activity with APC mutations, but other studies have suggested that p53 and Ki-ras mutations in tumors may be inversely related to physical activity (167, 168). Another study examined physical activity with colorectal adenomas and reported that people who were more active were more likely to have Ki-ras-negative rather than Ki-ras-positive tumors (169).

**3.2. Obesity
and Overweight**

Numerous cohort and case-control studies have consistently demonstrated a positive relationship between body size and colorectal cancer. This relationship has been observed in men and women, with the risk being stronger for men than women (*152*). In these studies, this relationship is stronger for those who are obese as compared with those who are overweight. In general, this relationship has also been proven to be stronger for cancer of the colon than the rectum, and for the distal rather than the proximal colon. Body size has also been shown to influence colorectal carcinogenesis: BMI has been found to be associated with colorectal adenoma, a precursor lesion of colorectal cancer, and large adenomas of the distal colon and rectum in several epidemiological studies (*170–177*). There is also evidence to suggest that abdominal or visceral adiposity is a risk factor for colorectal cancer independent of BMI. Recent studies have shown that higher waist-to-hip ratio (WHR) increases the risk for colorectal cancer (*178–180*).

The understanding of the biological mechanisms linking body size to colorectal cancer is evolving. One plausible mechanism is that a high BMI causes insulin resistance, which promotes colon carcinogenesis. The term insulin resistance refers to a state of cellular unresponsiveness to the effects of insulin, with higher levels of insulin required to normalize plasma glucose, which is associated with a high BMI (*181*). Diabetes mellitus type 2 is a disease that occurs when insulin resistance coincides with impaired pancreatic secretion of insulin, and is positively associated with colorectal cancer. Type 2 diabetic patients have a threefold increased risk for colorectal cancer compared with nondiabetic patients (*182*), and in general, non-obese colorectal cancer patients exhibit clinical manifestations of insulin resistance, with higher insulin and glucose levels compared with their control patients (*183*). Furthermore, serum levels of C-peptide (the cleaved product of proinsulin and a marker of insulin secretion), glycated hemoglobin, and glucose have all been positively associated with colorectal neoplasia (*184–188*). In addition, plasma levels of IGF-I, which can be increased by insulin, has been positively associated with colorectal cancer (*189*). Furthermore, several metabolic disturbances resulting from the insulin-resistant state, including hyperinsulinemia, hyperglycemia, hypertriglyceridemia, and increased levels of non-esterified fatty acids, have been found to be positively associated with colorectal cancer risk among fasting participants in prospective studies (*190, 191*). At least three mechanisms exist through which insulin resistance may cause colorectal cancer. The first is that insulin promotes the growth of colorectal tumors. Specifically, insulin has been shown to stimulate cellular proliferation and reduce cellular apoptosis in colorectal cancer cell lines (*192, 193*), and it promotes colorectal cancer growth in animal models (*194–196*). Second, insulin increases IGF-I levels, and high circulating levels of IGF-I have been associated with colorectal cancer risk (*189, 197,*

198). IGF-I has also been shown to promote the growth of colon cancers in a mouse model (*199*). In addition, obesity is associated with a state of chronic inflammation, thought to be induced by high circulating levels of lipids and glucose, both of which create a proinflammatory environment that contains a high free radical content (*200, 201*). It is well known that inflammatory bowel disease increases the risk for colorectal cancer (*202*). In addition, randomized clinical trials have shown that the use of the nonsteroidal anti-inflammatory drugs, celecoxib and aspirin, reduce colorectal cancer risk (*203, 204*), where a 45% risk reduction was noted with the use of aspirin for adenoma recurrence (*204*). Finally, there is some evidence that the association of body size with colorectal cancer may be mediated through other disease pathways. One study reported that an elevated BMI was associated with a mutation of Ki-*ras* in colorectal tumors, which was more likely to occur in women than men (*205*).

3.3. Diet

Although not entirely consistent, numerous case-control and cohort studies have reported a positive association between red meat consumption and processed meat in particular, with colon cancer risk that was not noted with poultry and fish intake. Red meat intake is thought to increase the risk for colorectal cancer due to its higher heme content compared with the white meats, poultry and fish (*206, 207*). Heme damages the colonic mucosa and stimulates epithelial cell proliferation in animal studies (*207*). Both the ingestion of red meat and heme iron supplementation have been found to increase fecal concentrations of *N*-nitroso compounds (*208*) and DNA adducts in human colonocytes (*208, 209*). The central role for DNA adducts in carcinogenesis has been established and confirmed as a biological fact for over 50 years (*210*). Nitrosamines have also been detected in foods with added nitrates or nitrites, such as processed meat (*211, 212*). A meta-analysis of case-control and cohort studies that were published during 1973–1999 assessed the hypothesis that the consumption of red meat and processed meat increases colorectal cancer risk. This study indicated that the RR (higher versus lowest category) for red meat was 1.27 and for processed meat was 1.59 (*213*). A recent prospective cohort study that included 148,610 adults also assessed the effect of long-term red meat and processed meat, as well as poultry and fish, consumption on colorectal cancer risk (*214*). In this study, the risk of distal colon cancer was positively associated with the consumption of processed meat (RR = 1.50), and the risk of rectal cancer was positively associated with the consumption of red meat (RR = 1.71). In contrast, a lower risk of proximal and distal colon cancer was noted with the long-term consumption of poultry and fish in this study (*213*).

Folic acid deficiency has long been known to cause tumors in animals, which is thought to be the result of altering gene expression through DNA methylation or by increasing the incorporation of uracil in DNA (*215*). There is considerable evidence from case-control and cohort studies that supports an inverse association between folate intake and colon cancer risk (216), with this association being stronger among alcohol users (217). A recent study indicated that the inverse association between dietary folate intake and colon cancer risk was stronger for ever smokers compared with never smokers (218). A positive association between a functional polymorphism in the folic acid metabolizing gene, methylene tetrahydrofolate reductase, and the incidence of colon cancer adds support to the potential casual relationship between folic acid deficiency and colon cancer (219).

3.4. Tobacco

In 2004, the US Surgeon General recently concluded that the evidence for the relationship of smoking with colorectal cancer was suggestive but not sufficient to infer a causal relationship (220). At the time of this report, 3 prospective cohort studies (221–223) and 13 case-control studies (224–235), with the exception of the study by Kato and colleagues, identified the RR estimates between smoking and colorectal adenomatous polyps to be between 1.5 and 3.8, after adjusting for age and other important covariates (236). However, in a more recent study (237), the tobacco use of 4,383 subjects with histologically verified benign (hyperplastic or adenomatous) polyps of the distal colon were compared with the tobacco use among 33,667 subjects who were endoscopy negative for distal colon tumors in the screening arm of a randomized trial of flexible sigmoidoscopy. In this study, the risk estimated by the odds ratio (OR) was 4.4 for hyperplastic polyps, 1.8 for adenomas polyps only, and 6.2 for both hyperplastic and adenomatous polyps, which provides stronger support for this relationship.

Prospective studies that have investigated the relationship between smoking and colon cancer have generally reported RR estimates of 1.2–1.4 for colon cancer and 1.4–2.0 for rectal cancer (238–244). To date, there has not been a meta-analysis that has evaluated this relationship across all studies that controlled for factors that influence colorectal cancer risk.

Recent studies indicate that variants of the metabolizing genes, NAT1, CYP1A1, GSTM1, and GSTT1, may interact with smoking to increase the risk of colorectal cancer (245–247).

4. Lung Cancer

Lung cancer is the leading cause of cancer death for men and women in the USA; 85% of patients who develop lung cancer will die from it within 5 years of diagnosis (248). Although more than 80% of lung cancer cases are attributable to cigarette smoking, recent studies have noted a protective effect for lung cancer with physical activity in men and women after adjusting for smoking (5). Past case-control and large cohort studies among men and women were encouraging as to the potential benefit of vegetable and fruit consumption reducing lung cancer risk (5), however, this inverse relationship has not held up in more recent studies (249). Thus, there is likely a major benefit for men and women for modifying their lifestyle related to cigarette exposure, and possibly physical activity and fruit and vegetable intake.

4.1. Tobacco

Cigarette smoking is more strongly associated with lung cancer than with any other cancer type. Cigarette smoking is also the strongest risk factor for lung cancer, increasing the risk of this disease by at least 10-fold and as much as 20-fold, depending on smoking habits and the medical history. There is also a dose-response relationship between smoking and lung cancer that relates to the number of cigarettes smoked, the deepness of the inhalation of cigarette smoke, and the duration of smoking (250). The median delay between the initiation of smoking and death from lung cancer is approximately 50 years (251). Cigarette smoking is more strongly associated with squamous and small cell lung carcinomas, but is increasingly becoming associated with adenocarcinoma and large cell carcinomas that are usually located in the periphery of the lung (252). The incidence of adenocarcinoma has increased in many industrialized countries since the 1970s, which is thought to be due to the introduction of filter-tip cigarettes and reconstructed tobacco in the 1950s (252). There is also increasing evidence suggesting that there are significant differences in lung cancer susceptibility and histological type between the sexes. It appears that women may be more susceptible to lung cancer development than men with and without cigarette smoke exposure, and that the histological distribution of lung cancer differs between men and women, with adenocarcinoma being more common in women than men. Studies are underway to determine if genetic variation, as well as biological factors, may play a role in these differences between the sexes related to lung cancer histological type and overall risk (253).

Tobacco products contain a diverse array of chemical carcinogens, which are responsible for the development of lung cancer and other cancers. More than 60 known carcinogens have been detected in cigarette smoke (254). These include polycyclic aromatic hydrocarbons (PAH); tobacco-specific nitrosamines and other nitrosamines; aromatic amines; aldehydes; volatile hydrocarbons such as benzene, 1,3-butadiene, and ethylene oxide; and inorganic compounds (254). Tobacco carcinogens and their metabolically activated forms induce gene mutations through the formation of DNA adducts, which disrupt cell cycle checkpoints and cause genetic instability that predisposes to the development of malignancy (255). It has been shown that activation of tobacco carcinogens via multiple forms of the cytochrome P450 enzyme system, which detoxifies drugs and toxic compounds primarily in the liver, leads to DNA adduct-forming intermediates that are detoxified further by additional steps in metabolism. Metabolizing genes that have been shown to activate or deactivate tobacco smoke constituents are: *CYP1A1, GSTM1, GSTT1, NAT2,* and *GSTP1* (*256*). Therefore, large studies have been undertaken to investigate the role of functional polymorphisms in these genes in lung cancer development (*257*). Also, as an extension of this approach, research is ongoing on the role of functional polymorphisms in DNA repair genes in the development of lung cancer (*258*). Furthermore, research is ongoing to determine whether the interaction of cigarette smoke with these genes increases the risk for lung cancer (*259*).

4.2. Vegetable and Fruit Consumption

Although an inverse relationship between high levels of consumption of fruits and vegetables and the risk of lung cancer has been observed in both case-control and large cohort studies (*260*), a recent meta-analysis that included more than 3,000 incident cases of lung cancer in men and women did not confirm these results (*249*). It is thought that this inverse relationship may have been due to counting an inverse association with one or a few foods as support for the benefit of fruits and vegetables, when this may have been the result of chance due to multiple comparisons. However, it is still possible that biologically active substances in fruits and vegetables do exist but in doses too small and not possible to estimate using food frequency questionnaires, and that measuring blood levels of candidate substances would be best for assessing these dietary exposures (*261*).

4.3. Physical Activity

A recent meta-analysis that evaluated the relationship between physical activity and lung cancer found that this was a statistically inverse relationship, in which several studies were able to adjust for smoking (*262*). The ORs were 0.87 for moderate leisure-time physical activity and 0.70 for high physical activity, with the inverse association occurring for both sexes, although it was somewhat stronger for women. Four more recent prospective cohort studies, which all adjusted for smoking, yielded mixed results; with three out of the four studies showing an inverse relationship between physical activity and lung cancer risk (*263–266*). In the study that only included women (n = 36,929), physical activity was only inversely related to lung cancer risk in former and never smokers (*266*).

5. Prostate Cancer

Prostate cancer is the most common and second deadliest cancer in US men (*267*). Clinical prostate cancer usually presents late in life, leaving much opportunity for preventive interventions.

Although microscopic evidence of prostate cancer occurs in more than 70% of all men by age 70 years (*268*), the progression to clinically manifest cancer of the prostate is significantly more frequent in regions such as North America when compared with Asian countries (*269*). There is also an increased incidence of clinical prostate cancer in Asian men who emigrate to the USA compared with men who remain in Asian countries (*270, 271*). This feature of this disease suggests that environmental factors are contributors to the progression of prostate cancer. Preventive measures for this disease are not established, however, there is evidence that lifestyle modification that includes a diet rich in tomato products and controlling weight may reduce the risk for prostate cancer progression.

5.1. Diet

Several reports have noted an inverse association between a diet rich in tomato products and prostate cancer risk. The key component in tomatoes that is believed to be responsible for this effect is lycopene, which is a carotenoid and is the most effective antioxidant of all of the carotenoids (*272*). As is the case with other micronutrients, most of the evidence for the protective effect of lycopene in humans is derived from observational studies. A recent review of the published epidemiological evidence suggested that there was a potential benefit of lycopene against the risk of prostate cancer, particularly the more aggressive forms of this cancer. Five of these studies supported a 30% to 40% reduction in this risk, and three were consistent with a 30% reduction in risk, but the results of these studies were not statistically significant, and seven studies were not supportive of an association between lycopene and prostate cancer risk (*273*). The largest dietary prospective cohort study, which was conducted in male professionals, found that the consumption of two to four servings of tomato sauce per week was associated with nearly a 35% risk reduction of prostate cancer and a 50% reduction of advanced (extraprostatic) prostate cancer. Of the three blood-based prospective cohort studies, all demonstrated an inverse association between lycopene and prostate cancer risk, however, this association was only statistically significant related to aggressive prostate cancers. Thus, although not definitive, the data from these observational studies collectively suggests that lycopene may be protective for prostate cancer, particularly for the aggressive form.

5.2. Obesity and Overweight

In a recent meta-analysis that involved case-control and cohort studies, obesity was found to be positively associated with an increased risk of prostate cancer, particularly in the advanced stage tumors. In these studies, the association was small, 5% on the average, across the categories for BMI, and the range of RR was 0.66–2.28. A similar risk was seen for height and prostate cancer incidence, but only among the cohort studies. There were also weak positive associations with height and waist circumference, but no notable relationship between WHR and the risk of prostate cancer. A methodological issue for many of the studies represented in this meta-analysis was recall bias due to study subjects recalling their height and weight (*274*). However, in a recent large prospective cohort study, BMI and adult weight gain was positively associated with prostate cancer mortality, with a RR of 2.12 for the highest BMI category ($\geq$35 kg/m^2) (*275*).

Despite the lack of an association between markers of obesity and prostate cancer from the above epidemiological studies, several biological markers that are related to obesity suggest an association of these markers with prostate cancer risk. Leptin, an adipocyte-derived hormone that regulates satiety and energy expenditure, has been shown to increase prostate cancer risk (*276*). In addition, higher serum insulin levels increase prostate cancer risk, independent of abdominal obesity (*277*). A meta-analysis of published studies on hormonal markers of prostate cancer risk also found that men with serum IGF-I levels in the upper quartile of the population distribution had a twofold higher prostate cancer risk (*278*). However, how BMI may play a role in the association of these markers with prostate cancer is complex and not well understood.

6. Summary and Conclusions

Although the underlying mechanisms that are operative in the association between lifestyle and these cancers has not been established (**Table 2.1**), there is now overwhelming evidence that lifestyle factors affect breast, colorectal, lung, and, likely, prostate cancer risk. Physical activity, weight loss, and a reduction in alcohol use can strongly be recommended for the reduction of breast cancer risk. In addition, weight loss, physical activity, and cessation of tobacco use are important behavior changes to reduce colorectal cancer risk, along with the potential benefit for the reduction of red meat consumption and the increase in folic acid intake. Smoking cessation is still the most important prevention intervention for reducing lung cancer risk, but recent evidence indicates that increasing physical activity may also be an important prevention intervention for this disease. The potential benefit of lifestyle change to reduce prostate cancer risk is growing, with recent evidence indicating the importance of a diet rich in tomato-based foods and weight loss. Also, in the cancers for which there are established lifestyle risk factors, such as physical inactivity, obesity, and tobacco use for colorectal cancer, there is emerging information on the role that genetics plays in interacting with these factors, as well as the interaction of combinations

Table 2.1
Biological mechanisms that may be involved in the association of lifestyle, genes, and cancer

Cancer	Possible mechanisms
Breast	

Physical activity

Decreased circulating estrogen levels due to a decrease in SHBG levels

Prevents silencing of tumor suppressor genes, such as *APC*, in breast tissue due to gene promoter hypermethylation

Reduced production of IGF-I that promotes cancer cell growth, due to lower circulating levels of estrogen

Obesity and overweight

Aromatization of high levels of androgens in adipose tissue leading to higher circulating estrogen levels

Higher estrogen levels increase the production of insulin-like growth factors, such as IGF-I, which increases cancer cell growth

Alcohol

Higher estrogen levels increase the production of insulin-like growth factors, such as IGF-I, which increases cancer cell growth

The combination of alcohol consumption and folate deficiency may alter folate metabolism that causes an imbalance in the DNA repair processes that promote cancer cell growth

Polymorphisms in the metabolizing genes for alcohol, *GSTM1* and *GSTT1*, in combination with alcohol consumption may promote cancer cell growth

Colorectal

Physical activity

Increases bowel transit time, which may reduce mucosal exposure to fecal carcinogens

Decreases levels of insulin-like growth factors, such as IGF-I, which increases cancer cell growth

May prevent mutations of genes that regulate cell growth and apoptosis, such as *APC*, *p*53, and Ki-*ras*

Obesity and overweight

May increase levels of leptin and insulin-like growth factors, such as IGF-I, which increase cancer cell growth

Obesity produces a state of chronic inflammation that increases the production of free radicals that may lead to gene mutations that promote cancer cell growth

Obesity may cause mutations in genes involved in regulating cell growth and apoptosis, such as Ki-Ras, which increases cancer cell growth

Folic acid deficiency

Folic acid deficiency may alter gene expression through DNA methylation or by increasing the incorporation of uracil in DNA causing cancer cell growth

(continued)

**Table 2.1
(continued)**

Cancer	Possible mechanisms
	Tobacco Tobacco carcinogens in combination with specific polymorphisms of the metabolizing genes, *NAT2*, *CYP1A1*, *GSTM1*, and *GSTT1*, may increase the risk for initiating colorectal cancer
Lung	*Tobacco* Tobacco carcinogens initiate lung cancer by inducing gene mutations and genetic instability through the production of DNA adducts Specific polymorphisms of the genes that metabolize tobacco carcinogens, *NAT2*, *CYP1A1*, *GSTM1*, and *GSTT1*, may increase the risk for tobacco-induced lung cancer
Prostate	*Lycopene* Lycopene may reduce the production of free radicals that may lead to gene mutations that promote cancer cell growth
	Obesity and overweight May increase levels of leptin, insulin, and insulin-like growth factors, such as IGF-I, which increase cancer cell growth

SHBG, Sex hormone-binding globulin; *IGF*-I, Insulin-like growth Factor

of lifestyle factors. Integration of genetic information into lifestyle factors can help to clarify the causal relationships between lifestyle and genetic factors and assist in better identifying cancer risk, ultimately leading to better informed choices about effective methods to enhance health and prevent cancer.

References

1. Cancer Facts and Figures 2007. (2007) National Home Office, American Cancer Society, Inc., 1599 Clifton Road, NE, Atlanta, GA 30239–34251.

2. Stein CJ, Colditz GA. (2004) Modifiable risk factors for cancer. Brit J Cancer. 90, 299–303.

3. Ezzati M, Lopez AD, Rodgers A, Vander Hoorn S, Murray CJ. (2002) Selected major risk factors and global and regional burden of disease. Lancet. 360, 1347–1360.

4. Colditz GA, DeJong W, Hunter DJ, Trichopoulos D, Willet WC (eds). (1996) Harvard report on cancer prevention. Cancer Causes Control. 7(Suppl), S1–S55.

5. Curry SJ, Byers T, Hewitt M. (2003) Fulfilling the Potential of Cancer Prevention and Early Detection. The National Academies Press, 500 Fifth Street, NW, Washington, DC 20001.

6. Parkin DM, Pisani P, Ferlay J. (1999) Estimates of the worldwide incidence of 25

major cancers in 1990. Int J Cancer. 80, 827–841.

7. Lacey JV, Devesa SS, Brinton LA. (2002) Recent trends in breast cancer incidence and mortality. Environ Mol Mutagen. 39, 82–88.

8. Key TJ, Verkasalo PK, Banks E. Epidemiology of breast cancer. (2001) Lancet. 2, 133.

9. McTiernan A. (2003) Behavioral risk factors in breast cancer, can risk be modified? The Oncologist. 8, 326–334.

10. Monninkhof EM, Elias SG, Vlems FA, van der Tweel I, Schuit AJ, Voskuil DW, et al. (2007) Physical activity and breast cancer a systematic review. Epidemiol. 18, 137–157.

11. Ueji M, Ueno E, Osei-Hyiaman D, Takahashi H, Kano K. (1997) Physical activity and the risk of breast cancer, a case-control study of Japanese women. J Epidemiol. 8(2), 115–122.

12. Adams-Campbell LL, Rosenberg L, Rao RS, Palmer JR. (2001) Strenuous physical activity and breast cancer risk in African-American women. J Natl Med Assoc. 93(7/8), 267–275.

13. Matthews CE, Shu XO, Jin F, Dai Q, Hebert JR, Ruan ZX, et al. (2001) Lifetime physical activity and breast cancer risk in the Shanghai Breast Cancer Study. Br J Cancer. 84(7), 994–1001.

14. Yang D, Bernstein L, Wu AH. (2003) Physical activity and breast cancer risk among Asian-American women in Los Angeles. Cancer. 97(10), 2565–2575.

15. John EM, Horn-Ross PL, Koo J. (2003) Lifetime physical activity and breast cancer risk in a multiethnic population, The San Francisco Bay Area Breast Cancer Study. Cancer Epidemiol Biomarkers Prev. 12, 1143–1152.

16. King MC, Marks JH, Mandell JB. (2003) Breast and ovarian cancer risks due to inherited mutations in BRCA1 and BRCA2. Science. 302, 643.

17. Holmes MD, Chen WY, Feskanich D, Kroenke CH, Colditz GA. (2005) Physical activity and survival after breast cancer diagnosis. JAMA. 293(20), 2479–2486.

18. Abrahamson PE, Gammon MD, Lund MJ, Britton JA, Marshall SW, Flagg EW, et al. (2006) Recreational physical activity and survival among young women with breast cancer. Cancer. 107, 1777–1785.

19. Nelson ME, Meredith CN, Dawson-Hughes B, Evans WJ. (1988) Hormone and bone mineral status in endurance-trained and sedentary postmenopausal women. J Clin Endocrinol Metab. 66, 927–933.

20. Jasienska G, Ziomkiewicz A, Thune I, Lipson SF, Ellison PT. (2006) Habitual physical activity and estradiol levels in women of reproductive age. Eur J Cancer Prev. 15, 439–445.

21. Cauley JA, Gutai JP, Kuller LH, LeDonne D, Powell JG. (1989) The epidemiology of serum sex hormones in postmenopausal women. Am J Epidemiol. 129, 1120–1131.

22. McTiernan A, Tworoger SS, Ulrich CM, Yasui Y, Irwin ML, Rajan KB, et al. (2004) Effect of exercise on serum estrogens in postmenopausal women, a 12-month randomized trial. Cancer Res. 64, 2923–2928.

23. The Endogeneous Hormones and Breast Cancer Collaborative Group. (2002) Endogenous sex hormones and breast cancer in postmenopausal women, reanalysis of nine prospective studies. J Natl Cancer Inst. 94, 606–616.

24. McTiernan A (Ed.) Cancer Prevention and Management Through Exercise and Weight Control. Boca Raton, CRC Press, Taylor & Francis Group, LLC, 2006.

25. Lonning PE, Helle SI, Johannessen DC, Ekse D, Adlercreutz H. (1996) Influence of plasma estrogen levels on the length of the disease-free interval in postmenopausal women with breast cancer. Breast Cancer Res Treat. 29, 335–341.

26. Combined Hormone Trialists' Group and the European Organization for Research and Treatment of Cancer. (2001) Combined tamoxifen and luteinizing hormone-releasing hormone (LHRH) agonist versus LHRH agonist along in premenopausal advanced breast cancer, a meta-analysis of four randomized trials. J Clin Oncol. 19, 343–353.

27. Clemons M, Gross P. (2001) Mechanisms of disease, estrogen and the risk of breast cancer. NEJM. 344, 276–285.

28. Byrne C, Colditz GA, Willet WC, Speizer FE, Pollak M, Hankinson SE. (2000) Plasma insulin-like growth factor (IGF) I, IGF-binding protein 3, and mammographic density. Cancer Res. 60, 3744–3748.

29. McCormack VA, dos Santos Silva I. (2006) Breast density and parenchymal patterns as markers of breast cancer risk, a meta-analysis. Cancer Epidemiol Biomarkers Prev. 15, 1159–1169.

30. Peyrat JP, Bonneterre J, Hecquest B, Vennein P, Louchez MM, Fournier C, Lefebvre J, Demaille A. (1993) Plasma insulin-like growth-factor (IGF-I) concentrations in human breast cancer. Eur J Cancer. 29A, 492–497.

31. Bruning PF, Van Doorn J, Bonfrer JMG, Van Noord PA, Korse CM, Linders TC, Hart AA. (1995) Insulin-like growth-factor-binding protein 3 is decreased in early-stage operable pre-menopausal breast cancer. Int J Cancer. 62, 266–270.

32. Hankinson SE, Willett WC, Colditz GA, Hunter DJ, Michaud DS, Deroo B, Rosner B, Speizer FE, Pollak M. (1998) Circulating concentrations of insulin-like growth factor-I and risk of breast cancer. Lancet. 351, 1393–1396.

33. Bohlke K, Cramer DW, Trichopoulos D, Manzoros CS. (1998) Insulin-like growth factor-I in relation to premenopausal ductal carcinoma in situ of the breast. Epidemiology. 9, 570–573.

34. Eliakim A, Scheett TP, Newcomb R, Mohan S, Cooper DM. (2001) Fitness, Training, and the Growth Hormone→Insulin-like Growth Factor I Axis in Prepubertal Girls. J Clin Endocrinol Metab. 86, 2797–2802.

35. Eliakim A, Brasel JA, Mohan S, Barstow TJ, Berman N, Cooper DM. (1996) Physical fitness, endurance training, and the growth hormone-insulin-like growth factor I system in adolescent females. J Clin Endocrinol Metab. 81, 3986–3992.

36. Fairey AS, Courneya KS, Field CJ, Bell G, Jones LW, Macky JR. (2003) Effects of exercise training on fasting insulin, insulin resistance, insulin-like growth factors, and insulin-like growth factor binding proteins in postmenopausal breast cancer survivors, a randomized controlled trial. Cancer Epidemiol Biomarkers Prev. 12, 721–727.

37. Milliken LA, Going SB, Houtkooper LB, Flint-Wagner HG, Figueroa A, Metcalfe LL, Blew RM, Sharp SC, Lohman, TG. (2003) Effects of exercise training on bone remodeling, insulin-like growth factors, and bone mineral density in postmenopausal women with and without hormone replacement therapy. Calcif Tissue Int. 72, 478–484.

38. Schmitz KH, Ahmed RL, Hannan PJ, Yee D. (2005) Safety and efficacy of weight training in recent breast cancer survivors to alter body composition, insulin, and insulin-like growth factor axis proteins. Cancer Epidemiol Biomarkers Prev. 14, 1672–1680.

39. Schmitz KH, Ahmed RL, Yee D. (2002) Effects of a 9-month strength training intervention on insulin, insulin-like growth factor (IGF)-I, IGF-binding protein (IGFBP)-1, and IGFBP-1 in 30–50-year-old women. Cancer Epidemiol Biomarkers Prev. 11, 1597–1604.

40. Russo J, Hu Y-F, Yang X, Russo IH. (2000) Chapter 1, Developmental, cellular, and molecular basis of human breast cancer. J Natl Cancer Inst Monogr. 27, 17–37.

41. Klein CB, Costa M. (1997) DNA methylation, heterochromatin and epigenetic carcinogens. Mutation Res. 386, 163–180.

42. Klein CB, Leszczynska J. (2005) Estrogen-induced DNA methylation of E-cadherin & p16 in non-tumor breast cells. Proc Amer Assoc Cancer Res. 46, 2744.

43. Fernandez SV, Wu Y-Z, Russo IH, Plass C, Russo J. (2006) The role of DNA methylation in estrogen-induced transformation of human breast epithelial cells. Proc Amer Assoc Cancer Res. 47, 1590.

44. Shames DS, Minna JD, Gazdar AF. (2007) DNA methylation in health, disease, and cancer. Curr Mol Med. 7, 85–102.

45. Widschwendter M, Jones PA. (2001) DNA methylation and breast carcinogenesis. Oncogene. 21, 5462–5482.

46. Russo J, Russo IH. (2006) The role of estrogen in the initiation of breast cancer. J Steroid Biochem Mol Biol. 102, 89–96.

47. Li S, Ma L, Chiang TC, Burow M, Newbold RR, Negishi M, Barrett JC, McLachlan JA. (2001) Promoter CpG methylation of Hox-a10 and Hox-a11 in mouse uterus not altered upon neonatal diethylstilbestrol exposure. Mol Carcinogenesis. 32, 213–219.

48. Alworth LC, Howdeshell KL, Ruhlen RL, Day JK, Lubahn DB, Huang TH, Besch-Williford CL, vom Saal FS. (2002) Uterine responsiveness to estradiol and DNA methylation are altered by fetal exposure to diethylstilbestrol and methoxychlor in CD-1 mice, effects of low versus high doses. Toxicol Appl Pharmacol. 183, 10–22.

49. Jin Z, Tamura G, Tsuchiya T, Sakata K, Kashiwaba M, Osakabe M, Motoyama T. (2001) Adenomatous polyposis coli (APC) gene promoter hypermethylation in primary breast cancers. Br J Cancer. 85(1), 69–73.

50. Virmani AK, Rathi A, Sathyanarayana UG, Padar A, Huang CX, Cunnigham HT, Farinas AJ, Milchgrub S, Euhus DM, Gilcrease M, Herman J, Minna JD, Gazdar AF. (2001) Aberrant methylation of the adenomatous polyposis coli (APC) gene promoter 1A in breast and lung carcinomas. Clin Cancer Res. 7, 1998–2004.

51. Burbee DG, Forgacs E, Zochbauer-Muller S, Shivakumar L, Fong K, Gao B, Randle D, Kondo M, Virmani A, Bader S, Sekido Y, Latif F, Milchgrub S, Toyooka S, Gazdar AF, Lerman MI, Zabarovsky E, White M,

Minna JD. (2001) Epigenetic inactivation of RASSF1A in lung and breast cancers and malignant phenotype suppression. J Natl Cancer Inst. 93, 691–699.

52. Dammann R, Yang G, Pfeifer GP. (2001) Hypermethylation of the CpG island of ras association domain family 1A (RASSF1A), a putative tumor suppressor gene from the 3p21.3 locus, occurs in a large percentage of human breast cancers. Cancer Res. 61, 3105–3109.

53. Honorio S, Agathanggelou A, Schuermann M, Pankow W, Viacava P, Maher ER, Latif F. (2003) Detection of RASSF1A aberrant promoter hypermethylation in sputum from chronic smokers and ductal carcinoma in situ from breast cancer patients. Oncogene. 22, 147–150.

54. Pu RT, Laitala LE, Alli PM, Fackler MJ, Sukumar S, Clark DP. (2003) Methylation profiling of benign and malignant breast lesions and its application to cytopathology. Mod Pathol. 16(11), 1095–1101.

55. Fackler MJ, McVeigh M, Mehrotra J, Blum MA, Lange J, Lapides A, Garrett E, Argani P, Sukumar S. (2004) Quantitative multiplex methylation-specific PCR assay for the detection of promoter hypermethylation in multiple genes in breast cancer. Cancer Res. 64, 442–452.

56. Lewis CM, Cler LR, Bu DW, Zochbauer-Muller S, Milchgrub S, Naftalis EZ, Leitch AM, Minna JD, Euhus DM. (2005) Promoter hypermethylation in benign breast epithelium in relation to predicted breast cancer risk. Clin Cancer Res. 11, 166–172.

57. Gail MH, Brinton LA, Byar DP, Corle DK, Green SB, Schairer C, Mulvihill JJ. (1989) Projecting individualized probabilities of developing breast cancer for white females who are being examined annually. J Natl Cancer Inst. 81, 1879–1886.

58. Sirchia SM, Ferguson AT, Sironi E, Subramanyan S, Orlandi R, Sukumar S, Sacchi N. (2000) Evidence of epigenetic changes affecting the chromatin state of the retinoic acid receptor β2 promoter in breast cancer cells. Oncogene. 19, 1556–1563.

59. Yang Q, Shan L, Yoshimura G, Nakamira M, Nakamura Y, Suzuma T, Umemura T, Mori I, Sakurai T, Kakudo K. (2002) 5-aza-2′-deoxycytidine induces retinoic acid receptor beta 2 demethylation, cell cycle arrest and growth inhibition in breast carcinoma cells. Anticancer Res. 22, 2753–2756.

60. Widschwendter M, Berger J, Hermann M, Muller HM, Amberger A, Zeschnigk M, Widschwendter A, Abendstein B, Zeimet AG, Daxenbichler G, Marth C. (2000) Methylation and silencing of the retinoic acid receptor-β2 gene in breast cancer. J Natl Cancer Inst. 92, 826–832.

61. Coyle YM, Xie X-J, Lewis CM, Bu D, Milchgrub S, Euhus D. (2006) Role of physical activity in modulating breast cancer risk as defined by *APC* and *RASSF1A* promoter hypermethylation in non-malignant breast tissue. Cancer Epidemiol Biomarkers Prev. 16, 192–196.

62. IARC Working Group on the Evaluation of Cancer-Preventive Agents. (2002) Weight Control and Physical Activity, IARC Handbooks of Cancer Prevention, Volume 6. Lyon, France, IARC.

63. Friedenreich CM. (2001) Review of anthropometric factors and breast cancer risk. Eur J Cancer Prev. 10, 15–32.

64. van den Brandt PA, Spiegelman D, Yaun SS, Adami HO, Beeson L, Folsom AR, et al. (2000) Pooled analysis of prospective cohort studies on height, weight, and breast cancer risk. Am J Epidemiol. 152, 514–527.

65. Bergstrom A, Pisani P, Tenet V, Wolk A, Adami HO. (2001) Overweight as an avoidable cause of cancer in Europe. Int J Cancer. 91, 421–430.

66. Huang Z, Hankinson SE, Colditz GA, Stampfer MJ, Hunter DJ, Manson JE, Hennekens CH, Rosner B, Speizer FE, Willett WC. (1997) Dual effects of weight and weight gain on breast cancer risk. JAMA. 278, 1407–1411.

67. Evans DJ, Hoffman RG, Kalkhoff RK, Kissebah AH. (1984) Relationship of body fat topography to insulin sensitivity and metabolic profiles in premenopausal women. Metabolism. 33, 68–75.

68. Haffner SM, Katz MS, Stern MP, Dunn JF. (1989) Relationship of sex hormone binding globulin to overall adiposity and body fat distribution in a biethnic population. Int J Obes. 13, 1–9.

69. Kirschner MA, Samojlik E, Drejka M, Szmal E, Schneider G, Ertel N. (1990) Androgen-estrogen metabolism in women with upper body versus lower body obesity. J Clin Endocrinol Metab. 70, 473–479.

70. Kaye SA, Folsom AR, Soler JT, Prineas RJ, Potter JD. (1991) Associations of body mass and fat distribution with sex hormone concentrations in post menopausal women. Int J Epidemiol. 20, 151–156.

71. Bruning PF, Bonfrer JM, van Noord PA, Hart AA, Jong-Bakker M, Nooijen WJ.

(1992) Insulin resistance and breast-cancer risk. Int J Cancer. 52, 511–516.

72. Bruning PF, Bonfrer JM, Hart AA, van Noord PA, van der Hoeven H, Collette HJ, Battermann JJ, Jong-Bakker M, Nooijen WJ, de Waard F. (1992) Body measurements, estrogen availability and the risk of human breast cancer, A case-control study. Int J Cancer. 51, 14–19.

73. Potischman N, Swanson CA, Siiteri P, Hoover RN. (1996) Reversal of relation between body mass and endogenous estrogen concentrations with menopausal status. J Natl Cancer Inst. 88, 456–758.

74. Key TJ, Pike MC. (1988) The dose-effect relationship between "unopposed" oestrogens and endometrial mitotic rate, its central role in explaining and predicting endometrial cancer risk. Br J Cancer. 57, 205–212.

75. Key TJ, Pike MC. (1988) The roles of oestrogens and progestagens in the epidemiology and prevention of breast cancer. Eur J Cancer Clin Oncol. 24, 29–43.

76. Kirschner MA, Ertel N, Schneider G. (1981) Obesity, hormones and cancer. Cancer Res. 41, 3711–3717.

77. Bruning PF. (1987) Endogenous estrogens and breast cancer a possible relationship between body fat distribution and estrogen availability. J Steroid Biochem. 27, 487–492.

78. Moore JW, Key TJ, Bulbrook RD, Clark GM, Allen DS, Wang DY, Pike MC. (1987) Sex hormone binding globulin and risk factors for breast cancer in a population of normal women who had never used exogenous sex hormones. Br J Cancer. 56, 661–666.

79. Clayton SJ, May FE, Westley BR. (1997) Insulin-like growth factors control the regulation of oestrogen and progesterone receptor expression by oestrogens. Mol Cell Endocrinol. 128, 57–68.

80. Peyrat JP, Bonneterre J, Hecquet B, Vennin P, Louchez MM, Fournier C, Lefebvre J, Demaille A. (1993) Plasma insulin-like growth factor-1 (IGF-1) concentrations in human breast cancer. Eur J Cancer. 29A, 492–497.

81. Bruning PF, Van Doorn J, Bonfrer JM, van Noord PA, Korse CM, Linders TC, Hart AA. (1995) Insulin-like growth-factor-binding protein 3 is decreased in early-stage operable pre-menopausal breast cancer. Int J Cancer. 62, 266–270.

82. Del Giudice ME, Fantus IG, Ezzat S, McKeown-Eyssen G, Page D, Goodwin PJ. (1998) Insulin and related factors in pre-menopausal breast cancer risk. Breast Cancer Res Treat. 47, 111–120.

83. Hankinson SE, Willett WC, Colditz GA, Hunter DJ, Michaud DS, Deroo B, Rosner B, Speizer FE, Pollak M. (1998) Circulating concentrations of insulin-like growth factor-I risk of breast cancer. Lancet. 351, 1393–1396.

84. Toniolo B, Bruning PF, Akhmedkhanov A, Bonfrer JM, Koenig KL, Lukanova A, Shore RE, Zeleniuch-Jacquotte A. (2000) Serum insulin-like growth factor-1 and breast cancer. Int J Cancer. 88, 828–832.

85. Jernstrom H, Barrett-Connor E. (1999) Obesity weight change, fasting insulin, proinsulin, C-peptide and insulin-like growth factor-1 levels in women with and without breast cancer, The Rancho Bernardo Study. J Womens Health Gend Based Med. 8, 1265–1272.

86. Yang G, Lu G, Jin F, Dai Q, Best R, Shu XO, Chen JR, Pan XY, Shrubsole M, Zheng W. (2001) Population-based, case-control study of blood C-peptide level and breast cancer risk. Cancer Epidemiol Biomarkers Prev. 10, 1207–1211.

87. Yu H, Rohan T. (2000) Role of the insulin-like growth factor family in cancer development and progression. J Natl Cancer Inst. 92, 1472–1489.

88. Hu X, Juneja SC, Maihle NJ, Cleary MP. (2002) Leptin-a growth factor in normal and malignant breast cells and for normal mammary gland development. J Natl Cancer Inst. 94, 1704–1711.

89. Laud K, Gourdou I, Pessemesse L, Peyrat JP, Djiane J. (2002) Identification of leptin receptors in human breast cancer, functional activity in the T47-D breast cancer cell line. Mol Cel Endocrinol. 188, 219–226.

90. Dieudonne MN, Machinal-Quelin F, Serazin-Leroy V, Leneveu MC, Pecquery R, Giudicelli Y. (2002) Leptin mediates a proliferative response in human MCF7 breast cancer cells. Biochem Biophys Res Commun. 293, 622–628.

91. Okumura M, Yamamoto M, Sakuma H, Kojima T, Maruyama T, Jamali M, Cooper DR, Yasuda K. (2002) Leptin and high glucose stimulate cell proliferation in MCF-7 human breast cancer cells, reciprocal involvement of PKC-alpha and PPAR expression. Biochimica et Biophysica Acta. 1592, 107–116.

92. Mantzoros CS, Bolhke K, Moschos S, Cramer DW. (1999) Leptin in relation to carcinoma in situ of the breast, a study of pre-menopausal cases and controls. Int J Cancer. 80, 523–526.

93. Malin A, Matthews CE, Shu XO, Cai H, Dai Q, Jin F, Gao YT, Zheng W. (2005) Energy balance and breast cancer risk. Cancer Epidemiol Biomarkers Prev. 14(6), 1496–1501.

94. Singletary KW, Gapstur SM. (2001) Alcohol and breast cancer, review of epidemiologic and experimental evidence and potential mechanisms. JAMA. 286, 2143–2151.

95. Smith-Warner SA, Spiegelman D, Yaun SS, Van Den Brandt PA, Folsom AR, Goldbohm A, Graham S, Holmberg L, Howe GR, Marshall JR, Miller AB, Potter JD, Speizer FE, Willet WC, Wolk A, Hunter DJ. (1998) Alcohol and breast cancer in women. A pooled analysis of cohort studies. JAMA. 270, 535–540.

96. Mezzetti M, La Vecchia C, Decarli A, Boyle P, Talamini R, Franceschi S. (1998) Population attributable risk for breast cancer, diet, nutrition and physical exercise. J Natl Cancer Inst. 90, 389–394.

97. Byers T, Funch DF. (1982) Alcohol and breast cancer. Lancet. 1, 799–800.

98. Baumgartner KB, Anneggers JF, McPherson RS, Frankowski RF, Gilliland FD, Samet JM. (2002) Is alcohol intake associated with breast cancer in Hispanic women? The New Mexico Women's Health Study. Ethn Dis. 12, 460–469.

99. Reichman ME, Judd JT, Longcope C, Schatzkin A, Clevidence BA, Nair PP, et al. (1993) Effects of alcohol consumption on plasma and urinary hormone concentrations in pre-menopausal women. J Natl Cancer Inst. 85, 722–727.

100. Muti P, Trevisan M, Micheli A, Krogh V, Bolelli G, Sciajno R, et al. (1998) Alcohol consumption and total estradiol in premenopausal women. Cancer Epidemiol Biomarkers Prev. 7, 189–193.

101. Sarkola T, Makisalo H, Fukunaga T, Eriksson C. (1999) Acute effect of alcohol on estradiol, estrone, progesterone, prolactin, cortisol and luteinizing hormone in premenopausal women. Alcohol Clin Exp Res. 23, 976–982.

102. Dorgan JF, Reichman ME, Judd JT, Brown C, Longcope C, Schatzkin A, et al. (1994) The relation of reported alcohol ingestion to plasma levels of estrogens and androgens in pre-menopausal women (Maryland, United States). Cancer Causes Control 1994. 5, 53–60.

103. Sarkola T, Fukunaga T, Makisalo H, Eriksson C. (2000) Acute effect of alcohol on androgens in pre-menopausal women. Alcohol Alcohol. 35, 84–90.

104. Verkasalo P, Thomas H, Appleby P, Davey G, Key T. (2001) Circulating levels of sex hormones and their relation to risk factors for breast cancer, a cross-sectional study in 1092 pre- and postmenopausal women (United Kingdom). Cancer Causes Control. 12, 47–59.

105. Martin C, Mainous A, Curry T, Martin D. (1999) Alcohol use in adolescent females, correlated with estradiol and testosterone. Am J Addict. 8, 9–14.

106. Stevens R, Davis S, Mirick D, Kheifets L, Kaune W. (2000) Alcohol consumption and urinary concentration of 6-sulfatoxymelatonin in healthy women. Epidemiology. 11, 660–665.

107. Purohit V. (1998) Moderate alcohol consumption and estrogen levels in postmenopausal women, a review. Alcohol Clin Exp Res. 22, 994–997.

108. Dorgan JF, Baer DJ, Albert PS, Judd JT, Brown ED, Corle DK, et al. (2001) Serum hormones and the alcohol-breast cancer association in postmenopausal women. J Natl Cancer Inst. 93, 710–715.

109. Longnecker M, Tseng M. (1998) Alcohol, hormones and postmenopausal women. Alcohol Health Res World. 22, 185–189.

110. Boyd N, McGuire V, Fishell E, Kuriov V, Lockwood G, Tritchler D. (1989) Plasma lipids in premenopausal women with mammographic dysplasia. Br J Cancer. 59, 766–771.

111. Herrington L, Saftlas A, Stanford J, Brinton L, Wolfe J. (1993) Do alcohol intake and mammographic densities interact in regard to the risk of breast cancer? Cancer. 71, 3029–3035.

112. Funkhouser E, Waterbor J, Cole P, Rubin E. (1993) Mammographic patterns and breast cancer risk factors among women having elective screening. South Med J. 86, 177–180.

113. Boyd NF, Connelly P, Byng J, Yaffe M, Draper H, Little L, et al. (1995) Plasma lipids, lipoproteins and mammographic densities. Cancer Epidemiol Biomarkers Prev. 4, 727–733.

114. Vachon C, Kushi L, Cerhan J, Kuni C, Sellers T. (2000) Association of diet and mammographic breast density in the Minnesota Breast Cancer Family cohort. Cancer Epidemiol Biomarkers Prev. 9, 151–160.

115. Vachon C, Kuni C, Anderson K, Anderson V, Sellers T. (2000) Association of mammographically defined breast density with epidemiologic risk factors for breast cancer (United States). Cancer Causes Control. 11, 653–662.

116. Byrne C, colditz G, Willett W, Speizer F, Pollak M, Hankinson S. (2000) Plasma insulin-like growth factor (IGF)-1, IGF-binding protein 3 and mammographic density. Cancer Res. 60, 3744–3748.

117. Boyd N, Jensen H, Cooke G, Han N, Lockwood G, Miller A. (2000) Mammographic densities and the prevalence and incidence of histological types of benign breast disease, Reference Pathologists of the Canadian National Breast Screening Study. Eur J Cancer Prev. 9, 15–24.

118. Lee M, Petrakis N, Wrensch M, King E, Miike R, Sickles E. (1994) Association of abnormal nipple aspirate cytology and mammographic pattern and density. Cancer Epidemiol Biomarkers Prev. 3, 33–36.

119. Boyd N, Lockwood G, Byng J, Tritchler D, Yaffe M. (1998) Mammographic densities and breast cancer risk. Cancer Epidemiol Biomarkers Prev. 7, 1133–1144.

120. Zhang S, Hunter DJ, Hankinson SE, Giovannucci EL, Rosner BA, Colditz GA, et al. (1999) A prospective study of folate intake and the risk of breast cancer. JAMA. 281, 1632–1637.

121. Rohan T, Jain M, Howe G, Miller A. (2000) Dietary folate consumption and breast cancer risk. J Natl Cancer Inst. 92, 266–269.

122. Negri E, LaVecchia C, Franceschi S. (2000) Dietary folate consumption and breast cancer risk. J Natl Cancer Inst. 92, 1270–1271.

123. Sellers T, Kushi L, Cerhan J, et al. (2001) Dietary folate mitigates alcohol associated risk of breast cancer in a prospective study of postmenopausal women. Epidemiology. 12, 420–428.

124. Hillman R, Steinberg S. (1982) The effects of alcohol on folate metabolism. Annu Rev Med. 33, 345–354.

125. Jacques P, Sulsky S, Hartz S, Russell R. (1989) Moderate alcohol intake and nutritional status in nonalcoholic elderly subjects. Am J Clin Nutr. 50, 875–883.

126. Bailey L. (1990) Folate status assessment. J Nutr. 120(suppl 11), 1508–1511.

127. Giovanucci E, Stampfer M, Colditz G, Rimm E, Trichopoulos D, Rosner B, et al. (1993) Folate, methionine and alcohol intake and risk of colorectal adenoma. J Natl Cancer Inst. 85, 875–884.

128. Choi S, Mason J. (2000) Folate and carcinogenesis, an integrated scheme. J Nutr. 130, 129–132.

129. Kim Y. (1999) Folate and carcinogenesis, evidence, mechanisms and implications. J Nutr Biochem. 10, 66–88.

130. Duthie S. (1999) Folic acid deficiency and cancer, mechanisms of DNA instability. Br Med Bull. 55, 578–592.

131. Fenech M, Aitken C, Rinaldi J. (1998) Folate, vitamin B12, homocysteine status and DNA damage in young Australian adults. Carcinogenesis. 19, 1163–1171.

132. Smith S, Crocitto L. (1999) DNA methylation in eukaryotic chromosome stability revisited, DNA methyltransferase in the management of DNA conformation space. Mol Carcinog. 25, 1–9.

133. Drewnowski A, Rock CL, Henderson SA, Shore AB, Fischler C, Galan P, et al. (1997) Serum beta-carotene and vitamin C as biomarkers of vegetable and fruit intakes in a community-based sample of French adults. Am J Clin Nutr. 65, 1706–1802.

134. Forman MR, Beecher GR, Lanza E, Reichman ME, Graubard BI, Campbell WS, et al. (1995) Effect of alcohol consumption on plasma carotenoid concentrations in premenopausal women, a controlled dietary study. Am J Clin Nutr. 62, 131–135.

135. Park SK, Yoo KY, Lee SJ, Kim SU, Ahn SH, Noh DY, et al. (2000) Alcohol consumption, glutathione S-transferase M1 and T1 genetic polymorphisms and breast cancer risk. Pharmacogenetics. 10, 301–309.

136. Willett WC. (2001) Diet and cancer, one view at the start of the millennium. Cancer Epidemiol Biomarkers Prev. 10, 3–8.

137. Howe GR, Hirohata T, Hislop TG, Iscovich JM, Yuan JM, Katsouyanni K, et al. (1990) Dietary factors and risk of breast cancer, combined analysis of 12 case-control studies. J Natl Cancer Inst. 82, 561–569.

138. Hunter DJ, Spiegelman D, Adami HO, Beeson L, van den Brandt PA, Folsom AR, et al. (1996) Cohort studies of fat intake and the risk of breast cancer, a pooled analysis. N Eng J Med. 334, 356–361.

139. Smith-Warner SA, Spiegelman D, Adami HO, Beeson WL, van den Brandt PA, Folsom AR, et al. (2001a) Types of dietary fat and breast cancer, a pooled analysis of cohort studies. Int J Cancer. 92, 767–774.

140. Prentice RL, Caan B, Chlebowski RT, Patterson R, Kuller LH, Ockene JK, Margolis KL, Limacher MC, Manson JE, et al. (2006) Low-fat dietary pattern and risk of invasive breast cancer; the Women's Health Initiative Randomized Controlled Dietary Modification Trial. JAMA. 295, 629–642.

141. World Cancer Research Fund Panel (Potter JD Chair). Food, Nutrition and the Prevention of Cancer, a Global Perspective. Washington, DC, American Institute for Cancer Research, 1997.

142. Smith-Warner SA, Spiegelman D, Yaun SS, Adami HO, Beeson WL, van den Brandt PA, et al. (2001) Intake of fruits and vegetables and risk of breast cancer, a pooled analysis of cohort studies. JAMA. 285, 769–776.

143. van Gils CH, Peeters PH, Bueno-de-Mesquita HB, Boshuizen HC, Lahmann PH, Clavel-Chapelon F, et al. (2005) Consumption of vegetables and fruits and risk of breast cancer. JAMA. 293(2), 183–193.

144. Ahn J, Gammon MD, Santella RM, Gaudet MM, Britton JA, Teitelbaum SL, Terry MB, Neugut AI, Josephy PD, Ambrosone CB. (2004) Myeloperoxidase genotype, fruit and vegetable consumption and breast cancer risk. Cancer Res. 64(20), 7634–7639.

145. Wu AH, Ziegler RG, Nomura AM, West DW, Kolonel LN, Horn-Ross PL, et al. (1998) Soy intake and risk of breast cancer in Asians and Asian Americans. Am J Clin Nutr. 68(suppl 6), 1437S–1443S.

146. Greenwald P. (2002) Cancer prevention clinical trials. J Clin Oncol. 20(suppl 18), 14S–22S.

147. Jones JL, Daley BJ, Enderson BL, Zhou JR, Karlstad MD. (2002) Genistein inhibits tamoxifen effects on cell proliferation and cell cycle arrest in T47D breast cancer cells. Am Surg. 68, 575–577.

148. JU YH, Doerge DR, Allred KF, Allred CD, Helferich WG. (2002) Dietary genistein negates the inhibitory effect of tamoxifen on growth of estrogen-dependent human breast cancer (MCF-7) cells implanted in athymic mice. Cancer Res. 62, 2474–2477.

149. Dorgan JF, Sowell A, Swanson CA, Potischman N, Miller R, Schussler N, et al. (1998) Relationships of serum carotenoids, retinol, alpha-tocopherol and selenium with breast cancer risk, results from a prospective study in Columbia, Missouri (United States). Cancer Causes Control. 9, 89–97.

150. Hulten K, Van Kappel AL, Winkvist A, Kaaks R, Hallmans G, Lenner P, et al. (2001) Carotenoids, alpha-tocopherols and retinol in plasma and breast cancer risk in northern Sweden. Cancer Causes Control. 12, 529–537.

151. Sato R, Helzlsouer KJ, Alberg AJ, Hoffman SC, Norkus EP, Comstock GW. (2002) Prospective study of carotenoids, tocopherols and retinoid concentrations and the risk of breast cancer. Cancer Epidemiol Biomarkers Prev. 11, 451–457.

152. IARC. (2002) Weight control and physical activity. IARC Handbooks of Cancer Prevention, vol. 6. Lyon, France, IARC Press.

153. Colditz GA. (1997) Epidemiology-future directions. Int J Epidemiol. 26(4), 693–697.

154. Marrett LD, Theis B, Ashbury FD. (2000) Workshop report, physical activity and cancer prevention. Chronic Dis Can. 21(4), 143–149.

155. Slattery M. (2004) Physical activity and colorectal cancer. Sports Med. 34, 239–252.

156. Calton BA, Lacey JV Jr, Schatzkin A, Schairer C, Colbert LH, Albanes D, Leitzmann MF. (2006) Physical activity and the risk of colon cancer among women, a prospective cohort study (United States). Int J Cancer. 119, 385–291.

157. Larsson SC, Rutegard J, Bergkvist L, Wolk A. (2006) Physical activity, obesity and risk of colon and rectal cancer in a cohort of Swedish men. Eur J Cancer. 42, 2590–2597.

158. Friedenreich C, Norat T, Steindorf K, Boutron-Ruault MC, Pischon T, Mazuir M, et al. (2006) Physical activity and risk of colon and rectal cancers, the European prospective investigation into cancer and nutrition. Cancer Epidemiol Biomarkers Prev. 15(12), 2398–2407.

159. Lee KJ, Inoue M, Otani T, Iwasaki M, Sasazuki S, Tsugane S. (2007) Physical activity and risk of colorectal cancer in Japanese men and women, the Japan Public Health Center-based prospective study. Cancer Causes Control. 18, 199–209.

160. Rosenberg L, Boggs D, Wise LA, Palmer JR, Roltsch MH, Makambi KH, Adams-Campbell LL. (2006) A follow-up study of physical activity and incidence of colorectal polyps in African-American women. Cancer Epidemiol Biomarkers Prev. 15(8), 1438–1442.

161. Hill MJ, Morson BC, Bussey HJ. (1978) Aetiology of adenoma-carcinoma sequence in large bowel. Lancet. 1, 245–247.

162. McTiernan A, Yasui Y, Sorensen B, Irwin ML, Morgan A, Rudolph RE, Surawicz C, Lampe JW, Ayub K, Potter JD, Lampe PD. (2006) Effect of a 12-month exercise intervention on patterns of cellular proliferation in colonic crypts, A randomized controlled trial. Cancer Epidemiol Biomarkers Prev. 15(9), 1588–1597.

163. Bostick RM, Fosdick L, Lillemoe TJ, Overn P, Wood JR, Grambsch P, et al. (1997) Methodological findings and considerations in measuring colorectal epithelial cell proliferation in humans. Cancer Epidemiol Biomarkers Prev. 6, 931–842.

164. Quadrilatero J, Hoffman-Goetz L. (2003) Physical activity and colon cancer, A systematic

review of potential mechanisms. J Sports Med Phys Fitness. 43, 121–138.

165 Kaaks R, Toniolo P, Akhmedkhanov A, Lukanova A, Biessy C, Dechaud H, et al. (2000) Serum C-peptide, insulin-like growth factor (IGF)-I, IGF-binding proteins, and colorectal cancer risk in women. J Natl Cancer Inst. 92(19), 1592–1600.

166. Ma J, Pollak MN, Giovannucci E, Chan JM, Tao Y, Hennekens CH, et al. (1999) Prospective study of colorectal cancer risk in men and plasma levels of insulin-like growth factor (IGF)-I and IGF-binding proteins-3. J Natl Cancer Inst. 91(7), 620–625.

167. Slattery ML, Curtin K, Ma K, Edwards S, Schaffer D, Anderson K, et al. (2002) Diet activity and lifestyle associations with p53 mutation in colon tumors. Cancer Epidemiol Biomarkers Prev. 11(6), 541–548.

168. Slattery ML, Anderson K, Curtin K, Ma K, Schaffer D, Edwards S, et al. (2001) Lifestyle factors and Ki-ras mutations in colon cancer tumors. Mutat Res. 483(12), 73–81.

169. Martinez ME, Maltzman T, Marshall JR, Einspahr J, Reid ME, Sampliner R, et al. (1999) Risk factors for Ki-ras protooncogene mutation in sporadic colorectal adenomas. Cancer Res. 59(20), 5181–5185.

170. Boutron-Rualt MC, Senesse P, Meance S, Belghiti C, Faivre J. (2001) Energy intake, body mass index, physical activity and the colorectal adenoma-carcinoma sequence. Nutr Cancer. 39, 50–57.

171. Neugut AI, Lee WC, Garbowski GC, Waye JD, Forde KA, Treat MR, et al. (1991) Obesity and colorectal adenomatous polyps. J Natl Cancer Inst. 83, 359–361.

172. Shinchi K, Kono S, Honjo S, Todoroki I, Sakurai Y, Imanishi K, et al. (1994) Obesity and adenomatous polyps of the sigmoid colon. Jpn J Cancer Res. 85, 479–484.

173. Davidow AL, Neugut AI, Jacobson JS, Ahsan H, Garbowski GC, Forde KA, et al. (1996) Recurrent adenomatous polyps and body mass index. Cancer Epidemiol Biomarkers Prev. 5, 313–315.

174. Giovannucci E, Colditz GA, Stampfer MJ, Willett WC. (1996) Physical activity, obesity and risk of colorectal adenoma in women (United States). Cancer Causes Control. 7, 253–263.

175. Bird CL, Frankl HD, Lee ER, Haile RW. (1998) Obesity, weight gain, large weight changes and adenomatous polyps of the left colon and rectum. Am J Epidemiol. 147, 670–680.

176. Kono S, Handa K, Hayabuchi H, Kiyohara C, Inoue H, Marugame T, et al. (1999) Obesity, weight gain and risk of colon adenomas in Japanese men. Jpn J cancer Res. 90, 801–811.

177. Lukanova A, Bjor O, Kaaks R, Lenner P, Lindahl B, Hallmans G, Stattin P. (2006) Body mass index and cancer. Results from the northern Sweden health and disease cohort. Int J Cancer. 118, 458–466.

178. Moore LL, Bradlee ML, Singer MR, Splansky GL, Proctor MH, Ellison RC, et al. (2004) BMI and waist circumference as predictors of lifetime colon cancer risk in Framingham Study adults. Int J Obes Relat Metab Disord. 28, 559–567.

179. MacInnis RJ, English DR, Hopper JL, Haydon AM, Gertiz DM, Giles GG. (2004) Body size and composition and colon cancer risk in men. Cancer Epidemiol Biomarkers Prev. 13, 553–559.

180. Pischon T, Lahmann PH, Boeing H, Friedenreich C, Norat T, Tjonneland A, et al. (2006) Body size and risk of colon and rectal cancer in the European prospective investigation into cancer and nutrition (EPIC). J Natl Cancer Inst. 98, 920–931.

181. Gunter MJ, Leitzmann MF. (2006) Obesity and colorectal cancer, epidemiology, mechanisms and candidate genes. J Nutr Biochem. 17, 145–156.

182. Khaw KT, Wareham N, Bingham S, Luben R, Welch A, Day N. (2004) Preliminary communication, glycated hemoglobin, diabetes and incident colorectal cancer in men and women, a prospective analysis from the European prospective investigation into cancer. Norfolk study. Cancer Epidemiol Biomarkers Prev. 13, 915–919.

183. Yam D, Fink A Mashia A, Ben-Hur E. (1996) Hyperinsulinemia in colon, stomach and breast cancer patients. Cancer Lett. 104, 129–132.

184. Nilsen TI, Vatten LJ. (2001) Prospective study of colorectal cancer risk and physical activity, diabetes, blood glucose and BMI, exploring the hyperinsulinaemia hypothesis. Br J Cancer. 84, 417–422.

185. Platz EA, Hankinson SE, Rifai N, Colditz GA, Speizer FE, Giovannucci E. (1999) Glycosylated hemoglobin and risk of colorectal cancer and adenoma (United States). Cancer Causes Control. 10, 379–386.

186. Kaaks R, Toniolo P, Akhmedkhanov A, Lukanove A, Biessy C, Dechaud H, et al. (2000) Serum C-peptide, insulin-like growth factor (IGF)-I, IGF-binding proteins, and colorectal cancer risk in women. J Natl Cancer Inst. 92, 1592–1600.

187. Jee SH, Ohrr H, Sull JW, Yun JE, Ji M, Samet JM. (2005) Fasting serum glucose level and cancer risk in Korean men and women. JAMA. 293, 194–202.

188. Saydah SH, Platz EA, Rifai N, Pollak MN, Brancati FL, Helzlsour KJ. (2003) Association of markers of insulin and glucose control with subsequent colorectal cancer risk. Cancer Epidemiol Biomarkers Prev. 12, 412–418.

189. Ma J, Pollak MN, Giovannucci E, Chan JM, Tao Y, Hennekens CH, et al. (1999) Prospective study of colorectal cancer risk in men and plasma levels of insulin-like growth factor (IGF)-I and IGF-binding protein-3. J Natl Cancer Inst. 91, 620–625.

190. Yamada K, Araki S, Tamura M, Sakai I, Takahashi Y, Kashihara H, et al. (1998) Relation of serum total cholesterol, serum triglycerides and fasting plasma glucose to colorectal carcinoma in situ. Int J Epidemiol. 27, 794–798.

191. Schoen RE, Tangen CM, Kuller LH, Burke GL, Cushman M, Tracy RP, et al. (1999) Increased blood glucose and insulin, body size and incident colorectal cancer. J Natl Cancer Inst. 91, 1147–1154.

192. Koenuma M, Yamori T, Sururo T. (1989) Insulin and insulin-like growth factor I stimulate proliferation of metastatic variants of colon carcinoma 26. Jpn J Cancer Res. 80, 51–58.

193. Wu X, Fan Z, Masui H, Rosen N, Mendelsohn J. (1995) Apoptosis induced by an anti-epidermal growth factor receptor monoclonal antibody in a human colorectal carcinoma cell line and its delay by insulin. J Clin Invest. 95, 1897–1905.

194. Bjork J, Nilsson J, Hultcrantz R, Johansson C. (1993) Growth-regulatory effects of sensory neuropeptides, epidermal growth factor, insulin, and somatostatin on the non-transformed intestinal epithelial cell line IEC-6 and the colon cancer cell line HT 29. Scand J Gastroenterol. 28, 879–884.

195. Tran TT, Medline A, Bruce WR. (1995) Insulin promotion of colon tumors in rats. Cancer Epidemiol Biomarkers Prev. 5, 1013–1015.

196. Corpet DE, Jacquinet C, Peiffer G, Tache S. (1997) Insulin injections promote the growth of aberrant crypt foci in the colon of rats. Nutr Cancer. 27, 316–320.

197. Giovannucci E. (2001) Insulin, insulin-like growth factors and colon cancer, a review of the evidence. J Nutr. 131, 3109S–3120S.

198. DeLellis K, Rinoldi S, Kaaks FJ, Kolonel LN, Henderson B, Le Marchand L. (2004) Dietary and lifestyle correlates of plasma insulin-like growth factor-I (IGF-I) and IGF finding protein-3 (IGFBP-3), The Multiethnic Cohort. Cancer Epidemiol Biomarkers Prev. 13(9), 1444–1451.

199. Wu Y, Yakar S, Zhao L, Hennighausen L, LeRoith D. (2002) Circulating insulin-like growth factor-I levels regulate colon cancer growth and metastasis. Cancer Res. 62, 1030–1035.

200. Esposito K, Nappo F, Marfella R, Giugliano G, Giugliano F, Ciotola M, et al. (2002) Inflammatory cytokine concentrations are acutely increased by hyperglycemia in humans, role of oxidative stress. Circulation. 106, 2067–2072.

201. Mohanty P, Hamouda W, Garg R, Aljada A, Ghanim H, Dandona P. (2000) Glucose challenge stimulates reactive oxygen species (ROS) generation by leukocytes. J Clin Endocrinol Metab. 85, 2970–2973.

202. Eaden JA, Abrams KR, Mayberry JF. (2001) The risk of colorectal cancer in ulcerative colitis, a meta-analysis. Gut. 48, 526–535.

203. Steinbach G, Lynch PM, Phillips RK, Wallace M, Hawk E, Gordon G, et al. (2000) The effect of celecoxib, a cyclooxygenase-2 inhibitor, in familial adenomatous polyposis. New Engl J Med. 342, 1946–1952.

204. Baron JA, Cole BF, Sandler RS, Haile RW, Ahnen D, Bresalier R, et al. (2003) A randomized trial of aspirin to prevent colorectal adenomas. New Engl J Med. 348, 891–899.

205. Slattery ML, Anderson K, Curtin K, Ma KN, Schaffer D, Edwards S, Samowitz W. (2001) Lifestyle factors and Ki-ras mutation in colon cancer tumors. Mut Res. 483, 73–81.

206. Cross AJ, Pollock JRA, Bingham SA. (2003) Haem, not protein or inorganic iron, is responsible for endogenous intestinal N-nitrosation arising from red meat. Cancer Res. 63, 2358–2360.

207. Sesink AL, Termont DS, Kleibeuker JH, Van der Meer R. (1999) Red meat and colon cancer: the cytotoxic and hyperproliferative effects of dietary heme. Cancer Res. 59, 5704–5709.

208. Hughes R, Pollock JRA, Bingham S. (2002) Effect of vegetables, tea, and soy on endogenous N-nitrosation, fecal ammonia, and fecal water genotoxicity during a high meat diet in humans. Nutr Cancer. 42, 70–77.

209. Hughes R, Cross AJ, Pollock JRA, Bingham S. (2001) Dose-dependent effect of dietary meat on endogenous colonic N-nitrosation. Carcinogenesis 22, 199–202.

210. Miller JA. (1994) Research in chemical carcinogenesis with Elizabeth Miller a trail of discovery with our associates. Drug Metabol Dispos. 26, 1–36.

211. Scanlan RA. (1983) Formation and occurrence of nitrosamines in food. Cancer Res. 43, 2435S–2440S.

212. Hothckiss JH. (1989) Preformed N-nitroso compounds in foods and beverages. Cancer Surv. 8, 295–321.

213. Norat T, Lukanova A, Ferrari P, Riboli E. (2002) Meat consumption and colorectal cancer risk, dose-response meta-analysis of epidemiological studies. Int J Cancer. 98, 241–256.

214. Chao A, Thun MJ, Connell CJ, McCullough ML, Jacobs EJ, Flanders WD, et al. (2005) Meat consumption and risk of colorectal cancer. JAMA. 293(2), 172–182.

215. Blount BC, Ames BN. (1994) Analysis of uracil in DNA by gas chromatography-mass spectrometry. Anal Biochem. 219, 195–200.

216. Giovannucci E. (2002a) Epidemiologic studies of folate and colorectal neoplasia, A review. J Nutr. 132, 2350S–2355S.

217. Giovannucci E, Rimm EB, Ascherio A, Stampfer MJ, Colditz GA, Willett WC. (1995) Alcohol, low-methionine-low-folate diets and risk or colon cancer in men. J Natl Cancer Inst. 87, 265–273.

218. Larsson SC, Giovannucci E, Wolk A. (2005) A prospective study of dietary folate intake and risk of colorectal cancer, Modification by caffeine intake and cigarette smoking. Cancer Epidemiol Biomarkers Prev. 14(3), 740–743.

219. Jiang Q, Chen K, Ma X, Li Q, Yu W, Shu G, Yao K. (2005) Diets, polymorphisms of methylenetetrahydrofolate reductase, and the susceptibility of colon cancer and rectal cancer. Cancer Detection and Prev. 29, 146–154.

220. Department of Health and Human Services. (2004) The Health Consequences of Tobacco Use, A Report of the Surgeon General. Atlanta, U.S. Department of Health and Human Services, Centers for Disease Control and Prevention, National Center for Chronic Disease Prevention and Health Promotion, Office on Smoking and Health.

221. Giovannucci E, Colditz GA, Stampfer MJ, Hunter D, Rosner BA, Willett WC, et al. (1994) A prospective study of cigarette smoking and risk of colorectal adenoma and colorectal cancer in U.S. women. J Natl Cancer Inst. 86, 192–199.

222. Giovannucci E, Rimm EB, Ascherio A, Colditz GA, Spiegelman D, Stampfer MJ, et al. (1999) Smoking and risk of total and fatal prostate cancer in United States health professionals. Cancer Epidemiol Biomarkers Prev. 8, 277–282.

223. Nagata C, Shimizu H, Kametani M, Takeyema N, Ohnuma T, Matsushita S. (1999) Cigarette smoking, alcohol use, and colorectal adenoma in Japanese men and women. Dis Colon Rectum. 42, 337–342.

224. Kikendall JW, Bowen PE, Burgess MB, Magnetti C, Woodward J, Langenberg P. (1989) Cigarettes and alcohol as independent risk factors for colonic adenomas. Gastroenterology. 97, 660–664.

225. Cope GF, Wyatt JI, Pinder IF, Lee PN, Heatley RV, Kelleher J. (1991) Alcohol consumption in patients with colorectal adenomatous polyps. Gut. 32, 70–72.

226. Monnet E, Allemand H, Farina H, Carayon P. (1991) Cigarette smoking and the risk of colorectal adenoma in men. Scand J Gastroenterol. 26, 758–762.

227. Zahm S, Cocco P, Blair A. (1991) Tobacco smoking as a risk for colon polyps. Am J. Public Health. 81, 846–849.

228. Longnecker MP, Chen MJ, Probst-Hensch NM, Harper JM, Lee ER, Frankl HD, et al. (1996) Alcohol and smoking in relation to the prevalence of adenomatous colorectal polyps at sigmoidoscopy. Epidemiology. 7, 275–280.

229. Olsen J, Kronborg O. (1993) Coffee, tobacco and alcohol as risk factors for cancer and adenoma of the large intestine. Int J Epidemiol. 22, 398–402.

230. Boutron MC, Faivre J, Dop MC, Quipourt V, Senesse P. (1995) Tobacco, alcohol and colorectal tumors, a multistep process. Am J Epidemiol. 141, 1038–1046.

231. Breuer-Katschinski B, Nemes K, Marr A, Rump B, Leiendecker B, Breuer N, et al. (2000) Alcohol and cigarette smoking and the risk of colorectal adenomas. Dig Dis Sci. 45, 487–493.

232. Almendingen K, Hofstad B, Trygg K, Hoff G, Hussain A, Vatn MH. (2000) Smoking and colorectal adenomas, a case-control study. Eur J Cancer Prev. 9, 193–203.

233. Hisako I, Chikako K, Tomomi M, Sachiko S, Emiko T, Koichi H, et al. (2000) Cigarette smoking, CYPIA1 MspI and GSTM1 genotypes, and colorectal adenomas. Cancer Res. 60, 3749–3752.

234. Martinez ME, McPherson RS, Annegers JF, Levin B. (1995) Cigarette smoking and alcohol consumption as risk factors for colorectal adenomatous polyps. J Natl Cancer Inst. 87, 274–279.

235. Potter JD, Bigler J, Fosdick L, Bostick RM, Kampman E, Chen C, et al. (1999) Colorectal adenomatous and hyper-plastic polyps, smoking and N-acetyltransferase 2 polymorphisms. Cancer Epidemiol Biomarkers Prev. 8, 69–75.

236. Kato I, Tominaga S, Matsuura A, Yoshii Y, Shirai M, Kobayashi S. (1990) A comparative case-control study of colorectal cancer and adenoma. Jpn J Cancer Res. 81, 1101–1108.

237. Ji BT, Weissfeld JL, Chow WH, Huang WY, Schoen RE, Hayes RB. (2006) Tobacco smoking and colorectal hyperplastic and adenomatous polyps. Cancer Epidemiol Biomarkers Prev. 15(5), 897–901.

238. Chute C, Willet W, Colditz G, Stampfer MJ, Baron JA, Rosner B, et al. (1991) A prospective study of body mass, height, and smoking and risk of colorectal cancer in women. Cancer Causes Control. 2, 117–224.

239. Chyou P-H, Nomura A, Stemmermann G. (1996) A prospective study of colon and rectal cancer among Hawaii Japanese men. Ann Epidemiol. 6, 276–282.

240. Doll R, Peto R, Wheatley K, Gray R, Sutherland I. (1994) Mortality in relation to smoking, 40 years' observations on male British doctors. BMJ. 309, 901–911.

241. Engeland A, Andersen A, Haldorsen T, Tretli S. (1996) Smoking habits and risk of cancers other than lung cancer, 28 years' follow-up of 26,000 Norwegian men and women. Cancer Causes Control. 7, 497–506.

242. Heineman E, Zahm S, McLaughlin J, Vaught J. (1994) Increased risk of colorectal cancer among smokers, results of a 26-year follow-up of US veterans and a review. Int J Cancer. 59, 728–738.

243. Nyren O, Bergstrom R, Nystrom L, Engholm G, Ekbom A, Adami HO, et al. (1996) Smoking and colorectal cancer, a 20-year follow-up study of Swedish construction workers. J Natl Cancer Inst. 88, 1302–1307.

244. Tverdal A, Thelle D, Stensvold I, Leren P, Bjartveit K. (1993) Mortality in relation to smoking history, 13 years' follow-up of 68,000 Norwegian men and women 35–49 years. J Clin Epidemiol. 46, 475–487.

245. Slattery ML, Samowtiz W, Ma K, Murtaugh M, Sweeney C, Levin TR, Neuhausen S. (2004) CYP1A1, cigarette smoking and colon and rectal cancer. Am J Epidemiol. 160, 842–852.

246. Huang K, Sandler RS, Milikan RC, Schroeder JC, North KE, Hu J. (2006) GSTM1 and GSTT1 polymorphisms, cigarette smoking and risk of colon cancer, a population-based case-control study in North Carolina (United States). Cancer Causes Control. 17, 385–394.

247. van der Hel OL, de Mesquita HBB, Sandkuijl L, van Noord PA, Pearson PL, Grobbee DE, et al. (2003) Rapid N-acetyltransferase 2 imputed phenotype and smoking may increase risk of colorectal cancer in women (Netherlands). Cancer Causes Control. 14, 293–298.

248. Report of the Lung Cancer Progress Review Group. National Cancer Institute. Publication No. 01-5025. August 2001.

249. Smith-Warner S, Spiegelman D, Yaun S-S, Albanes D, Beeson W, van den Brandt PA, et al. (2003) Fruits, vegetables and lung cancer, a pooled analysis of cohort studies. Int J Cancer. 107, 1001–1011.

250. US Department of Health and Human Services. (2004) The Health Consequences of Tobacco Use, A Report of the Surgeon General, Atlanta, US Department of Health and Human Services, Center for Disease Control and Prevention, National Center for Chronic Disease Prevention and Health Promotion, Office of Smoking and Health.

251. Thun M, Henley S, Calle E. (2002) Tobacco use and cancer, an epidemiologic perspective for geneticists. Oncogene. 21, 7307–7325.

252. Thun M, Lally C, Flannery J, Calle E, Flanders W, Heath C. (1997b) Cigarette smoking and changes in the histopathology of lung cancer. J Natl Cancer Inst. 89, 1580–1586.

253. Patel JD. (2005) Lung cancer in women. J Clin Oncol. 23, 3212–3218

254. Hecht SS. (2003) Tobacco carcinogens, their biomarkers and tobacco-induced cancer. Nature Rev Cancer. 3, 733–744.

255. Osada H, Takahashi T. (2002) Genetic alterations of multiple tumor suppressors and oncogenes in the carcinogenesis and progression of lung cancer. Oncogene. 21, 7421–7434.

256. Smits KM, Benhamou S, Garte S, Weijenberg MP, Alamanos Y, Ambrosone C, et al. (2004) Association of metabolic gene polymorphisms with tobacco consumption in healthy controls. Int J Cancer. 110, 266–270.

257. Kiyohara C, Otsu A, Shirakawa T, Fukuda S, Hopkin JM. (2002) Genetic polymorphisms and lung cancer susceptibility, a review. Lung Cancer. 37, 241–256.

258. Goode EL, Ulrich CM, Potter JD. (2002) Polymorphisms in DNA repair genes and associations with cancer risk. Cancer Epidemiol Biomarkers. 11, 1513–1530.

259. Christiani DC. (2000) Smoking and the molecular epidemiology of lung cancer. Clinics Chest Med. 21(1), 87–93.

260. World Cancer Research fund and American Institute for Cancer Research, 1997. Food,

nutrition and prevention of cancer, A global prospective. Washington, DC, American Institute for Cancer Research.

261. Kristal AR, Potter JD. (2006) Not the time to abandon the food frequency questionnaire, Counterpoint. Cancer Epidemiol Biomarkers Prev. 15(10), 1759–1764.

262. Tardon A, Lee WJ, Delgado-Rodriguez M, Dosemeci M, Albanes D, Hoover R, Blair A. (2005) Leisure-time physical activity and lung cancer, a meta-analysis. Cancer Causes Control. 16, 389–397.

263. Alfano CM, Klesges RC, Murray DM, Bowen DJ, McTiernan A, Vander Weg MW, et al. (2004) Physical activity in relation to all-site and lung cancer incidence and mortality in current and former smokers. Cancer Epidemiol Biomarkers Prev. 13(12), 2233–2241.

264. Bak H, Christensen J, Thomsen BL, Tjonneland A, Overvad K, Loft S, Raaschou-Nielsen O. (2005) Physical activity and risk for lung cancer in a Danish cohort. Int J Cancer. 116, 439–445.

265. Steindorf K, Friedenreich, Linseisen J, Rohrmann S, Rundle A, Veglia F, et al. (2006) Physical activity and lung cancer risk in the European prospective investigation into cancer and nutrition cohort. Int J Cancer. 119, 2389–2397.

266. Sinner P, Folsom AR, Harnack L, Eberly LE, Schmitz KH. (2006) The association of physical activity with lung cancer incidence in a cohort of older women. The Iowa women's health study. Cancer Epidemiol Biomarkers Prev. 15, 2359–2363.

267. Jemal A, Murray T, Ward E, Samuels A, Tiwari RC, Ghafoor A, et al. (2005) Cancer statistics. CA Cancer J Clin. 55, 10–30.

268. Breslow N, Chan CW, Dhom G, (1977) Latent carcinoma of prostate of autopsy in seven areas. Int J Cancer. 20, 680.

269. Dhom G. (1983) Epidemiologic aspects of latent and clinically manifest carcinoma of the prostate. J Cancer Res Clin Oncol. 106, 210.

270. Haenszel W, Kurihara M. (1968) Studies of Japanese migrants. I. Mortality from cancer and other diseases among Japanese in the United States. J Natl Cancer Inst. 40, 43.

271. Shimizu H, Ross RK, Bernstein L, Yatani R, Henderson BE, Mack TM. (1991) Cancers of the prostate and breast among Japanese and white immigrants in Los Angeles County. Br J Cancer. 63, 963.

272. Di Mascio P, Kaiser S, Sies H. (1989) Lycopene as the most efficient biological carotenoid singlet oxygen quencher. Arch Biochem Biopys. 274, 532.

273. Giovannucci E. (2002) A review of epidemiologic studies of tomatoes, lycopene and prostate cancer. Exp Biol Med. 227, 852–859.

274. MacInnis RJ, English DR. (2006) Body size and composition and prostate cancer risk, systematic review and meta-regression analysis. Cancer Causes Control. 17, 989–1003.

275. Wright ME, Chang S-C, Schatzkin A, Albanes D, Kipnis V, Mouw T, et al. (2007) Prospective study of adiposity and weight change in relation to prostate cancer incidence and mortality. Cancer. 109, 675–684.

276. Hsing AW, Chua S Jr, Gao YT, Gentzschein E, Chang L, Deng J, et al. (2001) Prostate cancer risk and serum levels of insulin and leptin, a population based study. J Natl Cancer Inst. 93, 783–789.

277. Mantzoros CS, Tzonou A, Signorello LB, Stampfer M, Trichopoulos D, Adami HO. (1997) Insulin-like growth factor 1 in relation to prostate cancer and benign prostatic hyperplasia. Br J Cancer. 76, 1115–1118.

278. Shaneyfelt T, Husein R, Bubley G. (2000) Hormonal predictors of prostate cancer, a meta-analysis. J Clin Oncol. 18, 847–853.

Chapter 3

Energy Balance, Physical Activity, and Cancer Risk

Alecia Malin Fair and Kara Montgomery

Abstract

This chapter posits that cancer is a complex and multifactorial process as demonstrated by the expression and production of key endocrine and steroid hormones that intermesh with lifestyle factors (physical activity, body size, and diet) in combination to heighten cancer risk. Excess weight has been associated with increased mortality from all cancers combined and for cancers of several specific sites. The prevalence of obesity has reached epidemic levels in many parts of the world; more than 1 billion adults are overweight with a body mass index (BMI) exceeding 25. Overweight and obesity are clinically defined indicators of a disease process characterized by the accumulation of body fat due to an excess of energy intake (nutritional intake) relative to energy expenditure (physical activity). When energy intake exceeds energy expenditure over a prolonged period of time, the result is a positive energy balance (PEB), which leads to the development of obesity. This physical state is ideal for intervention and can be modulated by changes in energy intake, expenditure, or both.

Nutritional intake is a modifiable factor in the energy balance-cancer linkage primarily tested by caloric restriction studies in animals and the effect of energy availability. Restriction of calories by 10 to 40% has been shown to decrease cell proliferation, increasing apoptosis through anti-angiogenic processes. The potent anticancer effect of caloric restriction is clear, but caloric restriction alone is not generally considered to be a feasible strategy for cancer prevention in humans. Identification and development of preventive strategies that "mimic" the anticancer effects of low energy intake are desirable. The independent effect of energy intake on cancer risk has been difficult to estimate because body size and physical activity are strong determinants of total energy expenditure. The mechanisms that account for the inhibitory effects of physical activity on the carcinogenic process are reduction in fat stores, activity related changes in sex-hormone levels, altered immune function, effects in insulin and insulin-like growth factors, reduced free radical generation, and direct effect on the tumor. Epidemiologic evidence posits that the cascade of actions linking overweight and obesity to carcinogenesis are triggered by the endocrine and metabolic system. Perturbations to these systems result in the alterations in the levels of bioavailable growth factors, steroid hormones, and inflammatory markers. Elevated serum concentrations of insulin lead to a state of hyperinsulinemia. This physiological state causes a reduction in insulin-like growth factor-binding proteins and promotes the synthesis and biological activity of insulin-like growth factor (IGF)-I, which regulates cellular growth in response to available energy and nutrients from diet and body reserves. In vitro studies have clearly established that both insulin and IGF-I act as growth factors that promote cell proliferation and inhibit apoptosis. Insulin also affects on the synthesis and biological availability of the male and female sex steroids, including androgens, progesterone, and

M. Verma (ed.), *Methods of Molecular Biology, Cancer Epidemiology, vol. 472*
© 2009 Humana Press, a part of Springer Science+Business Media, Totowa, NJ
Book doi: 10.1007/978-1-60327-492-0

estrogens. Experimental and clinical evidence also indicates a central role of estrogens and progesterone in regulating cellular differentiation, proliferation, and apoptosis induction. Hyperinsulinemia is also associated with alterations in molecular systems such as endogenous hormones and adipokines that regulate inflammatory responses. Obesity-related dysregulation of adipokines has the ability to contribute to tumorigenesis and tumor invasion via metastatic potential. Given the substantial level of weight gain in industrialized countries in the last two decades, there is great interest in understanding all of the mechanisms by which obesity contributes to the carcinogenic process. Continued focus must be directed to understanding the various relationships between specific nutrients and dietary components and cancer cause and prevention. A reductionist approach is not sufficient for the basic biological mechanisms underlying the effect of diet and physical activity on cancer. The joint association between energy balance and cancer risk are hypothesized to share the same underlying mechanisms, the amplification of chemical mediators that modulate cancer risk depending on the responsiveness to those hormones to the target tissue of interest. Disentangling the connection between obesity, the insulin-IGF axis, endogenous hormones, inflammatory markers, and their molecular interaction is vital.

Key words: Adenocarcinoma, energy balance, insulin-like growth factor-1, nutrition, obesity, physical activity.

1. Introduction

Overweight and obesity are clinically defined indicators of a disease process characterized by the accumulation of body fat due to an excess of energy intake (nutritional intake) relative to energy expenditure (physical activity) *(1, 2)*. When energy intake exceeds energy expenditure over a prolonged period of time, the result is a positive energy balance (PEB), which leads to the development of obesity. This physical state is ideal for intervention and can be modulated by changes in energy intake, expenditure, or both *(3, 4)*.

The outcome of PEB, excess adipose tissue, has two main categories: subcutaneous and visceral. Subcutaneous adipose is defined as fat tissue between the skin and muscle, whereas visceral adipose tissue is found within the main cavities of the body, primarily in the abdominal cavity. Abdominal visceral adipocytes are more metabolically active and linked to a series of reactions leading to carcinogenesis. Several measures are used to define obesity. The most utilized parameter is body mass index (BMI) (weight in kilograms divided by height in meters squared), a measure of overall overweight status. The World Health Organization (WHO) defined an overweight status as a BMI of 25.0 or higher. The overweight category is then divided into four categories: preobese, 25.00 to 29.9 kg/m²; obese class I, 30.00 to 34.99 kg/m²; obese class II, 35.00 to 39.99 kg/m²; and obese class III, ≥40.00 kg/m² *(5)*. The many techniques of estimating BMI include underwater weighing (hydrodensitometry), dilution methods (hydrometry), dual-energy x-ray absorptiometry (DXA), measurement of skinfolds, bioimpedance analysis, and imaging methods. Only two techniques can distinguish between subcutaneous and visceral fat abdominal adipose tissue. They are computed tomography (CT) and magnetic resonance imaging (MRI). These two techniques are too costly and complex to be used in large-scale epidemiologic studies. Therefore, the waist-to-hip ratio (WHR), the circumference of the waist and hip, is used as a proxy measure of central adiposity.

The prevalence of obesity has reached epidemic levels in many parts of the world (6). Worldwide, more than 1 billion adults are overweight (BMI >25) and at least 300 million of them are obese (BMI >30). In the United States, 59 million adults (31%) are obese and 4.7% are considered morbidly obese (BMI ≥40) (7). The occurrence of obesity is reported to be associated with an increased risk for a number of chronic diseases and conditions, including diabetes, orthopedic conditions, and cardiovascular diseases. Excess adiposity has also been and associated with increased mortality from all cancers combined and for cancers of several specific sites (5). Epidemiologic studies have indicated that excess weight contributes to increased incidence for death from cancers of the colon, breast (in postmenopausal women), endometrium, kidney, prostate, esophagus (adenocarcinoma) ovaries, pancreas, and lungs, and possibly other cancers (1, 8). It has been estimated that 15–20% of all cancer deaths in the United States can be attributed to being overweight and obese (9). A recent analysis showed more than 70,000 of the 3.5 million new cases of cancer each year in the European Union are attributable to being overweight and obese (10).

Epidemiologic evidence posits that the cascade of actions linking overweight and obesity to carcinogenesis are triggered by the endocrine and metabolic system. Perturbations to these systems results in the alterations in the levels of bioavailable growth factor and steroid hormones. Given the substantial level of weight gain in industrialized countries in the last two decades (11, 12), there is great interest in understanding all of the mechanisms by which obesity contributes to the carcinogenic process and to developing preventive strategies that can effectively minimize excess risk.

2. Determinants of Energy Balance

2.1. Nutritional Intake

An expert panel of the American Institute of Cancer Research (AICR) and the World Cancer Research Fund (WCRF) estimate that achievable dietary practices could prevent up to 40% of world cancer cases (13). The risk for breast cancer is reported to have a significant association with obesity (14), and the majority of preclinical studies of the PEB risk hypothesis have been conducted using experimental models for breast cancer. Nutritional intake is a modifiable factor in the energy balance cancer linkage primarily tested by caloric restriction studies in animals and the effect of energy availability. Restriction of calories by 10 to 40% of *ad libitum* intake has been shown to inhibit mammary gland tumors in animal models by decreasing cell proliferation, increasing apoptosis, and possibly through anti-angiogenic processes.

There is evidence to suggest that a negative energy balance, or less energy intake compared with energy expenditure, is associated with a hormonal and metabolic milieu that mimics several features of caloric restriction and is consistent with a low risk for breast cancer. The effect of energy restriction on breast cancer risk has been examined in epidemiological studies with mixed results. Michaels et al. (2004) prospectively followed a cohort of Swedish women diagnosed and treated for anorexia prior to age 40 years and reported that they had nearly half the risk of breast cancer compared with age-matched controls *(15)*. Studies examining the influence of war-related famine on breast cancer have provided conflicting results. One study suggested decreased risk *(16)* and another increased risk *(17)* for women exposed to short-lived famine conditions. Lower levels of energy availability have been associated with luteal phase deficiency (i.e., shorter luteal phase, lower progesterone) in premenopausal women *(18)*, and among postmenopausal women, this exposure pattern would limit the accumulation of adipose tissue during adulthood and, subsequently, reduce postmenopausal estrogen exposure through aromatization of adrenal androgens *(19)*.

On the other hand, in a prospective cohort study of Canadian women, those who consumed in excess of 2,406 kcal/day had a higher risk of breast cancer (odds ratio (OR), 1.18; $p = 0.02$) in contrast to those women who consumed < 1,630 kcal/day *(20)*.

In addition, findings from the Shanghai Breast Cancer Study indicates that women with higher BMIs and lower levels of physical activity and those with lower physical activity levels and higher energy intakes were at increased risk of breast cancer when compared with women who consumed less calories or had a lower BMI *(21)*. When researchers examined the relationship between energy intake and rectal cancer in a case–control study of 2,157 men and women, they found a significant association between high levels of energy intake and rectal cancer *(22)*. Moreover, the relationship between energy intake and rectal cancer was stronger in those who were diagnosed at a younger age (OR = 3.9; 95% confidence interval (CI), 1.7–9.1 for men; and OR, 2.8; 95% CI, 1.1–7.1 for women) when comparing the highest quintile of energy intake with the lowest.

2.1.1. Protein Intake

A prospective study of almost 30,000 Danish women found that higher intakes of fish were associated with a higher incidence of breast cancer among postmenopausal women *(23)*. More research needs to be done to determine whether similar study results would be found in either a similar or diverse population group.

2.1.2. Fiber Intake

Having noticed the inconsistent results of studies focusing on a relationship between dietary fiber and risk of colorectal cancer, researchers examined 13 prospective cohort studies through the Pooling Project of Prospective Studies of Diet and Cancer. An age-adjusted model showed a statistically significant inverse association between dietary fiber intake in the highest quintile compared with the lowest (pooled age-adjusted relative risk (RR), 0.84; 95% CI, 0.77–0.92) *(24)*. However, after testing for other colorectal risk factors (red meat intake, total milk intake, and alcohol intake), the association was no longer statistically significant. Researchers have examined the relationship between fiber intake and breast cancer risk using 88,678 female participants in the Nurses' Health Study *(25)*. They found no statistically significant relationship between dietary fiber intake and risk of breast cancer. However, a case-control study of diet and ovarian cancer with 124 female subjects did find a relationship between fiber intake and reduced risk of ovarian cancer *(26)*. When comparing those subjects in the highest quintile of dietary fiber intake with those subjects in the lowest quintile, there was a statistically significant reduction in risk (OR, 0.43; CI, 0.20–0.94; $p < 0.05$). Overall, research has not shown dietary fiber intake to have a reduction on colon cancer *(27)*.

2.1.3. Total Fruit and Vegetable Intake

Other researchers have used the Nurses' Health Study to investigate the relationship between fruit and vegetable consumption and risk of bladder cancer *(28)*. The study did not establish a statistically significant relationship between fruit and vegetable consumption and risk of bladder cancer in the population of adult women. In addition, consumption of cruciferous vegetables was not related to bladder cancer risk in this population.

The Nurses' Health Study was also examined to determine any relationship between diet quality and risk of breast cancer *(29)*. The study population consisted of 3,580 postmenopausal women with breast cancer. Researchers found that when separating breast cancer cases into two groups, estrogen receptor positive (ER+) and estrogen receptor negative (ER–), diet quality had a statistically significant relationship only with the ER– group. Specifically, individual servings of vegetables were associated with a 6% decrease in ER– cases and individual servings of fruit were associated with a 12% decrease in ER– cases.

A meta-analysis of 16 research studies looking at fruit and vegetable intake and oral cancer found that there was a significant relationship between fruit and vegetable consumption and reduced risk of oral cancer *(30)*. For fruit, each portion consumed in a day was statistically significant in reducing the risk of oral cancer by 49% (OR, 0.51; CI, 0.40–0.65). For vegetables, each portion of primarily green vegetables was found to significantly reduce the risk of oral cancer by 50% (OR, 0.50; CI, 0.38–0.65).

2.1.4. Vegetable Intake

A case-control study of diet and ovarian cancer revealed statistically significant relationships between specific food group intake and ovarian cancer risk *(26)*. Women in the highest quintile of vegetable intake had a significantly lower risk when compared with women in the lowest quintile of vegetable intake (OR, 0.47; 95% CI, 0.23–0.97; $p < 0.05$).

2.1.5. Phytoestrogen Intake

Lignan is a phytoestrogen found in plant foods. Lignans are found in flaxseed, grains, nuts, fruits, and vegetables. A case-control study of the relationship between dietary intakes of lignans and risk of colorectal cancer showed that there was a significant reduction in colorectal cancer risk when comparing the highest intakes of lignan to the lowest (T3 v T1) = 0.71; 95% CI, 0.56–0.94, p value for trend = 0.01) *(31)*.

2.1.6. Dietary Fat Intake

A prospective cohort study of 17,035 Swedish adult females found that consuming a diet where 46.1% of the total daily energy came from fat resulted in a significantly higher risk of cancer mortality (RR, 1.46; CI, 1.04–2.04; $p = 0.029$) *(32)*. The RR was related to a lower percentage of total dietary fat coming from monounsaturated fat.

2.1.7. Folate Intake

A prospective cohort of more than 65,000 men revealed a lack of a statistically significant relationship between folate intake and risk of prostate cancer *(33)*. In addition, the study authors did not find any association between folate intake, alcohol consumption, and prostate cancer.

A study using a population of 481 women diagnosed with ovarian cancer from the Nurses' Health Study examined the relationship between folate intake and epithelial ovarian cancer *(34)*. Results revealed that there was a statistically significant inverse association with increasing dietary folate (RR, 0.66; 95% CI, 0.43, 1.03; p for trend = 0.09) when 75 cases were excluded that were diagnosed during the 4 years following the dietary intake assessment. Additionally, there was no association between either dietary or total folate intake, alcohol consumption, and ovarian cancer.

When considering nutrition and cancer, it is important to remember that individual dietary constituents probably do not affect all stages of cancer in the same way *(35)*. The potent anticancer effect of caloric restriction is clear, but caloric restriction alone is not generally considered to be a feasible strategy for cancer prevention in humans. However, the identification and development of preventive strategies that "mimic" the anticancer effects of low energy intake are desirable *(36)*. The independent effect of energy intake on cancer risk has been difficult to estimate because body size and physical activity are strong determinants of total energy expenditure *(37)*.

2.2. Physical Activity

There is substantial evidence supporting the existence of an inverse association between physical activity and cancer incidence/mortality. Epidemiologic studies of physical activity categorize energy expenditure by occupational or recreational; within these broad categories, physical activity is further described by its type, frequency, duration, and intensity. Physical activity has been measured using metabolic-equivalent tasks (METs), which summarize the intensity of energy exerted during the period of activity (MET-hours/week/year) *(38)*. The amount of intensity with which activities are performed may influence what is being measured in physical activity *(39)*. The time period during one's life when activity levels are measured may have a further impact on these associations. The primary mode of capturing physical activity measures in epidemiologic field studies has been survey questionnaires of self-report physical activity data. This type of methodology is still evolving in its ability to quantify the amount of physical activity in cumulative versus continuous bouts and the activities that are moderate versus vigorous in intensity, as to which maximize protective associations in the biological mechanisms involved in the disease process *(39)*. The mechanisms that account for the inhibitory effects of physical activity on the carcinogenic process are reduction in fat stores, activity related changes in sex-hormone levels, altered immune function, effects in insulin and insulin-like growth factors, reduced free radical generation, and direct effect on the tumor *(40)*.

Another inherent factor in epidemiologic physical activity measurement is the ability of the study participants to accurately recall activities performed in the past. Previous literature states that participants who perform vigorous activities on a regular basis are more likely to recall their activities than those subjects who do many different activities less frequently *(41)*.

3. Epidemiology of Energy Balance and Cancer Risk

The available literature on weight and cancer has contributed to the knowledge that a PEB or obese status is related to elevated cancer risk *(21, 42)*. The literature on the relationship between body size and the colon and rectal cancers has demonstrated a positive association between risk of colorectal cancer and body fat distribution as indicated by BMI or WHR. Studies that have examined association with obesity (BMI >30.0 kg/m²) found nearly twice the risk for colorectal cancer compared with those reporting association for overweight status or a BMI of over 25 *(1, 14, 39, 43)*.

The risk of colon cancer in men with a BMI > 30 increased up to 80% *(10)*. A gender difference, in which obese men are more likely to develop colorectal cancer than obese women, has been observed consistently across studies and populations. Obesity has been consistently associated with higher risk of colorectal cancer in men (RRs, ~1.5–2.0) and women (RRs, ~1.2–1.5) in both case-control and cohort studies (**Table 3.1**) *(14)*. The reasons for this gender difference are speculative. Some studies found that WHR or central adiposity, which occurs more frequently in men, is a stronger risk factor for colon cancer than peripheral adiposity or general overweight. Support for the role of central obesity in the development of colorectal cancer comes from studies reporting that waist circumference and the WHR are strongly related to risk of colorectal cancer and large adenomas in men *(44)*. However, several studies have reported that WHR is a strong

Table 3.1
Obesity-related cancers

Type of cancer	Relative risk[a] with BMI of 25–30 kg/m²	Relative risk[a] with BMI of ≥30 kg/m²	PAF (%) for US population[b]	PAF (%) for EU population[c]
Colorectal (men)	1.5	2.0	35.4	27.5
Colorectal (women)	1.2	1.5	20.8	14.2
Female breast (post-menopausal)	1.3	1.5	22.6	16.7
Endometrial	2.0	3.5	56.8	45.2
Kidney (renal cell)	1.5	2.5	42.5	31.1
Esophageal (adeno-carcinoma)	2.0	3.0	52.4	42.7
Pancreatic	1.3	1.7	26.9	19.3
Liver	ND	1.5–4.0	ND[d]	ND[d]
Gallbladder	1.5	2.0	35.5	27.1
Gastric cardia (adeno-carcinoma)	1.5	2.0	35.5	27.1

Relative risks (RRs) associated with overweight and obesity, and the percentage of cases attributable to overweight and obesity in the USA. *BMI*, body mass index; *ND*, not determined; *EU*, European Union; *PAF*, population attributable fraction. Adapted by permission from Macmillan Publishers Ltd. (Nature Review Cancer) ref. *(8)*, Copyright 2004. [a]RR estimates are summarized from the literature cited in the main text. [b]Data on prevalence of overweight and obesity are from the National Health and Nutrition Examination Survey (1999–2000) *(223)* for men and women from the United States aged from 50 to 69 years. [c]Data on prevalence of overweight and obesity are from a range of sources *(224)* of adult men and women residing in 15 European countries in the 1980s and 1990s. [d]PAFs were not estimated because the magnitude of the RRs across studies are not sufficiently consistent.

predictor (same strength as BMI) of colorectal cancer risk, especially in women *(45–52)*, leaving doubts as to whether body fat distribution completely explains the observed gender differences. This association has been observed more consistently for cancer of the distal colon and the proximal colon *(45–48)*.

The explanation of the effect of obesity on colorectal cancer risk in women has been inconsistent. Evidence suggests that exogenous estrogens (in the form of postmenopausal hormone therapy) reduce the risk of colorectal cancer in women *(49)*. However, this hypothesis is also very speculative, as circulating levels of endogenous estrogens are higher in obese men as well as obese women, compared with lean individuals *(50)*. Conversely, obese premenopausal women or women who use hormone-replacement therapy (HRT) have shown greater than a twofold risk for colon cancer versus postmenopausal women who were not taking HRT and who did not have an elevated risk *(22)*. Among postmenopausal women, this exposure pattern would increase the accumulation of adipose tissue during adulthood and subsequently reduce postmenopausal estrogen exposure through aromatization of adrenal androgens *(51)*.

In studies that were able to separately examine the colon and rectum, RRs were consistently higher for developing cancers of the colon *(14)*. Most studies evaluating the relationship between body size and adenoma occurrence have found associations similar to those observed for colon cancer *(52, 53)*. Studies of the association between body fatness and colorectal adenomas are necessary to provide evidence for the time (or times) in colorectal carcinogenesis when factors associated with body weight might be important in colorectal cancer *(54)*. Most studies have observed 1.5- to 2.5-fold increases in risk of adenomas among the group with the largest BMI. Similar relationships are seen for colon adenomas, with stronger associations between obesity and the incidence of larger (versus smaller) colon adenomas *(44, 53, 55–57)*.

A few studies have examined the relationship between body size and rectal cancer, but these studies were reported on results with few cases. From these studies, body size is not related with rectal cancer among men or women *(14, 22, 48, 58–61)*. In a large population study *(62)*, no difference was found in the risk of rectal cancer in overweight subjects with a BMI of >25 or obese subjects (BMI > 30).

The relationship between body fat and the risk of breast cancer has voluminous epidemiologic research dating to studies in the 1970s. Early studies established that the association between body size and risk of breast cancer varied based on menopausal status–that heavier women were at increased risk of developing postmenopausal, but not premenopausal, breast cancer *(14, 63)*. Such extensive research is necessary to examine the role of energy balance in breast cancer etiology during different periods of a woman's life cycle when weight status fluctuates: early childhood, adolescence, and adulthood. The most rigorous studies differentiate between premenopausal and postmenopausal breast cancer and the effect of weight gain, overall and central adiposity, and the differentiated effects of exposure to endogenous and exogenous hormones (birth control and HRT) *(64)*.

The effect of obesity on premenopausal breast cancer risk is inconsistent. Overall, obesity has a protective effect or a null association *(65, 66)* with premenopausal breast cancer risk *(14, 67–76)*. Among premenopausal women, there is consistent evidence of a modest reduction in risk among those with a high (≥ 28 kg/m^2) BMI. This reduction in risk could be because of the increased tendency for young obese women to have anovulatory menstrual cycles and lower levels of circulating steroid hormones, notably of progesterone and estradiol *(77)*. Yet, there is evidence to support that an obese status confers increased risk on premenopausal women *(21, 78–82)*. It is important to discern what type of body fat distribution has been linked to premenopausal breast cancer risk. Increased risk with higher central adiposity (WHR) but not overall adiposity (BMI) has been reported *(83–85)*, as has a higher BMI without a higher WHR *(86–88)*. The epidemiologic evidence on weight gain and premenopausal breast cancer risk has consistently shown either no association *(71, 89, 90)* or an inverse association *(81, 91–94)*.

Obesity has been consistently shown to increase rates of breast cancer in postmenopausal women by 30–50% **(Table 3.1)** *(8, 21, 95–98)*. Overweight status has been identified an independent predictor of postmenopausal breast cancer risk in numerous epidemiologic studies *(14, 17, 69, 81, 83, 87, 97, 99–119)*. However, adult weight gain has consistently been associated with a larger increase in risk of postmenopausal breast cancer than has BMI in studies that examined both factors *(78, 100, 119, 120)*. Both BMI and weight gain are more strongly related to risk of breast cancer among postmenopausal women who have never used HRT *(118, 121–123)* compared with women who have used hormones *(91, 119, 124)*. This finding lends support to the hypothesis that adiposity increases breast cancer risk through its estrogenic effects *(8)*. Postmenopausal women produce estrogen in fat through the aromatization of androgens to estrogens *(125)*. Estrogens are tumor promoters in vitro and in vivo. Women with high circulating levels of estrogens are at increased risk of developing breast cancer *(126)*.

Endometrial cancer (cancer of the uterine lining) was the first cancer to be recognized as being related to obesity. A linear increase in the risk of endometrial cancer with increasing weight or BMI has been observed in most studies *(9, 67, 127–135)* ranging from twofold to fivefold in premenopausal and postmenopausal and overweight and/or obese women (**Table 3.1**). Only two case-control studies observed no association between weight and endometrial cancer risk *(136, 137)*. The association of excess weight and endometrial cancer risk was equal or somewhat stronger for older *(130, 138)* as opposed to younger women *(133, 139)*. Other anthropometric measures of body fat distribution, such as WHR and skinfold thickness, displayed a positive association with endometrial cancer *(133, 140–145)* independent from BMI. Conversely, other studies found that this association attenuated once the results were adjusted for BMI *(140, 143)*.

Weight gain in early adulthood was not a strong factor in the prediction of endometrial risk *(133, 138, 141, 144–147)*. Weight gain as an adult illustrates increased endometrial cancer risk *(133, 137, 138, 141, 144–146)*, yet the association of risk with weight gain mitigated when adjusted for recent BMI or weight *(137, 138)*.

It is estimated that 27% of the renal cell cases among American men and 29% among women could be attributed to overweight and obesity *(148)*. Global studies of obesity and renal cell cancer reveal up to a threefold risk in renal cell cancer among overweight and obese individuals than in normal weight men and women *(14, 72, 148–150)*. Most studies show a linear dose response effect yet, with increasing weight or BMI, a stronger association of energy balance on the risk of renal cell cancer has been reported for women *(9, 151–157)*, although at present this finding remains unexplained *(148)*. A meta-analysis of 14 studies on both genders revealed no effect modification by sex and BMI as an equally strong predictor of the risk of renal cell cancer between men and women *(148)*.

Obesity has been linked with adenocarcinoma of the esophagus and gastric cardia independent of known risk factors, such as cigarette smoking and alcohol consumption *(158)*. Cases of adenocarcinomas of the esophagus and gastric cardia are more likely to have a history of gastroesophageal reflux disease (GERD), hiatal hernia, or Barrett's esophagus *(159–161)*. These conditions are precursors to esophageal adenocarcinomas and also prevalent among overweight and obese individuals *(162)*. The mechanisms by which obesity could increase the risk of esophageal adenocarcinoma are unclear, one hypothesis is that central obesity may prompt a series of events beginning with hiatal hernia and GERD, which targets the gastroesophageal junction *(163)*. Continuous irritation of the squamous cells in the lower esophagus may provoke a compensatory response leading to Barrett's metaplasia a precursor for esophageal adenocarcinoma. In this condition, the gastric and bile acids potentiate an inflamed esophagus, leading to low-grade cell hyperproliferation, then leading to premalignant high-grade dysplastic changes to the esophagus, resulting in esophageal adenocarcinoma *(164)*.

The incidence of adenocarcinoma of the esophagus has been rapidly increasing in Westernized countries in recent decades *(165, 166)* in parallel with an equally rapid increase in the prevalence of obesity *(167)*. Rates for the other main histological subtype of esophageal cancer, squamous cell carcinoma, have remained stable or decreased. As a result, an increasing proportion of all esophageal cancers in Western countries are adenocarcinomas. Obesity increases risk for adenocarcinoma of the esophagus by twofold to threefold *(14, 168)* (**Table 3.1**), but is not associated with an increased risk of squamous cell carcinoma of the esophagus *(159, 160, 169)*.

Risk for adenocarcinoma of the gastric cardia has been found to be related to obesity *(163, 169, 170)*, but the magnitude of the association is not as great as for adenocarcinoma of the esophagus. RRs are in the range of 1.5–2.0. It is unclear why risks associated with obesity are greater for esophageal adenocarcinoma than for gastric cardia adenocarcinoma. It is possible that reflux mechanisms are more closely related to adenocarcinoma of the esophagus than of the gastric cardia. Data are limited for noncardia cancers of the stomach, but there is no indication of increased risk with obesity *(169, 170)*.

Results from many recent studies indicate that obesity is associated with an almost twofold increased risk for pancreatic cancer in men and women (**Table 3.1**) *(9, 72, 129, 171–174)*. Earlier studies, however, reported either no association or a smaller association between the two, so further research is needed *(150, 175, 176)*. However, the rapidly fatal nature of pancreatic cancer and the use of case-controls studies to obtain data result in low participation rates and rely on proxy responders to obtain exposure data *(172, 177–180)*. In this situation, selection and recall bias could occur and underlie the lack of association reported between obesity and pancreatic cancer. Weight misclassification is apt to occur in case-controls studies of body weight and the risk of pancreatic cancer for several reasons. Recall of body weight several years prior to pancreatic cancer diagnosis is not a stable measurement of weight status. Weight loss is often a hallmark characteristic leading to the diagnosis of pancreatic cancer. Additionally, proxy responders may provide less accurate data on the patient's weight, particularly if the proxy consistently underestimates the patient's weight. This misclassification via proxy interview of weight status due to patient weight loss may explain why a null association is found between obesity and pancreatic cancer in case-control studies *(178, 180)*. Case-control studies using direct interviews revealed a positive association between body weight and pancreatic cancer risk in men and women *(172)*.

Cohort studies of pancreatic cancer are ideal to measure the association between adiposity and pancreatic cancer risk because weight information is collected prior to disease status and proxy interview information is not used. However, the sample size for these studies is problematic as pancreatic cancer is ranked 11th out of all cancers in the United States *(181)* and numerous years of follow-up are necessary to retain patients. Out of the cohort studies conducted on the relationship of pancreatic cancer and excess adiposity, significant elevated risks were found for obese individuals compared with those with normal body weight *(9, 172, 182, 183)*.

Epidemiologic studies of energy balance and ovarian cancer risk reveal inconsistent results, which may be attributed to women's overweight status during the life cycle as a risk modifier. Higher BMI during early adulthood has been associated with increased risk of ovarian cancer *(184–186)*. The pathogenesis of a higher BMI at age 18 years throughout adult life exhibited a significant increased risk of ovarian cancer *(186)*, versus the null association found between recent BMI and ovarian cancer risk *(187)*. Premenopausal women have been identified as high risk for frank and borderline ovarian cancer with a higher adult BMI *(122, 188–190)*.

Being overweight and obese are inconsistently associated with prostate cancer risk *(95)*. In some studies, no association or an inverse association has been found *(67, 68, 121, 128, 191–194)*. However, some studies show that a PEB can influence prostate cancer risk *(185, 195–198)*. BMI has been shown to be a strong predictor of metabolically active androgen concentrations. The conversion of androgens to estrogens and estrogens to more potent carcinogens is plausible *(72, 112, 197, 199–207)*. A higher BMI has been associated with higher-grade prostate tumors, disease progression, and poor prognosis *(206, 207)*.

The issue of BMI and its link to lung cancer risk is still contentious. Most epidemiologic studies have observed an inverse association between BMI and lung cancer risk *(9, 72, 195, 208–213)*. The inverse association may be explained by weight loss due to preclinical disease *(195, 208, 210)* or the residual confounding effect of smoking *(79, 127, 214–216)*. However, a positive association of BMI in never-smokers and former smokers has been found for lung cancer, as has a null association *(121, 217)*. Four studies have found an increased risk (1.5- to 4-fold) of liver cancer, or hepatocellular carcinoma (HCC), among obese individuals *(128, 129, 150, 218)*, whereas a fifth study did not *(72)*. Taken together, these studies indicate that obesity increases the risk of liver cancer, but the magnitude of the observed RR from existing studies is not consistent. There have also been a limited number of studies of gallbladder cancer and obesity, and most have been relatively small, as gallbladder cancer is very rare, especially in men. However, these few studies have consistently found that obesity increased risk by about twofold *(9, 128, 129, 150, 219)* **(Table 3.1)**. Obesity increases the risk of gallstones, which cause chronic inflammation and, therefore, increased risk of biliary tract cancer *(220)*.

Few studies have examined the relationship between hematopoietic cancers and BMI. The results from these studies are to be interpreted with caution due to the small number of cancer cases *(9, 128, 129, 150, 217, 221, 222)*. A significant positive association with obesity was observed for non-Hodgkin's lymphoma *(9, 72, 128)*, multiple myeloma *(72, 128)*, and leukemia *(9, 72, 128, 129, 150)*.

4. Mechanisms Related Energy Balance to Cancer Risk

4.1. Insulin-Resistance Hormones

Insulin is a peptide hormone secreted by the beta cells of the pancreas in response to elevated levels of glucose in the blood. Insulin controls the movement of glucose into muscle cells and suppresses the liver's production of glucose. Insulin also regulates the breakdown of fat cells in adipose tissue. Adipose tissue constitutes an active endocrine and metabolic organ that can have far-reaching effects on the pathophysiology of insulin resistance.

Weight gain resulting in being overweight and obese leads to insulin resistance because insulin resistance decreases the organ's sensitivity to the actions of insulin and the body compensates by secreting more insulin. Elevated serum concentrations of insulin lead to a state of hyperinsulinemia. Type II diabetes, which is usually associated with insulin resistance and increased pancreatic insulin secretion for long periods both before and after disease onset, is associated with increased risk of cancers of the colon *(44)*, breast *(225, 226)*, pancreas *(227, 228)*, endometrium *(229)*, and kidney *(230, 231)*.

Increased blood levels of insulin cause a reduction in insulin-like growth factor (IGF)-binding proteins (IGFBPs), which promotes the synthesis and biological activity of IGF-I–a peptide hormone that has a molecular structure very similar to that of insulin and that regulates cellular growth in response to available energy and nutrients from diet and body reserves **(Fig. 3.1)** *(8)*.

Insulin's tumorigenic effects may be direct, through the insulin receptor, or indirect, via insulin's influence on IGF-I and IGF-I receptor (IGF-IR) *(232)*. In vitro studies have clearly established that both insulin and IGF-I act as growth factors that promote cell proliferation and inhibit apoptosis *(233–243)*. Experiments with insulin-deficient (diabetic) animals have shown that insulin promotes tumor growth and development in xenograft models and in chemical models of carcinogenesis *(214, 215, 244, 245)*.

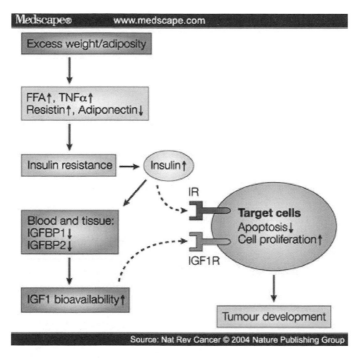

Fig. 3.1. Effects of obesity on growth-factor production. In obesity, increased release from adipose tissue of free fatty acids (*FFA*), tumor-necrosis factor-α (*TNFα*), and resistin, and reduced release of adiponectin lead to the development of insulin resistance and compensatory, chronic hyperinsulinemia. Increased insulin levels, in turn, lead to reduced liver synthesis and blood levels of insulin-like growth factor (IGF)-binding protein (IGFBP)-1 (*IGFBP1*), and probably also reduce IGFBP1 synthesis locally in other tissues. Increased fasting levels of insulin in the plasma are generally also associated with reduced levels of IGFBP2 in the blood. This results in increased levels of bioavailable IGF-I. Insulin and IGF-I signal through the insulin receptors (*IR*) and IGF-I receptor (*IGF1R*), respectively, to promote cellular proliferation and inhibit apoptosis in many tissue types. These effects might contribute to tumorigenesis. Adapted by permission from Macmillan Publishers Ltd. (Nature Review Cancer), ref. *(8)*, Copyright 2004.

There have been at least six IGFBPs identified in the IGF axis (IGFBP1, IGFBP2, IGFBP3, IGFBP4, IGFBP5, and IGFBP6). The most abundant of which is IGFBP-3. This binds to approximately >90% of circulating IGF-I *(246)*. The bioavailability of serum levels of IGF in absolute concentrations or relative to IGFBP-3 may be associated with an increased risk of breast cancer in women *(216, 247–249)*, particularly premenopausal breast cancer *(250–255)*, prostate cancer *(256–258)*, colon cancer *(259–264)*, and lung cancer *(265–267)*.

The exact role that circulating IGF-I levels play in cancer risk is not fully elucidated. One hypothesis postulates that high bioavailable IGF-I levels stimulate motility in human carcinoma cell lines enhancing a selective growth advantage and consequently migration and invasion *(268–270)* (**Fig. 3.1**).

4.2. Endogenous Sex Steroids

Insulin also affects on the synthesis and biological availability of the male and female sex hormones, including androgens, progesterone, and estrogens. Epidemiological studies have provided a substantial amount of evidence that adiposity-induced alterations in circulating levels of sex steroids are explained by the associations observed between anthropometric measures of excess weight and risks of cancers of the breast (postmenopausal women only), endometrium (both premenopausal and postmenopausal women), and prostate. Experimental and clinical evidence also indicates a central role of estrogens and progesterone in regulating cellular differentiation, proliferation, and apoptosis induction *(271–273)*.

The physical difference between men and premenopausal women and postmenopausal women profoundly affects the relationship between adiposity, circulating sex hormone levels, and cancer risk *(19)*. Adiposity affects the synthesis and bioavailability of the estrogens, the androgens, and progesterone. Adipose tissue expresses various sex steroid-metabolizing enzymes that promote the formation of estrogens from androgenic precursors *(51, 274)*. In men and premenopausal women, the formation of estrogen and androgen are secreted by the gonads or adrenal glands. In contrast, in postmenopausal women, estrogens are largely produced by conversion in the adipose tissue and other peripheral tissues from precursor androgens (largely androstenedione) secreted by the adrenal gland.

The interrelationship between estrogen, androgens, and sex hormone-binding globulin (SHBG), a glycoprotein synthesized in the liver that has specific binding sites for estrogens and androgens, is complex *(19)*. SHBG regulates the proportion of the sex steroids that are bound and free. The serum concentration of SHBG fluctuates with the level of BMI. When BMI is high, serum concentration of SHBG falls. This inverse relationship has been observed in premenopausal women, postmenopausal women, and in men. The average concentration of SHBG is double in thin individuals (BMI <20 kg/m²) than in obese individuals (BMI >30 kg/m²). The mechanism at work here is attributed to the risk in insulin levels with increasing BMI *(275)*.

In the case of breast cancer, excess adiposity is thought to favor breast tumor development by a change in endogenous sex hormone metabolism *(274)*. In premenopausal women, excess adiposity causes a reduction in SHBG and total estradiol, but does not affect the free, unbound estradiol. Consistent with the epidemiologic findings, premenopausal women who are overweight are not at increased risk for breast cancer. The decreased risk of breast cancer in premenopausal women is not well understood, but may be attributed to an increase in the frequency of anovular cycles and reduced exposure to progesterone and, partially, to a later diagnosis of tumors in obese women. In postmenopausal women, obesity increases breast cancer risk. This is probably due to the lower levels of SHBG resulting in an increase of the bioavailable fraction of testosterone and estradiol. Prospective cohort studies have shown approximately a twofold increase in breast cancer risk among postmenopausal women in the upper versus lower quintiles in production of various sex steroids, including pro hormone dehydroepiandrosterone (DHEA), testosterone, estrone, and total estradiol. Breast cancer risk was directly related to higher blood levels of bioavailable estradiol unbound to SHBG with increasing BMI *(274, 276)*. Risk for postmenopausal women was also found to be directly related to levels of estrone and total and bioavailable estradiol *(277, 278)*, with estimated RRs up to about 5.0 for women in the upper quartiles or quintiles of estradiol levels *(278)*.

Excess body weight is one of the key risk factors for endometrial cancer in premenopausal and postmenopausal women *(14, 148)* The relationship between an increasing BMI and endometrial cancer risk is linear, especially among postmenopausal women and premenopausal women with a BMI of 30 kg/m² or higher. Excess body weight has been estimated to account for about half of endometrial cancer incidence in Western Europe and the USA *(8)*. The relationship of endometrial cancer risk with blood levels of endogenous estrogens has been examined in several epidemiologic studies. Increased endometrial cancer risk has been observed among postmenopausal women with a low to high ratio of SHBG levels to levels of bioavailable estrogens *(146, 279–281)*. A prospective cohort study of endometrial cancer showed a sixfold risk for postmenopausal women in the top quintile of bioavailable unbound estradiol compared with their counterparts in the bottom quartile *(278)*. In postmenopausal women, the degree of adiposity is linearly related to plasma levels of estrone and estradiol, especially bioavailable estradiol unbound to SHBG *(282–285)*.

The sensitivity of endometrial cancer to the endogenous sex hormones can be explained by the "unopposed estrogen" theory and endometrial cancer *(273, 277)*, where endometrial cancer risk is increased by the mitogenic effects of estrogens insufficiently counterbalanced by progesterone. This theory is demonstrated by the striking behavior changes in endometrial cells during normal menstrual cycles with high levels of mitotic endometrial cell activity during exposure to estradiol alone during the follicular phase, but abrogated by progesterone during the luteal phase *(19)*.

Postmenopausal women with excess weight experience increased estrogen concentration from peripheral conversion of androgens to estrogens in adipose tissue by aromatase enzyme *(286, 287)*. The large increase in endometrial cancer risk is due to higher levels of unbound estradiol with the very low levels of progesterone *(19)*. The converse is true in premenopausal women, where excess weight has little effect on levels of total or bioavailable estradiol *(288–291)*. Compared with postmenopausal women who produce estrogen from their adipose tissue, premeno-pausal women produce estrogen from their ovaries. The increase in endometrial cancer risk be explained by the high incidence of anovular menstrual cycles in obese women and the consequent exposure to high levels of estradiol unopposed by progesterone *(19)*.

Among men, prostate cancer development is also thought to be related to endogenous hormone metabolism, such as by androgen production *(191, 192)*. Yet, the results of epidemiologic studies of BMI and prostate cancer risk have been inconsistent *(121, 198, 292)*. Large prospective study results reveal a null association between BMI and the risk for incident prostate cancer. The exception to this finding is with advanced disease, where a statistically significant increase in prostate cancer mortality was found with increasing BMI, intimating that obesity might reduce survival in men with prostate cancer *(198, 293, 294)*.

4.3. Adipokines and Inflammation Markers

The insulin cancer hypothesis is that chronic hyperinsulinemia is associated with increased availability of IGF-I and concomitant changes in the cellular environment that favor tumor formation *(295)*. Aside from the endocrine system's biological mechanisms that link adiposity to cancer risk, not much is known about other biomarkers and the causality of obesity in cancer risk. However, hyperinsulinemia is also associated with alterations in molecular systems such as endogenous hormones and adipokines, proteins secreted by adipose tissue that regulate inflammatory responses. Although this is an evolving area of research, obesity-related dysregulation of adipokines has the ability to contribute to tumorigenesis and tumor invasion via metastatic potential *(8)*. An increasing number of immune mediators produced from adipocytes found in adipose tissues are being identified. One adipocyte-produced immune-related protein, tumor necrosis factor (TNF)-α, has been identified as a potential link between obesity and diabetes. The release of TNF-α from the adipose tissue gives rise to insulin resistance *(237)*. The effects of insulin-resistance are believed to contribute to tumorigenesis *(296)*. Two other inflammatory mediators associated with obesity are C-reactive protein (CRP) and interleukin (IL)-6. CRP is produced in the liver and mediates activation of monocytes and macrophages *(297)*. CRP is regulated by IL-6, which influences antigen-specific immune responses and inflammatory responses. Recent data show an increase in obesity and heightened levels of CRP in both men and women *(298)*. Overweight and obese individuals experience low-grade systemic inflammation. IL-6 is secreted by visceral adipose tissue, in vivo, particularly in obese individuals. Long-term secretion of IL-6 dampens the production of TNF-α and stimulates CRP *(299)*.

Increased CRP levels via IL-6 signaling suggest that obesity may be a marker of an escalating immune response. This relationship may be a key factor in understanding how obesity increases the risk for cancer *(7)*. A recent cohort study conducted in older adults aged 70–79 years found that baseline levels of IL-6, CRP, and TNF-α were associated with the risk of cancer events. All three markers were associated with lung cancer risk. Colorectal cancer risk was associated with IL-6 and CRP, which is consistent with findings from a nested case-control study *(300, 301)*.

Cancer is a complex and multifactorial process. A reductionist approach is not sufficient for the basic biological mechanisms underlying the effect of diet and physical activity on cancer. The joint association between energy balance and cancer risk are hypothesized to share the same underlying mechanisms, the amplification of chemical mediators that modulate cancer risk depending on the responsiveness to those hormones of the target tissue of interest. As the prevalence of obesity increases, disentangling the connection between obesity, the insulin-IGF axis, endogenous hormones, inflammatory markers, and their molecular interaction is vital.

References

1. Mao, Y., Pan, S. Y., and Ugnat, A. M. (2006) Obesity as a cancer risk factor; Epidemiology. In *Nutrition and Cancer Prevention* (Awad, A. and Bradford, P., eds.), Taylor & Francis Group, Boca Raton, FL, pp. 541–564.

2. Rock, C. (2006) Energy balance and cancer prognosis: colon, prostate, and other cancers. In *Cancer Prevention and Management Through Exercise and Weight Control* (McTiernan, A., ed.), Taylor & Francis, Boca Raton, FL, pp. 437–446.

3. Thompson, H. J., Zhu, Z., and Jiang, W. (2003) Dietary energy restriction in breast cancer prevention. *J Mammary Gland Biol Neoplasia.* **8**, 133–142.

4. Wade, G. N., Schneider, J. E., and Li, H. Y. (1996) Control of fertility by metabolic cues. *Am J Physiol.* **270**, E1–19.

5. World Health Organization. (2000) Obesity: preventing and managing the global epidemic. Report of a WHO consultation. 894. Geneva, Switzerland, World Health Organization. WHO Technical Reports Series.

6. World Health Organization. (2003) World Cancer Report. Stewart, B. W. and Kleihues, P. Geneva, Switzerland, World Health Organization. IARC Nonserial Publication.

7. Power, C., Miller S.K., and Alpert, P. (2007) Promising new causal explanation for obesity and obesity-related diseases. *Biol Res Nurs.* **8**, 223–233.

8. Calle, E. E. and Kaaks, R. (2004) Overweight, obesity and cancer: epidemiological evidence and proposed mechanisms. *Nat Rev Cancer.* **4**, 579–591.

9. Calle, E. E., Rodriguez, C., Walker-Thurmond, K., and Thun, M. J. (2003) Overweight, obesity, and mortality from cancer in a prospectively studied cohort of U.S. adults. *N Engl J Med.* **348**, 1625–1638.

10. McMillan, D. C., Sattar, N., and McArdle, C. S. (2006) ABC of obesity. Obesity and cancer. *BMJ.* **333**, 1109–1111.

11. Mokdad, A. H., Bowman, B. A., Ford, E. S., Vinicor, F., Marks, J. S., and Koplan, J. P. (2001) The continuing epidemics of obesity and diabetes in the United States. *JAMA.* **286**, 1195–1200.

12. Paeratakul, S., Popkin, B. M., Keyou, G., Adair, L. S., and Stevens, J. (1998) Changes in diet and physical activity affect the body mass index of Chinese adults. *Int J Obes Relat Metab Disord.* **22**, 424–431.

13. Go, V. L., Wong, D. A., and Butrum, R. (2001) Diet, nutrition and cancer prevention: where are we going from here? *J Nutr.* **131**, 3121S–3126S.

14. International Agency for Research on Cancer. IARC Working Group on the Evaluation of

Cancer-Preventive Strategies. 2002. Lyon: France, IARC Press. IARC Handbooks of Cancer Prevention, vol 6. Weight Control and Physical Activity.

15. Michels, K. B. and Ekbom, A. (2004) Caloric restriction and incidence of breast cancer. *JAMA.* **291**, 1226–1230.

16. Elias, S. G., Peeters, P. H., Grobbee, D. E., and van Noord, P. A. (2004) Breast cancer risk after caloric restriction during the 1944–1945 Dutch famine. *J Natl Cancer Inst.* **96**, 539–546.

17. Tretli, S. and Gaard, M. (1996) Lifestyle changes during adolescence and risk of breast cancer: an ecologic study of the effect of World War II in Norway. *Cancer Causes Control.* **7**, 507–512.

18. DeSouza, M. J., Van Heest, J., Demers, L. M., and Lasley, B. L. (2003) Luteal phase deficiency in recreational runners: evidence for a hypometabolic state. *J Clin Endocrinol Metab.* **88**, 337–346.

19. Key, T. J., Allen, N. E., Verkasalo, P. K., and Banks, E. (2001) Energy balance and cancer: the role of sex hormones. *Proc Nutr Soc.* **60**, 81–89.

20. Silvera, S. A., Jain, M., Howe, G. R., Miller, A. B., and Rohan, T. E. (2005) Energy balance and breast cancer risk: a prospective cohort study. *Breast Cancer Res Treat.* 1–10.

21. Malin, A., Matthews, C. E., Shu, X. O., Cai, H., Dai, Q., Jin, F., Gao, Y. T., and Zheng, W. (2005) Energy balance and breast cancer risk. *Cancer Epidemiol Biomarkers Prev.* **14**, 1496–1501.

22. Slattery, M. L., Caan, B. J., Benson, J., and Murtaugh, M. (2003) Energy balance and rectal cancer: an evaluation of energy intake, energy expenditure, and body mass index. *Nutr Cancer.* **46**, 166–171.

23. Stripp, C., Overvad, K., Christensen, J., Thomsen, B. L., Olsen, A., Moller, S., et al. (2003) Fish intake is positively associated with breast cancer incidence rate. *J Nutr.* **133**, 3664–3669.

24. Park, Y., Hunter, D. J., Spiegelman, D., Bergkvist, L., Berrino, F., van den Brandt, P. A., et al. (2005). Dietary fiber intake and risk of colorectal cancer: a pooled analysis of prospective cohort studies. *JAMA.* **294**, 2849–2857.

25. Holmes, M. D., Liu, S., Hankinson, S. E., Colditz, G. A., Hunter, D. J., and Willett, W. C. (2004). Dietary carbohydrates, fiber, and breast cancer risk. *Am J Epidemiol.* **159**, 732–739.

26. McCann, S. E., Freudenheim, J. L., Marshall, J. R., and Graham, S. (2003). Risk of

human ovarian cancer is related to dietary intake of selected nutrients, phytochemicals and food groups. *J Nutr.* **133**, 1937–1942.

27. Willett, W. C. (2000) Diet and cancer. *Oncologist.* **5**, 393–404.

28. Holick, C. N., De, V., I, Feskanich, D., Giovannucci, E., Stampfer, M., Michaud, D. S. (2005) Intake of fruits and vegetables, carotenoids, folate, and vitamins A, C, E and risk of bladder cancer among women (United States). *Cancer Causes Control.* **16**, 1135–1145.

29. Fung, T. T., Hu, F. B., McCullough, M. L., Newby, P. K., Willett, W. C., Holmes, M. D. (2006) Diet quality is associated with the risk of estrogen receptor-negative breast cancer in postmenopausal women. *J Nutr.* **136**, 466–472.

30. Pavia, M., Pileggi, C., Nobile, C. G., and Angelillo, I. F. (2006) Association between fruit and vegetable consumption and oral cancer: a meta-analysis of observational studies. *Am J Clin Nutr.* **83**, 1126–1134.

31. Cotterchio, M., Boucher, B. A., Manno, M., Gallinger, S., Okey, A., Harper, P. (2006) Dietary phytoestrogen intake is associated with reduced colorectal cancer risk. *J Nutr.* **136**, 3046–3053.

32. Leosdottir, M., Nilsson, P. M., Nilsson, J. A., Mansson, H., Berglund, G. (2005) Dietary fat intake and early mortality patterns—data from The Malmo Diet and Cancer Study. *J Intern Med.* **258**, 153–165.

33. Stevens, V. L., Rodriguez, C., Pavluck, A. L., McCullough, M. L., Thun, M. J., Calle, E. E. (2006) Folate nutrition and prostate cancer incidence in a large cohort of US men. *Am J Epidemiol.* **163**, 989–996.

34. Tworoger, S. S., Hecht, J. L., Giovannucci, E., and Hankinson, S. E. (2006) Intake of folate and related nutrients in relation to risk of epithelial ovarian cancer. *Am J Epidemiol.* **163**, 1101–1111.

35. Kritchevsky, D. (2003) Diet and cancer: what's next? *J Nutr.* **133**, 3827S–3829S.

36. Hursting, S. D., Lavigne, J. A., Berrigan, D., Perkins, S. N., and Barrett, J. C. (2003) Calorie restriction, aging, and cancer prevention: mechanisms of action and applicability to humans. *Annu Rev Med.* **54**, 131–152.

37. Ravussin, E., Lillioja, S., Anderson, T. E., Christin, L., and Bogardus, C. (1986) Determinants of 24-hour energy expenditure in man. Methods and results using a respiratory chamber. *J Clin Invest.* **78**, 1568–1578.

38. Matthews, C. E., Shu, X. O., Yang, G., Jin, F., Ainsworth, B. E., Liu, D., et al. (2003) Repro-

ducibility and validity of the Shanghai Women's Health Study physical activity questionnaire. *Am J Epidemiol.* **158**, 1114–1122.

39. Slattery, M. L. (2006) Physical activity and colon cancer. In *Cancer Prevention and Management Through Exercise and Weight Control* (McTiernan, A., ed.), Taylor & Francis, Boca Raton, FL, pp. 75–87.

40. Thompson, H. J., Jiang, W., and Zhu, Z. (2006) Obesity as a cancer risk factor: potential mechanisms. In *Nutrition and Cancer Prevention* (Awad, A. and Bradford, P., eds.), Taylor & Francis, Boca Raton, FL, pp. 565–578.

41. Slattery, M. L. and Jacobs, D. R., Jr. (1995) Assessment of ability to recall physical activity of several years ago. *Ann Epidemiol.* **5**, 292–296.

42. Slattery, M.L., Potter, J., Caan, B., Edwards, S., Coates, A., Ma, K.N., and Berry T. D. (1997) Energy balance and colon cancer—beyond physical activity. *Cancer Res.* **57**, 75–80.

43. Kopelman, P. G. (2000). Obesity as a medical problem. *Nature.* **404**, 635–643.

44. Giovannucci, E., Ascherio, A., Rimm, E. B., Colditz, G. A., Stampfer, M. J., and Willett, W. C. (1995) Physical activity, obesity, and risk for colon cancer and adenoma in men. *Ann Intern Med.* **122**, 327–334.

45. MacInnis, R. J., English, D. R., Hopper, J. L., Haydon, A. M., Gertig, D. M., and Giles, G. G. (2004) Body size and composition and colon cancer risk in men. *Cancer Epidemiol Biomarkers Prev.* **13**, 553–559.

46. Terry, P. D., Miller, A. B., and Rohan, T. E. (2002) Obesity and colorectal cancer risk in women. *Gut.* **51**, 191–194.

47. Martinez, M. E., Giovannucci, E., Spiegelman, D., Hunter, D. J., Willett, W. C., and Colditz, G. A. (1997) Leisure-time physical activity, body size, and colon cancer in women. Nurses' Health Study Research Group. *J Natl Cancer Inst.* **89**, 948–955.

48. Le Marchand, L., Wilkens, L. R., Kolonel, L. N., Hankin, J. H., and Lyu, L. C. (1997) Associations of sedentary lifestyle, obesity, smoking, alcohol use, and diabetes with the risk of colorectal cancer. *Cancer Res.* **57**, 4787–4794.

49. Calle, E. E., Mervis, C. A., Wingo, P. A., Thun, M. J., Rodriguez, C., and Heath, C. W., Jr. (1995) Spontaneous abortion and risk of fatal breast cancer in a prospective cohort of United States women. *Cancer Causes Control.* **6**, 460–468.

50. Tchernof, A. and Despres, J. P. (2000). Sex steroid hormones, sex hormone-binding

globulin, and obesity in men and women. *Horm Metab Res.* **32**, 526–536.

51. Key, T. J., Allen, N. E., Verkasalo, P. K., and Banks, E. (2001) Energy balance and cancer: the role of sex hormones. *Proc Nutr Soc.* **60**, 81–89.

52. Davidow, A. L., Neugut, A. I., Jacobson, J. S., Ahsan, H., Garbowski, G. C., Forde, et al. (1996) Recurrent adenomatous polyps and body mass index. *Cancer Epidemiol Biomarkers Prev.* **5**, 313–315.

53. Giovannucci, E., Colditz, G. A., Stampfer, M. J., and Willett, W. C. (1996) Physical activity, obesity, and risk of colorectal adenoma in women (United States). *Cancer Causes Control.* **7**, 253–263.

54. Boutron-Ruault, M. C., Senesse, P., Meance, S., Belghiti, C., and Faivre, J. (2001) Energy intake, body mass index, physical activity, and the colorectal adenoma-carcinoma sequence. *Nutr Cancer.* **39**, 50–57.

55. Honjo, S., Kono, S., Shinchi, K., Wakabayashi, K., Todoroki, I., Sakurai, Y. et al. (1995) The relation of smoking, alcohol use and obesity to risk of sigmoid colon and rectal adenomas. *Jpn J Cancer Res.* **86**, 1019–1026.

56. Shinchi, K., Kono, S., Honjo, S., Todoroki, I., Sakurai, Y., Imanishi, K., et al. (1994) Obesity and adenomatous polyps of the sigmoid colon. *Jpn J Cancer Res.* **85**, 479–484.

57. Kono, S., Handa, K., Hayabuchi, H., Kiyohara, C., Inoue, H., Marugame, T., et al. (1999) Obesity, weight gain and risk of colon adenomas in Japanese men. *Jpn J Cancer Res.* **90**, 805–811.

58. Dietz, A. T., Newcomb, P. A., Marcus, P. M., and Storer, B. E. (1995) The association of body size and large bowel cancer risk in Wisconsin (United States) women. *Cancer Causes Control.* **6**, 30–36.

59. Russo, A., Franceschi, S., La Vecchia, C., Dal Maso, L., Montella, M., Conti, E., et al. (1998) Body size and colorectal-cancer risk. *Int J Cancer.* **78**, 161–165.

60. Graham, S., Dayal, H., Swanson, M., Mittelman, A., and Wilkinson, G. (1978) Diet in the epidemiology of cancer of the colon and rectum. *J Natl Cancer Inst.* **61**, 709–714.

61. Terry, P., Giovannucci, E., Bergkvist, L., Holmberg, L., and Wolk, A. (2001) Body weight and colorectal cancer risk in a cohort of Swedish women: relation varies by age and cancer site. *Br J Cancer.* **85**, 346–349.

62. Slattery, M. L., Caan, B. J., Benson, J., and Murtaugh, M. (2003). Energy balance

and rectal cancer: an evaluation of energy intake, energy expenditure, and body mass index. *Nutr Cancer.* **46**, 166–171.

63. de Waard, F. and Baanders-van Halewijn, E. A. (1974) A prospective study in general practice on breast-cancer risk in postmenopausal women. *Int J Cancer.* **14**, 153–160.

64. Ballard-Barbash, R. (2006) Obesity, weight change, and breast cancer incidence. In *Cancer Prevention and Management Through Exercise and Weight Control* (McTiernan, A., ed.), Taylor & Francis, Boca Raton, FL, pp. 219–232.

65. Hayes, T. M., Underhill, C. R., Clarke, K., and Tattersall, M. H. (2003) Hormone replacement therapy after a diagnosis of breast cancer: cancer recurrence and mortality. *Med J Aust.* **178**, 412–413.

66. Slattery, M. L. (2001) Does an apple a day keep breast cancer away? *JAMA.* **285**, 799–801.

67. Bianchini, F., Kaaks, R., and Vainio, H. (2002) Overweight, obesity, and cancer risk. *Lancet Oncol.* **3**, 565–574.

68. Bergstrom, A., Pisani, P., Tenet, V., Wolk, A., and Adami, H. O. (2001) Overweight as an avoidable cause of cancer in Europe. *Int J Cancer.* **91**, 421–430.

69. Yoo, K., Tajima, K., Park, S., Kang, D., Kim, S., Hirose, K., et al. (2001) Postmenopausal obesity as a breast cancer risk factor according to estrogen and progesterone receptor status (Japan). *Cancer Lett.* **167**, 57–63.

70. Hirose, K., Tajima, K., Hamajima, N., Takezaki, T., Inoue, M., Kuroishi, T., et al. (2001) Association of family history and other risk factors with breast cancer risk among Japanese premenopausal and postmenopausal women. *Cancer Causes Control.* **12**, 349–358.

71. Shu, X. O., Jin, F., Dai, Q., Shi, J. R., Potter, J. D., Brinton, L. A., et al. (2001) Association of body size and fat distribution with risk of breast cancer among Chinese women. *Int J Cancer.* **94**, 449–455.

72. Pan, S. Y., Johnson, K. C., Ugnat, A. M., Wen, S. W., and Mao, Y. (2004) Association of obesity and cancer risk in Canada. *Am J Epidemiol.* **159**, 259–268.

73. Stephenson, G. D. and Rose, D. P. (2003) Breast cancer and obesity: an update. *Nutr Cancer.* **45**, 1–16.

74. Jonsson, H., Tornberg, S., Nystrom, L., and Lenner, P. (2003) Service screening with mammography of women aged 70–74 years in Sweden. Effects on breast cancer mortality. *Cancer Detect Prev.* **27**, 360–369.

75. Tornberg, S., Carstensen, J., Hakulinen, T., Lenner, P., Hatschek, T., and Lundgren, B. (1994) Evaluation of the effect on breast cancer mortality of population based mammography screening programmes. *J Med Screen.* **1**, 184–187.

76. Lam, P. B., Vacek, P. M., Geller, B. M., and Muss, H. B. (2000) The association of increased weight, body mass index, and tissue density with the risk of breast carcinoma in Vermont. *Cancer.* **89**, 369–375.

77. Potischman, N., Swanson, C. A., Siiteri, P., and Hoover, R. N. (1996) Reversal of relation between body mass and endogenous estrogen concentrations with menopausal status. *J Natl Cancer Inst.* **88**, 756–758.

78. Huang, Z., Hankinson, S. E., Colditz, G. A., Stampfer, M., Hunter, D. J., Manson, J.E., et al. (1997) Dual effects of weight and weight gain on breast cancer risk. *JAMA.* **278**, 1407–1411.

79. Ziegler, R. G., Hoover, R. N., Nomura, A. M., West, D. W., Wu, A. H., Pike, M. C., et al. (1996) Relative weight, weight change, height, and breast cancer risk in Asian-American women. *J Natl Cancer Inst.* **88**, 650–660.

80. Mayberry, R. M. (1994) Age-specific patterns of association between breast cancer and risk factors in black women, ages 20 to 39 and 40 to 54. *Ann Epidemiol.* **4**, 205–213.

81. Chu, K. C., Kramer, B. S., and Smart, C. R. (1991) Analysis of the role of cancer prevention and control measures in reducing cancer mortality. *J Natl Cancer Inst.* **83**, 1636–1643.

82. Wenten, M., Gilliland, F. D., Baumgartner, K., and Samet, J. M. (2002) Associations of weight, weight change, and body mass with breast cancer risk in Hispanic and non-Hispanic white women. *Ann Epidemiol.* **12**, 435–444.

83. Shu, X.-O., Jin, F., Dai, Q., Shi, J. R., Potter, J. D., Brinton, L. A., et al. (2001) Association of body size and fat distribution with risk of breast cancer among Chinese women. *Int J Cancer.* **94**, 449–454.

84. Sonnenschein, E., Toniolo, P., Terry, M. B., Bruning, P. F., Kato, I., Koenig, K. L., et al. (1999) Body fat distribution and obesity in pre- and postmenopausal breast cancer. *Int J Epidemiol.* **28**, 1026–1031.

85. Mannisto, S., Pietinen, P., Pyy, M., Palmgren, J., Eskelinen, M., and Uusitupa, M. (1996) Body-size indicators and risk of breast cancer according to menopause and estrogen-receptor status. *Int J Cancer.* **68**, 8–13.

86. Swanson, C. A., Coates, R. J., Schoenberg, J. B., Malone, K. E., Gammon, M. D., Stanford, J. L., et al. (1996) Body size and breast cancer risk among women under age 45 years. *Am J Epidemiol.* **143**, 698–706.

87. Franceschi, S., Favero, A., LaVecchia, C., Baron, A. E., Negri, E., Dal Maso, L., et al. (1996). Body size indices and breast cancer risk before and after menopause. *Int J Cancer.* **67**, 181–186.

88. Bruning, P. F., Bonfrer, J. M., van Noord, P. A., Hart, A. A., Jong-Bakker, M., and Nooijen, W. J. (1992) Insulin resistance and breast-cancer risk. *Int J Cancer.* **52**, 511–516.

89. Franceschi, S., Favero, A., La Vecchia, C., Baron, A. E., Negri, E., Dal Maso, L. et al. (1996) Body size indices and breast cancer risk before and after menopause. *Int J Cancer.* **67**, 181–186.

90. Hirose, K., Tajima, K., Hamajima, N., Takezaki, T., Inoue, M., Kuroishi, T., et al. (1999) Effect of body size on breast-cancer risk among Japanese women. *Int J Cancer.* **80**, 349–355.

91. Huang, Z., Hankinson, S. E., Colditz, G. A., Stampfer, M. J., Hunter, D. J., Manson, J. E., et al (1997) Dual effects of weight and weight gain on breast cancer risk. *JAMA.* **278**, 1407–1411.

92. Coates, R. J., Uhler, R. J., Hall, H. I., Potischman, N., Brinton, L. A., Ballard-Barbash, R., et al. (1999) Risk of breast cancer in young women in relation to body size and weight gain in adolescence and early adulthood. *Br J Cancer.* **81**, 167–174.

93. Peacock, S. L., White, E., Daling, J. R., Voigt, L. F., and Malone, K. E. (1999) Relation between obesity and breast cancer in young women. *Am J Epidemiol.* **149**, 339–346.

94. Brinton, L. A. and Swanson, C. A. (1992) Height and weight at various ages and risk of breast cancer. *Ann Epidemiol.* **2**, 597–609.

95. Ballard-Barbash, R. and Swanson, C. A. (1996) Body weight: estimation of risk for breast and endometrial cancers. *Am J Clin Nutr.* **63**, 437S–441S.

96. Galanis, D. J., Kolonel, L. N., Lee, J., and Le Marchand, L. (1998) Anthropometric predictors of breast cancer incidence and survival in a multi-ethnic cohort of female residents of Hawaii, United States. *Cancer Causes Control.* **9**, 217–224.

97. Trentham-Dietz, A., Newcomb, P. A., Storer, B. E., Longnecker, M. P., Baron, J. A., Greenberg, E. R., et al. (1997) Body size and risk of breast cancer. *Am J Epidemiol.* **145**, 1011–1019.

98. Harvie, M., Hooper, L., and Howell, A. H. (2003) Central obesity and breast cancer risk: a systematic review. *Obes Rev.* **4**, 157–173.

99. Choi, N. W., Howe, G. R., Miller, A. B., Matthews, V., Morgan, R. W., Munan, L., et al. (1978) An epidemiologic study of breast cancer. *Am J Epidemiol.* **107**, 510–521.

100. Folsom, A. R., Kaye, S. A., Prineas, R. J., Potter, J. D., Gapstur, S. M., and Wallace, R. B. (1990) Increased incidence of carcinoma of the breast associated with abdominal adiposity in postmenopausal women. *Am J Epidemiol.* **131**, 794–803.

101. Harris, R. E., Namboodiri, K. K., and Wynder, E. L. (1992) Breast cancer risk: effects of estrogen replacement therapy and body mass. *J Natl Cancer Inst.* **84**, 1575–1582.

102. Hislop, T. G., Coldman, A. J., Elwood, J. M., Skippen, D. H., and Kan, L. (1986) Relationship between risk factors for breast cancer and hormonal status. *Int J Epidemiol.* **15**, 469–476.

103. Le Marchand, L., Kolonel, L. N., Earle, M. E., and Mi, M.-P. (1988) Body size at different periods of life and breast cancer risk. *Am J Epidemiol.* **128**, 137–152.

104. Paffenbarger, R. S., Jr., Kampert, J. B., Chang, H. G. (1980) Characteristics that predict risk of breast cancer before and after the menopause. *Am J Epidemiol.* **112**, 258–268.

105. Sellers, T. A., Alberts, S. R., Vierkant, R. A., Grabrick, D. M., Cerhan, J. R., Vachon, C. M., et al. (2002) High-folate diets and breast cancer survival in a prospective cohort study. *Nutr Cancer.* **44**, 139–144.

106. Magnusson, C., Colditz, G., Rosner, B., Bergstrom, R., and Persson, I. (1998) Association of family history and other risk factors with breast cancer risk (Sweden). *Cancer Causes Control.* **9**, 259–267.

107. Enger, S. M., Ross, R. K., Paganini-Hill, A., Carpenter, C. L., and Bernstein, L. (2000) Body size, physical activity, and breast cancer hormone receptor status: results from two case-control studies. *Cancer Epidemiol Biomarkers Prev.* **9**, 681–687.

108. Wenten, M., Gilliland, F. D., Baumgartner, K., and Samet, J. M. (2002) Associations of weight, weight change, and body mass with breast cancer risk in Hispanic and non-Hispanic white women. *Ann Epidemiol.* **12**, 435–444.

109. Morimoto, L. M., White, E., Chen, Z., Chlebowski, R. T., Hays, J., Kuller, L., et al. (2002) Obesity, body size, and risk of post-menopausal breast cancer: the Women's Health Initiative (United States). *Cancer Causes Control.* **13**, 741–751.

110. Tretli, S. (1989) Height and weight in relation to breast cancer morbidity and mortality. A prospective study of 570,000 women in Norway. *Int J Cancer.* **44**, 23–30.

111. Hall, I. J., Newman, B., Millikan, R. C., and Moorman, P. G. (2000) Body size and breast cancer risk in black women and white women: the Carolina Breast Cancer Study. *Am J Epidemiol.* **151**, 754–764.

112. Friedenreich, C. M. and Orenstein, M. R. (2002) Physical activity and cancer prevention: etiologic evidence and biological mechanisms. *J Nutr.* **132**, 3456S–3464S.

113. Kolonel, L. N., Nomura, A. M., Lee, J., and Hirohata, T. (1986). Anthropometric indicators of breast cancer risk in postmenopausal women in Hawaii. *Nutr Cancer.* **8**, 247–256.

114. Negri, E., La Vecchia, C., Bruzzi, P., Dardanoni, G., Decarli, A., Palli, D., et al. (1988) Risk factors for breast cancer: pooled results from three Italian case-control studies. *Am J Epidemiol.* **128**, 1207–1215.

115. Lubin, F., Ruder, A.M., Wax, Y., and Modan, B. (1985) Overweight and changes in weight throughout adult life in breast cancer etiology. *Am J Epidemiol.* **122**, 579–588.

116. Yong, L. C., Brown, C. C., Schatzkin, A., and Schairer, C. (1996) Prospective study of relative weight and risk of breast cancer: The Breast Cancer Detection Demonstration Project follow-up study, 1979 to 1987–1989. *Am J Epidemiol.* **143**, 985–995.

117. Ziegler, R. G., Hoover, R. N., Nomura, A. M. Y., West, D. W., Wu, A. H., Pike, M. C., et al. (1996) Relative weight, weight change, height, and breast cancer risk in Asian-American women. *J Natl Cancer Inst.* **88**, 650–660.

118. Lahmann, P. H., Lissner, L., Gullberg, B., Olsson, H., and Berglund, G. (2003) A prospective study of adiposity and post-menopausal breast cancer risk: the Malmo diet and cancer study. *Int J Cancer.* **103**, 246–252.

119. Feigelson, H. S., Jonas, C. R., Teras, L. R., Thun, M. J., and Calle, E. E. (2004) Weight gain, body mass index, hormone replacement therapy, and postmenopausal breast cancer in a large prospective study. *Cancer Epidemiol Biomarkers Prev.* **13**, 220–224.

120. Barnes-Josiah, D., Potter, J. D., Sellers, T. A., and Himes, J. H. (1995) Early body size and subsequent weight gain as predictors of breast cancer incidence (Iowa, United States). *Cancer Causes Control.* **6**, 112–118.

121. Nomura, A., Heilbrun, L. K., and Stemmermann, G. N. (1985) Body mass index as a predictor of cancer in men. *J Natl Cancer Inst.* **74**, 319–323.

122. Harris, R., Whittemore, A. S., and Itnyre, J. (1992) Characteristics relating to ovarian cancer risk: collaborative analysis of 12 US case-control studies. III. Epithelial tumors of low malignant potential in white women. Collaborative Ovarian Cancer Group. *Am J Epidemiol.* **136**, 1204–1211.

123. van den Brandt, P. A., Spiegelman, D., Yaun, S. S., Adami, H. O., Beeson, L., Folsom, A. R., et al. (2000). Pooled analysis of prospective cohort studies on height, weight, and breast cancer risk. *Am J Epidemiol.* **152**, 514–527.

124. Schairer, C., Mink, P. J., Carroll, L., and Devesa, S. S. (2004) Probabilities of death from breast cancer and other causes among female breast cancer patients. *J Natl Cancer Inst.* **96**, 1311–1321.

125. Meldrum, D.R., Davidson, B.J., Tataryn, I.V., and Judd, H. L. (1981) Changes in circulating steroids with aging in postmenopausal women. *Obstet Gynecol.* **57**, 624–628.

126. Key, T., Appleby, P., Barnes, I., and Reeves, G. (2002). Endogenous sex hormones and breast cancer in postmenopausal women: reanalysis of nine prospective studies. *J Natl Cancer Inst.* **94**, 606–616.

127. Bergstrom, A., Pisani, P., Tenet, V., Wolk, A., and Adami, H. O. (2001). Overweight as an avoidable cause of cancer in Europe. *Int J Cancer.* **91**, 421–430.

128. Wolk, A., Gridley, G., Svensson, M., Nyren, O., McLaughlin, J. K., Fraumeni, J. F., and Adami, H. O. (2001) A prospective study of obesity and cancer risk (Sweden). *Cancer Causes Control.* **12**, 13–21.

129. Moller, H., Mellemgaard, A., Lindvig, K., and Olsen, J. H. (1994) Obesity and cancer risk: a Danish record-linkage study. *Eur J Cancer.* **30A**, 344–350.

130. Furberg, A. S. and Thune, I. (2003) Metabolic abnormalities (hypertension, hyperglycemia and overweight), lifestyle (high energy intake and physical inactivity) and endometrial cancer risk in a Norwegian cohort. *Int J Cancer.* **104**, 669–676.

131. Horn-Ross, P. L., John, E. M., Canchola, A. J., Stewart, S. L., and Lee, M. M. (2003)

Phytoestrogen intake and endometrial cancer risk. *J Natl Cancer Inst.* **95**, 1158–1164.

132. Augustin, L. S., Gallus, S., Bosetti, C., Levi, F., Negri, E., Franceschi, S., et al. (2003) Glycemic index and glycemic load in endometrial cancer. *Int J Cancer.* **105**, 404–407.

133. Xu, W., Dai, Q., Ruan, Z., Cheng, J., Jin, F., and Shu, X. (2002) Obesity at different ages and endometrial cancer risk factors in urban Shanghai, China. *Zhonghua Liu Xing Bing Xue Za Zhi.* **23**, 347–351.

134. Newcomer, L. M., Newcomb, P. A., Trentham-Dietz, A., and Storer, B. E. (2001) Hormonal risk factors for endometrial cancer: modification by cigarette smoking (United States). *Cancer Causes Control.* **12**, 829–835.

135. Niwa, K., Imai, A., Hashimoto, M., Yokoyama, Y., Mori, H., Matsuda, Y., et al.(2000) A case-control study of uterine endometrial cancer of pre- and post-menopausal women. *Onco Rep.* **7**, 89–93.

136. Parslov, M., Lidegaard, O., Klintorp, S., Pedersen, B., Jonsson, L., and Eriksen, P. S. (2000) Risk factors among young women with endometrial cancer: a Danish case-control study. *Am J Obstet Gynecol.* **182**, 23–29.

137. Terry, P., Baron, J. A., Weiderpass, E., Yuen, J., Lichtenstein, P., and Nyren, O. (1999) Lifestyle and en dometrial cancer risk: a cohort study from the Swedish Twin Registry. *Int J Cancer.* **82**, 38–42.

138. La Vecchia, C., Franceschi, S., Decarli, A., Gallus, G., and Tognoni, G. (1984) Risk factors for endometrial cancer at different ages. *J Natl Cancer Inst.* **73**, 667–671.

139. Tornberg, S. A. and Carstensen, J. M. (1994) Relationship between Quetelet's index and cancer of breast and female genital tract in 47,000 women followed for 25 years. *Br J Cancer.* **69**, 358–361.

140. Swanson, C. A., Potischman, N., Wilbanks, G. D., Twiggs, L. B., Mortel, R., Berman, M. et al. (1993) Relation of endometrial cancer risk to past and contemporary body size and body fat distribution. *Cancer Epidemiol Biomarkers Prev.* **2**, 321–327.

141. Shu, X. O., Brinton, L. A., Zheng, W., Swanson, C. A., Hatch, M. C., Gao, Y. T., et al. (1992) Relation of obesity and body fat distribution to endometrial cancer in Shanghai, China. *Cancer Res.* **52**, 3865–3870.

142. Austin, H., Austin, J. M., Jr., Partridge, E. E., Hatch, K. D., and Shingleton, H. M. (1991) Endometrial cancer, obesity, and body fat distribution. *Cancer Res.* **51**, 568–572.

143. Olson, S. H., Trevisan, M., Marshall, J. R., Graham, S., Zielezny, M., Vena, J. E., et al (1995) Body mass index, weight gain, and risk of endometrial cancer. *Nutr Cancer.* **23**, 141–149.

144. Weiderpass, E., Adami, H. O., Baron, J. A., Wicklund-Glynn, A., Aune, M., Atuma, S., et al. (2000) Organochlorines and endometrial cancer risk. *Cancer Epidemiol Biomarkers Prev.* **9**, 487–493.

145. Hirose, K., Tajima, K., Hamajima, N., Kuroishi, T., Kuzuya, K., Miura, S., et al. (1999). Comparative case-referent study of risk factors among hormone-related female cancers in Japan. *Jpn J Cancer Res.* **90**, 255–261.

146. Austin, H., Austin, J. M., Jr., Partridge, E. E., Hatch, K. D., and Shingleton, H. M. (1991) Endometrial cancer, obesity, and body fat distribution. *Cancer Res.* **51**, 568–572.

147. Levi, F., La Vecchia, C., Negri, E., Parazzini, F., and Franceschi, S. (1992) Body mass at different ages and subsequent endometrial cancer risk. *Int J Cancer.* **50**, 567–571.

148. Bergstrom, A., Pisani, P., Tenet, V., Wolk, A., and Adami, H. O. (2001) Overweight as an avoidable cause of cancer in Europe *Int J Cancer.* **91**, 421–430.

149. Hu, J., Mao, Y., and White, K. (2003) Overweight and obesity in adults and risk of renal cell carcinoma in Canada. *Soz Praventivmed.* **48**, 178–185.

150. Samanic, C., Chow, W. H., Gridley, G., Jarvholm, B., and Fraumeni, J. F., Jr. (2006) Relation of body mass index to cancer risk in 362,552 Swedish men. *Cancer Causes Control.* **17**, 901–909.

151. Heath, C. W., Jr., Lally, C. A., Calle, E. E., McLaughlin, J. K., and Thun, M. J. (1997) Hypertension, diuretics, and antihypertensive medications as possible risk factors for renal cell cancer. *Am J Epidemiol.* **145**, 607–613.

152. Chow, W. H., McLaughlin, J. K., Mandel, J. S., Wacholder, S., Niwa, S., and Fraumeni, J. F., Jr. (1996) Obesity and risk of renal cell cancer. *Cancer Epidemiol Biomarkers Prev.* **5**, 17–21.

153. Mellemgaard, A., Lindblad, P., Schlehofer, B., Bergstrom, R., Mandel, J. S., McCredie, et al. (1995) International renal-cell cancer study. III. Role of weight, height, physical activity, and use of amphetamines. *Int J Cancer.* **60**, 350–354.

154. Kreiger, N., Marrett, L. D., Dodds, L., Hilditch, S., and Darlington, G. A. (1993)

Risk factors for renal cell carcinoma: results of a population-based case-control study. *Cancer Causes Control.* **4**, 101–110.

155. Benhamou, S., Lenfant, M. H., Ory-Paoletti, C., and Flamant, R. (1993) Risk factors for renal-cell carcinoma in a French case-control study. *Int J Cancer.* **55**, 32–36.

156. McLaughlin, J. K., Gao, Y. T., Gao, R. N., Zheng, W., Ji, B. T., Blot, W. J., et al. (1992) Risk factors for renal-cell cancer in Shanghai, China. *Int J Cancer.* **52**, 562–565.

157. Wolk, A., Lindblad, P., and Adami, H. O. (1996) Nutrition and renal cell cancer. *Cancer Causes Control.* **7**, 5–18.

158. Hoyo, C. and Gammon, M. D. (2006) Obesity and overweight in relation to adenocarcinoma of the esophagus, in *Cancer Prevention and Management Through Exercise and Weight Control* (McTiernan, A., ed.), Taylor & Francis, Boca Raton, FL, pp. 269–282.

159. Lagergren, J., Bergstrom, R., and Nyren, O. (1999) Association between body mass and adenocarcinoma of the esophagus and gastric cardia. *Ann Intern Med.* **130**, 883–890.

160. Tretli, S. and Robsahm, T. E. (1999) Height, weight and cancer of the oesophagus and stomach: a follow-up study in Norway. *Eur J Cancer Prev.* **8**, 115–122.

161. Farrow, D. C., Vaughan, T. L., Hansten, P. D., Stanford, J. L., Risch, H. A., Gammon, M. D., et al. (1998) Use of aspirin and other nonsteroidal anti-inflammatory drugs and risk of esophageal and gastric cancer. *Cancer Epidemiol Biomarkers Prev.* **7**, 97–102.

162. Nilsson, M., Johnsen, R., Ye, W., Hveem, K., and Lagergren, J. (2003) Obesity and estrogen as risk factors for gastroesophageal reflux symptoms. *JAMA.* **290**, 66–72.

163. Ji, B. T., Chow, W. H., Yang, G., McLaughlin, J. K., Gao, R. N., Zheng, W., et al. (1997) Body mass index and the risk of cancers of the gastric cardia and distal stomach in Shanghai, China. *Cancer Epidemiol Biomarkers Prev.* **6**, 481–485.

164. Knudson, A. G., Jr. (1971) Mutation and cancer: statistical study of retinoblastoma. *Proc Natl Acad Sci USA.* **68**, 820–823.

165. Devesa, S. S., Blot, W. J., and Fraumeni, J. F., Jr. (1998) Changing patterns in the incidence of esophageal and gastric carcinoma in the United States. *Cancer.* **83**, 2049–2053.

166. Wild, C. P. and Hardie, L. J. (2003) Reflux, Barrett's oesophagus and adenocarcinoma: burning questions. *Nat Rev Cancer.* **3**, 676–684.

167. Mokdad, A. H., Ford, E. S., Bowman, B. A., Dietz, W. H., Vinicor, F., Bales, V. S., et al. (2003). Prevalence of obesity, diabetes, and obesity-related health risk factors, 2001. *JAMA.* **289**, 76–79.

168. Wu, A. H., Wan, P., and Bernstein, L. (2001). A multiethnic population-based study of smoking, alcohol and body size and risk of adenocarcinomas of the stomach and esophagus (United States). *Cancer Causes Control.* **12**, 721–732.

169. Vaughan, T. L., Davis, S., Kristal, A., and Thomas, D. B. (1995) Obesity, alcohol, and tobacco as risk factors for cancers of the esophagus and gastric cardia: adenocarcinoma versus squamous cell carcinoma. *Cancer Epidemiol Biomarkers Prev.* **4**, 85–92.

170. Chow, W. H., Blot, W. J., Vaughan, T. L., Risch, H. A., Gammon, M. D., Stanford, J. L., et al. (1998) Body mass index and risk of adenocarcinomas of the esophagus and gastric cardia. *J Natl Cancer Inst.* **90**, 150–155.

171. Gapstur, S. M., Gann, P. H., Lowe, W., Liu, K., Colangelo, L., and Dyer, A. (2000) Abnormal glucose metabolism and pancreatic cancer mortality. *JAMA.* **283**, 2552–2558.

172. Michaud, D. S., Giovannucci, E., Willett, W. C., Colditz, G. A., Stampfer, M. J., and Fuchs, C. S. (2001) Physical activity, obesity, height, and the risk of pancreatic cancer. *JAMA.* **286**, 921–929.

173. Silverman, D. T., Swanson, C. A., Gridley, G., Wacholder, S., Greenberg, R. S., Brown, L. M., et al. (1998) Dietary and nutritional factors and pancreatic cancer: a case-control study based on direct interviews. *J Natl Cancer Inst.* **90**, 1710–1719.

174. Hanley, A. J., Johnson, K. C., Villeneuve, P. J., and Mao, Y. (2001) Physical activity, anthropometric factors and risk of pancreatic cancer: results from the Canadian enhanced cancer surveillance system. *Int J Cancer.* **94**, 140–147.

175. Berrington, D. G., Sweetland, S., and Spencer, E. (2003) A meta-analysis of obesity and the risk of pancreatic cancer. *Br J Cancer.* **89**, 519–523.

176. Lee, I. M., Sesso, H. D., Oguma, Y., and Paffenbarger, R. S., Jr. (2003) Physical activity, body weight, and pancreatic cancer mortality. *Br J Cancer.* **88**, 679–683.

177. Zatonski, W., Przewozniak, K., Howe, G. R., Maisonneuve, P., Walker, A. M., and Boyle, P. (1991) Nutritional factors and pancreatic cancer: a case-control study from south-west Poland. *Int J Cancer.* **48**, 390–394.

178. Howe, G. R., Jain, M., and Miller, A. B. (1990) Dietary factors and risk of pancreatic cancer: results of a Canadian population-based case-control study. *Int J Cancer.* **45**, 604–608.

179. Ghadirian, P., Boyle, P., Simard, A., Baillargeon, J., Maisonneuve, P., and Perret, C. (1991) Reported family aggregation of pancreatic cancer within a population-based case-control study in the Francophone community in Montreal, Canada. *Int J Pancreatol.* **10**, 183–196.

180. Bueno de Mesquita, H. B., Moerman, C. J., Runia, S., and Maisonneuve, P. (1990) Are energy and energy-providing nutrients related to exocrine carcinoma of the pancreas? *Int J Cancer.* **46**, 435–444.

181. Amercian Cancer Society. (2007) ACS Cancer Facts and Figures. Atlanta: Georgia, American Cancer Society.

182. Friedman, G. D. and van den Eeden, S. K. (1993) Risk factors for pancreatic cancer: an exploratory study. *Int J Epidemiol.* **22**, 30–37.

183. Patel, A. V., Rodriguez, C., Bernstein, L., Chao, A., Thun, M. J., and Calle, E. E. (2005) Obesity, recreational physical activity, and risk of pancreatic cancer in a large U.S. Cohort. *Cancer Epidemiol Biomarkers Prev.* **14**, 459–466.

184. Anderson, J. P., Ross, J. A., and Folsom, A. R. (2004) Anthropometric variables, physical activity, and incidence of ovarian cancer: The Iowa Women's Health Study. *Cancer.* **100**, 1515–1521.

185. Engeland, A., Tretli, S., and Bjorge, T. (2003) Height, body mass index, and ovarian cancer: a follow-up of 1.1 million Norwegian women. *J Natl Cancer Inst.* **95**, 1244–1248.

186. Lubin, F., Chetrit, A., Freedman, L. S., Alfandary, E., Fishler, Y., Nitzan, H., et al. (2003) Body mass index at age 18 years and during adult life and ovarian cancer risk. *Am J Epidemiol.* **157**, 113–120.

187. Fairfield, K. M., Willett, W. C., Rosner, B. A., Manson, J. E., Speizer, F. E., and Hankinson, S. E. (2002) Obesity, weight gain, and ovarian cancer. *Obstet Gynecol.* **100**, 288–296.

188. Kuper, H., Cramer, D. W., and Titus-Ernstoff, L. (2002) Risk of ovarian cancer in the United States in relation to anthropometric measures: does the association depend on menopausal status? *Cancer Causes Control.* **13**, 455–463.

189. Dal Maso, L., Franceschi, S., Negri, E., Conti, E., Montella, M., Vaccarella, S., et al. (2002) Body size indices at different ages and epithelial ovarian cancer risk. *Eur J Cancer.* **38**, 1769–1774.

190. Riman, T., Dickman, P. W., Nilsson, S., Correia, N., Nordlinder, H., Magnusson, C. M., et al. (2001) Risk factors for epithelial borderline ovarian tumors: results of a Swedish case-control study. *Gynecol Oncol.* **83**, 575–585.

191. Giovannucci, E., Rimm, E. B., Liu, Y., Leitzmann, M., Wu, K., Stampfer, M. J. et al. (2003). Body mass index and risk of prostate cancer in U.S. health professionals. *J Natl Cancer Inst.* **95**, 1240–1244.

192. Lee, I. M., Sesso, H. D., and Paffenbarger, R. S., Jr. (2001) A prospective cohort study of physical activity and body size in relation to prostate cancer risk (United States). *Cancer Causes Control.* **12**, 187–193.

193. Habel, L. A., van den Eeden, S. K., and Friedman, G. D. (2000) Body size, age at shaving initiation, and prostate cancer in a large, multiracial cohort. *Prostate.* **43**, 136–143.

194. Sung, J. F., Lin, R. S., Pu, Y. S., Chen, Y. C., Chang, H. C., and Lai, M. K. (1999) Risk factors for prostate carcinoma in Taiwan: a case-control study in a Chinese population. *Cancer.* **86**, 484–491.

195. Chyou, P. H., Nomura, A. M., and Stemmermann, G. N. (1994) A prospective study of weight, body mass index and other anthropometric measurements in relation to site-specific cancers. *Int J Cancer.* **57**, 313–317.

196. Rodriguez, C., Freedland, S. J., Deka, A., Jacobs, E. J., McCullough, M. L., and Patel, A. V., et al. (2007) Body mass index, weight change, and risk of prostate cancer in the Cancer Prevention Study II Nutrition Cohort. *Cancer Epidemiol Biomarkers Prev.* **16**, 63–69.

197. Putnam, S. D., Cerhan, J. R., Parker, A. S., Bianchi, G. D., Wallace, R. B., Cantor, K. P., et al. (2000) Lifestyle and anthropometric risk factors for prostate cancer in a cohort of Iowa men. *Ann Epidemiol.* **10**, 361–369.

198. Andersson, S. O., Wolk, A., Bergstrom, R., Giovannucci, E., Lindgren, C., Baron, J., et al. (1996) Energy, nutrient intake and prostate cancer risk: a population-based case-control study in Sweden. *Int J Cancer.* **68**, 716–722.

199. Thompson, M. M., Garland, C., Barrett-Connor, E., Khaw, K. T., Friedlander, N. J., Wingard, D. L. (1989) Heart disease risk factors, diabetes, and prostatic cancer in an adult community. *Am J Epidemiol.* **129**, 511–517.

200. Snowdon, D. A., Phillips, R. L., and Choi, W. (1984) Diet, obesity, and risk of fatal prostate cancer. *Am J Epidemiol.* **120**, 244–250.

201. MacInnis, R. J., English, D. R., Gertig, D. M., Hopper, J. L., and Giles, G. G. (2003) Body size and composition and prostate cancer risk. *Cancer Epidemiol Biomarkers Prev.* **12**, 1417–1421.

202. Thune, I. and Lund, E. (1994) Physical activity and the risk of prostate and testicular cancer: a cohort study of 53,000 Norwegian men. *Cancer Causes Control.* **5**, 549–556.

203. Gronberg, H., Damber, L., and Damber, J. E. (1996) Familial prostate cancer in Sweden. A nationwide register cohort study. *Cancer.* **77**, 138–143.

204. Talamini, R., La Vecchia, C., Decarli, A., Negri, E., and Franceschi, S. (1986) Nutrition, social factors and prostatic cancer in a Northern Italian population. *Br J Cancer.* **53**, 817–821.

205. Key, T. J., Silcocks, P. B., Davey, G. K., Appleby, P. N., and Bishop, D. T. (1997) A case-control study of diet and prostate cancer. *Br J Cancer.* **76**, 678–687.

206. Neugut, A. I., Chen, A. C., and Petrylak, D. P. (2004) The "skinny" on obesity and prostate cancer prognosis. *J Clin Oncol.* **22**, 395–398.

207. Furuya, Y., Akimoto, S., Akakura, K., and Ito, H. (1998) Smoking and obesity in relation to the etiology and disease progression of prostate cancer in Japan. *Int J Urol.* **5**, 134–137.

208. Henley, S. J., Flanders, W. D., Manatunga, A., and Thun, M. J. (2002) Leanness and lung cancer risk: fact or artifact? *Epidemiology.* **13**, 268–276.

209. Kark, J. D., Yaari, S., Rasooly, I., and Goldbourt, U. (1995) Are lean smokers at increased risk of lung cancer? The Israel Civil Servant Cancer Study. *Arch Intern Med.* **155**, 2409–2416.

210. Drinkard, L. C., Hoffman, P. C., Samuels, B. L., Watson, S., Bitran, J. D., Golomb, H. M., et al. (1995) Dose intensification—a phase I study of ifosfamide with vinorelbine (Navelbine): rationale and study design in advanced non-small cell lung cancer. *Semin Oncol.* **22**, 30–37.

211. Knekt, P., Heliovaara, M., Rissanen, A., Aromaa, A., Seppanen, R., Teppo, L., et al. (1991) Leanness and lung-cancer risk. *Int J Cancer.* **49**, 208–213.

212. Goodman, G. E., Omenn, G. S., Thornquist, M. D., Lund, B., Metch, B., and Gylys-Colwell, I. (1993) The Carotene and Retinol Efficacy Trial (CARET) to prevent lung cancer in high-risk populations: pilot study with cigarette smokers. *Cancer Epidemiol Biomarkers Prev.* **2**, 389–396.

213. Kabat, G. C. and Wynder, E. L. (1992) Body mass index and lung cancer risk. *Am J Epidemiol.* **135**, 769–774.

214. Shafie, S. M. and Grantham, F. H. (1981) Role of hormones in the growth and regression of human breast cancer cells (MCF-7) transplanted into athymic nude mice. *J Natl Cancer Inst.* **67**, 51–56.

215. Heuson, J. C. and Legros, N. (1970) Effect of insulin and of alloxan diabetes on growth of the rat mammary carcinoma in vivo. *Eur J Cancer.* **6**, 349–351.

216. Peyrat, J. P., Bonneterre, J., Hecquet, B., Vennin, P., Louchez, M. M., Fournier, C., et al. (1993) Plasma insulin-like growth factor-1 (IGF-1) concentrations in human breast cancer. *Eur J Cancer.* **29A**, 492–497.

217. Pan, W., Hindler, K., Lee, V. V., Vaughn, W. K., and Collard, C. D. (2006) Obesity in diabetic patients undergoing coronary artery bypass graft surgery is associated with increased postoperative morbidity. *Anesthesiology.* **104**, 441–447.

218. Zatonski, W. A., Lowenfels, A. B., Boyle, P., Maisonneuve, P., Bueno de Mesquita, H. B., et al. (1997) Epidemiologic aspects of gallbladder cancer: a case-control study of the SEARCH Program of the International Agency for Research on Cancer. *J Natl Cancer Inst.* **89**, 1132–1138.

219. Strom, B. L., Soloway, R. D., Rios-Dalenz, J. L., Rodriguez-Martinez, H. A., West, S. L., Kinman, J. L., et al. (1995) Risk factors for gallbladder cancer. An international collaborative case-control study. *Cancer.* **76**, 1747–1756.

220. World Cancer Research Fund. 1997.

221. Holly, E. A., Lele, C., Bracci, P. M., McGrath, M. S. (1999) Case-control study of non-Hodgkin's lymphoma among women and heterosexual men in the San Francisco Bay Area, California. *Am J Epidemiol.* **150**, 375–389.

222. Cerhan, J. R., Torner, J. C., Lynch, C. F., Rubenstein, L. M., Lemke, J. H., Cohen, M. B., et al. (1997) Association of smoking, body mass, and physical activity with risk of prostate cancer in the Iowa 65+ Rural Health Study (United States). *Cancer Causes Control* **8**, 229–238.

223. National Center for Health Statistics, C. F. D. C. A. P. National Health and Nutrition

Examination Survey 1999–2000 [online]. *Nat Rev Cancer.* 2004.

224. Bergstrom, A., Pisani, P., Tenet, V., Wolk, A., and Adami, H. O. (2001) Overweight as an avoidable cause of cancer in Europe. *Int J Cancer.* **91**, 421–430.

225. Kaaks, R., Van Noord, P. A. H., Den Tonkelaar, I., Peeters, P. H. M., Riboli, E., and Grobbee, D. E. (1998) Breast-cancer incidence in relation height, weight and body-fat distribution in the Dutch "DOM" cohort. *Int J Cancer.* **76**, 647–651.

226. Stoll, B. A. (1999) Premalignant breast lesions: role for biological markers in predicting progression to cancer. *Eur J Cancer.* **35**, 693–697.

227. Weiderpass, E., Partanen, T., Kaaks, R., Vainio, H., Porta, M., Kauppinen, T., et al. (1998) Occurrence, trends and environment etiology of pancreatic cancer. *Scand J Work Environ Health.* **24**, 165–174.

228. Everhart, J. and Wright, D. (1995) Diabetes mellitus as a risk factor for pancreatic cancer. A meta-analysis. *JAMA.* **273**, 1605–1609.

229. Kaaks, R., Lundin, E., Rinaldi, S., Manjer, J., Biessy, C., Soderberg, S., et al. (2002) Prospective study of IGF-I, IGF-binding proteins, and breast cancer risk, in northern and southern Sweden. *Cancer Causes Control.* **13**, 307–316.

230. Wideroff, L., Gridley, G., Mellemkjaer, L., Chow, W. H., Linet, M., Keehn, S., et al. (1997) Cancer incidence in a population-based cohort of patients hospitalized with diabetes mellitus in Denmark. *J Natl Cancer Inst.* **89**, 1360–1365.

231. Lindblad, P., Chow, W. H., Chan, J., Bergstrom, A., Wolk, A., Gridley, G., et al. (1999) The role of diabetes mellitus in the aetiology of renal cell cancer. *Diabetologia.* **42**, 107–112.

232. Moschos, S. J. and Mantzoros, C. S. (2002) The role of the IGF system in cancer: from basic to clinical studies and clinical applications. *Oncology.* **63**, 317–332.

233. Lawlor, M. A. and Alessi, D. R. (2001) PKB/Akt: a key mediator of cell proliferation, survival and insulin responses? *J Cell Sci.* **114**, 2903–2910.

234. Prisco, M., Romano, G., Peruzzi, F., Valentinis, B., and Baserga, R. (1999) Insulin and IGF-I receptors signaling in protection from apoptosis. *Horm Metab Res.* **31**, 80–89.

235. Ish-Shalom, D., Christoffersen, C. T., Vorwerk, P., Sacerdoti-Sierra, N., Shymko, R. M., Naor, D., et al. (1997) Mitogenic properties of insulin and insulin analogues mediated by the insulin receptor. *Diabetologia.* **40 Suppl 2**, S25–S31.

236. Le Roith, D. (2000). Regulation of proliferation and apoptosis by the insulin-like growth factor I receptor. *Growth Horm IGF Res.* **10 Suppl A**, S12–S13.

237. Khandwala, H. M., McCutcheon, I. E., Flyvbjerg, A., and Friend, K. E. (2000) The effects of insulin-like growth factors on tumorigenesis and neoplastic growth. *Endocr Rev.* **21**, 215–244.

238. Yu, H., Jin, F., Shu, X. O., Li, B. D., Dai, Q., Cheng, J. R., et al. (2002) Insulin-like growth factors and breast cancer risk in Chinese women. *Cancer Epidemiol Biomarkers Prev.* **11**, 705–712.

239. Ibrahim, Y. H. and Yee, D. (2004) Insulin-like growth factor-I and cancer risk. *Growth Horm IGF Res.* **14**, 261–269.

240. Goodwin, P. J., Ennis, M., Pritchard, K. I., Trudeau, M. E., Koo, J., Madarnas, Y., et al. (2002) Fasting insulin and outcome in early-stage breast cancer: results of a prospective cohort study. *J Clin Oncol.* **20**, 42–51.

241. Papa, V. and Belfiore, A. (1996) Insulin receptors in breast cancer: biological and clinical role. *J Endocrinol Invest.* **19**, 324–333.

242. Werner, H. and LeRoith, D. (1996) The role of the insulin-like growth factor system in human cancer. *Adv Cancer Res.* **68**, 183–223.

243. Pollak, M. N., Schernhammer, E. S., and Hankinson, S. E. (2004) Insulin-like growth factors and neoplasia. *Nat Rev Cancer.* **4**, 505–518.

244. Shafie, S. M. and Hilf, R. (1981) Insulin receptor levels and magnitude of insulin-induced responses in 7,12-dimethylbenz(a)anthracene-induced mammary tumors in rats. *Cancer Res.* **41**, 826–829.

245. Cocca, C., Gutierrez, A., Nunez, M., Croci, M., Martin, G., Cricco, G., et al. (2003) Suppression of mammary gland tumorigenesis in diabetic rats. *Cancer Detect Prev.* **27**, 37–46.

246. Allen, N. E., Roddam, A. W., Allen, D. S., Fentiman, I. S., Dos Santos Silva, I., Peto, J., et al . (2005) A prospective study of serum insulin-like growth factor-I (IGF-I), IGF-II, IGF-binding protein-3 and breast cancer risk. *Br J Cancer.* **92**, 1283–1287.

247. Loucks, A. B., Vaitukaitis, J., Cameron, J. L., Rogol, A. D., Skrinar, G., Warren, M. P., et al. (1992) The reproductive system and exercise in women. *Med Sci Sports Exerc.* **24**, S288–S293.

248. Bruning, P. F., Van Doorn, J., Bonfrer, J. M., Van Noord, P. A., Korse, C. M., Linders, T. et al. (1995) Insulin-like growth-factor-binding protein 3 is decreased in early-stage operable pre-menopausal breast cancer. *Int J Cancer.* **62**, 266–270.

249. Bohlke, K., Cramer, D. W., Trichopoulos, D., and Mantzoros, C. S. (1998) Insulin-like growth factor-I in relation to premenopausal ductal carcinoma in situ of the breast. *Epidemiology.* **9**, 570–573.

250. Hankinson, S. E., Willett, W. C., Colditz, G. A., Hunter, D. J., Michaud, D. S., Deroo, et al. (1998) Circulating concentrations of insulin-like growth factor-I and risk of breast cancer. *Lancet.* **351**, 1393–1396.

251. Muti, P., Quattrin, T., Grant, B. J., Krogh, V., Micheli, A., Schunemann, H. J., et al. (2002) Fasting glucose is a risk factor for breast cancer: a prospective study. *Cancer Epidemiol Biomarkers Prev.* **11**, 1361–1368.

252. Toniolo, P., Bruning, P. F., Akhmedkhanov, A., Bonfrer, J. M., Koenig, K. L., Lukanova, A., et al. (2000) Serum insulin-like growth factor-I and breast cancer. *Int J Cancer.* **88**, 828–832.

253. Keinan-Boker, L., Bueno De Mesquita, H. B., Kaaks, R., Van Gils, C. H., Van Noord, P. A., Rinaldi, S., et al. (2003) Circulating levels of insulin-like growth factor I, its binding proteins -1,-2, -3, C-peptide and risk of postmenopausal breast cancer. *Int J Cancer.* **106**, 90–95.

254. Malin, A., Dai, Q., Yu, H., Shu, X. O., Jin, F., Gao, Y. T., et al. (2004) Evaluation of the synergistic effect of insulin resistance and insulin-like growth factors on the risk of breast carcinoma. *Cancer.* **100**, 694–700.

255. Kaaks, R. and Lukanova, A. (2001) Energy balance and cancer: the role of insulin and insulin-like growth factor-I. *Proc Nutr Soc.* **60**, 91–106.

256. Chan, J. M., Giovannucci, E., Andersson, S. O., Yuen, J., Adami, H. O., and Wolk, A. (1998) Dairy products, calcium, phosphorous, vitamin D, and risk of prostate cancer (Sweden). *Cancer Causes Control.* **9**, 559–566.

257. Stattin, P., Adlercreutz, H., Tenkanen, L., Jellum, E., Lumme, S., Hallmans, G., et al. (2002) Circulating enterolactone and prostate cancer risk: a Nordic nested case-control study. *Int J Cancer.* **99**, 124–129.

258. Lacey, J. V., Jr., Deng, J., Dosemeci, M., Gao, Y. T., Mostofi, F. K., Sesterhenn, I. A., et al. (2001) Prostate cancer, benign prostatic hyperplasia and physical activity in Shanghai, China. *Int J Epidemiol.* **30**, 341–349.

259. DeLellis, K., Rinaldi, S., Kaaks, R. J., Kolonel, L. N., Henderson, B., and Le Marchand, L. (2004) Dietary and lifestyle correlates of plasma insulin-like growth factor-I (IGF-I) and IGF binding protein-3 (IGFBP-3): the multiethnic cohort. *Cancer Epidemiol Biomarkers Prev.* **13**, 1444–1451.

260. Kaaks, R., Toniolo, P., Akhmedkhanov, A., Lukanova, A., Biessy, C., Dechaud, H., et al. (2000) Serum C-peptide, insulin-like growth factor (IGF)-I, IGF-binding proteins, and colorectal cancer risk in women. *J Natl Cancer Inst.* **92**, 1592–1600.

261. Palmqvist, R., Stenling, R., Oberg, A., and Landberg, G. (1999) Prognostic significance of p27(Kip1) expression in colorectal cancer: a clinico-pathological characterization. *J Pathol.* **188**, 18–23.

262. Ma, J., Pollak, M. N., Giovannucci, E., Chan, J. M., Tao, Y., Hennekens, C. H., et al. (1999) Prospective study of colorectal cancer risk in men and plasma levels of insulin-like growth factor (IGF)-I and IGF-binding protein-3. *J Natl Cancer Inst.* **91**, 620–625.

263. Probst-Hensch, N. M., Yuan, J. M., Stanczyk, F. Z., Gao, Y. T., Ross, R. K., and Yu, M. C. (2001) IGF-1, IGF-2 and IGFBP-3 in prediagnostic serum: association with colorectal cancer in a cohort of Chinese men in Shanghai. *Br J Cancer.* **85**, 1695–1699.

264. Giovannucci, E., Pollak, M. N., Platz, E. A., Willett, W. C., Stampfer, M. J., Majeed, N., et al. (2000) A prospective study of plasma insulin-like growth factor-1 and binding protein-3 and risk of colorectal neoplasia in women. *Cancer Epidemiol Biomarkers Prev.* **9**, 345–349.

265. Lukanova, A., Toniolo, P., Akhmedkhanov, A., Biessy, C., Haley, N. J., Shore, R. E., et al. (2001) A prospective study of insulin-like growth factor-I, IGF-binding proteins-1, -2 and -3 and lung cancer risk in women. *Int J Cancer.* **92**, 888–892.

266. London S. J., Colditz, G. A., Stampfer, M., Willet, W. C., Rosner, B., and Speizer, F. E. (1989) Prospective study of relative weight. *JAMA.* **262**, 2853–2858.

267. Spitz, M. R., Barnett, M. J., Goodman, G. E., Thornquist, M. D., Wu, X., and Pollak, M. (2002) Serum insulin-like growth factor (IGF) and IGF-binding protein levels and risk of lung cancer: a case-control study nested in the beta-carotene and retinol efficacy trial cohort. *Cancer Epidemiol Biomarkers Prev.* **11**, 1413–1418.

268. Sachdev, D. and Yee, D. (2001) The IGF system and breast cancer. *Endocr Relat Cancer.* **8**, 197–209.

269. Macaulay, V. M. (1992) Insulin-like growth factors and cancer. *Br J Cancer.* **65**, 311–320.

270. Yee, D. (2001) Are the insulin-like growth factors relevant to cancer? *Growth Horm IGF Res.* **11**, 339–345.

271. Dickson, R. B. and Stancel, G. M. (2000) Estrogen receptor-mediated processes in normal and cancer cells. *J Natl Cancer Inst Monogr.* 135–145.

272. Flototto, T., Djahansouzi, S., Glaser, M., Hanstein, B., Niederacher, D., Brumm, C., et al. (2001) Hormones and hormone antagonists: mechanisms of action in carcinogenesis of endometrial and breast cancer. *Horm Metab Res.* **33**, 451–457.

273. Key, T. J. and Pike, M. C. (1988) The role of oestrogens and progestagens in the epidemiology and prevention of breast cancer. *Eur J Cancer Clin Oncol.* **24**, 29–43.

274. Key, T. J., Appleby, P. N., Reeves, G. K., Roddam, A., Dorgan, J. F., Longcope, C., et al. (2003) Body mass index, serum sex hormones, and breast cancer risk in postmenopausal women. *J Natl Cancer Inst.* **95**, 1218–1226.

275. Franks, S., Kiddy, D. S., Hamilton-Fairley, D., Bush, A., Sharp, P. S., and Reed, M. J. (1991) The role of nutrition and insulin in the regulation of sex hormone binding globulin. *J Steroid Biochem Mol Biol.* **39**, 835–838.

276. Zeleniuch-Jacquotte, A., Adlercreutz, H., Shore, R. E., Koenig, K. L., Kato, I., Arslan, A., et al. (2004) Circulating enterolactone and risk of breast cancer: a prospective study in New York. *Br J Cancer.* **91**, 99–105.

277. Kaaks, R., Lukanova, A., and Kurzer, M. S. (2002) Obesity, endogenous hormones, and endometrial cancer risk: a synthetic review. *Cancer Epidemiol Biomarkers Prev.* **11**, 1531–1543.

278. Lukanova, A., Lundin, E., Zeleniuch-Jacquotte, A., Muti, P., Mure, A., Rinaldi, S., et al. (2004) Body mass index, circulating levels of sex-steroid hormones, IGF-I and IGF-binding protein-3: a cross-sectional study in healthy women. *Eur J Endocrinol.* **150**, 161–171.

279. Aleem, F. A., Moukhtar, M. A., Hung, H. C., and Romney, S. L. (1976) Plasma estrogen in patients with endometrial hyperplasia and carcinoma. *Cancer.* **38**, 2101–2104.

280. Nyholm, H. C., Nielsen, A. L., Lyndrup, J., Dreisler, A., Hagen, C., and Haug, E. (1993) Plasma oestrogens in postmenopausal women with endometrial cancer. *Br J Obstet Gynaecol.* **100**, 1115–1119.

281. Potischman, N., Hoover, R. N., Brinton, L. A., Siiteri, P., Dorgan, J. F., Swanson, C. A., et al. (1996) Case-control study of endogenous steroid hormones and endometrial cancer. *J Natl Cancer Inst.* **88**, 1127–1135.

282. Katsouyanni, K., Boyle, P., and Trichopoulos, D. (1991) Diet and urine estrogens among postmenopausal women. *Oncology.* **48**, 490–494.

283. Toniolo, P. G., Levitz, M., Zeleniuch-Jacquotte, A., Banerjee, S., Koenig, K. L., Shore, R. E., et al. (1995) A prospective study of endogenous estrogens and breast cancer in postmenopausal women. *J Natl Cancer Inst.* **87**, 190–197.

284. Bruning, P. F., Bonfrer, J. M., Hart, A. A., van Noord, P. A., van der, H. H., Collette, H. J., et al. (1992) Body measurements, estrogen availability and the risk of human breast cancer: a case-control study. *Int J Cancer.* **51**, 14–19.

285. Zeleniuch-Jacquotte, A., Bruning, P. F., Bonfrer, J. M., Koenig, K. L., Shore, R. E., Kim, M. Y., et al. (1997) Relation of serum levels of testosterone and dehydroepiandrosterone sulfate to risk of breast cancer in postmenopausal women. *Am J Epidemiol.* **145**, 1030–1038.

286. Siiteri, P. K. (1987) Adipose tissue as a source of hormones. *Am J Clin Nutr.* **45**, 277–282.

287. Longcope, C., Pratt, J. H., Schneider, S. H., and Fineberg, S. E. (1978) Aromatization of androgens by muscle and adipose tissue in vivo. *J Clin Endocrinol Metab.* **46**, 146–152.

288. Verkasalo, P. K., Thomas, H. V., Appleby, P. N., Davey, G. K., and Key, T. J. (2001) Circulating levels of sex hormones and their relation to risk factors for breast cancer: a cross-sectional study in 1092 pre- and postmenopausal women (United Kingdom). *Cancer Causes Control.* **12**, 47–59.

289. Dorgan, J. F., Reichman, M. E., Judd, J. T., Brown, C., Longcope, C., Schatzkin, A., et al. (1995) The relation of body size to plasma levels of estrogens and androgens in premenopausal women (Maryland, United States). *Cancer Causes Control.* **6**, 3–8.

290. Nagata, C., Kaneda, N., Kabuto, M., and Shimizu, H. (1997) Factors associated with serum levels of estradiol and sex hormone-binding globulin among premenopausal Japanese women. *Environ Health Perspect.* **105**, 994–997.

291. Thomas, H. V., Key, T. J., Allen, D. S., Moore, J. W., Dowsett, M., Fentiman, I. S., et al. (1997) Re: reversal of relation between body mass and endogenous estrogen concentrations with menopausal status. *J Natl Cancer Inst.* **89**, 396–398.

292. Giovannucci, E., Rimm, E. B., Stampfer, M. J., Colditz, G. A., and Willett, W. C. (1997) Height, body weight, and risk of prostate cancer. *Cancer Epidemiol Biomarkers Prev.* **6**, 557–563.

293. Kaaks, R., Lukanova, A., and Sommersberg, B. (2000) Plasma androgens, IGF-1, body size, and prostate cancer risk: a synthetic review. *Prostate Cancer Prostatic. Dis.* **3**, 157–172.

294. Hsing, A. W., Chokkalingam, A. P., Gao, Y. T., Wu, G., Wang, X., Deng, J., et al. (2002) Polymorphic CAG/CAA repeat length in the AIB1/SRC-3 gene and prostate cancer risk: a population-based case-control study. *Cancer Epidemiol Biomarkers Prev.* **11**, 337–341.

295. Renehan, A. G., Frystyk, J., and Flyvbjerg, A. (2006) Obesity and cancer risk: the role of the insulin-IGF axis. *Trends Endocrinol Metab.* **17**, 328–336.

296. Khandwala, H. M., McCutcheon, I. E., Flyvbjerg, A., and Friend, K. E. (2000) The effects of insulin-like growth factors on tumorigenesis and neoplastic growth. *Endocr Rev.* **21**, 215–244.

297. Priest, E. L. and Church, T. S. (2006) Obesity, cytokines, and other inflammatory markers. In *Cancer Prevention and Management Through Exercise and Weight Control* (McTiernan, A., ed.), Taylor & Francis, Boca Raton, FL, pp. 317–324.

298. Visser, M., Bouter, L. M., McQuillan, G. M., Wener, M. H., and Harris, T. B. (1999) Elevated C-reactive protein levels in overweight and obese adults. *JAMA.* **282**, 2131–2135.

299. Vgontzas, A. N., Tsigos, C., Bixler, E. O., Stratakis, C. A., Zachman, K., Kales, A.V., et al. (1998) Chronic insomnia and activity of the stress system: a preliminary study. *J Psychosom Res.* **45**, 21–31.

300. Il'yasova, D., Colbert, L. H., Harris, T. B., Newman, A. B., Bauer, D. C., Satterfield, S., et al. (2005) Circulating levels of inflammatory markers and cancer risk in the health aging and body composition cohort. *Cancer Epidemiol Biomarkers Prev.* **14**, 2413–2418.

301. Erlinger, T. P., Platz, E. A., Rifai, N., and Helzlsouer, K. J. (2004) C-reactive protein and the risk of incident colorectal cancer. *JAMA.* **291**, 585–590.

Chapter 4

Genetic Epidemiology Studies in Hereditary Non-Polyposis Colorectal Cancer

Rodney J. Scott and Jan Lubinski

Abstract

Genetic epidemiology studies in hereditary non-polyposis colorectal cancer (HNPCC) have the potential to radically improve assessment of disease risk such that more individualised information can be provided to patients susceptible to developing disease. Studies of HNPCC initially focused on disease associations and the definition of the disease and its association with different cancers within the context of an inherited predisposition. With the identification of the genetic basis of HNPCC, new insights into the disease have been forthcoming and many advances in our understanding have been made. There have been many reports examining potential modifier genes in HNPCC, yet the results remain controversial as many findings have not been replicated and therefore no clear consensus as to the role of specific modifier genes has been reached. This review focuses on some of the factors associated with disease risk in HNPCC and where some of the difficulties lie in assessing the value of genetic epidemiology studies in this disorder.

Key words: HNPCC, Lynch syndrome, genetic epidemiology, modifier genes.

1. Introduction

Hereditary non-polyposis colorectal cancer (HNPCC), or Lynch syndrome, is a hereditary condition that predisposes to a variety of epithelial malignancies that include, as its name suggests, colorectal cancer as well as a variety of other cancers, such as endometrial cancer, stomach cancer, brain tumours, and ovarian cancer (1). The presence of colorectal cancer alone within a family has been termed Lynch syndrome I, and those with a spectrum of malignancies, Lynch syndrome II (2). The genetic basis of the disease (mutations in the *hMSH2* gene) was identified in 1993 (3) and found to be associated with an inherited deficiency in

M. Verma (ed.), *Methods of Molecular Biology, Cancer Epidemiology, vol. 472*
© 2009 Humana Press, a part of Springer Science+Business Media, Totowa, NJ
Book doi: 10.1007/978-1-60327-492-0

DNA mismatch repair. A second gene also involved in DNA mismatch repair was reported in 1994, termed *hMLH1*, and a further three genes (*hPMS1*, *hPMS2*, and *hMSH6*) were subsequently found to be involved in the same process and linked to HNPCC *(4–6)*. The actual role of *hPMS1* in HNPCC has, however, been called into question since there have been no subsequent reports of its involvement in this disorder and indeed the original family has been shown to harbour a causative *hMSH2* mutation *(7, 8)*. Approximately 60% of families fulfilling the Amsterdam criteria harbour mutations in *hMSH2* or *hMLH1* and up to 10% can be accounted for by mutations in *hPMS2* and *hMSH6* *(9, 10)*. Initially, it was thought that bi-allelic mutations in DNA mismatch repair genes was incompatible with development, but two reports on Turcot's Syndrome demonstrating bi-allelic mutations in *hPMS2* indicated otherwise *(11, 12)*. Since those first two cases of bi-allelic mutations in *hPMS2*, a series of reports have been forthcoming demonstrating the presence of bi-allelic mutations in both *hMSH2* and *hMLH1*, which have been reviewed by Felton et al. *(13)*. The phenotype observed in persons with bi-allelic mutations in DNA mismatch repair gene carriers does appear to be different to mono-allelic carriers as there is a preponderance of early onset haematological malignancies and brain tumours, which has been proposed to be termed Lynch Syndrome III *(14)*.

Mutations in any of the four genes (*hMSH2*, *hMLH1*, *hPMS2*, and *hMSH6*) that either result in a loss of or change in function of DNA mismatch repair are characterised by high levels of DNA microsatellite instability (MSI), which is best assessed by examining changes in the sizes of mononucleotide or dinucleotide repeat microsatellite DNA *(15, 16)*. MSI is considered a phenotypic hallmark of HNPCC.

2. Epidemiology of HNPCC

Unlike other predispositions to colorectal cancer, such as familial adenomatous polyposis and Peutz–Jeghers Syndrome, HNPCC is difficult to diagnose in the absence of disease because there is no premalignant marker by which to identify persons at risk. For this reason, a set of criteria were established primarily to standardise the classification of cancer families into a defined group to aid in the identification of the genetic basis of the disease. This classification, known as the Amsterdam criteria, state that there must be at least three relatives with colorectal cancer; one affected person must be a first-degree relative of the other two; at least two successive generations have to be affected; at least one person must be diagnosed under the age of 50 years; and familial adenomatous polyposis must have been excluded *(17)*.

This classification scheme has remained in use for the identification of HNPCC families although it has been through several reiterations and appears in the literature under the guises of the Amsterdam II criteria (which takes into account other malignancies such as cancers of the endometrium, small bowel, ureter, or renal pelvis, but not those of the stomach, ovary, brain, bladder, or skin) *(18)*. The Bethesda Criteria are defined as persons from families that meet the Amsterdam Criteria; patients with two HNPCC-associated cancers including synchronous and metachronous colorectal cancer or associated extra-colonic cancers; patients with colorectal cancer and a first-degree relative with colorectal cancer and/or a HNPCC-related extra-colonic cancer and/or a colorectal adenoma diagnosed younger than the age of 40 years; colorectal cancer or endometrial cancer patients diagnosed younger than 45 years of age; patients younger than the age of 45 years diagnosed with right-sided colorectal cancer with an undifferentiated pattern (solid or cribriform) on histopathology; patients with signet ring cell-type colorectal cancer diagnosed younger than 45 years of age; and persons with adenomas diagnosed at younger than 40 years of age *(19)*. The revised Bethesda criteria are colorectal cancer diagnosed in individuals younger than the age of 50 years; presence of synchronous, metachronous colorectal, or other HNPCC-associated tumors, regardless of age; colorectal cancer with MSI-H histology (presence of tumor-infiltrating lymphocytes, Crohn's-like lymphocytic reaction, mucinous/signet ring differentiation, or medullary growth pattern) in patients 60 years of age; colorectal cancer in one or more 1st-degree relatives with an HNPCC-related tumor, with one of the cancers being diagnosed at younger than age 50 years; and colorectal cancer diagnosed in two or more first- or second-degree relatives with HNPCC-related tumors, regardless of age *(20)*.

The use of defined selection criteria for the identification of HNPCC families has proved extremely useful in countries where extensive family records have been kept for some time, but they become difficult to apply in countries where family structures have broken down. In families where there is only limited information available about the extended kindred, an effective mechanism by which to identify HNPCC families is to select potential patients using nuclear pedigrees where the proband has been diagnosed with colorectal cancer and a second relative has an associated HNPCC malignancy *(21)*.

The frequency of HNPCC is not precisely known but it appears to account for approximately 1.7% of all colorectal cancer cases, which increases to 14.7% if patients younger than 50 years of age only are considered, based on Danish colorectal cancer population statistics *(22)*. This overall frequency of HNPCC has been corroborated in the German population *(23)*, but variance does exist between other populations, ranging from 1% to approximately 6% *(24)*. The observed frequency of HNPCC in different populations is probably a result of ascertainment, genetic, and environmental variance as there has been no standardised collection of HNPCC patient data across different countries.

There have been relatively few systematic studies undertaken to assess cancer risk in HNPCC families. It is generally accepted that the overall disease risk in HNPCC is somewhere in the order of 90% by 70 years of age *(25)*. Colorectal cancer risk has been studied in more detail than any other malignancy in HNPCC and the lifetime risk of this disease is estimated to be approximately 80% *(26–28)*. Colorectal cancer risk is, however significantly greater in men, 74% by 70 years of age, compared with women, where it is estimated to be between 30% and 52% by 70 years of age *(25, 29, 30)*. In women, the major cancer risk is endometrial cancer, which is somewhere between 42% and 54% by 70 years of age *(25, 29)*. Several recent studies however, suggest that cancer risks in HNPCC are significantly over-estimated as a result of ascertainment bias *(31–33)*. Consistent with these reports is a recent analysis of disease risk in HNPCC families using a genotype-restricted likelihood method, which is a function of the observed genotypes, phenotypes, and ascertainment within a family. The results of this type of analysis indicate that colorectal cancer penetrance at 70 years of age is approximately 45% and for endometrial cancer only 14% *(34)*.

There remains some question about what cancers actually comprise the entity HNPCC. Studies from North America and Holland suggest that breast cancer is a malignancy that is not over-represented in these HNPCC populations *(1, 30, 35)* but appears to be in the Australian and Brazilian families *(9, 36)*. When MSI is assessed in breast tumours derived from women harbouring germ-line DNA mismatch repair gene mutations, it is invariably observed *(30, 35, 37, 38)*. Given that there are several reports suggesting that MSI occurs in breast tumours derived from patients harbouring germline mismatch repair gene mutations, it appears as suggested by Vasen et al. *(39)* that the underlying mechanisms of disease involve loss of DNA mismatch repair capacity. What cannot be so readily reconciled is the relative percentage of breast cancer cases observed in HNPCC families from Australia and Brazil compared with those reported from Finland, North America, and Holland. The final answer as to whether breast cancer is over-represented in HNPCC will have to await larger prospective studies.

Other malignancies that occur with increased frequency in HNPCC compared with the general population have not been accurately assessed with respect to their disease penetrance as they do not occur at sufficient frequency to allow for meaningful analysis. Indeed, the presence of rare cancer types within HNPCC has lead to some confusion in defining what is and is not part of the tumour spectrum in HNPCC. Prior to the identification of the genetic basis of HNPCC, it was accepted that tumours occurring within families at incidence rates greater than the general population were part of the syndrome. Since the ability to test for the hallmark of HNPCC (MSI in tumour tissue) it has become apparent that rarer cancers can also display MSI *(40)*, suggesting that they too are part of the syndrome *(41)*. In summary, cancer risk in HNPCC remains to be precisely defined and the influence of environmental and other genetic factors needs to be taken into account before accurate and robust estimates can be made.

As the majority of families have been found to harbour mutations in either *hMSH2* or *hMLH1*, most penetrance estimates are determined using families that harbour mutations in either one of these genes. Some information has been ascertained with respect to differences in disease penetrance for *hMSH2* mutation carriers compared with *hMLH1* mutation carriers. Studies of Dutch HNPCC kindreds indicate that there is greater disease penetrance for *hMSH2* mutations carriers compared with *hMLH1* mutation carriers *(42)*. Other detailed confirmatory reports are lacking but there is a growing body of evidence to suggest that there are subtle differences in disease expression between the two groups *(9, 10, 43, 44)*. Little penetrance information is available for hPMS2, which is probably a result of the difficulties in screening this gene due to the presence of highly homologous pseudogenes neighbouring it *(45, 46)*.

More information is known about *hMSH6* mutation positive families as there is now a larger body of evidence indicating more precisely disease risks conferred by mutations in this gene *(47)*. More marked differences in disease expression have been observed in families harbouring *hMSH6* compared with *hMSH2* or *hMLH1* mutations. There appears to be a decreased likelihood of colorectal cancer in *hMSH6*-associated families compared with those with *hMSH2* or *hMLH1* mutations and an increased likelihood of endometrial cancer *(48–50)*, although this remains controversial.

Notwithstanding the differences in disease expression between patients who harbour mutations in different genes, it has also become apparent that patients with germline changes in the same gene and indeed even those with the same mutation can present with very different disease symptoms and with vastly different ages of cancer diagnosis *(27, 51–53)*. Colorectal cancer is considered to be a disease that is a result of a combination of environmental and genetic factors, and this is also true for the development of this malignancy within the context of HNPCC. Individuals harbouring mutations in DNA mismatch repair genes do not have any premalignant symptoms or signs that distinguish them from their mutation-free relatives, nor can any single individual who develops colorectal cancer be used to predict disease onset in a sibling, parent, or child. Examination of any extended pedigree reveals the presence of a range of disease onset ages and phenotypes, which could be explained by environmental factors, genetic factors, or both (26). An obvious point to investigate with respect to differences in disease expression in HNPCC is to examine the functions of the DNA mismatch repair genes that have identified to determine whether they can be used to predict disease variability (44). Inspection of the functions of each of the DNA mismatch repair genes implicated in HNPCC reveals that each of the genes encodes specific attributes that are important in orchestrating the DNA mismatch repair process. Mutations occurring in functionally distinct regions of these genes, therefore, are likely to be associated with differential facets of disease that are manifest as phenotypic variation.

The identification of causative mutations in three of the DNA mismatch repair genes has been categorically associated with HNPCC, but little additional information is available at this time that specifically indicates what role polymorphisms in other DNA mismatch repair genes may have on disease expression. It remains to be seen whether variability in DNA mismatch repair genes can be used to better define genotype/phenotype correlations in HNPCC. It is to be expected that any change in the interaction between any of the DNA mismatch repair genes will result in more subtle alterations in the overall mismatch repair process (44). At this time, however, evidence remains to be collected to prove whether such an association exists.

Apart from the genetic variability of DNA mismatch repair genes themselves, there remains a considerable amount of variability in HNPCC disease expression that cannot be readily explained by genetic variance occurring solely within DNA mismatch repair genes. Since the identification of the genetic basis of HNPCC, several studies have tried to determine whether there are any genetic modifying factors that could be associated with an increased likelihood of developing disease (52, 54–58). Most studies aimed at investigating modifier genes have focused on candidate markers chosen on the basis of biological plausibility, identified primarily by epidemiological research into large cohorts of unselected colorectal cancer patients or from similar investigations examining other tumour types. Such genes identified by these studies include those associated with xenobiotic metabolism, which include N-acetyl transferase 1 (NAT1) and N-acetyl transferase 2 (NAT2), the glutathione-S-transferase (GST) genes, and the cytochrome P450 (CYP) genes. Since there is considerable variation in the phase 1 and phase 2 metabolising enzyme genes that confer differences in the kinetics of their gene products, they make excellent candidate modifier genes. Other candidate genes have also been examined and these include genes involved with control of the cell cycle, DNA repair proteins other than DNA mismatch repair genes, cytokine polymorphisms, and genes coding for proteins involved in cell migration.

3. Xenobiotic Metabolising Enzymes

Most initial studies examining the role of modifier genes in HNPCC suffered from small sample sizes and were therefore subject to type 1 statistical errors and indeed re-examination of potential modifier genes in larger patient collections has often failed to verify initial reports. For example, several studies have focused on *NAT1* and *NAT2 (52, 55, 59–61)*, enzymes that are involved in the acetylation of aromatic amines, in HNPCC. In 1999, an association between the age of colorectal cancer onset in HNPCC and polymorphisms in *NAT2* was reported *(59)*, which was based on 78 samples that comprised 63 *hMLH1* and 15 *hMSH2* mutation carriers. This result was confirmed in another small study *(61)*, which was based on 86 individuals harbouring mutations in either *hMSH2*, *hMLH1*, or *hPMS1*.

Re-investigation of larger collections of patients has failed to confirm the original reports, suggesting that *NAT2* alleles were not associated with colorectal cancer risk in HNPCC *(55, 60)*. The failure to recapitulate the original studies could be due to population differences but the evidence seems unlikely, since in the reports by Talseth et al. *(55)* and Pistorius et al. *(60)*, three separate populations were examined, one from Poland, one from Australia, and one from Germany, all yielding very similar results.

A second xenobiotic enzyme that has received considerable attention is GST because it has consistently been associated with cancer risk. This super-family of genes has been shown to be important for the conjugation of reactive chemical intermediates to form soluble glutathione derivative for excretion *(62)*. Null alleles for *GSTT1* and *GSTP1* have been identified that presumably confer a loss of *GSTM1* and *GSTP1* activity in persons who are homozygote null carriers, and a polymorphism in *GSTT1* appears to be associated with an alteration in the kinetics of the enzyme *(63)*. Studies investigating the relationship between *GST* alleles and disease risk in HNPCC have been controversial as some reports indicate a relationship *(64)* whereas others do not. In studies examining patients of European descent, there appears to be no obvious relationship between *GSTT1*, *GSTP1*, and cancer risk *(59)*, whereas studies from Korea suggest that there is an association *(56)*. Similar to the earlier studies on *NAT2*, the

HNPCC populations were small and subject to type 1 statistical errors. More latterly, other larger investigations have been undertaken that do not support the original observations (55). Taken together these results suggest the presence of type 1 errors, something that is highly likely given the size of the initial populations under study. An alternative explanation that could account for the reported differences between the Korean and European studies are differences in the polymorphism frequencies between the two populations. Clearly, to determine precisely the relationship between GST polymorphisms and disease risk in HNPCC, additional larger studies are required.

There are other xenobiotic clearance enzymes that represent good candidates that warrant further study but as yet not much has been reported in the literature. The CYP enzymes represent another excellent series of candidate modifier genes, consisting of 18 families and 43 sub-families of genes, since they are important for sex steroid synthesis and degradation, the synthesis of cholesterol, and the conversion of procarcinogens to carcinogens by hydroxylation. Several studies have examined the relationship between polymorphic variants of the CYP enzymes and cancer risk in HNPCC (55, 65, 66). There is some evidence to suggest that a polymorphism in CYP1A1 (T3810C) is associated with an increased risk of colorectal cancer (55) and a C4887T polymorphism with endometrial cancer (66). This suggests that these two polymorphisms and in functionally different outcomes, each of which results in a specific site dependent change in disease risk. Other polymorphic genes that are involved in steroid synthesis or degradation remain attractive candidates for determining endometrial and possibly breast cancer risk in HNPCC.

4. Cell Cycle Control

Another potential group of genes that could explain differences in disease expression in HNPCC are those that are associated with cell cycle control. Several studies had examined the role of a common polymorphism in TP53 in cancer risk and found a correlation with disease severity for individuals harbouring the R72P polymorphism (67, 68). In 2005, a report appeared using an American group of HNPCC patients that suggested the common R72P polymorphism in TP53 was associated with a decreased age of colorectal cancer onset in patients with HNPCC. This was tested in three separate groups of HNPCC patients from Australia, Poland, and Finland and found to be unsubstantiated (69–71). The difference in results could be due to the mutation spectrum in each of the groups and/or the relative numbers of hMLH1 mutations carriers compared with *hMSH2* carriers. In relation to *TP53*, there does not appear to be any difference between the role of the R72P polymorphism in *hMSH2* compared with *hMLH1* mutation carriers, since in the study by Talseth et al. no differences between the two groups were observed *(69)*.

In a study examining the role of *cyclin D1*, an intriguing relationship is emerging, which suggests there are different molecular attributes associated with *hMSH2* compared with *hMLH1*. In a report from Texas, an association was observed in the age of onset of disease in HNPCC patients harbouring a single nucleotide polymorphism (SNP) in the *CyclinD1* gene *(72)*. The relationship between the *cyclinD1* SNP and age of disease onset was also tested in the Finnish population and no association was seen *(57)*. The major difference between the two populations was the frequency of *hMSH2* mutation carriers in the first study (66.3%) compared with that of the Finnish study (3.4%). A third study was undertaken in a very large group of German HNPCC patients, which confirmed the Finnish study suggesting that the original finding was a type 1 error *(73)*. In the latest report on the association between the *cyclin* D1 SNP and age of disease onset in HNPCC, an Australian study found that overall there was no association between the SNP and age of disease onset but if the population was stratified by gene (i.e. *hMSH2* or *hMLH1*), a clear association was observed between the *cyclin D1* SNP and age of disease onset in patients harbouring *hMSH2* mutations *(74)*. The most striking difference between the four studies was the numbers of cases examined. In the American study, 86 patients were included; in the Finnish report, 146 patients were studied; in the Australian/Polish investigation, 220 patients were examined; and in the German study, 406 patients were investigated. This raises again the possibility of a type 1 statistical error occurring in the smallest study, however, since there appears to be some consensus between three of the studies (the American, Finnish, and Australian/Polish reports) the results are more likely to be a true reflection of the influence of the polymorphism in *cyclin D1* on the age of disease diagnosis in *hMSH2* mutation carriers.

Another gene that has also been examined to determine its role as a modifier of disease expression in HNPCC is the cell cycle checkpoint control gene, *ATM*. One report suggests that the D1853N polymorphism modulates the age of onset of disease in HNPCC *(75)*. This result has not been repeated by others *(76)* and it remains to be seen if there is an association. Similar to other studies examining the role of modifier genes in HNPCC, the numbers of patients required for robust statistical assessment are lacking and at present, confirmation of these findings await studies of sufficient statistical power to accurately and robustly determine any association. In searching for modifier genes that influence disease characteristics in HNPCC, many studies have been performed and many more positive associations have been published compared with those that are negative. Publication bias remains a problem in reporting associations between modifier genes and disease risk since it is as important to rule out potential modifier genes as it is to accept them as bone fide disease risk modifiers.

5. Future Directions

Currently modifier genes are being identified as a result of selection of candidate genes that have some plausible biological role in the disease. Most studies are now capable of selecting large sets of potential modifier genes using new assay platforms for any single experiment and from these types of study, many additional associations will be identified. With the widespread introduction of single nucleotide polymorphism (SNP) arrays that contain hundreds of thousands of SNPs, it is inevitable that new types of analyses will be performed where multiple polymorphisms in a variety of genes can be assessed in a single assay thereby providing an individual profile of disease risk. The challenge at this present point in time is to obtain sufficient numbers of samples from HNPCC patients that have been well characterised at the clinical and molecular levels for the identification and assessment of modifier genes.

References

1. Watson, P. and H.T. Lynch, *Extracolonic cancer in hereditary nonpolyposis colorectal cancer.* Cancer, 1993. **71**(3): p. 677–685.

2. Lynch, H.T., S. Lanspa, T. Smyrk, B. Boman, P. Watson, and J. Lynch, *Hereditary nonpolyposis colorectal cancer (Lynch syndromes I & II). Genetics, pathology, natural history, and cancer control, Part I.* Cancer Genet Cytogenet, 1991. **53**(2): p. 143–160.

3. Fishel, R., M.K. Lescoe, M.R. Rao, N.G. Copeland, N.A. Jenkins, J. Garber, M. Kane, and R. Kolodner, *The human mutator gene homolog MSH2 and its association with hereditary nonpolyposis colon cancer.* Cell, 1993. **75**(5): p. 1027–1038.

4. Nicolaides, N.C., N. Papadopoulos, B. Liu, Y.F. Wei, K.C. Carter, S.M. Ruben, C.A. Rosen, W.A. Haseltine, R.D. Fleischmann, C.M. Fraser, et al., *Mutations of two PMS homologues in hereditary nonpolyposis colon cancer.* Nature, 1994. **371**(6492): p. 75–80.

5. Bronner, C.E., S.M. Baker, P.T. Morrison, G. Warren, L.G. Smith, M.K. Lescoe, M. Kane, C. Earabino, J. Lipford, A. Lindblom, et al., *Mutation in the DNA mismatch repair gene homologue hMLH1 is associated with hereditary non-polyposis colon cancer.* Nature, 1994. **368**(6468): p. 258–261.

6. Miyaki, M., M. Konishi, K. Tanaka, R. Kikuchi-Yanoshita, M. Muraoka, M. Yasuno, T. Igari, M. Koike, M. Chiba, and T. Mori, *Germline mutation of MSH6 as the cause of hereditary nonpolyposis colorectal cancer.* Nat Genet, 1997. **17**(3): p. 271–272.

7. Liu, T., H. Yan, S. Kuismanen, A. Percesepe, M.L. Bisgaard, M. Pedroni, P. Benatti, K.W. Kinzler, B. Vogelstein, M. Ponz de Leon, P. Peltomaki, and A. Lindblom, *The role of hPMS1 and hPMS2 in predisposing to colorectal cancer.* Cancer Res, 2001. **61**(21): p. 7798–7802.

8. Peltomaki, P., *Role of DNA mismatch repair defects in the pathogenesis of human cancer.* J Clin Oncol, 2003. **21**(6): p. 1174–1179.

9. Scott, R.J., M. McPhillips, C.J. Meldrum, P.E. Fitzgerald, K. Adams, A.D. Spigelman, D. du Sart, K. Tucker, and J. Kirk, *Hereditary nonpolyposis colorectal cancer in 95 families: differences and similarities between mutation-positive and mutation-negative kindreds.* Am J Hum Genet, 2001. **68**(1): p. 118–127.

10. Wijnen, J.T., H.F. Vasen, P.M. Khan, A.H. Zwinderman, H. van der Klift, A. Mulder, C. Tops, P. Moller, and R. Fodde, *Clinical findings with implications for genetic testing in families with clustering of colorectal cancer.* N Engl J Med, 1998. **339**(8): p. 511–518.

11. De Rosa, M., C. Fasano, L. Panariello, M.I. Scarano, G. Belli, A. Iannelli, F. Ciciliano, and P. Izzo, *Evidence for a recessive inheritance of Turcot's syndrome caused by compound heterozygous mutations within the PMS2 gene.* Oncogene, 2000. **19**(13): p. 1719–1723.

12. Hamilton, S.R., B. Liu, R.E. Parsons, N. Papadopoulos, J. Jen, S.M. Powell, A.J. Krush, T. Berk, Z. Cohen, B. Tetu, et al., *The molecular basis of Turcot's syndrome.* N Engl J Med, 1995. **332**(13): p. 839–847.

13. Felton, K.E., D.M. Gilchrist, and S.E. Andrew, *Constitutive deficiency in DNA mismatch repair.* Clin Genet, 2007. **71**(6): p. 483–498.

14. Felton, K.E., D.M. Gilchrist, and S.E. Andrew, *Constitutive deficiency in DNA mismatch repair: is it time for Lynch III?* Clin Genet, 2007. **71**(6): p. 499–500.

15. Peltomaki, P., *Deficient DNA mismatch repair: a common etiologic factor for colon cancer.* Hum Mol Genet, 2001. **10**(7): p. 735–740.

16. Vasen, H.F., Y. Hendriks, A.E. de Jong, M. van Puijenbroek, C. Tops, A.H. Brocker-Vriends, J.T. Wijnen, and H. Morreau, *Identification of HNPCC by molecular analysis of colorectal and endometrial tumors.* Dis Markers, 2004. **20**(4–5): p. 207–213.

17. Vasen, H.F., J.P. Mecklin, P.M. Khan, and H.T. Lynch, *The International Collaborative Group on Hereditary Non-Polyposis Colorectal Cancer (ICG-HNPCC).* Dis Colon Rectum, 1991. **34**(5): p. 424–425.

18. Fornasarig, M., A. Viel, E. Bidoli, E. Campagnutta, A.M. Minisini, R. Cannizzaro, L. Della Puppa, and M. Boiocchi, *Amsterdam criteria II and endometrial cancer index cases for an accurate selection of HNPCC families.* Tumori, 2002. **88**(1): p. 18–20.

19. Rodriguez-Bigas, M.A., C.R. Boland, S.R. Hamilton, D.E. Henson, J.R. Jass, P.M. Khan, H. Lynch, M. Perucho, T. Smyrk, L. Sobin, and S. Srivastava, *A National Cancer Institute Workshop on Hereditary Nonpolyposis Colorectal Cancer Syndrome: meeting highlights and Bethesda guidelines.* J Natl Cancer Inst, 1997. **89**(23): p. 1758–1762.

20. Umar, A., C.R. Boland, J.P. Terdiman, S. Syngal, A. de la Chapelle, J. Ruschoff, R. Fishel, N.M. Lindor, L.J. Burgart, R. Hamelin, S.R. Hamilton, R.A. Hiatt, J. Jass, A. Lindblom, H.T. Lynch, P. Peltomaki, S.D. Ramsey, M.A. Rodriguez-Bigas, H.F. Vasen, E.T. Hawk, J.C. Barrett, A.N. Freedman, and S. Srivastava, *Revised Bethesda Guidelines for hereditary nonpolyposis colorectal cancer (Lynch syndrome) and microsatellite instability.* J Natl Cancer Inst, 2004. **96**(4): p. 261–268.

21. Kladny, J., G. Moeslein, T. Myrhoj, G. Kurzawski, A. Jakubowska, T. Debniak, W. Petriczko, M. Kozlowski, T. Al-Amawi, M. Brzosko, J. Flicinski, A. Jawien, Z. Banaszkiewicz, P. Rychter, and J. Lubinski, *Nuclear Pedigree Criteria of Suspected HNPCC.* Hereditary Cancer in Clinical Practice, 2003. **1.0**(1): p. 34–38.

22. Katballe, N., M. Christensen, F.P. Wikman, T.F. Orntoft, and S. Laurberg, *Frequency of hereditary non-polyposis colorectal cancer in Danish colorectal cancer patients.* Gut, 2002. **50**(1): p. 43–51.

23. Lamberti, C., E. Mangold, C. Pagenstecher, M. Jungck, D. Schwering, M. Bollmann, J. Vogel, D. Kindermann, R. Nikorowitsch, N. Friedrichs, B. Schneider, F. Houshdaran, I.G. Schmidt-Wolf, W. Friedl, P. Propping, T. Sauerbruch, R. Buttner, and M. Mathiak, *Frequency of hereditary nonpolyposis colorectal cancer among unselected patients with colorectal cancer in Germany.* Digestion, 2006. **74**(1): p. 58–67.

24. Lynch, H.T. and A. de la Chapelle, *Hereditary colorectal cancer.* N Engl J Med, 2003. **348**(10): p. 919–932.

25. Dunlop, M.G., S.M. Farrington, A.D. Carothers, A.H. Wyllie, L. Sharp, J. Burn, B. Liu, K.W. Kinzler, and B. Vogelstein, *Cancer risk associated with germline DNA mismatch repair gene mutations.* Hum Mol Genet, 1997. **6**(1): p. 105–110.

26. Aarnio, M., J.P. Mecklin, L.A. Aaltonen, M. Nystrom-Lahti, and H.J. Jarvinen, *Lifetime risk of different cancers in hereditary non-polyposis colorectal cancer (HNPCC) syndrome.* Int J Cancer, 1995. **64**(6): p. 430–433.

27. Vasen, H.F., J.T. Wijnen, F.H. Menko, J.H. Kleibeuker, B.G. Taal, G. Griffioen, F.M. Nagengast, E.H. Meijers-Heijboer, L. Bertario, L. Varesco, M.L. Bisgaard, J. Mohr, R. Fodde, and P.M. Khan, *Cancer risk in families with hereditary nonpolyposis colorectal cancer diagnosed by mutation analysis.* Gastroenterology, 1996. **110**(4): p. 1020–1027.

28. Voskuil, D.W., H.F. Vasen, E. Kampman, and P. van't Veer, *Colorectal cancer risk in HNPCC families: development during lifetime and in successive generations. National Collaborative Group on HNPCC.* Int J Cancer, 1997. **72**(2): p. 205–209.

29. Hampel, H., J.A. Stephens, E. Pukkala, R. Sankila, L.A. Aaltonen, J.P. Mecklin, and A. de la Chapelle, *Cancer risk in hereditary nonpolyposis colorectal cancer syndrome: later age of onset.* Gastroenterology, 2005. **129**(2): p. 415–421.

30. Aarnio, M., R. Sankila, E. Pukkala, R. Salovaara, L.A. Aaltonen, A. de la Chapelle, P. Peltomaki, J.P. Mecklin, and H.J. Jarvinen, *Cancer risk in mutation carriers of DNA-mismatch-repair genes.* Int J Cancer, 1999. **81**(2): p. 214–218.

31. Carayol, J., M. Khlat, J. Maccario, and C. Bonaiti-Pellie, *Hereditary non-polyposis colorectal cancer: current risks of colorectal cancer largely overestimated.* J Med Genet, 2002. **39**(5): p. 335–339.

32. Parc, Y., C. Boisson, G. Thomas, and S. Olschwang, *Cancer risk in 348 French MSH2 or MLH1 gene carriers.* J Med Genet, 2003. **40**(3): p. 208–213.

33. Quehenberger, F., H.F. Vasen, and H.C. van Houwelingen, *Risk of colorectal and endometrial cancer for carriers of mutations of the hMLH1 and hMSH2 gene: correction for ascertainment.* J Med Genet, 2005. **42**(6): p. 491–496.

34. Alarcon, F., C. Lasset, J. Carayol, V. Bonadona, H. Perdry, F. Desseigne, Q. Wang, and C. Bonaiti-Pellie, *Estimating cancer risk in HNPCC by the GRL method.* Eur J Hum Genet, 2007. **15**(8): p. 831–836.

35. Vasen, H.F., H. Morreau, and J.W. Nortier, *Is breast cancer part of the tumor spectrum of hereditary nonpolyposis colorectal cancer?* Am J Hum Genet, 2001. **68**(6): p. 1533–1535.

36. Oliveira Ferreira, F., C.C. Napoli Ferreira, B.M. Rossi, W. Toshihiko Nakagawa, S. Aguilar, Jr., E.M. Monteiro Santos, M.L. Vierira Costa, and A. Lopes, *Frequency of extra-colonic tumors in hereditary nonpolyposis colorectal cancer (HNPCC) and familial colorectal cancer (FCC) Brazilian families: An analysis by a Brazilian Hereditary Colorectal Cancer Institutional Registry.* Fam Cancer, 2004. **3**(1): p. 41–47.

37. Risinger, J.I., J.C. Barrett, P. Watson, H.T. Lynch, and J. Boyd, *Molecular genetic evidence of the occurrence of breast cancer as an integral tumor in patients with the hereditary nonpolyposis colorectal carcinoma syndrome.* Cancer, 1996. **77**(9): p. 1836–1843.

38. Boyd, J., E. Rhei, M.G. Federici, P.I. Borgen, P. Watson, B. Franklin, B. Karr, J. Lynch, S.J. Lemon, and H.T. Lynch, *Male breast cancer in the hereditary nonpolyposis colorectal cancer syndrome.* Breast Cancer Res Treat, 1999. **53**(1): p. 87–91.

39. de Leeuw, W.J., M. van Puijenbroek, R.A. Tollenaar, C.J. Cornelisse, H.F. Vasen, and H. Morreau, *Correspondence re: A. Muller et al., Exclusion of breast cancer as an integral tumor of hereditary nonpolyposis colorectal cancer. Cancer Res., 62: 1014–1019, 2002.* Cancer Res, 2003. **63**(5): p. 1148–1149.

40. Watson, P. and B. Riley, *The tumor spectrum in the Lynch syndrome.* Fam Cancer, 2005. **4**(3): p. 245–248.

41. den Bakker, M.A., C. Seynaeve, M. Kliffen, and W.N. Dinjens, *Microsatellite instability in a pleomorphic rhabdomyosarcoma in a patient with hereditary non-polyposis colorectal cancer.* Histopathology, 2003. **43**(3): p. 297–299.

42. Vasen, H.F., A. Stormorken, F.H. Menko, F.M. Nagengast, J.H. Kleibeuker, G. Griffioen, B.G. Taal, P. Moller, and J.T. Wijnen, *MSH2 mutation carriers are at higher risk of cancer than MLH1 mutation carriers: a study of hereditary nonpolyposis colorectal cancer families.* J Clin Oncol, 2001. **19**(20): p. 4074–4080.

43. Bandipalliam, P., J. Garber, R.D. Kolodner, and S. Syngal, *Clinical presentation correlates with the type of mismatch repair gene involved in hereditary nonpolyposis colon cancer.* Gastroenterology, 2004. **126**(3): p. 936–937.

44. Bandipalliam, P., *Variability in the clinical phenotype among families with HNPCC—the potential importance of the location of the mutation in the gene.* Int J Cancer, 2007. **120**(10): p. 2275–2277; author reply 2278.

45. Hayward, B.E., M. De Vos, E. Sheridan, and D.T. Bonthron, *PMS2 mutations in HNPCC.* Clin Genet, 2004. **66**(6): p. 566–567; author reply 568.

46. De Vos, M., B.E. Hayward, S. Picton, E. Sheridan, and D.T. Bonthron, *Novel PMS2*

pseudogenes can conceal recessive mutations causing a distinctive childhood cancer syndrome. Am J Hum Genet, 2004. **74**(5): p. 954–964.

47. Hendriks, Y.M., A. Wagner, H. Morreau, F. Menko, A. Stormorken, F. Quehenberger, L. Sandkuijl, P. Moller, M. Genuardi, H. Van Houwelingen, C. Tops, M. Van Puijenbroek, P. Verkuijlen, G. Kenter, A. Van Mil, H. Meijers-Heijboer, G.B. Tan, M.H. Breuning, R. Fodde, J.T. Wijnen, A.H. Brocker-Vriends, and H. Vasen, *Cancer risk in hereditary nonpolyposis colorectal cancer due to MSH6 mutations: impact on counseling and surveillance.* Gastroenterology, 2004. **127**(1): p. 17–25.

48. Kolodner, R.D., J.D. Tytell, J.L. Schmeits, M.F. Kane, R.D. Gupta, J. Weger, S. Wahlberg, E.A. Fox, D. Peel, A. Ziogas, J.E. Garber, S. Syngal, H. Anton-Culver, and F.P. Li, *Germ-line msh6 mutations in colorectal cancer families.* Cancer Res, 1999. **59**(20): p. 5068–5074.

49. Plaschke, J., C. Engel, S. Kruger, E. Holinski-Feder, C. Pagenstecher, E. Mangold, G. Moeslein, K. Schulmann, J. Gebert, M. von Knebel Doeberitz, J. Ruschoff, M. Loeffler, and H.K. Schackert, *Lower incidence of colorectal cancer and later age of disease onset in 27 families with pathogenic MSH6 germline mutations compared with families with MLH1 or MSH2 mutations: the German Hereditary Nonpolyposis Colorectal Cancer Consortium.* J Clin Oncol, 2004. **22**(22): p. 4486–4494.

50. Wijnen, J., W. de Leeuw, H. Vasen, H. van der Klift, P. Moller, A. Stormorken, H. Meijers-Heijboer, D. Lindhout, F. Menko, S. Vossen, G. Moslein, C. Tops, A. Brocker-Vriends, Y. Wu, R. Hofstra, R. Sijmons, C. Cornelisse, H. Morreau, and R. Fodde, *Familial endometrial cancer in female carriers of MSH6 germline mutations.* Nat Genet, 1999. **23**(2): p. 142–144.

51. Mary, J.L., T. Bishop, R. Kolodner, J.R. Lipford, M. Kane, W. Weber, J. Torhorst, H. Muller, M. Spycher, and R.J. Scott, *Mutational analysis of the hMSH2 gene reveals a three base pair deletion in a family predisposed to colorectal cancer development.* Hum Mol Genet, 1994. **3**(11): p. 2067–2069.

52. Moisio, A.L., P. Sistonen, J.P. Mecklin, H. Jarvinen, and P. Peltomaki, *Genetic polymorphisms in carcinogen metabolism and their association to hereditary nonpolyposis colon cancer.* Gastroenterology, 1998. **115**(6): p. 1387–1394.

53. Brown, S.R., P.J. Finan, and D.T. Bishop, *Are relatives of patients with multiple HNPCC spectrum tumours at increased risk of cancer?* Gut, 1998. **43**(5): p. 664–668.

54. Talseth, B.A., C. Meldrum, J. Suchy, G. Kurzawski, J. Lubinski, and R.J. Scott, *Lack of association between genetic polymorphisms in cytokine genes and disease expression in patients with hereditary non-polyposis colorectal cancer.* Scand J Gastroenterol, 2007. **42**(5): p. 628–632.

55. Talseth, B.A., C. Meldrum, J. Suchy, G. Kurzawski, J. Lubinski, and R.J. Scott, *Genetic polymorphisms in xenobiotic clearance genes and their influence on disease expression in hereditary nonpolyposis colorectal cancer patients.* Cancer Epidemiol Biomarkers Prev, 2006. **15**(11): p. 2307–2310.

56. Shin, J.H., J.L. Ku, K.H. Shin, Y.K. Shin, S.B. Kang, and J.G. Park, *Glutathione S-transferase M1 associated with cancer occurrence in Korean HNPCC families carrying the hMLH1/hMSH2 mutation.* Oncol Rep, 2003. **10**(2): p. 483–486.

57. Bala, S. and P. Peltomaki, *CYCLIN D1 as a genetic modifier in hereditary nonpolyposis colorectal cancer.* Cancer Res, 2001. **61**(16): p. 6042–6045.

58. Chen, J., S. Sen, C.I. Amos, C. Wei, J.S. Jones, P. Lynch, and M.L. Frazier, *Association between Aurora-A kinase polymorphisms and age of onset of hereditary nonpolyposis colorectal cancer in a Caucasian population.* Mol Carcinog, 2007. **46**(4): p. 249–256.

59. Heinimann, K., R.J. Scott, P. Chappuis, W. Weber, H. Muller, Z. Dobbie, and P. Hutter, *N-acetyltransferase 2 influences cancer prevalence in hMLH1/hMSH2 mutation carriers.* Cancer Res, 1999. **59**(13): p. 3038–3040.

60. Pistorius, S., H. Goergens, C. Engel, J. Plaschke, S. Krueger, R. Hoehl, H.D. Saeger, and H.K. Schackert, *N-Acetyltransferase (NAT) 2 acetylator status and age of tumour onset in patients with sporadic and familial, microsatellite stable (MSS) colorectal cancer.* Int J Colorectal Dis, 2007. **22**(2): p. 137–143.

61. Frazier, M.L., F.T. O'Donnell, S. Kong, X. Gu, I. Campos, R. Luthra, P.M. Lynch, and C.I. Amos, *Age-associated risk of cancer among individuals with N-acetyltransferase 2 (NAT2) mutations and mutations in DNA mismatch repair genes.* Cancer Res, 2001. **61**(4): p. 1269–1271.

62. Ketterer, B., *Protective role of glutathione and glutathione transferases in mutagenesis and carcinogenesis.* Mutat Res, 1988. **202**(2): p. 343–361.

63. Helzlsouer, K.J., O. Selmin, H.Y. Huang, P.T. Strickland, S. Hoffman, A.J. Alberg, M. Watson, G.W. Comstock, and D. Bell, *Association between glutathione S-transferase M1, P1, and T1 genetic polymorphisms and development of breast cancer.* J Natl Cancer Inst, 1998. **90**(7): p. 512–518.

64. Felix, R., W. Bodmer, N.S. Fearnhead, L. van der Merwe, P. Goldberg, and R.S. Ramesar, *GSTM1 and GSTT1 polymorphisms as modifiers of age at diagnosis of hereditary nonpolyposis colorectal cancer (HNPCC) in a homogeneous cohort of individuals carrying a single predisposing mutation.* Mutat Res, 2006. **602**(1–2): p. 175–181.

65. Campbell, P.T., L. Edwards, J.R. McLaughlin, J. Green, H.B. Younghusband, and M.O. Woods, *Cytochrome P450 17A1 and catechol O-methyltransferase polymorphisms and age at Lynch syndrome colon cancer onset in Newfoundland.* Clin Cancer Res, 2007. **13**(13): p. 3783–3788.

66. Esteller, M., A. Garcia, J.M. Martinez-Palones, J. Xercavins, and J. Reventos, *Germ line polymorphisms in cytochrome-P450 1A1 (C4887 CYP1A1) and methylenetetrahydrofolate reductase (MTHFR) genes and endometrial cancer susceptibility.* Carcinogenesis, 1997. **18**(12): p. 2307–2311.

67. Zhang, Z.W., P. Newcomb, A. Hollowood, R. Feakins, M. Moorghen, A. Storey, M.J. Farthing, D. Alderson, and J. Holly, *Age-associated increase of codon 72 Arginine p53 frequency in gastric cardia and non-cardia adenocarcinoma.* Clin Cancer Res, 2003. **9**(6): p. 2151–2156.

68. Bougeard, G., S. Baert-Desurmont, I. Tournier, S. Vasseur, C. Martin, L. Brugieres, A. Chompret, B. Bressac-de Paillerets, D. Stoppa-Lyonnet, C. Bonaiti-Pellie, and T. Frebourg, *Impact of the MDM2 SNP309 and p53 Arg72Pro polymorphism on age of tumour onset in Li-Fraumeni syndrome.* J Med Genet, 2006. **43**(6): p. 531–533.

69. Talseth, B.A., C. Meldrum, J. Suchy, G. Kurzawski, J. Lubinski, and R.J. Scott, *Age of diagnosis of colorectal cancer in HNPCC patients is more complex than that predicted by R72P polymorphism in TP53.* Int J Cancer, 2006. **118**(10): p. 2479–2484.

70. Talseth, B.A., C. Meldrum, J. Suchy, G. Kurzawski, J. Lubinski, and R.J. Scott, *MDM2 SNP309 T>G alone or in combination with the TP53 R72P polymorphism does not appear to influence disease expression and age of diagnosis of colorectal cancer in HNPCC patients.* Int J Cancer, 2007. **120**(3): p. 563–565.

71. Sotamaa, K., S. Liyanarachchi, J.P. Mecklin, H. Jarvinen, L.A. Aaltonen, P. Peltomaki, and A. de la Chapelle, *p53 codon 72 and MDM2 SNP309 polymorphisms and age of colorectal cancer onset in Lynch syndrome.* Clin Cancer Res, 2005. **11**(19 Pt 1): p. 6840–6844.

72. Kong, S., C.I. Amos, R. Luthra, P.M. Lynch, B. Levin, and M.L. Frazier, *Effects of cyclin D1 polymorphism on age of onset of hereditary nonpolyposis colorectal cancer.* Cancer Res, 2000. **60**(2): p. 249–252.

73. Kruger, S., C. Engel, A. Bier, E. Mangold, C. Pagenstecher, M.K. Doeberitz, E. Holinski-Feder, G. Moeslein, G. Keller, E. Kunstmann, W. Friedl, J. Plaschke, J. Ruschoff, and H.K. Schackert, *Absence of association between cyclin D1 (CCND1) G870A polymorphism and age of onset in hereditary nonpolyposis colorectal cancer.* Cancer Lett, 2006. **236**(2): p. 191–197.

74. Talseth, B.A., K.A. Ashton, C. Meldrum, J. Suchy, G. Kurzawski, J. Lubinski, and R.J. Scott. *Aurora-A and Cyclin D1 polymorphisms and the age of onset of colorectal cancer in hereditary nonpolyposis colorectal cancer.* Int. J. Cancer, 2008. **122**: p1273–1277.

75. Maillet, P., P.O. Chappuis, G. Vaudan, Z. Dobbie, H. Muller, P. Hutter, and A.P. Sappino, *A polymorphism in the ATM gene modulates the penetrance of hereditary nonpolyposis colorectal cancer.* Int J Cancer, 2000. **88**(6): p. 928–931.

76. Jones, J.S., X. Gu, P.M. Lynch, M. Rodriguez-Bigas, C.I. Amos, and M.L. Frazier, *ATM polymorphism and hereditary nonpolyposis colorectal cancer (HNPCC) age of onset (United States).* Cancer Causes Control, 2005. **16**(6): p. 749–753.

Chapter 5

Parental Smoking and Childhood Leukemia

Jeffrey S. Chang

Abstract

Childhood leukemia is the most common cancer among children, representing 31% of all cancer cases occurring in children younger than the age of 15 years in the USA. There are only few known risk factors of childhood leukemia (sex, age, race, exposure to ionizing radiation, and certain congenital diseases, such as Down syndrome and neurofibromatosis), which account for only 10% of the childhood leukemia cases. Several lines of evidence suggest that childhood leukemia may be more due to environmental rather than genetic factors, although genes may play modifying roles. Human and animal studies showed that the development of childhood leukemia is a two-step process that requires a prenatal initiating event(s) plus a postnatal promoting event(s).

Despite a substantial public health effort to reduce cigarette smoking, a large proportion of the US and world population still smoke. Tobacco smoke contains at least 60 known human or animal carcinogens, with the major chemical classes being volatile hydrocarbons, aldehydes, aromatic amines, polycyclic aromatic hydrocarbons, and nitrosamines; among these chemicals, only benzene is an established leukemogen, although other chemicals in the tobacco could interact with one another in a complex way to jointly attain a significant carcinogenic effect on the development of leukemia.

Although tobacco smoke is an established risk factor for adult myeloid leukemia, the studies of association between parental smoking and childhood leukemia have produced inconsistent results. The majority of the studies on maternal smoking and childhood leukemia did not find a significant positive association and some even reported an inverse association. In contrast to studies of maternal smoking, studies of paternal smoking and childhood leukemia reported more positive associations but only by less than half of the studies.

Future directions to be considered for improving the study of parental smoking and childhood leukemia are: 1) consider all sources of benzene exposure in addition to smoking, including occupational exposure and traffic exhausts; 2) childhood leukemia is a heterogeneous disease and epidemiologic studies of childhood leukemia can be greatly improved by grouping childhood leukemia into more homogeneous groups by molecular techniques (e.g., structural and numerical chromosomal changes); and 3) assess gene-environment interaction.

It is hoped that through the continual effort, more will be uncovered regarding the causes of childhood leukemia. In the meantime, more effort should be spent on educating the parents to quit smoking, because parental smoking is known to affect many childhood diseases (e.g., asthma, respiratory tract infection, and otitis media) that are much more prevalent than childhood leukemia.

M. Verma (ed.), *Methods of Molecular Biology, Cancer Epidemiology, vol. 472*
© 2009 Humana Press, a part of Springer Science+Business Media, Totowa, NJ
Book doi: 10.1007/978-1-60327-492-0

Key words: Childhood leukemia, acute lymphoblastic leukemia, ALL, acute myeloid leukemia, AML, parental smoking, gene-environment interaction.

1. Childhood Leukemia

1.1. Incidence

Childhood leukemia is the most common cancer among children, representing 31% of all cancer cases occurring in children younger than the age of 15 years (1). Approximately 3,250 cases of leukemia are diagnosed among children and adolescents younger than the age of 20 years in the USA each year (1). Childhood leukemia is a heterogeneous disease and consists of 75–80% acute lymphoblastic leukemia (ALL), 20% acute myeloid leukemia (AML), 2% chronic myeloid leukemia (CML), and rarely chronic lymphocytic leukemia (CLL) (2).

The two major types of childhood leukemia, ALL and AML, have distinct demographic distributions. Childhood ALL has a peak incidence at age 2–3 years, is more likely to occur among boys than girls (male:female ratio = 1.2), and occurs more among white children than black children (white:black ratio = 1.6) (1). Childhood AML incidence peaks in the first 2 years of life, decreases after the first 2 years, and slowly increases during the adolescent period (1). There is no gender or racial (white versus black) difference in the incidence of AML (1).

The incidence of childhood ALL varies by and within countries, with the lowest rates observed by the African countries (from 4.5 per million to 14.3 per million), followed by Asian countries (from 9.2 per million to 40.6 per million), with the highest rates observed by European, American (North, Central, and South), and Oceania (Australia and New Zealand) countries (from 16.1 per million to 48 per million) (3). In contrast, the differences in the incidence of childhood AML among different countries are not as distinct (3). In addition, the ratio of ALL to AML also varies by region, with the lower ratios observed in most African and Asian countries, and higher ratios observed in the European, American, and Oceania countries (3).

According to the Surveillance, Epidemiology, and End Results (SEER) program of the National Cancer Institute, the incidence of childhood leukemia among those aged 0 to 15 years in the USA increased an average of 0.6% per year between 1975 and 2003 (4). This increasing trend occurred mostly between 1975 and 1988, during which the incidence increased an average of 1.3% per year (4). The incidence of childhood leukemia in the USA stabilized between 1988 and 2002, during which time the annual percent change was 0.1% (4).

1.2. Established Risk Factors

There are few known causes of childhood leukemia. As previously mentioned, sex, age, and race are associated with the risk of childhood ALL. Exposure to ionizing radiation and congenital diseases (e.g., Down syndrome and neurofibromatosis) are also known to be associated with an increased risk of childhood leukemia *(1)*; however, these risk factors account for only 10% of the childhood leukemia cases *(5)*.

1.3. Gene Versus Environment

Studies to date suggest that environmental factors may play a larger role in childhood leukemia than genetic factors. South Asian (India, Pakistan, and Bangladesh) children residing in the United Kingdom have a similar or higher incidence of childhood leukemia compared with non-South Asian Children *(6, 7)*, even though the incidence of childhood leukemia in India is much lower than that of the United Kingdom *(3)*. Chinese children residing in Hong Kong and Singapore have a higher incidence of ALL (40.6 and 39.5 per million, respectively) than Chinese in Tianjin, China (17.4 per million) *(3)*, suggesting factors associated with Westernization of lifestyles may play an important role.

Apart from rare familial cancer syndromes, siblings and parents of a child with leukemia do not have an increased risk of developing leukemia *(8, 9)*. Studies showed that the concordance rates of leukemia among identical twins range from 5 to 26% for leukemia in monozygotic twins *(10–12)*. The concordance of leukemia among identical twins, however, has a physiological basis rather than genetic basis. Studies showed that twins concordant for childhood leukemia share the same breakpoints in the translocated genes observed in the leukemic cells *(13, 14)*. Because these sequences are not inherited, the only explanation is that the preleukemic clone first occurs in one twin and then spreads to another twin via intraplacental anastomoses *(11)*. This observation supports the dominant effect of environmental risk factors in the development of childhood leukemia.

1.4. Current Hypothesis

Chromosomal translocations are commonly present in childhood leukemia. The most frequent translocations associated with ALL and AML are *TEL-AML1* (t(12;21); 20% of ALL) and *AML1-ETO* (t(8;21), 15% of AML), respectively *(15)*. Screening of dried fetal blood spots showed that many of the chromosomal translocations were present before birth *(15)*. It has been shown that the occurrence of *TEL-AML1* fusion gene is approximately 1% in the fetal cord blood sample, which is 100 times higher than the lifetime occurrence of ALL with *TEL-AML1* (1 in 10,000) *(16)*. In vitro and animal studies have shown that either expression of *TEL-AML1* or *AML1-ETO* fusion protein alone can establish a covert preleukemic clone *(17, 18)*; however, neither the expression of *TEL-AML1* or *AML1-ETO* fusion protein alone is sufficient to transform hematopoietic cell lines into leukemic cells

(19, 20). Other animal studies have shown that *TEL-AML1* or *AML1-ETO* together with a second mutation in other genes may induce acute leukemia *(21–24)*. These data strongly suggest that in addition to the prenatal initiating events, postnatal promoting events are necessary in the development of childhood leukemia as described by Greaves as a "two-hit" model *(25)*.

2. Tobacco Smoke

2.1. Prevalence of Tobacco Smoking in the USA and in the World

Tobacco smoke is known to cause at least nine cancers (lung, pancreas, esophagus, urinary bladder, oral cavity, nasopharynx, liver, cervix, and myeloid leukemia) *(26)*. Despite a substantial public health effort to reduce cigarette smoking, a large proportion of the USA and world population still smoke. According to the 2002 Behavioral Risk Factor Surveillance System (BRFSS) survey, the prevalence of current smoker among adults 18 years or older ranged from 12.7% in Utah to 32.6% in Kentucky, with a median of 23.7% *(27)*. The Pregnancy Risk Assessment Monitoring (PRAM) system 2000–2001 reports that the prevalence of maternal smoking during the last 3 months of pregnancy ranged from 9% in Hawaii to 17.4% in Maine *(17)*. Among mothers younger than 20 years of age, the prevalence of smoking during the last 3 months of pregnancy ranged from 11.1% in Florida to 34.6% in Maine *(17)*.

Although the prevalence of smokers has been decreasing in some countries such as USA, Japan, and United Kingdom, the overall cigarette consumption in the world has been increasing *(28)*. In countries such as China, Turkey, and Russia, more than 60% of men are smokers and over 15 billion cigarettes are smoked worldwide everyday *(28)*. In countries such as Argentina, Poland, and Cuba, more than 60% of the children are exposed to passive smoking at home *(28)*.

2.2. Carcinogens in Tobacco Smoke and Their Association with Leukemia

Tobacco smoke contains at least 60 known human or animal carcinogens, with the major chemical classes being volatile hydrocarbons, aldehydes, aromatic amines, polycyclic aromatic hydrocarbons (PAHs), and nitrosamines (**Table 5.1**) *(29)*.

2.2.1. Volatile Hydrocarbons
2.2.1.1. Benzene

Benzene is a volatile hydrocarbon and is one of the major carcinogens contained in mainstream tobacco smoke. Benzene is a well-established leukemogen and is classified by the International Agency for Research on Cancer (IARC) as a group 1 (carcinogenic) chemical *(30)*. A smoker is exposed to approximately 2 mg of benzene per day (89% from active smoking, 4% from outdoor air other than automobiles, 3% from indoor air other than passive

Table 5.1
Major carcinogens in tobacco smoke

Chemical class	Most representative carcinogens of the chemical class	International Agency for Research on Cancer (IARC) classification[a]	Quantity in mainstream smoke (ng per cigarette)
Volatile hydrocarbons	Benzene	1	59,000
	1,3-Butadiene	2A	52,000
Aldehydes	Formaldehyde	1	16,000
	Acetaldehyde	2B	819,000
Aromatic amines	2-Naphthylamine	1	10
	4-Aminobiphenyl	1	1.4
Polycyclic aromatic hydrocarbons	Benzo(a)pyrene	2A	9
Phenols	Catechol	2B	68,000
Nitro compound	Nitromethane	2B	500
Nitrosamines	NNN	2B	179
	NNK	2B	123
Other organic compounds	Ethylene oxide	1	7,000
	Acrylonitrile	2B	10,000
Inorganic compounds	Cadmium	1	132

[a]Group 1, the agent (mixture) is carcinogenic to humans; Group 2A, the agent (mixture) is probably carcinogenic to humans; Group 2B, the agent (mixture) is possibly carcinogenic to humans; Group 3, the agent is not classifiable in terms of its carcinogenicity; Group 4, the agent is not carcinogenic to humans. Source: International Agency for Research on Cancerhttp://www-cie.iarc.fr/monoeval/grlist.html (adapted from (29))

smoking, 2% from passive smoking, and 2% from automobiles) (31). A nonsmoker is exposed to approximately 0.2 mg of benzene per day (40% from outdoor air other than automobiles, 31% from indoor air other than passive smoking, 19% from automobiles, and 10% from passive smoking) (31).

The toxicity of benzene is mainly due to its metabolites. The ultimate carcinogen of benzene metabolism is benzoquinone.

Benzoquinone can damage DNA either through covalent binding or by entering redox cycling, which can generate free radicals to cause oxidative damage of DNA *(32)*.

Epidemiologic studies (both cohort and case-control studies) consistently indicate a strong association between occupational exposure of benzene and AML with a positive dose response *(33)*. Zhang et al. observed AML-specific aberrations in chromosomes 5 and 7 in cultured human lymphocytes treated with benzene metabolites (hydroquinone and 1,2,4-benzenetriol) *(34)*. Similarly, the same AML-specific aberrations in chromosomes 5 and 7 of peripheral blood lymphocytes were significantly increased in Chinese factory workers exposed to benzene compared with those not exposed *(35)*. Among the same group of Chinese workers, the peripheral blood lymphocytes of benzene-exposed subjects had significantly increased frequencies of hyperdiploidy of chromosomes 8 and 21, and also translocation between chromosomes 8 and 21, which are all chromosomal aberrations commonly associated with AML *(36)*. Data on the association between occupational exposure of benzene and ALL are limited and the results are inconclusive *(33)*.

2.2.1.2. 1,3-Butadiene

1,3-Butadiene is another volatile hydrocarbon present in high quantity in tobacco smoke. It has been classified as a group 2A (probably carcinogenic) chemical by IARC due to sufficient evidence in animal studies but limited evidence from epidemiologic studies *(37)*.

1,3-Butadiene is first oxidized by cytochrome P450 to form 1,2-epoxy-3-butene (EB). EB can then be: 1) detoxified through conjugation with glutathione; 2) hydrolyzed by epoxide hydrolase to 3-butene-1,2-diol, which can be eliminated directly in the urine, conjugated with glutathione, or oxidized by cytochrome P450 to 3,4-epoxy-1,2-butanediol (EBdiol); and 3) oxidized further by cytochrome P450 to 1,2:3,4-diepoxybutane (DEB), which is the most carcinogenic of all 1,3-butadiene metabolites *(38)*. In humans, the major metabolic pathway of 1,3-butadiene occurs through epoxide hydrolase *(38, 39)*.

Limited human data come from studies of occupational exposure among styrene-butadiene rubber workers and 1,3-butadiene production workers. A study of 13,130 men employed in a synthetic rubber factory showed a positive association between 1,3-butadiene and leukemia; however, the independent effect of 1,3-butadiene cannot be confirmed due to its correlation with other chemical exposures *(40)*. In a cohort of 614 petrochemical workers who were exposed to 1,3-butadiene, there were no reported cases of leukemia *(41)*. Another cohort study of 2,800 workers in a 1,3-butadiene monomer facility showed an increased risk of leukemia in the short-term workers but not among the workers with the longest period of exposure; therefore, the evidence was not convincing *(42)*. Overall, the data from epidemiologic studies are lacking to reach any definite conclusion regarding the association between 1,3-butadiene and leukemia.

2.2.2. Polycyclic Aromatic Hydrocarbons

PAHs are products of combustion processes. Examples of PAHs in the order of increasing carcinogenicity are benzo(a)pyrene (B(*a*)P), 7,12-dimethyl-benz(a)anthracene (DMBA), and dibenzo(*a,l*)-pyrene (DB(*a,l*)P) *(43)*. The metabolic activation of PAHs involves cytochrome P450 enzymes (mainly CYP1A1 and CYP1B1) and epoxide hydrolase, with the formation of diol epoxide being the ultimate carcinogen capable of binding DNA *(43)*.

There are a few animal studies suggesting PAHs as a possible cause of leukemia. Heidel et al. showed that DMBA induced the appearance of myelodysplastic cells, an indication of a pre-leukemic state, in the bone marrow of wild-type mice but not in CYP1B1-null mice *(44)*. Others have demonstrated the ability of DMBA to induce leukemia in rats *(45)*.

Besides smoking, the major sources of human exposure to PAHs are occupational and urban air pollution (from vehicle emissions and other sources). Occupational exposures to PAHs have been consistently associated with an elevated risk in bladder and lung cancer; however, little evidence links occupational exposure to PAHs to an increased risk of leukemia *(46)*. Exposure to PAHs in traffic has been associated with an increased risk of childhood leukemia by some studies *(47–49)*, while others reported no such associations *(50, 51)*. Although vehicle emissions are a major source of PAHs, they also contain other carcinogens, including benzene, thus, it is difficult to attribute the association between traffic and childhood leukemia entirely to PAHs.

2.2.3. Aromatic Amines

Aromatic amines (e.g., 4-aminobiphenyl (4-ABP) and 2-naphthylamine (2-NA)) are well-recognized carcinogens that can be found mainly in cigarette smoke, combustion of fossil fuels, in industries involved in the production of rubber, coal, textile, and in the printing process. Numerous studies have established the causal association between aromatic amines and bladder cancer *(52–55)*.

Both 4-ABP and 2-NA first undergo *N*-hydroxylation in the liver to produce *N*-hydroxyaromatic amines, which then undergo glucuronidation and are excreted in the urine *(56)*. The glucuronides are very unstable in the acidic environment of the urinary bladder and are hydrolyzed to form *N*-hydroxyaromatic amines, which cause the formation of bladder tumor by direct binding to DNA *(56)*, commonly occurring in the *p53* gene *(57)*, or oxidative damage of DNA *(58)*.

Although aromatic amines are established carcinogens, there has been no evidence to support their roles in the cause of leukemia.

2.2.4. Nitrosamines

Two major nitrosamines, *N*-nitrosonornicotine (NNN) and 4-(methylnitrosamino)-1-(3-pyridyl)-1-butanone (NNK), are present in tobacco smoke. Both NNN and NNK are classified by IARC as group 2B (possibly carcinogenic) chemicals *(30)*. NNN is recognized as a carcinogen for esophageal and oral cancer, whereas NNK is known to cause lung, pancreatic, and oral cancer *(59)*. To date, there is no evidence to support the association between nitrosamines and leukemia.

In summary, the only established leukemogen in tobacco smoke is benzene; however, the chemicals in the tobacco could interact with one another in a complex way to jointly attain a significant carcinogenic effect on the development of leukemia.

3. Genotoxicity of Tobacco Smoke on Fetus and Child

3.1. Paternal-Mediated Process

There is a growing body of literature suggesting that paternal smoking has the potential for initiating a carcinogenic process in offspring thorough its genotoxic effect on sperm. Fraga et al. showed that sperm of smoking men have a higher level of oxo[8]dG, an oxidative product of DNA damage, compared with those of nonsmoking men *(60)*. Similarly, Shen et al. also showed that sperm DNA of smoking men contain a higher level of 8-hydroxydeoxyguanosine (8-OHdG) than that of nonsmoking men, and the level of 8-OHdG is closely correlated with seminal cotinine concentration *(61)*. Shi et al. showed that cigarette smoking may increase the risk of aneuploidy for certain chromosomes in human sperm *(62)*. Zenzes et al. showed that benzo(a)pyrene diol epoxide-DNA (BPDE-DNA) adducts in sperm cells are increased by smoking *(63)*, and these BPDE-DNA adducts are transmitted to embryos by spermatozoa *(64)*.

3.2. Maternal-Mediated Process

Studies have suggested that in utero exposure to tobacco smoke can have genotoxic effects on the fetus. Ammenheuser et al. reported that the cord blood of fetuses of smoking mothers have significantly higher frequencies of lymphocytes containing mutations at the hypoxanthine phosphoribosyltransferase (hprt) locus than the cord blood of fetuses of nonsmoking mothers *(65)*. De la Chica et al. showed that amniocytes from fetuses of mothers who smoked have a significantly higher proportion of structural chromosomal abnormalities compared with those of fetuses of nonsmoking mothers. In addition, they found that band 11q23, commonly involved in leukemogenesis, is particularly prone to the genotoxic effect of tobacco *(66)*. An animal study by Ng et al. showed that offspring of mice exposed to mainstream cigarette smoke during pregnancy were less resistant to tumor challenge and had a greater increase in tumor incidence, possibly by reducing the activity of cytotoxic T lymphocytes *(67)*.

3.3. Postnatal Passive Smoking

Children exposed to passive smoke have also been shown to have increased genetic damage. Crawford et al. reported that children exposed to passive smoking had a higher level of PAH-albumin level compared with those not exposed, after accounting for diet and home environment *(68)*. Tang et al. showed a higher level of 4-aminobiphenyl-hemoglobin adducts, PAH-albumin, and sister chromatid exchanges in peripheral blood of children exposed to passive smoke compared with those who were not exposed *(69)*.

4. Tobacco Smoke and Leukemia

4.1. Adult Leukemia

4.1.1. Cohort Studies

In the past 20 years (1985–2006), a total of ten cohort studies on the association between smoking and adult leukemia have been published *(70–79)*. Cohort studies have the advantage of being less prone to recall bias compared with case-control studies, as the exposure status is ascertained before the occurrence of disease, and temporality can be more readily established to determine causality. Of the ten cohort studies, nine had information on all leukemia combined *(70, 71, 73–79)*. Five of the nine studies reported a positive association between smoking and adult leukemia *(73, 74, 76, 77, 79)*, while four reported a null association *(70, 71, 75, 78)*. Six of the ten cohort studies reported separate data on lymphatic leukemia *(70, 72–76)*, and only one reported a positive association between smoking and lymphoid leukemia *(74)*. Seven of the ten cohort studies had separate data on myeloid leukemia *(70, 72–77)* and five of them reported that smoking was associated with an increased risk with all myeloid leukemia *(73, 74, 76, 77)* or AML only *(72)*, while two reported a null association *(70, 75)*.

4.1.2. Case-Control Studies

Between 1985 and 2006, a total of 12 case-control studies on the association between smoking and adult leukemia have been published (**Table 5.2**) *(80–91)*. Of the five studies with information on all leukemia combined *(81–84, 91)*, two reported a positive association between smoking and adult leukemia *(81, 84)*, while three reported a null association *(82, 83, 91)*. Of the seven case-control studies with data on lymphoid leukemia *(81–85, 88, 91)*, one reported a positive association between smoking and chronic lymphoblastic leukemia (CLL) *(81)*, one reported a positive

Table 5.2
Studies on tobacco smoking and risk of childhood leukemia from 1985 to 2006

Cohort studies

Author, year (location) (reference)	Source of subjects	Data collection	Adjusted variables	Primary results (risk ratios)
Pershagen et al., 1992 (Sweden) (94)	497,051 live births from 1982–1987 identified from Swedish Medical Birth Registry	Interviews were performed by midwife during the first prenatal visit, usually 2–3 months into the pregnancy. Leukemia outcomes from January 1, 1982 to December 31, 1987 were ascertained from the Swedish Cancer Registry	Year and county of birth, birth order, and maternal age	Mother smoked during pregnancy (Yes vs. No) Lymphatic leukemia (84 cases): 0.76 (0.46–1.25) Myeloid leukemia (15 cases): 1.64 (0.56–4.79)
Klebanoff et al., 1996 (USA) (92)	54,795 children born of 44,621 mothers who enrolled in the Collaborative Perinatal Project cohort. Pregnant women were enrolled from 1959 to 1966 and children followed for up to 8 years	Mothers were interviewed at registration (17–24 weeks) and again at each visit thereafter. Women who reported smoking at any visit were considered to be smokers and their maximum daily consumption was used in analysis of dose response	None	All leukemia Mother smoked during pregnancy: 0.8 (0.3–2.1)
Mucci et al., 2004 (Sweden) (93)	All live births in Sweden between January 1, 1983 and December 31, 1997. (N=1,440,542)	During the first antenatal visit (8–12 weeks of gestation) information from a standardized questionnaire is recorded by a nurse midwife. Follow-up data on cancer outcome were obtained through linkage of the Birth Registry with the Swedish Cancer Registry and the National Cause if Death Registry	Maternal age, maternal education, parental status, residence at birth, maternal birthplace, parity, birth year, and gender	Maternal smoking during pregnancy **ALL** No: Reference Yes: 0.75 (0.60–0.93) 1–9 cpd: 0.69 (0.52–0.91) ≥10 cpd: 0.84 (0.61–1.15) *p* for trend: 0.043 **AML** No: Reference Yes: 1.28 (0.65–2.49) 1–9 cpd: 0.75 (0.29–1.96) ≥10 cpd: 2.20 (1.00–4.83) *p* for trend: 0.13

Case-Control Studies

Buckley et al., 1986 (USA, Canada) (96)	1,814 childhood cancer cases, including 742 cases of ALL, were identified from the study regions covered by the Children's Cancer Study Group. 720 healthy control children were identified randomly from approximately the same geographic regions	Questionnaire	Matched: Geographic location Adjusted: Birth year of the child, maternal age, illness during the pregnancy, and socioeconomic factors	ALL Mother smoked during pregnancy None: Reference 1–9 cpd: 0.97 (0.61–1.52) 10+ cpd: 0.85 (0.66–1.11)
McKinney et al., 1986 (United Kingdom) (103)	555 childhood cancer cases, including 171 cases of leukemia, were identified from the study regions covered by Inter-Regional Epidemiological Study of Childhood Cancer. 2 controls (1 from hospital admission for minor conditions and 1 from general practitioner) for every case were identified	Interview	Matched: Age and sex Adjusted: None	All leukemia Mother smoked during pregnancy None: Reference 1–10 cpd: 1.02 (0.62–1.68) 11+ cpd: 0.61 (0.36–1.02)
Stjernfeldt et al., 1986 (Sweden) (114)	National case-control study on childhood cancer was conducted between 1978 and 1981. 305 children with cancer (cases) and 340 children with insulin-dependent diabetes mellitus (controls), aged 0–16 years, who were treated at 37 pediatric departments	Structured questionnaire for self-assessment was given to families by their physicians	Matched: Year of diagnosis and sex Adjusted: Maternal age at the index pregnancy, illness during pregnancy, occupation, and place of residence	Maternal smoking during pregnancy ALL (132 cases) None-smoker: Reference 1–9 cpd: 1.34 10+ cpd: 2.07, $p < 0.01$ P for trend < 0.01

(continued)

**Table 5.2
(continued)**

Author, year (location) (reference)	Source of cases and controls	Data collection	Matched and adjusted variables	Primary results (odds ratios)
Magnani et al., 1990 (Italy) (102)	Cases (142 ALL, and 22 AnLL) were those diagnosed during the study period from 1981–1984 in the main Pediatric Hospital in Turin plus those diagnosed in the period of 1974–1980 who were still under observation. Controls were a random sample of children hospitalized in the medical or surgical ward of the same hospital	Face-to-face interview	Matched: None Adjusted: SES	ALL Mother smoked up to child's birth: 0.7 (0.5–1.1) 1–15 cpd: 0.6 (0.4–1.0) 16+ cpd: 1.0 (0.4–2.7) Father smoked up to child's birth: 0.9 (0.6–1.5) 1–15 cpd: 0.9 (0.5–1.6) 16+ cpd: 0.9 (0.6–1.5) AML Mother smoked up to child's birth: 2.0 (0.8–4.8) Father smoked up to child's birth: 0.9 (0.3–2.1)
John et al., 1991 (USA) (101)	Incident cancer cases (including 73 leukemia cases) diagnosed from 1976 to 1983, aged 0–14 years, and residing in the Denver Standard Metropolitan Statistical Area at the time of diagnosis were identified from the Colorado Central Cancer Registry and review of medical records of hospitals that did not provide data to the registry. 196 controls were selected through random digit dialing	Structured in-home interview or telephone interview	Matched: Age, sex, and telephone exchange area Adjusted: Father's education	ALL Mother 3 months before conception: No: Reference Yes: 2.1 (1.0–4.3) 1–10 cpd: 2.0 (0.8–5.0) 11+ cpd: 2.2 (1.0–4.9) During first trimester of pregnancy: No: Reference Yes: 2.3 (1.1–5.0) 1–10 cpd: 1.9 (0.7–5.6) 11+ cpd: 2.6 (1.1–6.3)

				During three trimesters of pregnancy:
				No: Reference
				Yes: 2.5 (1.2–5.4)
				1–10 cpd: 2.0 (0.7–5.9)
				11+ cpd: 2.9 (1.2–6.8)
				Father
				During the 12 months before child's birth:
				No: Reference
				Yes: 1.9 (1.0–3.7)
				1–10 cpd: 2.6 (0.9–7.9)
				11–20 cpd: 1.6 (0.7–3.7)
				21+ cpd: 1.6 (0.7–4.0)
				Mother and Father
				Mother smoked during the first trimester alone: 2.9 (0.8–10.3)
				Father smoked during the 12 months before child's birth alone: 1.7 (0.7–3.8)
				Mother smoked during the first trimester plus father smoked during the 12 months before child's birth: 2.2 (1.0–5.0)
Severson et al., 1993 (USA, Canada) (108)	187 AML cases were identified by 100 primary and affiliate institution of the Children Cancer Group.	Telephone interview	Matched: Date of birth, race, telephone area code and exchange	All FAB types (187 cases)
				Mother current smoker: 0.91 (0.58–1.43)
				Mother ever smoked: 1.32 (0.85–2.09)
				Mother smoked during pregnancy: 1.20 (0.77–1.86)
	187 controls were ascertained by random digit dialing		Adjusted: None	M1/M2 FAB types (107 cases)
				Mother current smoker: 0.89 (0.49–1.60)
				Mother ever smoked: 1.30 (0.73–2.35)
				Mother smoked during pregnancy: 1.39 (0.79–2.49)

(continued)

Table 5.2
(continued)

Author, year (location) (reference)	Source of cases and controls	Data collection	Matched and adjusted variables	Primary results (odds ratios)
				M3 FAB types (14 cases) Mother current smoker: 1.25 (0.27–6.30) Mother ever smoked: 0.50 (0.05–3.49) Mother smoked during pregnancy: 1.00 (0.19–5.37) M4 FAB types (37 cases) Mother current smoker: 1.17 (0.34–4.20) Mother ever smoked: 2.67 (0.64–15.61) Mother smoked during pregnancy: 1.33 (0.41–4.66) M5 FAB types (25 cases) Mother current smoker: 0.80 (0.16–3.72) Mother ever smoked: 1.60 (0.46–6.22) Mother smoked during pregnancy: 0.83 (0.20–3.28) Results for fathers were similar to those for mothers, although data not shown
Cnattingius et al., 1995 (Sweden) (98)	A nested case-control design. 613 lymphatic leukemia cases were identified in successive birth cohort from 1973 to 1989.	Smoking data were collected during the antenatal visit	Matched: Sex, birth year, and birth month	All age combined Maternal daily smoking reported at the first antenatal visit: 0.7 (0.5-1.1)
	For each case, 5 controls were selected from the source population		Adjusted: Age at delivery, parity, infertility, and spontaneous abortion	Age at diagnosis 0-1 year Maternal daily smoking reported at the first antenatal visit: 1.0 (0.4-2.1)

Study	Study description	Exposure assessment	Matched/Adjusted	Results
				Age at diagnosis 2–4 year Maternal daily smoking reported at the first antenatal visit: 0.6 (0.3–0.95) Age at diagnosis >5 year Maternal daily smoking reported at the first antenatal visit: 2.0 (0.6–7.1)
Chattingius et al., 1995 (Sweden) (97)	A nested case-control design. 98 myeloid leukemia cases were identified in successive birth cohort from 1973 to 1989. For each case, 5 controls were selected from the source population	Smoking data were collected during the antenatal visit	Matched: Sex, birth year, and birth month Adjusted: None	Maternal smoking reported at the first antenatal visit: 2.4 (0.9–6.5)
Sorahan et al., 1995 (England, Wales) (110)	Cases were 1,641 children who died with cancer in England and Wales during the period 1977 to 1981. 1,641 controls were obtained from the birth register of the local authority area in which the case parents were living at the time of the interview	In-person interview	Matched: Sex and date of birth Adjusted: None	ALL Prenatal daily consumption of cigarettes (Nonsmoker, <10 cpd, 10–19 cpd, 20–29 cpd, 30–39 cpd, 40+ cpd): Father (371 pairs): 1.16 (1.06–1.27) Mother (400 pairs): 0.94 (0.83–1.05) Myeloid leukemia Prenatal daily consumption of cigarettes (Nonsmoker, <10 cpd, 10–19 cpd, 20–29 cpd, 30–39 cpd, 40+ cpd): Father (147 pairs): 1.02 (0.89–1.16) Mother (151 pairs): 0.93 (0.79–1.10)
Cocco et al., 1996 (Italy) (99)	9 cases of ALL diagnosed between 1980 and 1989 in the town of Carbonia. 36 controls were identified from Carbonia	In-person interview	Matched: Gender and date of birth Adjusted: SES, family history of cancer, and parental birth outside Carbonia	ALL Maternal smoking: 1.8 (0.4–9.5)

(continued)

Table 5.2 (continued)

Author, year (location) (reference)	Source of cases and controls	Data collection	Matched and adjusted variables	Primary results (odds ratios)
Shu et al., 1996 (USA, Canada, Australia) (109)	Cases were children who were 18 months of age or younger, newly diagnosed with leukemia between January 1, 1983 and December 31, 1988, identified from 100 collaborating institutions of the Children Cancer Group. Controls were randomly selected by random digit dialing	Telephone interviews	Matched: Year of birth, telephone area code, and exchange number Adjusted: Sex, maternal (paternal) age, education, and maternal alcohol consumption during pregnancy	Total leukemia (302 cases) Maternal smoking The month prior to pregnancy: 0.71 (0.51–1.01) During pregnancy: 0.66 (0.46–0.94) 1–10 cpd: 0.66 (0.41–1.04) 11–20 cpd: 0.64 (0.39–1.06) >20 cpd: 0.62 (0.22–1.79) Test for trend: p = 0.03 Nursing period: 0.49 (0.29–0.83) Paternal smoking The month prior to pregnancy: 1.28 (0.90–1.81) 1–10 cpd: 1.39 (0.69–2.82) 11–20 cpd: 1.15 (0.74–1.80) >20 cpd: 1.36 (0.81–2.28) Test for trend: p = 0.23 ALL (203 cases) Maternal smoking The month prior to pregnancy: 0.84 (0.51–1.28) During pregnancy: 0.78 (0.51–1.18) 1–10 cpd: 0.78 (0.47–1.11) 11–20 cpd: 0.79 (0.46–1.17) >20 cpd: 0.48 (0.12–1.90) Test for trend: p = 0.18 Nursing period: 0.49 (0.26–0.93)

				Paternal smoking The month prior to pregnancy: 1.56 (1.03–2.36) 1–10 cpd: 2.40 (1.00–5.72) 11–20 cpd: 1.33 (0.79–2.34) >20 cpd: 1.51 (0.82–2.77) Test for trend: p = 0.12 AML (88 cases) Maternal smoking The month prior to pregnancy: 0.48 (0.22–1.05) During pregnancy: 0.45 (0.21–0.96) 1–10 cpd: 0.46 (0.16–1.31) 11–20 cpd: 0.41 (0.15–1.13) >20 cpd: 0.69 (0.08–5.78) Test for trend: p = 0.07 Nursing period: 0.61 (0.23–1.57) Paternal smoking The month prior to pregnancy: 0.75 (0.35–1.62) 1–10 cpd: 0.42 (0.09–1.95) 11–20 cpd: 0.73 (0.27–1.94) >cpd: 1.29 (0.44–3.74) Test for trend: p = 0.98
Ji et al., 1997 (China) (115)	A population-based case-control study. Cases of newly diagnosed cancer, who were permanent residents of urban Shanghai, younger than the age of 15 years.	In-person interview	Matched: Sex and year of birth Adjusted: Birth weight, income, paternal age, education, and alcohol drinking	Acute leukemia Pack-years before conception 0: reference ≤2: 0.7 (0.3–1.8) >2 to <5: 1.0 (0.4–2.1) ≥5: 2.4 (1.1–5.6) p for trend: 0.02

(continued)

**Table 5.2
(continued)**

Author, year (location) (reference)	Source of cases and controls	Data collection	Matched and adjusted variables	Primary results (odds ratios)
	Controls were selected from the general population of urban Shanghai using a household group as the primary sampling unit			**Pack-years after birth** 0: Reference ≤2: 1.3 (0.6–2.6) >2 to <5: 1.6 (0.7–3.5) ≥5: 1.0 (0.4–2.4) *p* for trend: 0.94 **ALL** Pack-years before conception 0: Reference ≤2: 0.8 (0.2–2.5) >2 to <5: 1.0 (0.4–2.7) ≥5: 3.8 (1.3–12.3) *p* for trend: 0.01 **Pack-years after birth** 0: Reference ≤2: 1.1 (0.4–2.8) >2 to <5: 1.8 (0.6–5.2) ≥5: 1.8 (0.6–5.5) *p* for trend: 0.33 **AML** Pack-years before conception 0: Reference ≤2: 0.9 (0.1–7.3) >2 to <5: 0.6 (0.1–3.1) ≥5: 2.3 (0.4–14.8) *p* for trend: 0.36

Reference (location)	Study description	Exposure assessment	Matched/Adjusted	Results
				Pack-years after birth 0: Reference ≤2: 5.0 (0.8–32.5) >2 to <5: 6.1 (0.8–45.1) ≥5: 0.5 (0.1–2.7) p for trend: 0.24
Petridou et al., 1997 (Greece) *(106)*	153 incident cases of childhood leukemia were identified through a nationwide network of childhood hematologist/oncologist during 1993–1994. Controls were selected from hospitals	Interviewer-administered questionnaire	Matched: Time of hospitalization, gender, age, area of residence Adjusted: Maternal alcohol consumption, maternal coffee drinking, breast feeding, pet ownership	**All leukemia** Maternal smoking during pregnancy: 1.19 (0.73–1.93)
Sorahan et al., 1997a (England, Wales, Scotland) *(111)*	Cases were 1,549 children who died with cancer in England, Wales, and Scotland during the period 1953 to 1955. 1,549 controls were obtained from the birth register of the local authority area in which the case child died	In-person interview	Matched: Sex and date of birth	**ALL** Daily consumption of cigarettes (<1 cpd, 1–9 cpd, 10–20 cpd, 20+ cpd): Father (371 pairs): 1.08 (0.91–1.27) Mother (400 pairs): 1.24 (1.01–1.52)
			Adjusted: None	**Myeloid leukemia** Daily consumption of cigarettes (<1 cpd, 1–9 cpd, 10–20 cpd, 20+ cpd): Father (147 pairs): 0.98 (0.73–1.32) Mother (151 pairs): 1.20 (0.85–1.68)
Sorahan et al., 1997b (England, Wales, Scotland) *(113)*	Cases were 2,587 children who died with cancer in England, Wales, and Scotland during the period 1971 to 1976. 2,587 controls were obtained from the birth register of the local authority area in which the case child died.	In-person interview	Matched: Sex and date of birth	**ALL (573 pairs from 1971 to 1976)** Daily consumption of cigarettes (1–9 cpd, 10–19 cpd, 20–29 cpd, 30–39 cpd, 40+ cpd): Father: 1.07 (0.99–1.16) Mother: 0.98 (0.89–1.07)

(continued)

**Table 5.2
(continued)**

Author, year (location) (reference)	Source of cases and controls	Data collection	Matched and adjusted variables	Primary results (odds ratios)
	In addition data were combined with two previous published studies (1953–1955 and 1977–1981)		Adjusted: None for 1971–1976 data. For combined data, analysis was adjusted for social class, age of father at birth of the child, age of birth of mother at birth of the child, sibship position, and obstetric radiography	**Myeloid leukemia (190 pairs from 1971 to 1976)** Daily consumption of cigarettes (1–9 cpd, 10–19 cpd, 20–29 cpd, 30–39 cpd, 40+ cpd): Father: 1.27 (1.10–1.47) Mother: 1.00 (0.83–1.20) **All leukemia (combined data, 2,364 pairs)** Father (smoker vs. nonsmoker): 1.20 (1.05–1.37) Mother (smoker vs. nonsmoker): 1.02 (0.90–1.16)
Brondum et al., 1999 (USA) (95)	Cases (1,842 ALL and 517 AML) were identified by Children's cancer group and affiliate member institution. Controls were identified by random digit dialing		Matched: Age, race, telephone area code, and exchange Adjusted: Annual income, parent's race, and education	**ALL Father** Never smoked: Reference Current smoker: 1.06 (0.90–1.25) Ever smoked: 1.04 (0.90–1.20) 1 month before pregnancy: 1.07 (0.90–1.27) <10 cpd: 1.16 (0.88–1.51) 10–20 cpd: 1.04 (0.83–1.31) 20+ cpd: 1.06 (0.88–1.26) p for trend: 0.56 **Mother** Never smoked: Reference Current smoker: 1.02 (0.87–1.79) Ever smoked: 1.04 (0.91–1.19) 1 month before pregnancy: 1.02 (0.87–1.20) 1st trimester: 0.96 (0.81–1.14) 2nd trimester: 1.00 (0.83–1.20)

3rd trimester: 0.99 (0.82–1.19)
<10 cpd: 1.02 (0.83–1.26)
10–20 cpd: 1.04 (0.86–1.26)
20+ cpd: 1.04 (0.87–1.26)
p for trend: 0.59

Father and Mother
Neither parent ever smoked: Reference
Both ever smoked: 1.09 (0.91–1.30)
Father ever smoked only: 1.04 (0.86–1.26)
Mother ever smoked only: 1.10 (0.88–1.38)

AML

Father Never smoked: Reference
Current smoker: 0.91 (0.67–1.24)
Ever smoked: 0.88 (0.67–1.16)
1 month before pregnancy: 0.87 (0.64–1.18)
<10 cpd: 1.04 (0.62–1.74)
10–20 cpd: 0.92 (0.61–1.37)
20+ cpd: 0.81 (0.58–1.14)
p for trend: 0.22

Mother
Never smoked: Reference
Current smoker: 0.97 (0.73–1.30)
Ever smoked: 0.95 (0.74–1.22)
1 month before pregnancy: 0.95 (0.74–1.21)
1st trimester: 0.95 (0.74–1.21)
2nd trimester: 0.95 (0.74–1.21)
3rd trimester: 0.95 (0.74–1.21)
<10 cpd: 1.25 (0.88–1.76)
10–20 cpd: 0.87 (0.61–1.24)
20+ cpd: 0.73 (0.30–1.07)
p for trend: 0.13

Father and Mother
Neither parent ever smoked: Reference
Both ever smoked: 0.85 (0.59–1.22)
Father ever smoked only: 1.32 (0.91–1.93)
Mother ever smoked only: 1.78 (1.15–2.75)

(continued)

**Table 5.2
(continued)**

Author, year (location) (reference)	Source of cases and controls	Data collection	Matched and adjusted variables	Primary results (odds ratios)
Schüz et al., 1999 (Germany) *(107)*	Cancer cases, including 650 acute leukemia cases, diagnosed between October 1992 and September 1994 were identified the nationwide cancer registry.	Questionnaire and telephone interview	Matched: Gender, date of birth, and district (smallest administrative unit in Germany)	**All acute leukemia** **Maternal smoking during pregnancy** None: Reference 1–10 cpd: 0.8 (0.6–1.1) 11–20 cpd: 0.5 (0.2–1.0) >20 cpd: 0.5 (0.1–2.7)
	Controls were selected from complete files of local offices for registrations of residents		Adjusted: Urbanization, SES	**Paternal smoking before pregnancy** None: Reference 1–10 cpd: 1.2 (0.9–1.8) 11–20 cpd: 1.0 (0.8–1.3) >20 cpd: 0.8 (0.5–1.2)
Infante-Rivard et al., 2000 (Canada) *(100)*	491 incident cases of childhood ALL cases, aged 0–9 years were recruited from tertiary care centers in the province of Québec between 1980 and 1993.	Telephone interview	Matched: Age, sex, and region of residence	**ALL** **Maternal smoking** First trimester of pregnancy None: Reference 1–20 cpd: 1.1 (0.8–1.6) >20 cpd: 1.0 (0.7–1.6) Second trimester of pregnancy None: Reference 1–20 cpd: 1.2 (0.8–1.6) >20 cpd: 1.2 (0.7–1.9)
	491 population-based controls were identified based on administrative and geographical regions determined by government		Adjusted: Maternal age and level of schooling	Third trimester of pregnancy None: Reference 1–20 cpd: 1.2 (0.8–1.6) >20 cpd: 1.2 (0.8–2.0)

Between birth and date of diagnosis
None: Reference
1–20 cpd: 1.0 (0.7–1.4)
>20 cpd: 1.0 (0.6–1.3)

Paternal smoking
Between birth and date of diagnosis
None: Reference
1–20 cpd: 1.0 (0.7–1.4)
>20 cpd: 1.0 (0.7–1.3)

Sorahan et al., 2001 (UK) (112)

761 children who were resident of Yorkshire, West Midland, and North Western Regional Health Authority area, diagnosed with cancer between January 1980 and January 1983.

Controls were selected from the lists of the case general practitioners

In-person interview

Matched: Sex and date of birth

Adjusted: Maternal or paternal age at the birth of the child, SES, and ethnic origin

ALL (140 cases)
Maternal smoking before pregnancy
Lifelong nonsmoker: Reference
<10 cpd: 1.34 (0.46–3.87)
10–19 cpd: 1.11 (0.59–2.08)
20–29 cpd: 0.98 (0.51–1.85)
30+ cpd: 0.26 (0.03–2.38)
p value for trend: 0.56

Paternal smoking before pregnancy
Lifelong nonsmoker: Reference
<10 cpd: 0.99 (0.35–2.85)
10–19 cpd: 1.34 (0.62–2.91)
20–29 cpd: 1.32 (0.72–2.45)
30–39 cpd: 2.33 (0.71–7.63)
40+ cpd: 5.29 (1.31–21.30)
p value for trend: 0.06

Pang et al., 2003 (UK) (105)

Cases were children under the age of 15 years, diagnosed with cancer between 1991–1994 in Scotland, and 1992–1994 in England and Wales.

Face-to-face structured interview

Matched: Sex, date of birth, and geographical area of residence at diagnosis

All leukemia (1,723 cases)
Paternal preconception smoking
Lifelong nonsmoker: Reference
1–19 cpd: 1.12 (0.96–1.32)
20+ cpd: 1.01 (0.87–1.17)
p for trend: 0.74

(continued)

Table 5.2
(continued)

Author, year (location) (reference)	Source of cases and controls	Data collection	Matched and adjusted variables	Primary results (odds ratios)
	For each case, two controls were randomly selected from Family Health Services Authorities list in England and Wales and Health Boards in Scotland		Adjusted: Parental age at birth of the child and deprivation score	**Maternal smoking during pregnancy** Lifelong nonsmoker: Reference 1–19 cpd: 0.93 (0.80–1.08) 20+ cpd: 0.76 (0.60–0.98) p for trend: 0.029 **ALL (1,449 cases)** Paternal preconception smoking: 1.04 (0.91–1.18) Maternal smoking during pregnancy: 0.89 (0.77–1.03) **AML (249 cases)** Paternal preconception smoking: 1.07 (0.80–1.43) Maternal smoking during pregnancy: 0.76 (0.54–1.07)
Menegaux et al., 2005 (France) (104)	Cases were all children diagnosed with acute leukemia before the age of 15 years in hospitals in Paris, Lille, Lyon, and Nancy between January 1995 and December 1999.	Face-to-face interviews with the mothers	Matched: Age, gender, hospital, and ethnic origin	**ALL** **Maternal smoking during pregnancy:** 0.9 (0.6–1.4) <5 cpd: 0.9 (0.5–1.8) 5–9 cpd: 0.8 (0.4–1.6) 10+ cpd: 1.3 (0.7–2.7) First trimester: 1.0 (0.7–1.6) Second trimester: 1.0 (0.6–1.6) Third trimester: 1.0 (0.6–1.5)

Controls were children hospitalized in the same hospital for
diseases other than cancer or
birth defects

Adjusted: None

Maternal smoking during breastfeeding: 0.7
(0.3–1.5)
Maternal smoking from birth to interview: 1.1
(0.7–1.6)
Paternal smoking from birth to interview: 1.1
(0.7–1.5)

ANLL
Maternal smoking during pregnancy: 1.0
(0.4–2.3)
<5 cpd: 1.5 (0.4–5.0)
5–9 cpd: 1.4 (0.4–4.8)
10+ cpd: —
First trimester: 0.9 (0.4–2.2)
Second trimester: 0.9 (0.3–2.2)
Third trimester: 0.9 (0.3–2.3)
Maternal smoking during breastfeeding: 1.0
(0.3–4.1)
Maternal smoking from birth to interview: 1.0
(0.5–2.1)
Paternal smoking from birth to interview: 1.3
(0.6–2.7)

Chang et al., 2006
(USA) (116)

Cases were all children
diagnosed with acute
leukemia before the age of
15 years in hospitals in the
San Francisco Bay Area and
California Central Valley
between 1995 and 2002.
Controls were randomly selected
using birth certificates

Telephone and in-person interview
with mothers

Matched: Age, sex,
Hispanic ethnicity,
and maternal race

ALL (281 cases)
Paternal smoking
Ever smoked: 1.25 (0.85–1.82)
Preconception: 1.32 (0.86–2.04)
Per cpd: 1.03 (1.00–1.06)

Maternal smoking
Ever smoked: 1.12 (0.79–1.59)
Preconception: 0.88 (0.57–1.36)
Per cpd: 1.02 (0.98–1.06)
During pregnancy: 0.93 (0.58–1.51)
Per cpd: 1.01 (0.95–1.07)
Postnatal: 0.99 (0.64–1.52)
Per cpd: 1.02 (0.98–1.06)

(continued)

Table 5.2
(continued)

Author, year (location) (reference)	Source of cases and controls	Data collection	Matched and adjusted variables	Primary results (odds ratios)
				AML (46 cases)
				Paternal smoking
				Ever smoked: 2.64 (0.98–7.12)
				Preconception: 3.84 (1.04–14.17)
				Per cpd: 1.05 (0.98–1.13)
				Maternal smoking
				Ever smoked: 1.00 (0.41–2.44)
				Preconception: 0.79 (0.21–2.95)
				Per cpd: 1.02 (0.93–1.12)
				During pregnancy: 0.60 (0.15–2.44)
				Per cpd: 1.01 (0.92–1.11)
				Postnatal: 0.94 (0.32–2.81)
				Per cpd: 1.05 (0.94–1.17)

ALL, acute lymphoblastic leukemia; *AML*, acute myeloid leukemia; *ANLL*, Acute non-lymphocytic leukemia; *cpd*, cigarettes smoked per day; *SES*, socioeconomic status association between smoking and ALL only among subjects older than 60 years old *(88)*, while the rest reported a null association *(82–85, 91)*. Of the 12 studies with data on myeloid leukemia, 9 reported a positive association between smoking and AML *(80, 82, 84–90)*, 1 reported a positive association between smoking and either AML or CML *(81)*, and only 2 reported a null association *(83, 91)*. Three of these studies reported a positive association between smoking specifically with M2 subtype of AML *(87, 88)* or AML with t(8:21) translocation *(86)*.

In summary, a majority of the cohort and case-control studies found a positive association between smoking and myeloid leukemia while the results on lymphoid leukemia have been inconclusive; however, the reason for inconsistent results seen among lymphoid leukemia could be due to the small number of cases as most of the adult leukemia is of the myeloid type.

4.2. Childhood Leukemia

4.2.1. Maternal Smoking

Three cohort studies on the association between maternal smoking during pregnancy and childhood leukemia have been published *(92–94)*. Two of the three cohort studies found no significant association between maternal smoking during pregnancy and childhood leukemia *(92, 94)*. In contrast, Mucci et al. reported a significant inverse association between maternal smoking during pregnancy and childhood ALL and a significant positive association between maternal smoking during pregnancy and childhood AML *(93)*.

Twenty case-control studies on the association between maternal smoking during pregnancy and childhood leukemia have been published between 1985 and 2005 *(95–114)*. None of the six studies with data on all leukemia combined reported a positive association between maternal smoking and childhood leukemia *(103, 105–107, 109, 113)*. Of the 15 studies with data on ALL *(95, 96, 98–102, 104, 105, 109–114)*, only 3 reported a positive association between maternal smoking and childhood ALL *(101, 111, 114)*. Of the ten studies with data on AML *(95, 97, 102, 104, 105, 108–111, 113)*, only one reported a positive association between maternal smoking and childhood AML *(97)*.

4.2.2. Paternal Smoking

All 15 published studies on the association between paternal smoking and childhood leukemia are case-control studies *(95, 100–102, 104, 105, 107–113, 115, 116)*. Of the five studies with data on all leukemia combined *(105, 107, 109, 113, 115)*, two reported a positive association between paternal smoking and childhood leukemia *(113, 115)*. Of the 13 studies with data on ALL *(95, 100–102, 104, 105, 109–113, 115, 116)*, 6 reported a positive association between paternal smoking and childhood

ALL *(101, 109, 110, 112, 115, 116)*. Of the ten studies with data on AML *(95, 102, 105, 108–111, 113, 115, 116)*, two reported a positive association between paternal smoking and childhood AML *(113, 116)*.

4.2.3. Limitations of the Studies Published to Date

Although the studies published to date suggest a stronger association between child leukemia and paternal smoking than that between childhood leukemia and maternal smoking, the results are still inconclusive regarding the role parental smoking plays on the development of childhood leukemia. One major limitation of the previous studies is that the sequence of smoking exposures was not considered. The current hypothesis is that the development of childhood leukemia requires at least a prenatal initiating event and a postnatal promoting event; therefore it is important to study the joint influence between prenatal and postnatal smoking exposures. One study that examined the joint influence of prenatal and postnatal smoking showed that greater risks of childhood ALL were observed compared with the risk associated with exposure to only paternal preconception smoking when paternal preconception smoking was combined with maternal postnatal smoking or postnatal passive smoking exposure *(116)*.

Another major limitation is the lack of genetic information, which is important in determining individual ' s susceptibility to carcinogens.

4.2.4. Gene Environment Interaction

There is evidence showing that fetal susceptibility to in utero exposure to carcinogens may be influenced by their individual genetic make-up. Whyatt et al. reported that newborns with a CYP1A1 *Msp*I variant and a GSTP isoleucine/isoleucine genotype have a higher level of white blood cell PAH-DNA adduct compared with newborns with a CYP1A1 *Msp*I variant absent and a GSTP valine/valine genotype *(117)*. Similarly, Pluth et al. reported that newborns who are heterozygous for the CYP1A1 *Msp*I variant had higher chromosomal aberration frequencies compared with children who are homozygous for CYP1A1 wild type *(118)*.

Only two studies to date have examined the interaction between maternal smoking and metabolizing genes on the development of childhood leukemia *(100, 119)*. Using a case-only design, Infante-Rivard et al. showed that CYP1A1*2A or CYP1A1*4 alleles has a positive joint influence with maternal smoking during pregnancy on the development of childhood ALL, although the results were not significant presumably due to a small study population (n=158) *(100)*. In a study by Clavel et al., a significant positive joint influence was found between maternal smoking during pregnancy and *CYP1A1* or *GSTM1* gene on the development of childhood leukemia using the case-only analysis; however, the case-control analyses of the same data set did not reach the same conclusion *(119)*.

Although the existing evidence indicates a dominant effect of environmental risk factors in the development of leukemia, studies by both Infante-Rivard et al. and Clavel et al. suggest that genetics can be a modifying factor that confers a variable susceptibility to the environmental risk factors *(100, 119)*; therefore, more studies regarding the influence of one's genetic make-up are warranted.

4.3. Future Directions and Conclusion

In spite of the many studies conducted on the association between parental smoking and childhood leukemia, the results have been inconclusive. Future directions to be considered for improving the study of parental smoking and childhood leukemia are:

1. Although smoking is one of the major sources of benzene, an established leukemogen, other sources of benzene exposure including traffic and parental occupational exposure should also be considered to reduce the misclassification of subject's benzene exposure status.

2. Although not firmly established, more studies suggest the association between paternal preconception smoking and childhood leukemia compared with the studies with maternal smoking. More studies need to be conducted to investigate whether the association is real or is due to recall bias as all the studies with paternal smoking to date have been case-control in design. In addition, more animal and biological studies need to be conducted to determine whether there is a biological explanation for the association between paternal preconception smoking and childhood leukemia.

3. Childhood leukemia is a heterogeneous disease. In addition to categorization by histology (lymphoblastic versus myeloid), childhood leukemia can be further categorized by molecular techniques (e.g., structural and numerical changes) into more homogeneous subgroups, which will increase the power to establish the associations between specific environmental exposures and specific molecular changes.

4. The metabolic pathways of chemicals in tobacco require the actions of many different enzymes; therefore, examining the joint effect of multiple genes may be more informative than studying a single gene. In addition to the child's genetic information, it is also important to collect genetic information from the mother. Chemicals from maternal smoking first get into mother's bloodstream, where they can be detoxified or activated by mother's metabolizing enzymes before they cross the placenta and reach a child's bloodstream. Thus, for a more complete picture of a child's in utero exposure to carcinogens, it would be important to consider both the mother's and the child's genetic information.
   With the advancement of biotechnology, the completion of the Human Genome Project, and information from the

International Hapmap Project, epidemiologists now have more tools than ever to study disease etiology and progression. It is hoped that through the continual effort, more will be uncovered regarding the causes of childhood leukemia. In the meantime, more effort should be spent on educating the parents to quit smoking, because parental smoking is known to affect many childhood diseases (e.g., asthma, respiratory tract infection, and otitis media) that are much more prevalent than childhood leukemia *(120)*.

References

1. Ries, L.A.G., Smith, M.A., Gurney, J.G., Linet, M., Tamra, T., Young, J.L. and Bunin, G.R. (eds.) (1999) *Cancer Incidence and Survival among Children and Adolescents: United States SEER Program 1975–1995*. National Cancer Institute, SEER Program. NIH Pub. No. 99–4649, Bethesda, MD.
2. Pui, C.H. (1999) *Childhood Leukemia*. Cambridge University Press, New York.
3. Parkin, D.M., Kramarova, E., Draper, G.J., Masuyer, E., Michaelis, J., Neglia, J., Qureshi, S. and Stiller, C.A. (eds.) (1998) *International Incidence of Childhood Cancer, Vol II*. International Agency for Research on Cancer, Lyon, France.
4. Ries, L.A.G., Harkins, D., Krapcho, M., Mariotto, A., Miller, B.A., Feuer, E.J., Clegg, L., Eisner, M.P., Horner, M.J., Howlader, N., et al. (eds.) (2006) *SEER Cancer Statistics Review, 1975–2003*. National Cancer Institute, Bethesda, MD, http://seer.cancer.gov/csr/1975_2003/, based on November 2005 SEER data submission, posted to the SEER web site, 2006.
5. Greaves, M.F. and Alexander, F.E. (1993) An infectious etiology for common acute lymphoblastic leukemia in childhood? *Leukemia*, 7, 349–360.
6. Cummins, C., Winter, H., Maric, R., Cheng, K.K., Silcocks, P., Varghese, C., and Batlle, G. (2001) Childhood cancer in the south Asian population of England (1990–1992). *Br J Cancer*, 84, 1215–1218.
7. McKinney, P.A., Feltbower, R.G., Parslow, R.C., Lewis, I.J., Glaser, A.W., and Kinsey, S.E. (2003) Patterns of childhood cancer by ethnic group in Bradford, UK 1974–1997. *Eur J Cancer*, 39, 92–97.
8. Winther, J.F., Sankila, R., Boice, J.D., Tulinius, H., Bautz, A., Barlow, L., Glattre, E., Langmark, F., Moller, T.R., Mulvihill, J.J., et al. (2001) Cancer in siblings of children with cancer in the Nordic countries: a population-based cohort study. *Lancet*, 358, 711–717.
9. Olsen, J.H., Boice, J.D., Jr., Seersholm, N., Bautz, A., and Fraumeni, J.F., Jr. (1995) Cancer in the parents of children with cancer. *N Engl J Med*, 333, 1594–1599.
10. Buckley, J.D., Buckley, C.M., Breslow, N.E., Draper, G.J., Roberson, P.K., and Mack, T.M. (1996) Concordance for childhood cancer in twins. *Med Pediatr Oncol*, 26, 223–229.
11. Greaves, M.F., Maia, A.T., Wiemels, J.L., and Ford, A.M. (2003) Leukemia in twins: lessons in natural history. *Blood*, 102, 2321–2333.
12. Kadan-Lottick, N.S., Kawashima, T., Tomlinson, G., Friedman, D.L., Yasui, Y., Mertens, A.C., Robison, L.L., and Strong, L.C. (2005) The risk of cancer in twins: A report from the childhood cancer survivor study. *Pediatr Blood Cancer*.
13. Ford, A.M., Ridge, S.A., Cabrera, M.E., Mahmoud, H., Steel, C.M., Chan, L.C., and Greaves, M. (1993) In utero rearrangements in the trithorax-related oncogene in infant leukaemias. *Nature*, 363, 358–360.
14. Wiemels, J.L., Ford, A.M., Van Wering, E.R., Postma, A., and Greaves, M. (1999) Protracted and variable latency of acute lymphoblastic leukemia after TEL-AML1 gene fusion in utero. *Blood*, 94, 1057–1062.
15. Greaves, M.F. and Wiemels, J. (2003) Origins of chromosome translocations in childhood leukaemia. *Nat Rev Cancer*, 3, 639–649.
16. Mori, H., Colman, S.M., Xiao, Z., Ford, A.M., Healy, L.E., Donaldson, C., Hows, J.M., Navarrete, C., and Greaves, M. (2002) Chromosome translocations and covert leukemic clones are generated during normal fetal development. *Proc Natl Acad Sci U S A*, 99, 8242–8247.

17. Phares, T.M., Morrow, B., Lansky, A., Barfield, W.D., Prince, C.B., Marchi, K.S., Braveman, P.A., Williams, L.M., and Kinniburgh, B. (2004) Surveillance for disparities in maternal health-related behaviors--selected states, Pregnancy Risk Assessment Monitoring System (PRAMS), 2000–2001. *MMWR Surveill Summ*, **53**, 1–13.

18. Higuchi, M., O'Brien, D., Kumaravelu, P., Lenny, N., Yeoh, E.J., and Downing, J.R. (2002) Expression of a conditional AML1-ETO oncogene bypasses embryonic lethality and establishes a murine model of human t(8;21) acute myeloid leukemia. *Cancer Cell*, **1**, 63–74.

19. Andreasson, P., Schwaller, J., Anastasiadou, E., Aster, J., and Gilliland, D.G. (2001) The expression of ETV6/CBFA2 (TEL/AML1) is not sufficient for the transformation of hematopoietic cell lines in vitro or the induction of hematologic disease in vivo. *Cancer Genet Cytogenet*, **130**, 93–104.

20. Rhoades, K.L., Hetherington, C.J., Harakawa, N., Yergeau, D.A., Zhou, L., Liu, L.Q., Little, M.T., Tenen, D.G., and Zhang, D.E. (2000) Analysis of the role of AML1-ETO in leukemogenesis, using an inducible transgenic mouse model. *Blood*, **96**, 2108–2115.

21. Bernardin, F., Yang, Y., Cleaves, R., Zahurak, M., Cheng, L., Civin, C.I., and Friedman, A.D. (2002) TEL-AML1, expressed from t(12;21) in human acute lymphocytic leukemia, induces acute leukemia in mice. *Cancer Res*, **62**, 3904–3908.

22. Matsuno, N., Osato, M., Yamashita, N., Yanagida, M., Nanri, T., Fukushima, T., Motoji, T., Kusumoto, S., Towatari, M., Suzuki, R., et al. (2003) Dual mutations in the AML1 and FLT3 genes are associated with leukemogenesis in acute myeloblastic leukemia of the M0 subtype. *Leukemia*, **17**, 2492–2499.

23. Yuan, Y., Zhou, L., Miyamoto, T., Iwasaki, H., Harakawa, N., Hetherington, C.J., Burel, S.A., Lagasse, E., Weissman, I.L., Akashi, K., et al. (2001) AML1-ETO expression is directly involved in the development of acute myeloid leukemia in the presence of additional mutations. *Proc Natl Acad Sci U S A*, **98**, 10398–10403.

24. Schessl, C., Rawat, V.P., Cusan, M., Deshpande, A., Kohl, T.M., Rosten, P.M., Spiekermann, K., Humphries, R.K., Schnittger, S., Kern, W., et al. (2005) The AML1-ETO fusion gene and the FLT3 length mutation collaborate in inducing acute leukemia in mice. *J Clin Invest*, **115**, 2159–2168.

25. Greaves, M. (2002) Childhood leukaemia. *BMJ*, **324**, 283–287.

26. International Agency for Research on Cancer. (2004) *IARC monograph on the evaluation of carcinogenic risks to humans: tobacco smoke and involuntary smoking.* International Agency for Research on Cancer, Volume **83**, Lyon, France.

27. Centers for Disease Control and Prevention. (2004) State-specific prevalence of current cigarette smoking among adults—Unites States, 2002. *MMWR Morb Mortal Wkly Rep*, **52**, 1277–1280.

28. Mackay, J. and Eriksen, M. (2002) *The tobacco atlas.* World Health Organization, Geneva, Switzerland.

29. Hecht, S.S. (2003) Tobacco carcinogens, their biomarkers and tobacco-induced cancer. *Nat Rev Cancer*, **3**, 733–744.

30. International Agency for Research on Cancer. Lists of IARC Evaluations, 2004. http://www-cie.iarc.fr/monoeval/grlist.html.

31. Wallace, L. (1996) Environmental exposure to benzene: an update. *Environ Health Perspect*, **104 Suppl 6**, 1129–1136.

32. Snyder, R. and Hedli, C.C. (1996) An overview of benzene metabolism. *Environ Health Perspect*, **104 Suppl 6**, 1165–1171.

33. Schnatter, A.R., Rosamilia, K., and Wojcik, N.C. (2005) Review of the literature on benzene exposure and leukemia subtypes. *Chem Biol Interact*, **153–154**, 9–21.

34. Zhang, L., Wang, Y., Shang, N., and Smith, M.T. (1998) Benzene metabolites induce the loss and long arm deletion of chromosomes 5 and 7 in human lymphocytes. *Leuk Res*, **22**, 105–113.

35. Zhang, L., Rothman, N., Wang, Y., Hayes, R.B., Li, G., Dosemeci, M., Yin, S., Kolachana, P., Titenko-Holland, N., and Smith, M.T. (1998) Increased aneusomy and long arm deletion of chromosomes 5 and 7 in the lymphocytes of Chinese workers exposed to benzene. *Carcinogenesis*, **19**, 1955–1961.

36. Smith, M.T., Zhang, L., Wang, Y., Hayes, R.B., Li, G., Wiemels, J., Dosemeci, M., Titenko-Holland, N., Xi, L., Kolachana, P., et al. (1998) Increased translocations and aneusomy in chromosomes 8 and 21 among workers exposed to benzene. *Cancer Res*, **58**, 2176–2181.

37. Rice, J.M. and Boffetta, P. (2001) 1,3-Butadiene, isoprene and chloroprene: reviews by the IARC monographs programme, outstanding issues, and research priorities in epidemiology. *Chem Biol Interact*, **135–136**, 11–26.

38. Jackson, M.A., Stack, H.F., Rice, J.M., and Waters, M.D. (2000) A review of the genetic and related effects of 1,3-butadiene in rodents and humans. *Mutat Res*, **463**, 181–213.

39. Henderson, R.F., Thornton-Manning, J.R., Bechtold, W.E., and Dahl, A.R. (1996) Metabolism of 1,3-butadiene: species differences. *Toxicology*, **113**, 17–22.

40. Delzell, E., Macaluso, M., Sathiakumar, N., and Matthews, R. (2001) Leukemia and exposure to 1,3-butadiene, styrene and dimethyldithiocarbamate among workers in the synthetic rubber industry. *Chem Biol Interact*, **135–136**, 515–534.

41. Tsai, S.P., Wendt, J.K., and Ransdell, J.D. (2001) A mortality, morbidity, and hematology study of petrochemical employees potentially exposed to 1,3-butadiene monomer. *Chem Biol Interact*, **135–136**, 555–567.

42. Divine, B.J. and Hartman, C.M. (2001) A cohort mortality study among workers at a 1,3 butadiene facility. *Chem Biol Interact*, 135–136, 535–553.

43. Baird, W.M., Hooven, L.A., and Mahadevan, B. (2005) Carcinogenic polycyclic aromatic hydrocarbon-DNA adducts and mechanism of action. *Environ Mol Mutagen*, **45**, 106–114.

44. Heidel, S.M., MacWilliams, P.S., Baird, W.M., Dashwood, W.M., Buters, J.T., Gonzalez, F.J., Larsen, M.C., Czuprynski, C.J., and Jefcoate, C.R. (2000) Cytochrome P4501B1 mediates induction of bone marrow cytotoxicity and preleukemia cells in mice treated with 7,12-dimethylbenz(a)anthracene. *Cancer Res*, **60**, 3454–3460.

45. Sugiyama, T., Osaka, M., Koami, K., Maeda, S., and Ueda, N. (2002) 7,12-DMBA-induced rat leukemia: a review with insights into future research. *Leuk Res*, **26**, 1053–1068.

46. Boffetta, P., Jourenkova, N., and Gustavsson, P. (1997) Cancer risk from occupational and environmental exposure to polycyclic aromatic hydrocarbons. *Cancer Causes Control*, **8**, 444–472.

47. Pearson, R.L., Wachtel, H., and Ebi, K.L. (2000) Distance-weighted traffic density in proximity to a home is a risk factor for leukemia and other childhood cancers. *J Air Waste Manag Assoc*, **50**, 175–180.

48. Crosignani, P., Tittarelli, A., Borgini, A., Codazzi, T., Rovelli, A., Porro, E., Contiero, P., Bianchi, N., Tagliabue, G., Fissi, R., et al. (2004) Childhood leukemia and road traffic: A population-based case-control study. *Int J Cancer*, **108**, 596–599.

49. Visser, O., van Wijnen, J.H., and van Leeuwen, F.E. (2004) Residential traffic density and cancer incidence in Amsterdam, 1989–1997. *Cancer Causes Control*, **15**, 331–339.

50. Reynolds, P., Elkin, E., Scalf, R., Von Behren, J., and Neutra, R.R. (2001) A case-control pilot study of traffic exposures and early childhood leukemia using a geographic information system. *Bioelectromagnetics*, **Suppl 5**, S58–68.

51. Langholz, B., Ebi, K.L., Thomas, D.C., Peters, J.M., and London, S.J. (2002) Traffic density and the risk of childhood leukemia in a Los Angeles case-control study. *Ann Epidemiol*, **12**, 482–487.

52. Cassidy, L.D., Youk, A.O., and Marsh, G.M. (2003) The Drake Health Registry Study: cause-specific mortality experience of workers potentially exposed to beta-naphthylamine. *Am J Ind Med*, **44**, 282–290.

53. Veys, C.A. (2004) Bladder tumours in rubber workers: a factory study 1946–1995. *Occup Med (Lond)*, **54**, 322–329.

54. Vineis, P. and Pirastu, R. (1997) Aromatic amines and cancer. *Cancer Causes Control*, **8**, 346–355.

55. Skipper, P.L., Tannenbaum, S.R., Ross, R.K., and Yu, M.C. (2003) Nonsmoking-related arylamine exposure and bladder cancer risk. *Cancer Epidemiol Biomarkers Prev*, **12**, 503–507.

56. Klassen, C. (ed.) (2001) *Toxicology: the basic science of poisons*. McGraw-Hill, New York.

57. Feng, Z., Hu, W., Rom, W.N., Beland, F.A., and Tang, M.S. (2002) 4-aminobiphenyl is a major etiological agent of human bladder cancer: evidence from its DNA binding spectrum in human p53 gene. *Carcinogenesis*, **23**, 1721–1727.

58. Ohnishi, S., Murata, M., and Kawanishi, S. (2002) Oxidative DNA damage induced by a metabolite of 2-naphthylamine, a smoking-related bladder carcinogen. *Jpn J Cancer Res*, **93**, 736–743.

59. Hecht, S.S. (1998) Biochemistry, biology, and carcinogenicity of tobacco-specific N-nitrosamines. *Chem Res Toxicol*, **11**, 559–603.

60. Fraga, C.G., Motchnik, P.A., Wyrobek, A.J., Rempel, D.M., and Ames, B.N. (1996) Smoking and low antioxidant levels increase oxidative damage to sperm DNA. *Mutat Res*, **351**, 199–203.

61. Shen, H.M., Chia, S.E., Ni, Z.Y., New, A.L., Lee, B.L., and Ong, C.N. (1997) Detection of oxidative DNA damage in human sperm and the association with cigarette smoking. *Reprod Toxicol*, **11**, 675–80.

62. Shi, Q., Ko, E., Barclay, L., Hoang, T., Rademaker, A., and Martin, R. (2001) Cigarette smoking and aneuploidy in human sperm. *Mol Reprod Dev*, **59**, 417–421.

63. Zenzes, M.T., Bielecki, R., and Reed, T.E. (1999) Detection of benzo(a)pyrene diol epoxide-DNA adducts in sperm of men exposed to cigarette smoke. *Fertil Steril*, **72**, 330–335.

64. Zenzes, M.T., Puy, L.A., Bielecki, R., and Reed, T.E. (1999) Detection of benzo(a)pyrene diol epoxide-DNA adducts in embryos from smoking couples: evidence for transmission by spermatozoa. *Mol Hum Reprod*, **5**, 125–131.

65. Ammenheuser, M.M., Berenson, A.B., Stiglich, N.J., Whorton, E.B., Jr., and Ward, J.B., Jr. (1994) Elevated frequencies of hprt mutant lymphocytes in cigarette-smoking mothers and their newborns. *Mutat Res*, **304**, 285–294.

66. de la Chica, R.A., Ribas, I., Giraldo, J., Egozcue, J., and Fuster, C. (2005) Chromosomal instability in amniocytes from fetuses of mothers who smoke. *Jama*, **293**, 1212–1222.

67. Ng, S.P., Silverstone, A.E., Lai, Z.W., and Zelikoff, J.T. (2006) Effects of prenatal exposure to cigarette smoke on offspring tumor susceptibility and associated immune mechanisms. *Toxicol Sci*, **89**, 135–144.

68. Crawford, F.G., Mayer, J., Santella, R.M., Cooper, T.B., Ottman, R., Tsai, W.Y., Simon-Cereijido, G., Wang, M., Tang, D., and Perera, F.P. (1994) Biomarkers of environmental tobacco smoke in preschool children and their mothers. *J Natl Cancer Inst*, **86**, 1398–1402.

69. Tang, D., Warburton, D., Tannenbaum, S.R., Skipper, P., Santella, R.M., Cereijido, G.S., Crawford, F.G., and Perera, F.P. (1999) Molecular and genetic damage from environmental tobacco smoke in young children. *Cancer Epidemiol Biomarkers Prev*, **8**, 427–431.

70. Adami, J., Nyren, O., Bergstrom, R., Ekbom, A., Engholm, G., Englund, A., and Glimelius, B. (1998) Smoking and the risk of leukemia, lymphoma, and multiple myeloma (Sweden). *Cancer Causes Control*, **9**, 49–56.

71. Engeland, A., Andersen, A., Haldorsen, T., and Tretli, S. (1996) Smoking habits and risk of cancers other than lung cancer: 28 years' follow-up of 26,000 Norwegian men and women. *Cancer Causes Control*, **7**, 497–506.

72. Friedman, G.D. (1993) Cigarette smoking, leukemia, and multiple myeloma. *Ann Epidemiol*, **3**, 425–428.

73. Garfinkel, L. and Boffetta, P. (1990) Association between smoking and leukemia in two American Cancer Society prospective studies. *Cancer*, **65**, 2356–2360.

74. Kinlen, L.J. and Rogot, E. (1988) Leukaemia and smoking habits among United States veterans. *BMJ*, **297**, 657–659.

75. Linet, M.S., McLaughlin, J.K., Hsing, A.W., Wacholder, S., Co-Chien, H.T., Schuman, L.M., Bjelke, E., and Blot, W.J. (1991) Cigarette smoking and leukemia: results from the Lutheran Brotherhood Cohort Study. *Cancer Causes Control*, **2**, 413–417.

76. McLaughlin, J.K., Hrubec, Z., Linet, M.S., Heineman, E.F., Blot, W.J., and Fraumeni, J.F., Jr. (1989) Cigarette smoking and leukemia. *J Natl Cancer Inst*, **81**, 1262–1263.

77. Mills, P.K., Newell, G.R., Beeson, W.L., Fraser, G.E., and Phillips, R.L. (1990) History of cigarette smoking and risk of leukemia and myeloma: results from the Adventist health study. *J Natl Cancer Inst*, **82**, 1832–1836.

78. Nordlund, L.A., Carstensen, J.M., and Pershagen, G. (1997) Cancer incidence in female smokers: a 26-year follow-up. *Int J Cancer*, **73**, 625–628.

79. Tulinius, H., Sigfusson, N., Sigvaldason, H., Bjarnadottir, K., and Tryggvadottir, L. (1997) Risk factors for malignant diseases: a cohort study on a population of 22,946 Icelanders. *Cancer Epidemiol Biomarkers Prev*, **6**, 863–873.

80. Bjork, J., Albin, M., Mauritzson, N., Stromberg, U., Johansson, B., and Hagmar, L. (2001) Smoking and acute myeloid leukemia: associations with morphology and karyotypic patterns and evaluation of dose-response relations. *Leuk Res*, **25**, 865–872.

81. Brown, L.M., Gibson, R., Blair, A., Burmeister, L.F., Schuman, L.M., Cantor, K.P., and Fraumeni, J.F., Jr. (1992) Smoking and risk of leukemia. *Am J Epidemiol*, **135**, 763–768.

82. Brownson, R.C., Chang, J.C., and Davis, J.R. (1991) Cigarette smoking and risk of adult leukemia. *Am J Epidemiol*, **134**, 938–941.

83. Kabat, G.C., Augustine, A., and Hebert, J.R. (1988) Smoking and adult leukemia: a case-control study. *J Clin Epidemiol*, **41**, 907–914.

84. Kane, E.V., Roman, E., Cartwright, R., Parker, J., and Morgan, G. (1999) Tobacco and the risk of acute leukaemia in adults. *Br J Cancer*, **81**, 1228–1233.

85. Mele, A., Szklo, M., Visani, G., Stazi, M.A., Castelli, G., Pasquini, P., and Mandelli, F. (1994) Hair dye use and other risk factors for leukemia and pre-leukemia: a case-control study. Italian Leukemia Study Group. *Am J Epidemiol*, **139**, 609–619.

86. Moorman, A.V., Roman, E., Cartwright, R.A., and Morgan, G.J. (2002) Smoking and the risk of acute myeloid leukaemia in cytogenetic subgroups. *Br J Cancer*, **86**, 60–62.

87. Pogoda, J.M., Preston-Martin, S., Nichols, P.W., and Ross, R.K. (2002) Smoking and risk of acute myeloid leukemia: results from a Los Angeles County case-control study. *Am J Epidemiol*, **155**, 546–553.

88. Sandler, D.P., Shore, D.L., Anderson, J.R., Davey, F.R., Arthur, D., Mayer, R.J., Silver, R.T., Weiss, R.B., Moore, J.O., Schiffer, C.A., et al. (1993) Cigarette smoking and risk of acute leukemia: associations with morphology and cytogenetic abnormalities in bone marrow. *J Natl Cancer Inst*, **85**, 1994–2003.

89. Severson, R.K. (1987) Cigarette smoking and leukemia. *Cancer*, **60**, 141–144.

90. Severson, R.K., Davis, S., Heuser, L., Daling, J.R., and Thomas, D.B. (1990) Cigarette smoking and acute nonlymphocytic leukemia. *Am J Epidemiol*, 132, 418–422.

91. Stagnaro, E., Ramazzotti, V., Crosignani, P., Fontana, A., Masala, G., Miligi, L., Nanni, O., Neri, M., Rodella, S., Costantini, A.S., et al. (2001) Smoking and hematolymphopoietic malignancies. *Cancer Causes Control*, **12**, 325–334.

92. Klebanoff, M.A., Clemens, J.D., and Read, J.S. (1996) Maternal smoking during pregnancy and childhood cancer. *Am J Epidemiol*, **144**, 1028–1033.

93. Mucci, L.A., Granath, F., and Cnattingius, S. (2004) Maternal smoking and childhood leukemia and lymphoma risk among 1,440,542 Swedish children. *Cancer Epidemiol Biomarkers Prev*, **13**, 1528–1533.

94. Pershagen, G., Ericson, A., and Otterblad-Olausson, P. (1992) Maternal smoking in pregnancy: does it increase the risk of childhood cancer? *Int J Epidemiol*, **21**, 1–5.

95. Brondum, J., Shu, X.O., Steinbuch, M., Severson, R.K., Potter, J.D., and Robison, L.L. (1999) Parental cigarette smoking and the risk of acute leukemia in children. *Cancer*, **85**, 1380–1388.

96. Buckley, J.D., Hobbie, W.L., Ruccione, K., Sather, H.N., Woods, W.G., and Hammond, G.D. (1986) Maternal smoking during pregnancy and the risk of childhood cancer (Letter). 2, 519–520.

97. Cnattingius, S., Zack, M., Ekbom, A., Gunnarskog, J., Linet, M., and Adami, H.O. (1995) Prenatal and neonatal risk factors for childhood myeloid leukemia. *Cancer Epidemiol Biomarkers Prev*, **4**, 441–445.

98. Cnattingius, S., Zack, M.M., Ekbom, A., Gunnarskog, J., Kreuger, A., Linet, M., and Adami, H.O. (1995) Prenatal and neonatal risk factors for childhood lymphatic leukemia. *J Natl Cancer Inst*, **87**, 908–914.

99. Cocco, P., Rapallo, M., Targhetta, R., Biddau, P.F., and Fadda, D. (1996) Analysis of risk factors in a cluster of childhood acute lymphoblastic leukemia. *Arch Environ Health*, **51**, 242–244.

100. Infante-Rivard, C., Krajinovic, M., Labuda, D., and Sinnett, D. (2000) Parental smoking, CYP1A1 genetic polymorphisms and childhood leukemia (Quebec, Canada). *Cancer Causes Control*, **11**, 547–553.

101. John, E.M., Savitz, D.A., and Sandler, D.P. (1991) Prenatal exposure to parents' smoking and childhood cancer. *Am J Epidemiol*, **133,** 123–132.

102. Magnani, C., Pastore, G., Luzzatto, L., and Terracini, B. (1990) Parental occupation and other environmental factors in the etiology of leukemias and non-Hodgkin's lymphomas in childhood: a case-control study. *Tumori*, **76**, 413–419.

103. McKinney, P.A. and Stiller, C.A. (1986) Maternal smoking during pregnancy and the risk of childhood cancer (Letter). *Lancet*, 2, 519–520.

104. Menegaux, F., Steffen, C., Bellec, S., Baruchel, A., Lescoeur, B., Leverger, G., Nelken, B., Philippe, N., Sommelet, D., Hemon, D., et al. (2005) Maternal coffee and alcohol consumption during pregnancy, parental smoking and risk of childhood acute leukaemia. *Cancer Detect Prev*, **29**, 487–493.

105. Pang, D., McNally, R., and Birch, J.M. (2003) Parental smoking and childhood cancer: results from the United Kingdom Childhood Cancer Study. *Br J Cancer*, **88**, 373–381.

106. Petridou, E., Trichopoulos, D., Kalapothaki, V., Pourtsidis, A., Kogevinas, M., Kalmanti, M., Koliouskas, D., Kosmidis, H., Panagiotou, J.P., Piperopoulou, F., et al. (1997) The risk profile of childhood leukaemia in Greece: a nationwide case-control study. *Br J Cancer*, **76**, 1241–1247.

107. Schuz, J., Kaatsch, P., Kaletsch, U., Meinert, R., and Michaelis, J. (1999) Association of childhood cancer with factors related to pregnancy and birth. *Int J Epidemiol*, **28**, 631–639.

108. Severson, R.K., Buckley, J.D., Woods, W.G., Benjamin, D., and Robison, L.L. (1993) Cigarette smoking and alcohol consumption by parents of children with acute myeloid leukemia: an analysis within morphological subgroups--a report from the Childrens

Cancer Group. *Cancer Epidemiol Biomarkers Prev*, **2**, 433–439.

109. Shu, X.O., Ross, J.A., Pendergrass, T.W., Reaman, G.H., Lampkin, B., and Robison, L.L. (1996) Parental alcohol consumption, cigarette smoking, and risk of infant leukemia: a Childrens Cancer Group study. *J Natl Cancer Inst*, **88**, 24–31.

110. Sorahan, T., Lancashire, R., Prior, P., Peck, I., and Stewart, A. (1995) Childhood cancer and parental use of alcohol and tobacco. *Ann Epidemiol*, **5**, 354–359.

111. Sorahan, T., Lancashire, R.J., Hulten, M.A., Peck, I., and Stewart, A.M. (1997) Childhood cancer and parental use of tobacco: deaths from 1953 to 1955. *Br J Cancer*, **75**, 134–138.

112. Sorahan, T., McKinney, P.A., Mann, J.R., Lancashire, R.J., Stiller, C.A., Birch, J.M., Dodd, H.E., and Cartwright, R.A. (2001) Childhood cancer and parental use of tobacco: findings from the inter-regional epidemiological study of childhood cancer (IRESCC). *Br J Cancer*, **84**, 141–146.

113. Sorahan, T., Prior, P., Lancashire, R.J., Faux, S.P., Hulten, M.A., Peck, I.M., and Stewart, A.M. (1997) Childhood cancer and parental use of tobacco: deaths from 1971 to 1976. *Br J Cancer*, **76**, 1525–1531.

114. Stjerntfeldt, M., Berglund, K., Lindsten, J., and Ludvigsson, J. (1986) Maternal smoking during pregnancy and risk of childhood cancer. *Lancet*, **1**, 1350–1352.

115. Ji, B.T., Shu, X.O., Linet, M.S., Zheng, W., Wacholder, S., Gao, Y.T., Ying, D.M., and Jin, F. (1997) Paternal cigarette smoking and the risk of childhood cancer among offspring of nonsmoking mothers. *J Natl Cancer Inst*, **89**, 238–244.

116. Chang, J.S., Selvin, S., Metayer, C., Crouse, V., Golembesky, A., and Buffler, P.A. (2006) Parental smoking and the risk of childhood leukemia. *Am J Epidemiol*, **163**, 1091–1100.

117. Whyatt, R.M., Perera, F.P., Jedrychowski, W., Santella, R.M., Garte, S., and Bell, D.A. (2000) Association between polycyclic aromatic hydrocarbon-DNA adduct levels in maternal and newborn white blood cells and glutathione S-transferase P1 and CYP1A1 polymorphisms. *Cancer Epidemiol Biomarkers Prev*, **9**, 207–212.

118. Pluth, J.M., Ramsey, M.J., and Tucker, J.D. (2000) Role of maternal exposures and newborn genotypes on newborn chromosome aberration frequencies. *Mutat Res*, **465**, 101–111.

119. Clavel, J., Bellec, S., Rebouissou, S., Menegaux, F., Feunteun, J., Bonaiti-Pellie, C., Baruchel, A., Kebaili, K., Lambilliotte, A., Leverger, G., et al. (2005) Childhood leukaemia, polymorphisms of metabolism enzyme genes, and interactions with maternal tobacco, coffee and alcohol consumption during pregnancy. *Eur J Cancer Prev.*, **14**, 531–540.

120. DiFranza, J.R., Aligne, C.A., and Weitzman, M. (2004) Prenatal and postnatal environmental tobacco smoke exposure and children's health. *Pediatrics*, **113**, 1007–1015.

Chapter 6

Lung Cancer and Exposure to Metals:
The Epidemiological Evidence

Pascal Wild, Eve Bourgkard, and Christophe Paris

Abstract

Exposure to metallic compounds is ubiquitous, with its widespread use in industry and its presence, mostly in trace amounts, in the environment. This paper reviews the epidemiologic evidence of the relation between lung cancer and exposure to metallic compounds by building on and updating the corresponding International Agency for Research on Cancer (IARC) assessments. Given that most of the well-identified human populations with given metal exposure are in occupational settings, this review is mostly based on results in occupational epidemiology. The epidemiological evidence is shortly reviewed for accepted carcinogens: chromium, nickel, beryllium, cadmium, arsenic, and silicon, highlighting what is still unclear. We then review in more detail metals for which the evidence is less clear: lead, titanium, iron, and cobalt. There is scarce evidence for the human carcinogenicity of titanium. Exposure to titanium dioxide is associated with lung cancer excesses in one large study, but this excess may be due to confounders. The evidence for lead is contradictory. The lung cancer risk is presented as a function of a post hoc exposure ranking but no dose—response relationship is found. A weak but consistent lung cancer excess in many populations exposed to iron oxides but it is not possible to state on causality. Finally the evidence in the hard metal industry is presented, which suggests a possible carcinogenic effect of cobalt in presence of tungsten carbide. A short discussion presents the limitations of epidemiology in assessing the carcinogenicity of metals.

Key words: Carcinogens, environmental factors, lung cancer, metal carcinogens.

---

1. Introduction

Metals are defined in chemistry as elements that readily form positive ions and have metallic bonds. Although nonmetal elements are more commonplace on Earth than metallic elements, the latter constitute most of the periodic table of elements. Thus (including metalloids), over 80 different metallic elements exist, most of which exist with different chemical valences and in many compounds. However, many of these elements are very rare and

M. Verma (ed.), *Methods of Molecular Biology, Cancer Epidemiology, vol. 472*
© 2009 Humana Press, a part of Springer Science+Business Media, Totowa, NJ
Book doi: 10.1007/978-1-60327-492-0

do not correspond to a large enough group of exposed humans to allow any epidemiological investigation of their possible effect. Nevertheless, certain rare metals are used in specific industrial applications so that there are some occupationally exposed groups, in which an epidemiological follow-up is possible.

It must be noted that the highest and most specific metal exposures occurred and still occur in occupational settings or in the immediate environment of industrial sources. The metal exposure in environmental settings is widespread but, except in immediate environment of industrial sources, much lower, much less specific and usually impossible to quantify precisely. Thus most epidemiological evidence, which can be directly related to an exposure to one or several metals, comes from cohort studies in occupational exposure groups.

We shall first screen systematically all metallic elements from the periodic table. Doing this, a first issue for each element is to identify whether there are any numerous enough human groups that are exposed to this metal or to its basic salts and compounds or whether there is any indication that such a group will exist in the future. A second issue is whether a suspicion of carcinogenicity has been raised with respect to this metal. This suspicion can be based on epidemiological studies or on other scientific evidence.

Finally we shall review the epidemiological evidence for the metals thus selected. This review will not concentrate on metals that have been officially classified as carcinogens for humans by regulatory agencies like the International Agency for Research on Cancer (IARC) or the United States National Toxicology Program (NTP) through its Reports on Carcinogens (RoC), although the rationale for each classification will be presented. For a list of possible or probable carcinogens, see the website of the American Cancer Society (http://www.cancer.org/docroot/PED/content/PED_1_3x_Known_and_Probable_Carcinogens.asp?sitearea=PED). Carcinogenicity of radioactive elements will not be discussed either, as their possible specific effect will be confounded with the effect of radioactivity. This review will concentrate on elements and their immediate compounds for which a suspicion of carcinogenicity has been published and that are typically classified as "probably or possibly carcinogenic" (2A or 2B) by IARC or "reasonably anticipated to be carcinogenic" by the NTP.

2. Metals: An Overview

Figure 6.1 shows the periodic table of elements. Starting with bottom of the table, nearly all elements with an atomic number >86 are more or less radioactive and few human exposure groups exist. Possible exceptions with a low radioactivity and some human exposures are uranium-238 (depleted uranium) and thorium-232 dioxide. The group of lanthanides (scandium, yttrium, and the elements with atomic numbers between 57 and 71) also misnamed as rare earth elements (some lanthanides like, e.g., cerium, are quite common in the earth crust), have some industrial applications and some human exposure has been documented but no suspicion of carcinogenicity has been published to our knowledge (*see* **ref**. *(1)*). There is no suspected carcinogen within the group of alkali metals (except for an arsenic compound of lithium that has been classified as carcinogenic as an arsenic compound). Within the group of alkaline earth metals, beryllium (Be) is classified as carcinogenic to humans both by IARC and NTP. Contrary to its radioactive form, ^{90}Strontium, suspected to be a bone carcinogen because it substitutes easily for calcium, its stable isotopes seem innocuous. The same lack of suspicion is true for the other alkali earth metals (calcium, magnesium, and barium). Most of the problematic metals are members of the group of transition metals. Thus titanium, chromium, iron, cobalt, tungsten, nickel, platinum, and cadmium have all, at some time and in some form, been suspected of, or been classified as, being carcinogenic *(2)*. The human exposures to some others (scandium, vanadium, yttrium, zirconium, niobium, technetium, hafnium, tantalum, and rhenium) are too rare for any epidemiological investigation and these others have, to our knowledge, never been mentioned as carcinogenic. Exposure to manganese and molybdenum is less rare, and both play important biological roles as essential trace elements in enzymes. The platinum group of elements (ruthenium, osmium, rhodium, iridium, palladium, and platinum) is also composed of very rare elements but, by analogy to platinum, these elements might be suspected of being carcinogenic. Human exposure to gold (Au) and silver (Ag) is relatively widespread, but despite the toxicity of some of their compounds, there has never been any mention of carcinogenicity. Finally the possibility of mercury (Hg) being a carcinogen has been evaluated by the IARC in 1993 *(3)* and mercury is classified as a *possible carcinogen* but based on scant human evidence. In the last group of metals, the so-called poor metals, comprising aluminum, gallium, indium, tin, thallium, lead, and bismuth, only lead is considered as a potential carcinogen. Finally, within metalloids (boron, silicon, germanium, arsenic, antimony, tellurium, and polonium), which are not strictly metals, silicon (in the form of crystalline silica) and arsenic have been classified as human carcinogens both by IARC and NTP, but antimony has been considered as a possible carcinogen *(4)* based solely on animal data.

Following this brief overview of metallic elements, this chapter proceeds by shortly reviewing the epidemiological evidence of lung carcinogenicity of metals and metalloids classified as human carcinogens in one of their forms, i.e., chromium (Cr), nickel (Ni), cadmium (Cd), beryllium (Be), arsenic (As), and silicon (Si), insist-

1	2	3	4	5	6	7	8	9	10	11	12	13	14	15	16	17	18
1 H 1.008																	2 He 4.003
3 Li 6.941	4 Be 9.012											5 B 10.811	6 C 12.011	7 N 14.007	8 O 15.999	9 F 18.998	10 Ne 20.180
11 Na 22.99	12 Mg 24.305											13 Al 26.982	14 Si 28.086	15 P 30.974	16 S 32.066	17 Cl 35.453	18 Ar 39.948
19 K 39.098	20 Ca 40.078	21 Sc 44.956	22 Ti 47.867	23 V 50.942	24 Cr 51.996	25 Mn 54.938	26 Fe 55.845	27 Co 58.933	28 Ni 58.693	29 Cu 63.546	30 Zn 65.39	31 Ga 69.723	32 Ge 72.61	33 As 74.922	34 Se 78.96	35 Br 79.904	36 Kr 83.80
37 Rb 85.468	38 Sr 87.62	39 Y 88.906	40 Zr 91.224	41 Nb 92.906	42 Mo 95.94	43 Tc (98)	44 Ru 101.07	45 Rh 102.91	46 Pd 106.42	47 Ag 107.87	48 Cd 112.41	49 In 114.82	50 Sn 118.71	51 Sb 121.76	52 Te 127.60	53 I 126.90	54 Xe 131.29
55 Cs 132.91	56 Ba 137.33	see below	72 Hf 178.49	73 Ta 180.95	74 W 183.84	75 Re 186.21	76 Os 190.23	77 Ir 192.22	78 Pt 195.08	79 Au 196.97	80 Hg 200.59	81 Tl 204.38	82 Pb 207.2	83 Bi 208.98	84 Po (209)	85 At (210)	86 Rn (222)
87 Fr (223)	88 Ra (226)	see below	104 Rf (261)	105 Db (262)	106 Sg (263)	107 Bh (262)	108 Hs (265)	109 Mt (266)	110 * (269)	111 * (272)	112 * (277)	113 +	114 +	115 +	116 +	117 +	118 +

57 La 138.91	58 Ce 140.12	59 Pr 140.91	60 Nd 144.24	61 Pm (145)	62 Sm 150.36	63 Eu 151.96	64 Gd 157.25	65 Tb 158.93	66 Dy 162.50	67 Ho 164.93	68 Er 167.26	69 Tm 168.93	70 Yb 173.04	71 Lu 174.97
89 Ac (227)	90 Th 232.04	91 Pa 231.04	92 U 238.03	93 Np (237)	94 Pu (244)	95 Am (243)	96 Cm (247)	97 Bk (247)	98 Cf (251)	99 Es (252)	100 Fm (257)	101 Md (258)	102 No (259)	103 Lr (262)

alkali metals (+1)	alkaline earth metals (+2)	transition metals	other metals	other nonmetals
halogens (−1)	noble gases (0)	lanthanides	actinides	

(*) elements have been discovered but have not been named yet.
(+) elements have yet to be discovered.

Fig. 6.1. Periodic table of the elements. *Elements have been discovered but have not been named yet; +Elements have yet to be discovered.

ing on the remaining scientific uncertainties. It then summarizes the epidemiological evidence for titanium (Ti), iron (Fe), lead (Pb), cobalt (Co), and tungsten (W), for which no consensus has yet been reached. A short discussion will complete this review.

3. Metals Recognized as Carcinogens

3.1. Chromium

Hexavalent chromium [Cr (VI)] was first linked to respiratory cancer as early as in the late 19th century (5). Since then, several epidemiological studies were conducted, mostly in the chromate and chromate pigments production across the world, and consistently reported high risks of lung cancer and nasal sinus cancer. This literature was assessed by IARC in 1990 in its monograph on chromium and chromium compounds (6). It concluded that "Chromium [VI] is *carcinogenic to humans*" based on "*sufficient evidence* in humans for the carcinogenicity of chromium [VI] compounds as encountered in the chromate production, chromate pigment production and chromium plating industries." The situation is different with trivalent chromium, Cr [III], which is naturally occurring as chromic oxide in the mineral chromite. The main exposure to trivalent chromium and to metallic chromium occurs in the production of ferrochromium. Only three epidemiological studies are available within this industry, and were carried out in Sweden *(7)*, Norway *(8)*, and France *(9)*. The evidence was conflicting and the only statistically significant excess occurred in the French study, in which the exposure to chromium was more or less confounded with exposure to other carcinogens in particular benzo(a)pyrene. This was summarized in the IARC monograph *(6)* by "Metallic chromium and chromium [III] compounds *are not classifiable as to their carcinogenicity to humans*" because of "inadequate evidence in humans for the carcinogenicity of metallic chromium and of chromium[III] compounds." Since this IARC assessment, a number of epidemiological studies have been published *(10–23)*, mostly confirming the lung cancer risk with chromium [VI] exposure. The last study *(23)* was remarkable in that the exposure assessment was based on over 12,000 urinary chromium exposure measurements. The authors concluded that their "data suggest a possible threshold effect of occupational hexavalent chromium exposure on lung cancer." This suggestion was however strongly disputed by Michaels et al. *(24)*. Finally, a reanalysis *(25)* of the data published by Gibb et al. *(18)* investigated the hypothesis of a possible threshold and found limited evidence in favor of a low cumulative exposure threshold.

3.2. Nickel

The earliest evidence with respect to a carcinogenic effect of nickel [Ni] was published in 1958 *(26)*. In the following 30 years, several epidemiological studies were conducted in all sectors exposing workers to nickel compounds, i.e., mostly nickel extraction, refining, smelting, and use in stainless steel production. The main studies were conducted in Ontario (Canada), USA, Wales (UK), and Norway. In 1990, the International Committee on Nickel Carcinogenesis in Man (ICNCM), chaired by Sir Richard Doll, reported on the results of all the available studies, some of which had never been available in published form, in a comprehensive document *(27)*. It concluded that "more than one form of nickel gives rise to lung and nasal cancer" and "The evidence from this study suggests that respiratory cancer risks are primarily related to soluble nickel at concentrations in excess of 1 mg Ni/m^3 and to exposures to less soluble forms at concentrations > 10 mg Ni/m^3."

The IARC assessment *(6)* of the same year considered that "Nickel compounds are *carcinogenic to humans*" and "Metallic nickel is *possibly carcinogenic to humans*." The first statement was based on "*sufficient evidence* in humans for the carcinogenicity of nickel sulfate, and of the combinations of nickel sulfides and oxides encountered in the nickel refining industry," whereas the second statement was based on experimental animal studies. Since 1990, the published evidence with respect to carcinogenicity of nickel has been conflicting. Two studies conducted in New Caledonia (28, 29) did not find any increased risk of respiratory cancer among nickel workers despite a reasonable power. The lung cancer mortality among nickel platers (30) was not found to be in excess. Similarly Sorahan and Williams (31) confirmed only partially in a recent survey the initial lung cancer excess in the Clydach (Wales) refinery described in ref. (27). On the other hand, Andersen et al. (32), Anttila et al. (33), as well as Grimsrud (34, 35), confirmed high level risks of lung cancer with consistent dose–response relationships. Although the issue remains controversial, this risk seems to be restricted to water-soluble nickel compounds (36).

3.3. Cadmium

Human exposure to cadmium [Cd] occurs predominantly through consumption of food and tobacco because cadmium bio-accumulates in plants via the contamination of topsoil by industrial activities. Cadmium and its compounds are used in a variety of industrial applications (batteries, pigments, alloys, electroplating and coating, plastics). Nowadays its predominant use is the production of nickel/cadmium batteries. In its 1993 monograph (3), IARC stated that "Cadmium and cadmium compounds are *carcinogenic to humans*" based on "*sufficient evidence*" both in humans and experimental animals. This was reinforced by the sentence "In making the overall evaluation, the Working Group took into consideration the evidence that ionic cadmium causes genotoxic effects in a variety of types of eukaryotic cells, including human cells." The assessment of the human evidence was mostly based on several papers analyzing a US cohort of cadmium recovery workers, see, e.g., ref. (37), showing a dose–response relationship between lung cancer and cumulative cadmium exposure and a series of papers in a cohort of 17 UK cadmium processing plants, see e.g. ref. (38), in which there were suggested trends with duration and intensity of exposure to cadmium. The IARC reviewed also a series of smaller cohort for which results are contradictory. The new data with respect to cadmium and cancer have been reviewed recently (39). The US cohort was reanalyzed by Sorahan and Lancashire (40) using detailed job histories previously not taken into account. This paper confirmed the dose–response relationships between lung cancer and cumulative cadmium exposure. However, when stratifying on arsenic exposure, cadmium is only significantly related to lung cancer for subjects concomitantly exposed to arsenic. Three further cohorts have been updated since the IARC report (41–43), which did not show any increased lung cancer risk (in the absence of arsenic co-exposure). The authors of the last paper claim that these results "might indicate that the IARC evaluation is perhaps suitable for re-examination" and "that the claims that carcinogenic effects have been shown in humans ought to be treated with some skepticism." The 2005 11th NTP Report on Carcinogens reevaluated cadmium but confirmed cadmium as "*known to be a human carcinogen*." Finally, a recent prospective population-based study in the vicinity of industrial sites generating a cadmium exposure *(44)* showed an increased lung cancer risk in relation to previously measured urinary cadmium.

3.4. Beryllium

The uses of beryllium are relatively widespread: specialty ceramics for electric and electronic appliances, nuclear and aircraft industries, aluminum and magnesium production, but jewelry and dental prosthetic industry also use beryllium alloys or pure beryllium. High long-term human exposures are probably (or hopefully were) restricted to the beryllium production industry. Its acute and chronic respiratory toxicity has long been recognized *(45)*, even among relatively low-exposed workers. The lung carcinogenicity of beryllium is more controversial, despite the classification of beryllium by IARC *(3)* as a "*carcinogenic to humans*" based on "*sufficient evidence*" both in humans and experimental animals. The human evidence relied on a moderate but consistent lung cancer excess in a cohort of the seven US beryllium production facilities (*see* **ref**. *(46)* for the last paper describing this population considered by the IARC review) and a high lung cancer risk in a beryllium case registry, which included cases of beryllium-induced pneumonitis *(47)*. The follow-up of the largest facility included in the US cohort was extended and a nested case–control study was conducted *(48)*, which enabled a quantitative assessment of the exposure. This study could dismiss confounding by smoking and showed an increasing trend when the exposure was lagged by 10 years but a decreased risk in the upper quartile. Modeling this trend with log-transformed exposure metrics yielded a significant coefficient, but trends with nontransformed exposure metrics were not statistically significant *(49)*. This and alleged methodological weaknesses led the authors of the latter paper *(49)* to challenge the conclusions concerning beryllium–lung cancer associations.

3.5. Arsenic

The relation between arsenic and lung cancers is one of the best-documented ones. While in its first assessment *(50)*, IARC stated that "the causative role (of arsenic) is uncertain," in its 1980 assessment *(51)*, IARC concluded that there was "sufficient evidence that inorganic arsenic compounds are skin and lung carcinogens in humans," while its 1987 *(52)* assessment was "Arsenic and arsenic compounds are *carcinogenic to humans*" but "This evaluation applies to the group of chemicals as a whole and not necessarily to all individual chemicals within the group." This classification was based on consistent lung cancer excesses and observed dose–response relationships with arsenic exposure among copper smelter workers (e.g., ref. *(53)*), which was confirmed in later studies all over the world (e.g., refs. *(54–58)*), including some environmental risks around smelters (e.g., refs. *(59, 60)*). Increased lung cancer risks were also found in arsenic-exposed copper, gold, and tin miners *(61–63)*, and among workers involved in the manufacture of arsenical pesticides *(64, 65)*. A more complete list of references is available in ref. *(66)*. Finally, high lung cancer risks in relation to drinking water arsenic have been published in Taiwan *(67)*, Chile *(68)*, and Bangladesh *(69)*.

3.6. Silicon

Measured by mass, silicon makes up 25.7% of the Earth's crust. Pure silicon crystals are however only occasionally found in nature, so that there is no human exposure to speak of, except possibly in the semiconductor industry. Naturally occurring silicon is usually found in the form of silicon dioxide (also known as silica), and silicates. There are many silicates, which are complex compounds involving silicon, oxygen, and other metallic and nonmetallic elements, and considering silicates as silicon compounds is stretching this concept. Silica on the other hand, is the simplest and most common silicon compound. Moreover, human exposure is widespread and its health consequences have been studied in many studies. In its 1997 monograph *(70)*, IARC stated that "Crystalline silica inhaled in the form of quartz or cristobalite from occupational sources is carcinogenic to humans" based on "*sufficient evidence in humans* for the carcinogenicity of inhaled crystalline silica in the form of quartz or cristobalite from occupational sources," whereas "Amorphous silica is *not classifiable as to its carcinogenicity to humans.*" This classification, which was since confirmed by the NTP *(71)*, gave rise to heated discussions (*see*, e.g., **ref**. *(72)*), notably based on the fact that studies of coal miners, who are exposed to crystalline silica, have not generally demonstrated an increased lung cancer risk. This was certainly a reason why the IARC working group added the following cautionary remark "Carcinogenicity may be dependent on inherent characteristics of the crystalline silica or on external factors affecting its biological activity or distribution of its polymorphs." Recent studies seem both to confirm the fact that overall, crystalline silica is carcinogenic *(73, 74)*, and that it is not always so *(75, 76)*. The most important problem seems now to be to understand what causes these inconsistent findings on silica and lung cancer *(77)*.

4. Titanium

Titanium [Ti] is a light strong, corrosion-resistant metal with a white–silvery metallic color. Although it is quite common in the Earth's crust (its proportion in soils is approximately 0.5 to 1.5% *(78)*), it is always bonded to other elements in nature and it is very expensive to extract the metal from its ores. It can be alloyed with other elements, such as iron, aluminum, vanadium, molybdenum, and others, to produce strong lightweight alloys for aerospace (the Boeing 777 contains about 10% titanium), military, automotive, medical (prostheses), sporting goods (golf clubs), and other applications. However 95% of titanium ore extracted is destined for refinement into titanium dioxide (TiO_2), mostly used as a pigment. Thus human exposure to titanium and titanium compounds is mainly in the production and use of TiO_2, although some human exposure is likely to exist to titanium metal in its metallurgical industry. In 1983, NIOSH estimated that 2.7 million workers were potentially exposed to TiO_2. There have been some animal studies *(79, 80)* showing increases in malignant bronchiolar/alveolar and squamous cell tumors of the lung in rats exposed to high levels of TiO_2. Searching the scientific literature, we identified four cohort studies among TiO_2 production workers *(81–84)*, one of which *(82)* was a nested case–control study in a cohort presented in ref. *(81)* focused on titanium tetrachloride ($TiCl_4$) exposure. We also identified a reanalysis *(85)* targeted toward exposure to TiO_2 of an earlier population-based case–control study *(86)*. Finally, in the 2001 unpublished final report of the worldwide multicentric IARC study in the pulp and paper industry, the lung cancer mortality of subjects ever exposed to TiO_2 (212 cases versus 225.9 expected) or ever highly exposed to TiO_2 (82 cases versus 84.2 expected) was not in excess. No epidemiological results are available for titanium-exposed humans in other contexts. **Table 6.1** presents the main results of these papers. Overall, there is only one significant excess of lung cancer mortality, based on a fixed effect summary of the European study. However, the detailed exposure assessment in this cohort enabled the authors to show that this (23%) excess was not related to the TiO_2 exposure and was most likely due to other factors (smoking and other occupational exposures) and possibly to inadequate reference rates.

The recent 2006 IARC assessment, of which presently only the summary evaluation is available, concluded, based on the same studies (except the results of the pulp and paper cohort, and one US study, most likely the study focusing on $TiCl_4$), that "Titanium dioxide is *possibly carcinogenic* to humans" based on "*inadequate evidence* in humans" and "*sufficient evidence* in experimental animals."

5. Iron

Iron [Fe] is the 26th element of the periodic table. It is a ductile and malleable metal, unique with his magnetic properties. It is a very reactive element and oxidizes (rusts) very easily.

Table 6.1
Epidemiological studies on lung cancer in relation to titanium compounds

Author [reference]	Year	Study type and location	Study population and follow-up	Lung cancer cases	RR estimate	95% CI
Cohort studies: TiO_2 production and use						
Chen et al. [81]	1988	Mortality study in 2 US plants	n = 2,477 (1,576 exposed to TiO_2) 1935–1983	9	SMR = 0.52	0.27–0.99
Fayer-weather et al. [82]	1992	Nested case–control in the largest plant	1935–1983	24	OR ($TiCl_4$) = 1.1	0.4–3.2
Fryzek et al. [83]	2003	Mortality study in 4 US plants	3,892 men, 409 women 1960–2000	61	SMR (all) = 1.0	0.8–1.3
				11	SMR (high TiO_2) = 1.0	0.5–1.7
Boffetta [84]	2004	Mortality study in 11 European plants	14,331 men, 686 women 1927 to 1969– 1995–2001	306.5	SMR = 1.23	1.10–1.38
					RR (random effect) = 1.19	0.96–1.48
IARC	2001	Worldwide mortality cohort in pulp and paper industry	Ever exposed to TiO_2	212	SMR = 0.94	0.82– 1.07
			Ever highly exposed to TiO_2	82	SMR = 0.97	0.77–1.21
Population-based case–control studies						
Boffetta [85]	2001	Montreal (Canada) 857 cases	Ever exposed to TiO_2	33	OR = 0.9	0.5–1.5
			Substantial exposure to TiO_2	8	OR = 1.0	0.3–2.7

It is widespread in the Earth's crust (about 5%). The main ores of iron are hematite or ferric oxide (Fe_2O_3), magnetite or ferrous oxide (Fe_3O_4), and limonite ($HFeO_2$). In the experimental literature, the carcinogenic effect of iron oxides on lung has long been debated. Studies on animals show no conclusive effect of iron oxides if alone. A carcinogenic effect has however been suggested in association with benzo[a]pyrene (B[a]P), ferrous oxide particles being considered as cofactors (87–89).

Several epidemiological studies have been carried out on the risks of cancer in industries generating exposure to iron oxides: iron ore mining, iron and steel manufacturing, foundry processes, and welding processes, although few of the studies focused on iron oxides. In what follows, we shall consider each of these industries or processes. The respective findings will be discussed considering that few if any of the occupations present "pure" exposures to Fe oxides, most presenting decidedly mixed exposures.

5.1. Iron Ore Mines

Several epidemiological studies conducted among underground hematite miners showed an increased risk of lung cancer. Some of these studies, reviewed in the 1987 IARC monograph (90), attributed this risk to radon daughters because they observed a higher incidence of lung cancer among miners exposed to radon daughters than among surface miners. In a retrospective study conducted in Minnesota (91), no excess of lung cancer was found among either underground or aboveground miners compared with US white men. These results were attributed to low levels of exposure to both radon daughters and silica dust, a strict smoking prohibition underground, and the absence of underground diesel fuel use. Two French studies were carried out in iron ore miners in the Lorraine basin, where the exposure levels to radon daughters are low. A proportional mortality study (92) of 1,075 miners deceased between 1960 and 1976 showed a significant excess of lung cancer mortality 2.2 times higher than expected in reference to French male mortality, increasing with the duration of work underground (Proportional mortality rate [PMR] = 4.24 for subjects who worked underground for more than 30 years). This excess risk may have been partly due to smoking but it led to the classification of lung cancer as a recognized occupational disease in France as a complication of siderosis. In a prospective study conducted in the same area, Chau et al. (93) confirmed the excess of lung cancer among underground workers (standardized mortality ratio [SMR] = 3.89; $p < 0.001$). The authors showed that the lung cancer risk increased with the duration of work underground and that this increase became more important with increasing smoking. They concluded that the lung cancer risk in Lorraine iron ore miners was possibly related to cumulative levels of dust (consisting mostly of iron oxides) and diesel exhausts, although the role of a low exposure to radon daughters could not be totally excluded. In a retrospective study conducted among workers of two hematite mines in China, Chen et al. *(94)* found an excess risk of lung cancer among underground miners exposed to radon and radon daughters that increased with levels of dust exposure among smokers but also among subjects with silicosis and silicotuberculosis, indicating a significant quartz content of this dust. A cohort study published in 2006 carried out among iron ore miners in China showed an increased risk for lung cancer among dust-exposed workers *(95)*.

In summary, most studies conducted among iron ore miners reported an excess lung cancer risk. However, this excess is difficult to attribute to iron oxide exposure, given the numerous confounders among which radon and radon daughters, diesel fumes, and smoking are the most important. Based on these findings, IARC *(90)* classified "underground haematite mining with exposure to radon" as being "*carcinogenic to humans*" while for haematite and iron oxide, the evidence for carcinogenicity in humans was considered "*inadequate.*"

5.2. Iron and Steel Foundries

Iron and steel founding is an industrial process that has been considered by IARC as "*carcinogenic to humans*" *(96, 97)*. This IARC assessment remarked that "Despite the absence of information to specify definitely the carcinogenic substances in the work environment (e.g., polycyclic aromatic hydrocarbons [PAHs], silica, metal fumes, and formaldehyde), the consistency of the excess in studies from around the world shows that certain exposures in iron and steel founding can cause lung cancer in humans." We can note that exposure to iron oxides was not even considered as a potential carcinogen. Since this evaluation, we are aware of seven new studies considering lung cancer in iron foundries *(98–104)*. A Polish nested case–control study *(98)* reported a consistent gradient of lung cancer risk, adjusted on smoking, with increasing duration of employment in a foundry: odds ratio (OR) = 1.28 (1–20 years), 1.58 (20–30 years), and 2.66 (>30 years). Adzresen et al. *(104)* reported an increased lung cancer risk (SMR = 164; 95% confidence interval [CI], 124–223). Sorahan et al. *(101)* showed an increased lung cancer mortality in 10 UK foundries (SMR = 146; 95% CI, 134–158; 551 cases) with no clear trend with exposure estimates. On the other hand, Rotimi et al. *(99)* and Andjekovich et al. *(101)* did not find any lung cancer excess in the mortality follow-up of two American steel foundries, neither did Hansen *(102)* in a population-based cohort of foundry workers, despite a large excess in death from pneumoconiosis. Finally, in a Spanish nested case–control study *(103)* carried out in a steel-producing industrial complex, a twofold lung cancer risk (not significant, adjusted on smoking) was observed among workers having worked predominantly in the foundry.

Again lung cancer is often in excess in this industrial sector and again it is not clear whether this excess is attributable to iron oxides.

5.3. Welders

Welding fumes contain a wide variety of mostly metallic compounds depending welded metals and the welding technique. For example, exposure to hexavalent chromium and nickel is likely during welding of stainless steel. However, except for very specialized welding, these fumes always contain iron compounds. Moreover, relatively high asbestos exposure is likely to have occurred in shipyards and a lower asbestos exposure may have occurred because of the use of asbestos welding blankets.

In the late 1980s, a large multicentric European cohort of welders *(105)* was set up. Exposures to chromium, nickel, and others were assessed using an ad hoc job-exposure matrix. Overall lung cancer was in significant excess but no clear difference was observed between mild steel and stainless steel welders. Moreover, no dose–response relationship could be shown between lung cancer and exposure to hexavalent chromium or nickel. A recent meta-analysis of all epidemiological studies among welders published between 1954 and 2004 *(106)* confirmed both the overall lung cancer excess (combined relative risk [CRR] = 1.26; 95% CI, 1.20–1.32) and the absence of difference between mild steel welders (CRR = 1.32; 95% CI, 1.10–1.59) and stainless steel welders (CRR = 1.31; 95% CI, 1.06–1.61). The authors considered this risk as unlikely to be attributable to confounding by smoking. A possible confounder is asbestos exposure, but the shipyard welders (CRR = 1.32; 95% CI, 1.16–1.51), in which this exposure was considered to be much higher, showed a similar risk as other welders. This was also the point of view expressed in the 1990 IARC monograph *(6)*, which classified welding fumes (and not welding processes) as "*possibly carcinogenic to humans.*" These nonspecific lung cancer risks could, at least partly, be due to iron oxide exposure, but this is only one hypothesis among others.

5.4. Steel Industry

Steel production gives rise to exposure to total dust containing varying concentrations of iron between the different processes. The authors of a French study in a steel-producing factory *(107)* reported percentages of iron (including oxides) in total dust varying from 30% in the blast furnace plant or in the steel making plant to more than 75% in the sinter plant or in the hot rolling mill. This study was specifically aimed at assessing the possible association between iron oxide exposures and lung cancer mortality while taking into account the main possible occupational and non-occupational confounders. A factory specific job-exposure matrix assessed occupational exposures. High iron oxide exposures occurred at the floor level of the steel making plant or of the blast furnace before the installation of a ventilation system, close to the sinter strand, during hot scarfing at the heavy plate mill. No lung cancer excess was observed among workers exposed to iron oxides (relative risk [RR] adjusted on asbestos, silica, and PAHs, 0.80; 95% CI, 0.55–1.17) and no dose–response relationship was observed with intensity, duration of exposure, and cumulative exposure indices. A further, nested case–control study in a cohort of stainless and alloyed steel-producing workers *(108)*, targeted at assessing lung cancer risk in relation to metals and iron exposures, did not detect any effect of iron oxide exposure either: the iron-oxide OR adjusted for potential confounding factors, i.e., PAHs, silica, and smoking, was lower than 0.50. In contrast to the two preceding studies, the majority of studies carried out in iron and steel plants analyzed lung cancer mortality according to workshops or job categories, but not in term of exposures to iron oxides and cofactors. In order to detect a possible role of iron oxide exposure, we concentrate on those workshops or plants in which such an exposure is most likely, although still possibly associated with other carcinogens. These consist of blast furnace, smelting, hot-rolling, scarfing, but, e.g., not coke oven plants. **Table 6.2** summarizes the lung cancer risks in studies in which this detail was available. In all four processes, it appears that the lung cancer risk is increased quite consistently.

5.5. Summary

The carcinogenic effect of iron oxides on lung has been suggested in the literature because excess risks of lung cancer were observed in many occupational activities involving exposure to iron oxides. A potential lung cancer risk was reported in many studies carried out in iron ore mines, in iron and steel foundries, among mild steel and stainless steel welders, and in the steel industry. However only three studies, one study *(121)* considering "pure" and considerable exposure to iron oxides in relation to the production of Fe_2O_3 from pyrite, and two mortality cohort studies carried out in steel-producing factories, addressed specifically the effect of iron oxides on lung cancer. In none of these three studies, when taking into account possible confounders, was such an effect observed. Finally some studies showed excesses of a nonmalignant respiratory disease, usually considered as benign, called siderosis. This disease is specifically related to the exposure to iron oxides and it has been suggested that lung cancer may occur as a complication of siderosis *(88)*. However, the single study investigating this possible relation did not find any excess, but its power was very low *(122)*. In summary, lung cancers risks are observed in population exposed to iron oxides but effects of iron oxides were not confirmed when they were specifically studied.

6. Lead

Lead is a toxic metal. Its neurotoxic, nephrotoxic, and hematologic effects have long been recognized *(123)*. Nevertheless, the human exposure is quite widespread: citing the summary

Table 6.2
Lung cancer risks in blast furnace, smelting, hot-rolling, and scarfing plants

Author [reference]	Year	Study type and location	Lung cancer cases	RR estimate	95% CI
Blast furnace					
Hurley [109]	1990	Cohort study, UK	18	SMR = 1.69	1.00–2.67[a]
Moulin [110]	1995	Cohort study, France	26	SMR = 1.36	0.89–1.99
Finkelstein [111]	1994	Case–control study, Canada	11	OR = 1.38	0.61–3.06
Smelting					
Redmond [112]	1975	Cohort study, USA	112	SMR = 0.89[c]	0.73–1.07[a]
Finkelstein [113]	1990	Cohort study, Canada	7	SMR = 3.61[b]	1.48–7.59[a]
Hurley [109]	1990	Cohort study, UK	13	SMR = 0.90	0.48–1.54[a]
Finkelstein [114]	1991	Cohort study, Canada	15	SMR = 1.45[b]	0.81–2.39[a]
Moulin [115]	1993	Cohort study, France	7	SMR = 1.04b	0.42–2.15
Cao [116]	1995	Cohort study, Chine	118	SMR = 1.09	0.91–1.31[a]
Moulin [110]	1995	Cohort study, France	17	SMR = 1.25[c]	0.73–2.01
Moulin [110]	1995	Cohort study, France	5	SMR = 1.04[b]	0.34–2.43
Moulin [110]	1995	Cohort study, France	14	SMR = 1.75	0.96–2.94
Blot [117]	1983	Case–control study, USA	20	OR = 2.60[c]	1.20–5.80
Finkelstein [113]	1994	Case–control study, Canada	17	OR = 0.92	0.50–1.70
Xu [118]	1996	Case–control study, China	166	OR = 1.60	1.20–2.10
Hot rolling					
Mazumdar [119]	1975	Cohort study, USA	21	SMR = 1.14	0.71–1.74[a]
Hurley [109]	1990	Cohort study, UK	19	SMR = 0.86	0.53–1.37[a]
Moulin [115]	1993	Cohort study, France	17	SMR = 1.51	0.88–2.42
Moulin [110]	1995	Cohort study, France	41	SMR = 1.29	0.93–1.75
Moulin [110]	1995	Cohort study, France	28	SMR = 1.16	0.77–1.68
Scarfing					
Mazumdar [119]	1975	Cohort study, USA	2	SMR = 0.80	0.10–2.89[a]
Beaumont [120]	1987	Cohort study, USA	35	SMR = 1.64	1.14–2.28
Moulin [110]	1995	Cohort study, France	7	SMR = 1.62	0.65–3.33

[a] Not available in the original publication, computed from available data. [b] Electric furnace. [c] Open hearth furnace.

report of the 2004 IARC assessment of the carcinogenicity of lead *(124)*, "The widespread occurrence of lead in the environment is largely the result of anthropogenic activity, which has occurred since prehistoric times. Lead usage increased progressively with industrialization and rose dramatically with the use of lead-acid batteries and leaded fuel for automobiles in the twentieth century. The predominant use of lead is now in batteries and, to a lesser extent, in construction materials and lead-based chemicals. The use of lead in pipes, paints and gasoline has been or is being phased out in many countries. The important routes of human exposure from lead-contaminated air, dust, soil, water and food are through inhalation and ingestion. Recent human exposure has arisen predominantly from the widespread use of leaded gasoline. Also, areas near lead mines and smelters have high environmental concentrations of lead. Occupations in which the highest potential exposure to lead exists include mining, primary and secondary smelting, production of lead-acid batteries, pigment production, construction and demolition. In spite of the persistence of lead in the environment, exposures have decreased substantially in countries where lead control measures have been implemented over the past 10–30 years."

The possible carcinogenic effect of lead has received a lot of attention recently. In 1999 a conference was dedicated to "Lead Exposure, Reproductive Toxicity and Carcinogenicity," whose proceedings have been published in a special issue of the American Journal of Industrial Medicine (Vol 38, no. 3; 2000). Shortly afterward, the aforementioned IARC assessment reviewed the evidence and a group of French experts also reviewed the evidence *(125)*. IARC considered that there was "*limited evidence* for the carcinogenicity to humans of exposure to inorganic lead compounds. The available epidemiological data on occupational exposure to organic lead compounds were considered to provide *inadequate evidence* for carcinogenicity to humans." **Table 6.3** presents the results of a series of published epidemiological studies analyzed in an unpublished meta-analysis by Dr. Moulin and coworkers *(126)* presented at the 16th International Symposium on Epidemiology in Occupational Health, in which subgroups of study populations were ranked by increasing lead exposure level, based on the available published information. Although overall there appears to be an increased lung cancer risk, no increasing trend with lead exposure emerges from this table. The increased lung cancer risk seems therefore to be, at least partly, due to confounding exposures.

Since this meta-analysis, three studies were published. Lundström et al. *(144)* conducted a nested case–control study in the Swedish smelter cohort *(141)* and concluded that "cumulative

Table 6.3
Lung cancer risks by coded lead exposure in subpopulation of studies published before 2002

Author [reference]	Year	Study type and location	Lung cancer cases	RR estimate	95% CI
Lowest lead exposure level		All combined		CRR = 1.36	0.71–2.57
Cordioli [127]	1987	Glass industry, Italy	13	SMR = 2.09	1.11–3.57
Sankila [128]	1990	Glass industry, mechanical work-shop Finland	4	SIR = 1.60	0.44–4.10
Michaels [129]	1991	Printers, US	37	SMR = 0.89	0.62–1.22
Low-medium exposure levels		All combined		CRR = 1.07	0.81–1.41
Sankila [128]	1990	Glass industry, glass blowers, Finland	1	SIR = 0.29	0.01–1.64
Sankila [128]	1990	Glass industry, others, Finland	37	SIR = 1.33	0.93–1.83
Wingren [130]	1987	Glass industry, others, Sweden	11	OR = 1.90	0.97–3.72
Bertazzi [131]	1980	Printing industry, Italy	1	SMR = 0.50	0.02–2.79
Greene [132]	1979	Printing industry, US, whites	61	SMR = 0.83	0.64–1.07
Greene [132]	1979	Printing industry, US, non whites	23	SMR = 1.06	0.67–1.59
Anttila [133]	1995	Population based, Finland, men	25	SMR = 0.70	0.02–2.79
Anttila [133]	1995	Population based, Finland, women	1	SMR = 0.70	0.01–4.00
Wingren [134]	1990	Glass industry, Sweden	6	SMR = 2.36	0.86–5.14
Medium exposure levels		All combined		CRR = 1.45	1.15–1.84
Gerhardsson [135]	1986	Smelter workers, Sweden	3	SMR = 1.43	0.29–4.17
Wingren [130]	1987	Glass industry, Sweden	4	OR = 2.30	0.83–6.35
Gerhardsson [136]	1995	Smelter workers, Sweden	6	SMR = 1.32	0.49–2.88
Steenland [137]	1992	Smelter workers, US	23	SMR = 1.36	0.86–2.05

(continued)

**Table 6.3
(continued)**

Author [reference]	Year	Study type and location	Lung cancer cases	RR estimate	95% CI
Anttila [133]	1995	Population based, Finland, men	35	SIR = 1.40	1.00–1.90
Anttila [133]	1995	Population based, Finland, women	2	SIR = 4.50	0.50–16.00
High exposure levels		All combined		CRR = 1.29	1.09–1.54
Wong [138]	2000	Battery workers, US	210	SMR = 1.14	0.99–1.30
Wong [138]	2000	Smelter workers, US	107	SMR = 1.22	1.00–1.47
Gerhardsson [135]	1986	Smelter workers, Sweden	5	SMR = 1.72	0.56–4.02
Steenland [137]	1992	Smelter workers, US	49	SMR = 1.11	0.82–1.47
Ades [139]	1988	Smelter, UK	182	OR = 1.25	1.07–1.44
Cocco [140]	1997	Smelter workers, Italy	31	SMR = 0.82	0.56–1.16
Lundstrom [141]	1997	Smelter workers, Sweden	42	SMR = 2.90	2.10–4.00
Anttila [133]	1995	Population based, Finland, men	11	SIR = 1.10	0.60–2.00
Sheffet [142]	1982	Pigment industry, US	10	SIR = 1.33	0.67–2.37
Davies [143]	1984	Pigment industry, UK	4	SIR = 1.45	0.39–3.71

SIR, standardized incidence ratio

arsenic and smoking were identified as risk factors, ... lead exposure however was not." Wingren *(145)* updated the cohort published in 1990 *(134)*. The slight lung cancer excess of the earlier study was not confirmed in this update. On the other hand, lung cancer mortality increased significantly with increasing categories of lead exposure in a recent Italian study in a lead and zinc foundry *(146)*.

In summary, there is some evidence of a carcinogenic effect of (inorganic) lead compounds, but it is not compelling, at least with respect to lung cancer.

7. Cobalt and Tungsten

Cobalt is a relatively widespread element. It occurs naturally in the form of sulfides, oxides, and arsenides, but not in its metallic form. It is rarely mined alone and tends to be produced as a by-product of nickel and copper mining activities. Cobalt in small amounts is essential to many living organisms, including humans. It is a central component of the vitamin B-12. Its uses are in making wear-resistant alloys, notably for aircraft engines, in high-strength steels, and other alloys. One of its most important applications is in the hard metal industry in which it is added to metallic carbides, especially tungsten carbide, to produce metal-working tools. Occupational exposure to cobalt occurs predominantly during refining, in the alloy production, and in the hard-metal industry.

The mortality of a French cobalt production facility was studied in two successive studies (147, 148), but the initial excess of lung cancer was not confirmed in the follow-up study. The main evidence with respect to a possible carcinogenic risk of cobalt comes from four studies in the hard-metal industry (149–152). In one of the studies (152), an unadjusted twofold lung cancer risk was observed in a cobalt production workshop without exposure to tungsten carbide exposure, but the main evidence is in workers exposed simultaneously to cobalt and tungsten carbide. The first paper (149) described the mortality experience (1951 to 1982) of the workforce of three hard-metal producing plants (3,163 workers) in Sweden. Overall there was a nonsignificant excess in cancer of the lung (SMR = 1.34; 17 cases; 95% CI, 0.77–2.13), which was higher when restricted to subjects exposed for longer than 20 years since first exposure (SMR = 2.30; 4 cases; 95% CI, 0.62–5.9). This excess became statistically significant when considering subjects exposed for longer than 10 years and whose first exposure was longer than 20 years ago (SMR = 2.78; 7 cases; 95% CI, 1.11–5.72). Another mortality cohort study (1956–1990) of a hard-metal producing plant located in France was published by Lasfargues et al. (150). This small study included 709 male subjects. In this study, there was a significant excess for lung cancer (SMR = 2.13; 10 cases; 95% CI, 1.02–3.93), mainly due to a large excess in the highest exposure group (SMR = 5.03; 6 cases; 95% CI, 1.85–10.9). However, mortality did not increase with duration of employment and time since employment. Potential confounding was treated in some detail for smoking and is unlikely to explain the observed results. Other potential occupational carcinogens (asbestos, nickel, etc.) were not discussed. The third study was published by Moulin et al. (151) and describes the mortality experience (1968–1991) of the workforce of ten French hard-metal producing plant with a total of 5,777 male subjects showing a borderline significant excess for lung cancer (SMR = 1.30; 63 cases; 95% CI, 1.00–1.66). A nested case—control study was included using an industry-specific job-exposure matrix ranking exposures to sintered and unsintered hard metal dust, and identifying exposure to other carcinogens. Smoking habits were obtained for 82% of the cases and 79% of the controls. The OR for simultaneous exposure to cobalt and tungsten carbide rated as >2 (on a scale from 0 to 9) was equal to 1.93 (95% CI, 1.03–3.62) adjusted for all other cobalt exposures (alone or simultaneous with other agents). The OR increased significantly with duration of exposure and cumulative exposure reaching OR = 4.13 (95% CI, 1.49–11.5) in the highest exposure quartile. Adjusting on smoking did not change the ORs to any extent. The last study *(152)* described the mortality experience (1968–1992) of the workforce of the largest facility (2,860 subjects) included in the preceding study. Overall there was a statistically significant lung cancer excess (SMR = 1.70; 46 cases; 95% CI, 1.24–2.26) mostly in subjects having worked in hard metal production steps before sintering (SMR = 2.42; 9 cases; 95% CI, 1.10–8.63), while in the workshops after sintering, only a relatively small excess is observed (SMR = 1.28; 5 cases; 95% CI, 0.41–5.9). According to the job-exposure matrix, the SMR of all hard-metal exposure rated as higher than 2 was in statistically significant excess (SMR = 2.02; 26 cases; 95% CI, 1.32–2.96) and increased with duration and cumulative exposure. In an internal regression adjusted on smoking and IARC carcinogens, the RR increased significantly with duration of exposure to unsintered hard metal dust at a level rated as >2.

In summary, although the possibility of some residual confounding cannot be excluded, it seems unlikely that the increased lung cancer risks in hard-metal workers were due to smoking or other carcinogens. However, the epidemiological evidence is limited in that it is mostly restricted to the population of French workers. These epidemiological findings agree however with experimental data. Injection of cobalt salts in different animal species produced sarcomas at the injection points *(153)*. Recent studies have confirmed the genotoxic potential of these compounds both in vitro *(154, 155)* and in vivo *(156)*. Interestingly, these experiments showed that the association of cobalt salts and tungsten carbide presented higher mutagenic effects than cobalt salts alone when measured by the comet *(155)* or micronuclei assays *(156)*. Recently, IARC reviewed the evidence of the carcinogenicity of cobalt particle with or without tungsten carbide *(157)*. Cobalt metal with tungsten carbide was evaluated as *probably carcinogenic* to humans on the basis of *limited evidence in humans* for increased risk of lung cancer and *sufficient evidence* in experimental animals for the carcinogenicity of cobalt metal powder and cobalt sulfate. On the other hand, the evidence for the carcinogenicity of cobalt metal without tungsten carbide was considered *inadequate*. It was noted that "a number of the IARC working group members supported an evaluation in Group 1 (i.e. *carcino-genic to humans*) because: (1) they judged the epidemiological evidence to be sufficient … and/or (2) they judged the mechanistic evidence to be strong enough to justify upgrading the default evaluation from 2A to 1."

Finally, no epidemiological data are available with respect to exposure to tungsten alone, except in the paper by Wild et al. *(152)*, in which a relatively small group of workers employed solely in the tungsten carbide production workshop did not show any excess of lung cancer mortality.

8. Discussion

The epidemiological evidence with respect to the carcinogenic effect of metals has been reviewed several times in the past *(66, 158, 159)*. To a certain extent, our review is an update of the earlier review by Hayes *(66)*. On the other hand, our focus is different, as our aim was neither to review the overall carcinogenicity, as we concentrated on epidemiological studies of lung cancer, nor to review the toxicological evidence. Moreover, we presented in more detail the epidemiological studies for metals for which the evidence is either recent (TiO_2, cobalt/tungsten), is still uncertain (lead), or for which exposure is very widespread and there remains a doubt (iron).

Does this review allow statements to be made about the metals themselves? To ask the question is to answer it. The human exposure to the metallic elements in their metallic form is usually not the predominant exposure. For example, the three most common elements discussed here, silicon, titanium, and even iron, barely exist, as a human exposure, in their metallic form. The epidemiologic evidence is thus not for exposure to metals but to their basic compounds, in the case of these three elements, to their oxides. For titanium and silicon, their dioxide is the virtually unique compound for which large human exposure groups exist. But even for iron, it can be difficult to identify exposure to only one of its two most common oxides, corresponding respectively to its bivalent and trivalent form. For chromium, the epidemiological evidence seems clear, in that only its hexavalent chromium is carcinogenic. This result is based on studies among workers, most of whom are exposed to a series of chromium compounds, which may well vary in the carcinogenic potential. The fact that the carcinogenicity may depend on the specific compounds is, for instance, specifically recognized in the already cited IARC assessment of nickel *(6)*, which states that human data are only available for certain compounds, and that the overall assessment for nickel compounds is based on animal data. Another issue is the physical structure of the compounds. The fact that some compounds are water soluble, others not, seem to make a difference (Ni, As). The crystalline structure may also make a difference. For instance, quartz is a recognized carcinogen, whereas noncrystalline silica seems to be innocuous. One must therefore be very cautious about the potential carcinogenic effect of nano-structured compounds, whose industrial use is becoming more common. This caution was recently underlined in a draft NIOSH report on TiO_2, whose nano-structured habit is already used in some marketed sunscreens (http://www.cdc.gov/niosh/review/public/TIO2/default.html).

Last but not least, the carcinogenicity depends on the co-exposures, which are not necessarily carcinogenic by themselves. This seems to be the case for cobalt, as neither cobalt nor tungsten seem to be carcinogenic alone, but as discussed above, their joint exposure as hard-metal dusts is strongly suspected to be carcinogenic based both on human and animal data. At least, in this industry, the co-exposures are relatively well identified, whereas in other industrial settings, e.g., in the different metallurgical industries, often many known or suspected carcinogens coexist, to say nothing about personal exposures (smoking, drugs).

Another relevant consideration is to acknowledge that some potentially carcinogenic metals are necessary trace elements in life (*see* **ref**. *(159)* for a review) or can even be used in anticancer drugs *(160)*, which would tend to show that the carcinogenic effect of metals and metal compounds depends on the dose. To cite Duffus *(142)*, "Metal ions are needed by the human body as essential nutrients. It is likely that there are homeostatic mechanisms which must be overcome before any adverse effect such as cancer can occur. This implies the existence of thresholds for metal carcinogenicity." The same review cautions against overinterpreting epidemiological study results on exposure to metals for the reasons stated before and for lack of adequately measured occupational exposures. It is therefore clear that epidemiological results alone can only exceptionally provide a final proof of metal carcinogenicity and that a plausible mechanism supported by experimental data is necessary for a reliable assessment. Thus, the carcinogenicity of beryllium, cadmium, and the combination of cobalt and tungsten carbide relies only on limited epidemiological data but is supported by findings of cancer occurrence in experimental studies.

Another case is for lead, which has been shown to be weakly mutagenic, and genotoxic in humans, but the epidemiological evidence is contradictory. Conversely, the quite consistent, although relatively weak, lung cancer excesses in populations exposed to iron oxides cannot be interpreted causally for lack of such experimental confirmation. Finally, there are few doubts about the carcinogenicity of hexavalent chromium, nickel and arsenic compounds or crystalline silica, but nevertheless some issues remain which have been discussed in what precedes. Only further epidemiological studies in populations with precisely estimated exposure to specific compounds and co-exposures can resolve the remaining uncertainties.

References

1. Hirano, S. and Suuki, K. T. (1996) Exposure, metabolism, and toxicity of rare earths and related compounds. *Env. Health Persp.* **104**, 85–95.

2. Kazantzis, G. (1981) Role of cobalt, iron, lead, manganese, mercury, platinum, selenium, and titanium in carcinogenesis. *Env. Health Persp.* **40**, 143–161.

3. International Agency for Research on Cancer (IARC). (1993) Beryllium, cadmium, mercury and exposures in the glass manufacturing industry. IARC Monogr Eval Carcinog Risks Hum, Vol 58. Lyon, France: IARC.

4. De Boeck, M., Kirsch-Volders, M., and Lison, D. (2003) Cobalt and antimony: genotoxicity and carcinogenicity. *Mutat. Res.* **533**, 135–152.

5. Langard, S. (1990) One hundred years of chromium and cancer: a review of epidemiological evidence and selected case reports. *Am. J. Ind. Med.* **17**, 189–215.

6. International Agency for Research on Cancer (IARC). (1990) Chromium, nickel and welding fumes. IARC Monogr Eval Carcinog Risks Hum, Vol **49**. Lyon, France: IARC.

7. Axelsson, G., Rylander, R., and Schmidt, A. (1980) Mortality and incidence of tumours among ferrochromium workers. *Br. J. Ind. Med.* **37**, 121–127.

8. Langard, S., Andersen, A., and Ravnestad, J. (1990) Incidence of cancer among ferrochromium and ferrosilicon workers: an extended observation period. *Br. J. Ind. Med.* **47**, 14–19.

9. Moulin, J, J, Portefaix, P., Wild, P., Mur, J. M., Smagghe, G., and Mantout, B. (1990) Mortality study among workers producing ferroalloys and stainless steel in France. *Br. J. Ind. Med.* **47**, 537–543.

10. Horiguchi, S., Morinaga, K., and Endo, G. (1990) Epidemiological study of mortality from cancer among chromium platers. *Asia-Pacific J. Publ. Health* **4**, 169–174.

11. Davies, J., Easton, D., and Bidstrup, P. (1991) Mortality from respiratory cancer and other causes in United Kingdom chromate production workers. *Br. J. Ind. Med.* **48**:299–313.

12. Korallus, U. and Ulm, K. (1993) Steinmann-Steiner-Haldenstaett W. Bronchial carcinoma mortty in the German chromate-producing industry: the effects of process modification. *Int. Arch. Occup. Environ. Health* **65**, 171–178.

13. Kano, K., Horikawa, M., Utsunomiwa, T., Tati, M., Satoh, K., and Yamaguchi, S. (1993) Lung cancer mortality among a cohort of male chromate pigment workers in Japan. *Int. J. Epidemiol.* **22**, 16–22.

14. Pastides, H., Austin, R., Lemeshow, S., et al. (1994) A retrospective-cohort study of occupational exposure to hexavalent chromium. *Am. J. Ind. Med.* **25**, 663–675.

15. Deschamps, F., Moulin, J. J., Wild, P. et al. (1995) Mortality study among workers producing chromate pigments in France. *Int. Arch. Occup. Environ. Health* **67**, 147–152.

16. Sorahan, T., Burges, D., Hamilton, L., and Harrington, J. (1998) Lung cancer mortality in nickel/chromium platers, 1946–95. *Occup. Environ. Med.* **55**, 236–242.

17. Sorahan, T. and Harrington, J. (2000) Lung cancer in Yorkshire chrome platers, 1972–97. *Occup. Environ. Med.* **57**, 385–389.

18. Gibb, H., Lees, P., Pinsky, P., et al. (2000) Lung cancer among workers in chromium chemical production. *Am. J. Ind. Med.* **38**, 115–126.

19. Fryzek, J., Mumma, M., McLaughlin, J., Henderson, B., and Blot, W. (2001) Cancer mortality in relation to environmental chromium exposure. *J. Occup. Environ. Med.* **43**, 635–640.

20. Luippold, R. S., Mundt, K. A, Austin, R. P., et al. (2003) Lung cancer mortality among chromate production workers. *Occup. Environ. Med.* **60**, 451–457.

21. Stern, F. (2003) Mortality among chrome leather tannery workers: an update. *Am. J. Ind. Med.* **44**, 197–206.

22. Luippold, R., Mundt, K., Dell, L., and Birk, T. (2005) Low-level hexavalent chromium exposure and rate of mortality among US chromate production employees. *Occup. Environ. Med.* **47**, 381–385.

23. Birk, T., Mundt, K. A., Dell, L. D., Luippold, R. S., Miksche, L., Steinmann-Steiner-Haldenstaett, W., and Mundt, D. J. (2006) Lung cancer mortality in the German chromate industry, 1958 to 1998. *J. Occup. Environ. Med.* **48**, 426–433.

24. Michaels, D., Lurie, P., and Monforton, C. (2006) Comment on "Lung cancer mortality in the German chromate industry, 1958 to 1998." *J. Occup. Environ. Med.* **48**, 995–997.

25. Park, R. M. and Stayner, L. T. (2006) A search for thresholds and other nonlinearities in the relationship between hexavalent chromium and lung cancer. *Risk. Anal.* **26**, 79–88.

26. Morgan, J. G. (1958) Some observations on the incidence of respiratory cancer in nickel workers. *Br. J. Ind. Med.* **15**, 224–234.

27. Doll, R., Andersen, A., Cooper, W. C. et al. (1990) Report of the International Committee on Nickel Carcinogenesis in Man. Scand. *J. Work. Environ. Health* **16**, 1–82.

28. Goldberg, M., Goldberg, P., Leclerc, A., Chastang, J. F., Marne, M. J., and Dubourdieu, D. (1994) A 10-year incidence survey of respiratory cancer and a case-control study within a cohort of nickel mining and refining workers in New Caledonia. *Cancer Causes Control.* **5**, 15–25.

29. Goldberg, M. and Goldberg, P., (2003) Occupational exposures and lung cancer in New Caledonia. *Occup. Environ. Med.* **60**, 584–589.

30. Pang, D., Burges, D. C., and Sorahan, T. (1996) Mortality study of nickel platers with special reference to cancers of the stomach and lung, 1945–93. *Occup. Environ. Med.* **53**, 714–717.

31. Sorahan, T. and Williams S. P. (2005) Mortality of workers at a nickel carbonyl refinery, 1958–2000. *Occup. Environ. Med.* **62**, 80–85.

32. Andersen, A., Berge, S. R., Engeland, A., and Norseth, T. (1996) Exposure to nickel compounds and smoking in relation to incidence of lung and nasal cancer among nickel refinery workers. *Occup. Environ. Med.* **53**, 708–713.

33. Anttila, A., Pukkala, E., Aitio, A., Rantanen, T., and Karjalainen, S. (1998) Update of cancer incidence among workers at a copper/nickel smelter and nickel refinery. Int. Arch. *Occup. Environ. Health.* **71**, 245–250.

34. Grimsrud, T. K., Berge, S. R., Martinsen, J. I., and Andersen, A. (2003) Lung cancer incidence among Norwegian nickel-refinery workers 1953–2000. *J. Environ. Monit.* **5**, 190–197.

35. Grimsrud, T. K., Berge, S. R., Steinar, R., Haldorsen, T., and Andersen, A. (2005) Can lung cancer risk among nickel refinery workers be explained by occupational exposures other than nickel? *Epidemiology* **16**, 146–154.

36. Grimsrud, T. K., Berge, S. R., Haldorsen, T., and Andersen, A. (2002) Exposure to differ-

ent forms of nickel and risk of lung cancer. *Am. J. Epidemiol.* **156**, 1123–1132.

37. Stayner, L., Smith, R. L., Thun, M., Schnoor, T., and Lemen, R (1992). A dose-response analysis and quantitative assessment of lung cancer risk and occupational cadmium exposure. *Ann. Epidemiol.* **2**, 177–194.

38. Kazantzis, G., Lam, T. H., and Sullivan, K. R. (1988) Mortality of cadmium-exposed workers. A five-year update. Scand. *J. Work Environ. Health.* **14**, 220–23.

39. Verougstraete, V., Lison, D., and Hotz, P. (2003) Cadmium, lung and prostate cancer : a systematic review of recent epidemiological data. *J. Toxicol. Environ. Health Part B* **6**, 227–255.

40. Sorahan, T. and Lancashire, R. J. (1997) Lung cancer mortality in a cohort of workers employed at a cadmium recovery plant in the United States: an analysis with detailed job histories. *Occup. Environ. Med.* **54**, 194–201.

41. Jarup, L., Bellander, T., Hogstedt, C., and Spang, G. (1998) Mortality and cancer incidence in Swedish battery workers exposed to cadmium and nickel. *Occup. Environ. Med.* **55**, 755–759.

42. Sorahan, T., Lister, A., Gilthorpe,M. S., and Harrington, J.M. (1995) Mortality of copper-cadmium alloy workers with special reference to lung cancer and non-malignant diseases of the respiratory system, 1946–92. *Occup. Environ. Med.* **52**, 804–812.

43. Sorahan, T. and Esmen, N. A. (2004) Lung cancer mortality in UK nickel-cadmium battery workers, 1947–2000. *Occup. Environ. Med.* **61**, 108–116.

44. Nawrot, T., Plusquin, M., Hagervorst, J., Roels, H. A., Celis, H., Thijs, L., Vangronsveld, J., Van Hecke, E., and Staessen, J. A. (2006) Environmental exposure to cadmium and risk of cancer : a prospective population-based study. *Lancet. Oncol.* **7**, 119–126.

45. Mroz, M. M., Balkisson, R., and Newman, L. S.(2001). In: Bingham E., Cohrssen B., Powelll C. H., eds. Patty's Toxicology. New York: John Wiley and sons, pp. 177–220.

46. Ward, E., Okun, A., Ruder, A., Fingerhut, M., and Steenland, K. (1992) A mortality study of workers at 7 beryllium processing plants. *Am. J. Ind. Med.* **22**, 885–904.

47. Steenland, K. and Ward, E. (1991) Lung cancer incidence among patients with beryllium disease: a cohort mortality study. *J. Natl. Cancer Inst.* **83**, 1380–1385.

48. Sanderson, W. T., Ward, E. M., Steenland, K., and Peterson, M. R. (2001) Lung cancer case—control study of beryllium workers. *Am. J. Ind. Med.* **39**, 133–144.

49. Levy, P. S., Roth, H. D., and Deubner, D. C. (2007) Exposure to beryllium and occurrence of lung cancer: a reexamination of findings from a nested case—control study. *J. Occup. Environ. Med.* **49**, 96–101.

50. International Agency for Research on Cancer (IARC). (1973) Arsenic and inorganic arsenic compounds. IARC Monogr Eval Carcinog Risks Hum, Vol 2. Lyon, France: IARC.

51. International Agency for Research on Cancer (IARC). (1980) Arsenic and arsenic compounds. IARC Monogr Eval Carcinog Risks Hum, Vol 23. Lyon, France: IARC.

52. International Agency for Research on Cancer (IARC). (1987) Arsenic and arsenic compounds. IARC Monogr Eval Carcinog Risks Hum, Supplement 7. Lyon, France: IARC.

53. Lee-Feldstein, A. (1986) Cumulative exposure to arsenic and its relationship to respiratory cancer among copper smelter employees. *J. Occup. Med.* **28**, 296–302.

54. Henderson, V. L., Callahan, C. M., and Paik, M. (1987) Some effects of cigarette smoking, arsenic, and SO2 on mortality among US copper smelter workers. *J. Occup. Med.* **29**, 831–838.

55. Jarup, L., Pershagen, G., and Wall, S. (1989) Cumulative arsenic exposure and lung cancer in smelter workers: a dose-response study. *Am. J. Ind. Med* **15**, 31–41.

56. Xu, Z. Y., Blot, W. J., Xiao, H. P., Wu, A., Feng, Y. P., Stone, B. J., Sun, J., Ershow, A. G., Henderson, B. E., and Fraumeni, J. F. (1989) Smoking, air pollution, and the high rates of lung cancer in Shenyang, China. *J. Natl. Cancer Inst.* **81**, 1800–1806.

57. Enterline, P. E., Day, R., and Marsh, G. M. (1995) Cancers related to exposure to arsenic at a copper smelter. *Occup. Environ. Med.* **52**, 28–32.

58. Lundstrom, N. G., Englyst, V., Gerhardsson, L., Jin, T., and Nordberg, G. (2006) Lung cancer development in primary smelter workers: a nested case-referent study. *J. Occup. Environ. Med.* **48**, 376–380.

59. Cordier, S. and Theriault, I. H. (1983) Mortality patterns in a population living near a copper smelter. *Environ. Res.* **31**, 311–322.

60. Pershagen, G. (1985) Lung cancer mortality among men living near an arsenic-emit-ting copper smelter. *Am. J. Epidemiol.* . **122**, 311–322.

61. Chen, R., Wei, L., and Huang, H. (1993) Mortality from lung cancer among copper miners. *Br. J. Ind. Med.* **50**, 505–509

62. Simonato, L., Moulin, J. J., Javelaud, B., Ferro, G., Wild, P., Winkelmann, R., and Saracci, R. (1994) A retrospective mortality study of workers exposed to arsenic in a gold mine and refinery in France. *Am. J. Ind. Med.* **25**, 625–633.

63. Qiao, Y. L., Taylor, P. R., Yao, S. X., Erozan, Y. S., Luo, X. C., Barrett, M. J., Yan, Q. Y., Giffen, C. A., Huag, S. Q., Maher, M. M., Forman, M. R., and Tockman, M. S. (1997) Risk factors and early detection of lung cancer in a cohort of Chinese tin miners. *Ann. Epidemiol.* **7**, 533–541.

64. Mabuchi, K., Lilienfeld, A. M., and Snell, L. M. (1985) Cancer and occupational exposure to arsenic: a study of pesticides workers. *Prev. Med.* **9**, 119–123.

65. Sobel, W., Bond, G. G., Baldwin, C. L., and Ducommun, D. J. (1988) An update of respiratory cancer and occupational exposure to arsenicals. *Am. J. Ind. Med.* **13**, 263–270.

66. Hayes, R. B (1997) The carcinogenicity of metals in humans. *Cancer Causes Contr.* **8**, 3171–3385.

67. Chen, C. L., Hsu, L. I., Chiou, H. Y., Hsueh, Y. M., Chen, S. Y., Wu, M. M., and Chen, C. J. (2004) Ingested arsenic, cigarette smoking, and lung cancer risk: a follow-up study in arseniasis-endemic areas in Taiwan. *JAMA* **292**, 2984–2990.

68. Ferreccio, C., Gonzalez, C., Milosavlevic, V., Marshall, G., Sancha, A. M., and Smith, A. H. (2000) Lung cancer and arsenic concentrations in drinking water in Chile. *Epidemiology* **11**, 673–679. Erratum in: *Epidemiology* **12**, 283.

69. Chen, Y. and Ahsan, H. (2000) Cancer burden from arsenic in drinking water in Bangladesh. *Am. J. Public Health* **94**, 741–744.

70. International Agency for Research on Cancer (IARC). (1997) Silica and some silicates. IARC Monogr Eval Carcinog Risks Hum: Lyon, France: IARC.

71. The National Toxicology Program (NTP). (2005) Report on Carcinogens, 11th ed. U.S. Department of Health and Human Services, Public Health Service. January 31, 2005.

72. Soutar, C. A., Robertson, A., Miller, B. G., Searl, A., and Bignon, J. (2000) Epidemio-

logical evidence on the carcinogenicity of silica: factors in scientific judgement. *Ann. Occup. Hyg.* **44**, 3–14.

73. Pelucchi, C., Pira, E., Piolatto, G., Coggiola, M., Carta, P., and La Vecchia, C. (2005) Occupational silica exposure and lung cancer risk: a review of epidemiological studies 1996–2005. *Ann. Oncol.* **17**, 1039–1050.

74. Cassidy, A., 't Mannetje, A., van Tongeren, M., Field, J. K., Zaridze, D., Szeszenia-Dabrowska, N., Rudnai, P., Lissowska, J., Fabianova, E., Mates, D., Bencko, V., Foretova, L., Janout, V., Fevotte, J., Fletcher, T., Brennan, P., and Boffetta, P. Occupational exposure to crystalline silica and lung cancer risk: a multicenter case–control study in Europe. *Epidemiology* **18**, 36–43.

75. Brown, T. P. and Rushton, L. (2005) Mortality in the UK industrial silica sand industry: 2. A retrospective cohort study. *Occup. Environ. Med.* **62**, 446–452.

76. Chen, W., Bochmann, F., and Sun, Y. Effects of work related confounders on the association between silica-exposure and lung cancer: a nested case-control study among Chinese miners and pottery workers. *Int. Arch. Environ. Health* **80**, 320–326.

77. Cocco, P., Dosemeci, M., and Rice, C. (2007) Lung cancer among silica-exposed workers: the quest for truth between chance and necessity. *Med. Lav.* **98**, 3–17.

78. Barksdale, J. (1968). The Encyclopedia of the Chemical Elements. Hampel CA Ed. New-York: Reinhold Book Corporation, 732–38 "Titanium".

79. Lee, K. P., Trochimowicz, H. J., and Reinhardt, C. F. Pulmonary response of rats exposed to titanium dioxide (TiO2) by inhalation for two years. *Toxicol. Appl. Pharmacol.* **79**, 179–192.

80. Dungworth, D. L., Mohr, U., Heinrich, U., Ernst, H., and Kittel, B. (1994) Pathologic effects of inhaled articles in rat lungs: associations between inflammatory and neoplastic processes. In: Mohr U, Dungworth DL, Mauderly JL, Oberdoster G, eds. Toxic and Carcinogenic Effects of Solid Particles in the Respiratory Tract. Washington, DC: ILSI Press; pp 75–98.

81. Chen, J. L. and Fayerweather, W. (1988) E. Epidemiologic study of workers exposed to titanium dioxide. *J. Occup. Med.* **30**, 937–942.

82. Fayerweather, W. E., Karns, M. E., Gilby, P. G., and Chen, J. L. (1992) Epidemiologic study of lung cancer mortality in workers exposed to titanium tetrachloride. *J. Occup. Med.* **34**, 164–169.

83. Fryzek, J.P., Chadda, B., Marano, D., White, K., McLaughlin, J. K., and Blot, W. J. (2003) A cohort mortality study among titanium dioxide manufacturing workers in the United States. *J. Occup. Environ. Med.* **45**, 400–409.

84. Boffetta, P., Soutar, A., Cherrie, J.W., Granath, F., Andersen, A., Anttila, A., Blettner, M., Gaborieau, V., Klug, S. J., Langard, S., Luce, D., Merletti, F., Miller, B., Mirabelli, D., Pukkala, E., Adami, H. O., and Weiderpass, E. Mortality among workers employed in the titanium dioxide production industry in Europe. *Cancer Causes Control* **15**, 697–706.

85. Boffetta, P., Gaborieau, V., Nadon, L., Parent, M. F., Weiderpass, E., and Siemiatycki, J. (2001) Exposure to titanium dioxide and risk of lung cancer in a population-based study from Montreal. *Scan. J. Work Environ. Health.* **27**, 227–232.

86. Siemiatycki, J. (1991) Risk factors for cancer in the workplace. Boca Raton (FL): CRC Press, 1991.

87. Haguenoer, J. M., Shirali, P., Hannothiaux, M. H., and Nisse-Ramond, C. (1996) Interactive effects of polycyclic aromatic hydrocarbons and iron oxides particles. Epidemiological and fundamental aspects. *Cent. Eur. J. Public Health.* **4**, 41–45.

88. Stokinger, H. E. (1984) A review of world literature finds iron oxides noncarcinogenic. *Am. J. Ind. Med.* **45**, 127–133.

89 Garry, S., Nesslany, F., Aliouat el, M., Haguenoer, J. M., and Marzin, D. Potent genotoxic activity of benzo[a]pyrene coated onto hematite measured by unscheduled DNA synthesis in vivo in the rat. *Mutagenesis* **18**, 449–455.

90. International Agency for Research on Cancer (IARC). (1987) Haematite and iron oxide. IARC Monogr Eval Carcinog Risks Hum, Supplement 7. Lyon, France: IARC.

91. Lawler, A. B., Mandel, J. S., Schuman, L. M., and Lubin, J. H. (1985) A retrospective cohort mortality study of iron ore (hematite) miners in Minnesota. *J. Occup. Med.* **27**, 507–517.

92. Mur, J. M., Meyer-Bisch, C., Pham, Q. T., Massin, N., Moulin, J. J., and Cavelier, C. (1987) Risk of lung cancer among iron ore miners: a proportional mortality study of 1.075 deceased miners in Lorraine (France). *J. Occup. Med.* **29**, 762–768.

93. Chau, N., Benamghar, L., Pham, Q. T., Teculescu, D., Rebstock, E., and Mur, J.M. (1993) Mortality of iron miners in Lorraine (France): Relation between lung

function and respiratory symptoms and subsequent mortality. *Br. J. Ind. Med.* **50**, 1017–1031.

94. Chen, S. Y., Hayes, R. B., Liang, S. R., Li, Q. G., Stewart, P. A., and Blair A. (1990) Mortality experience of hematite mine workers in China. *Br. J. Ind. Med.* **47**, 175–181.

95. Su, L. P., Guan, H. Y., Zhao, L. F., Zhang, J. M., and Chen, W. H. (2006) Cohort mortality study of dust exposed miners in iron mine. Zhonghua Lao Dong Wei Sheng Zhi Ye Bing Za Zhi 2006; **4**, 360–363 (in Chinese).

96. International Agency for Research on Cancer (IARC). (1987) Iron and steel founding. IARC Monogr Eval Carcinog Risks Hum, Supplement 7. Lyon, France: IARC.

97. International Agency for Research on Cancer (IARC). (1984) Polynuclear aromatic compounds. Part III: Industrial exposures in aluminium production, coal gasification, coke production and iron and steel founding. IARC Monogr Eval Carcinog Risks Hum, Vol. 34. Lyon, France: IARC.

98. Becher, H., Jedrychowski, W., Flak, E., Gomola, K., and Wahrendorf, J. (1989) Lung cancer, smoking, and employment in foundries. Scan. *J. Work Environ. Health* **15**, 38–42.

99. Rotimi, C., Austin, H., Delzell, E., Day, C., Macaluso, M., and Honda, Y. (1993) Retrospective follow-up study of foundry and engine plant workers. *Am. J. Ind. Med.* **24**, 485–498.

100. Sorahan, T., Faux, A. M., and Cooke, M. A. (1994) Mortality among a cohort of United Kingdom steel foundry workers with special reference to cancers of the stomach and lung, 1946–90. *Occup. Environ. Med.* **51**, 316–322.

101. Andjelkovich, D. A., Janszen, D. B., Brown, M. H., Richardson, R. B., and Miller, F.J. (1995) Mortality of iron foundry workers: IV. Analysis of a subcohort exposed to formaldehyde. *J. Occup. Environ. Med.* **37**, 826–837.

102. Hansen, E. S. (1997) A cohort mortality study of foundry workers. *Am. J. Ind. Med.* **32**, 223–233.

103. Rodriguez, V., Tardon, A., Kogevinas, M., Prieto, C. S., Cueto, A., Garcia, M., Menedez, I. A., and Zaplana, J. (2000) Lung cancer risk in iron and steel foundry workers: A nested case-control study in Asturias, Spain. *Am. J. Ind. Med.* **38**, 644–650.

104. Adzresen, K. H., Becker, N., Steindorf, K., and Frentzel-Beyme, R. (2003) Cancer mortality in a cohort of male German iron foundry workers. *Am. J. Ind. Med.* **43**, 295–305.

105. Simonato, L., Fletcher, A. C., Andersen, A., Anderson, K., Becker, N., Chang-Claude, J., Ferro, G., Gérin, M., Gray, C. N., Hansen, K. S., et al. (1991). A historical prospective study of European stainless steel, mild steel and shipyard welders. *Br. J. Ind. Med.* **48**, 145–154.

106. Ambroise, D., Wild, P., and Moulin, J. J. (2006) Update of a meta-analysis on lung cancer and welding. *Scand. J. Work. Environ. Health.* **32**, 22–31.

107. Bourgkard, E., Wild, P., Courcot, B., Diss, M., Ettlinger, J., Goutet, P., Hémon, D., Marquis, N., Mur, J. M., Rigal, C., Rohn-Janssens, M. P., and Moulin. J. J. (2007) Lung cancer mortality and iron oxide exposure in a French steel-producing factory. Accepted for publication.

108. Moulin, J. J., Clavel, T., Roy, D., Dananché, B., Marquis, N., Févotte, J., et al. (2000) Risk of lung cancer in workers producing stainless steel and metallic alloys. *Int. Arch. Occup. Environ. Health.* **73**, 171–180.

109. Hurley, J. F., Miller, B. G., and Jacobsen, M. (1990) Mortality 1967–1977 of industrial workers and ex-workers from the British Steel Industry: further analyses. Institute of Occupational Medicine, Report N° TM/90/07, 1990 Aug.

110. Moulin, J. J., Lafontaine, M., Mantout, B., Belanger, A., Michel, M., Wild, P. et al. (1995) Mortality due to bronchopulmonary cancers in workers of 2 foundries. *Rev. Epidemiol. Santé Publ.* **43**, 107–121 (in French).

111. Finkelstein, M. M. (1994) Lung cancer among steelworkers in Ontario. *Am. J. Ind. Med.* **26**, 549–557.

112. Redmond, C. K., Gustin, J., and Kamon, E. (1975) Long-term mortality experience of steelworkers: Mortality patterns of open hearth steelworkers (a preliminary report). *J. Occup. Med.* **17**, 40–43.

113. Finkelstein, M. M. and Wilk, N. (1990) Investigation of a lung cluster in the melt shop of an Ontario steel producer. *Am. J. Ind. Med.* **17**, 483–491.

114. Finkelstein, M. M., Boulard, M., and Wilk, N. (1991) Increased risk of lung cancer in the melting department of a second Ontario steel manufacturer. *Am. J. Ind. Med.* **19**, 183–194.

115. Moulin, J. J., Wild, P., Mantout, B., Portefaix, P., Fournier-Betz, M., Mur, J. M., et al. (1993) Mortality from lung cancer and cardiovascular diseases among stain-

less steel producing workers. *Cancer Causes Control* **4**, 75–81.

116. Cao, R., Dong, D., and Dong, G. (1995) Mortality study of cancer among Anshan iron and steel workers. *Chung. Hua. Chung. Liu. Tsa. Chih.* **17**, 49–54 (in Chinese).

117. Blot, W. J., Morris Brown, L., Pottern, L. M., Stone. B. J., and Fraumeni, J. F. (1983) Lung cancer among long-term steel workers. *Am. J. Epidemiol.* **117**, 706–716.

118. Xu, Z., Morris Brown, L., Pan, G. W., Liu, T. F., Gao, G. S., Stone, B. J., et al. (1996) Cancer risk among iron and steel workers in Anshan, China, Part II: Case-control studies of lung and stomach cancer. *Am. J. Ind. Med.* **30**, 7–15.

119. Mazumdar, S., Lerer, T., and Redmond, C. K. (1975) Long-term mortality study of steelworkers: Mortality patterns among sheet and tin mill workers. *J. Occup. Med.* **17**, 551–555.

120. Beaumont, J. J., Leveton, J., Knox, K., Bloom, T., McQuinston, T., Young, M., et al. (1987). Lung cancer mortality in workers exposed to sulfuric acid mist and other acid mists. *J. Natl. Cancer Inst.* **79**, 911–921.

121. Axelson, O., and Sjöberg, A. (1979) Cancer incidence and exposure to iron oxide dust. *J. Occup. Med.* **21**, 419–422.

122. Danielsen, T. E., Langrd, S., and Andersen, A. (1998) Incidence of lung cancer among shipyard welders investigated for siderosis. *Int. J. Occup. Environ. Health* **4**, 85–88.

123. Hernberg, S. (2000) Lead poisoning from a historical perspective. *Am. J. Ind. Med.* **38**, 244–254.

124. International Agency for Research on Cancer (IARC). (2004) Inorganic and organic lead compounds. IARC Monogr Eval Carcinog Risks Hum, Vol 87. Lyon, France: IARC.

125. Institut National de Recherche et de Sécurité. (2004) The carcinogenic risk of lead: Evaluation in occupational settings. B Hervé-Bazin editor, EDP Sciences, Paris, France, 2004 (in French).

126. Moulin, J. J., Hervé-Bazin, B., Goutet, P., and Wild, P. (2002) Cancer risk and occupational lead compounds: a meta-analysis. *Med. Lav.* **93**, 388.

127. Cordioli, G., Cuoghi, L., Solari, P. L., Berrino, F., Crosignani, P., and Riboli, E. (1987) Tumor mortality in a cohort of glass industry workers. *Epidemiol. Prev.* **9**, 16–18 (in Italian).

128. Sankila, R., Karjalainen, S., Pukkala, E., Oksanen, H., Hakulinen, T., Teppo, L., and Hakama, M. (1990) Cancer risk among glass factory workers: an excess of lung cancer? *Br. J. Ind. Med.* **47**, 815–818.

129. Michaels, D., Zoloth, S. R., and Stern, F. B. (1991) Does low-level lead exposure increase risk of death? A mortality study of newspaper printers. *Int. J. Epidemiol.* **20**, 978–983.

130 Wingren, G. and Axelsson, O. Mortality in the Swedish glassworks industry. Scand. *J. Work Environ. Health.* **13**, 412–416.

131. Bertazzi, P. A. and Zocchetti, C. (1980) A mortality study of newspaper printing workers. *Am. J. Ind. Med.* **1**, 85–97.

132. Greene, M. H., Hoover, R. N., Eck, R. L., and Fraumeni, J. F. Jr. (1979) Cancer mortality among printing plant workers. *Environ. Res.* **20**, 66–73.

133. Anttila, A., Heikkila, P., Pukkala, E., Nykyri, E., Kauppinen, T., Hernberg, S., and Hemminki K. (1995) Excess Lung cancer among workers exposed to lead. *Scand. J. Work Environ. Health.* **21**, 460–469.

134. Wingren, G. and Englander, V. (1990) Mortality and cancer morbidity in a cohort of Swedish glassworkers. *Int. Arch. Occup. Environ. Health.* **62**, 253–257.

135. Gerhardsson, L., Lundstrom, N. G., Nordberg, G., and Wall, S. (1986) Mortality and lead exposure: a retrospective cohort study of Swedish smelter workers. *Br. J. Ind. Med.* **43**, 707–712.

136. Gerhardsson, L., Hagmar, L., Rylander, L., and Skerfving, S. (1995) Mortality and cancer incidence among secondary lead smelter workers. *Occup. Environ. Med.* **52**, 667–672.

137. Steenland, K., Selevan, S., and Landrigan, P. (1992) The mortality of lead smelter workers: an update. *Am. J. Public Health* **82**, 161–164. Erratum in: *Am. J. Public. Health* (1993) **83**, 60.

138. Wong, O. and Harris, F. (2000) Mortality among employees of lead battery plants and lead-producing plants, 1947–1995. *Am. J. Ind. Med.* **38**, 255–270.

139. Ades, A. E. and Kazantzis, G. (1988) Lung cancer in a non-ferrous smelter: the role of cadmium. *Br. J. Ind. Med.* **45**, 435–442.

140. Cocco, P., Hua, F., Boffetta, P., Carta, P., Flore, C., Flore, V., Onnis, A., Picchiri, G. F., and Colin, D. (1997) Mortality of Italian lead smelter workers. *Scand. J. Work Environ. Health.* **23**, 15–23.

141. Lundstrom, N. G., Nordberg, G., Englyst, V., Gerhardsson, L., Hagmar, L., Jin, T., Rylander, L., and Wall, S. (1997) Cumulative lead exposure in relation to mortality and lung cancer morbidity in a cohort of primary smelter workers. Scand. *J. Work Environ. Health* **23**, 24–30.

142. Sheffet, A., Thind, I., Miller, A. M., and Louria, D. B. (1982) Cancer mortality in a pigment plant utilizing lead and zinc chromates. *Arch. Environ. Health.* **37**, 44–52.

143. Davies, J. M. (1984) Long term mortality study of chromate pigment workers who suffered lead poisoning. *Br. J. Ind. Med.* **41**, 170–178.

144. Lundström, N. G., Englyst, V., Gerhardsson, L., Jin, T., and Nordberg, G. (2006) Lung cancer development in primary smelter workers: a nested case-referent study. *J. Occup. Environ. Med.* **48**, 376–380.

145. Wingren, G. (2004) Mortality and cancer incidence in a Swedish art glassworks—an updated cohort study. *Int. Arch. Occup. Environ. Health.* **77**, 599–603.

146. Davies, J. M. (2005) Study on mortality by specific cause among workers at a lead and zinc foundry in Sardinia. *G. Ital. Med. Lav. Ergon.* **27**, 43–45 (in Italian).

147. Mur. J. M., Moulin, J. J., Charruyer-Seinerra, M. P., and Lafitte, J. (1987) A cohort mortality study among cobalt and sodium workers in an electrochemical plant. *Am. J. Ind. Med.* **11**, 75–81.

148. Moulin, J. J., Wild, P., Mur, J. M., Fournier-Betz, M., and Mercier-Gallay, M. (1993) A mortality study of cobalt production workers: an extension of the follow-up. *Am. J. Ind. Med.* **23**, 281–288.

149. Hogstedt, C. and Alexandersson, R (1990). Mortality among hard-metal workers. *Arbete Hälsa* **21**, 3–26 (in Swedish).

150. Lasfargues, G., Wild, P., Moulin, J. J., Hammon, B., Rosmorduc, B., Rondeau du Noyer, C., Lavandier, M, and Moline, J. (1994) Lung cancer mortality in a French cohort of hard-metal workers. *Am. J. Ind. Med.* **26**, 585–595.

151. Moulin, J. J., Wild, P., Romazini, S., Lasfargues, G., Peltier, A., Bozec, C., Deguerry, P., Pellet, F., and Perdrix, A. (1998) Lung cancer risk in hard-metal workers. *Am. J. Epidemiol.* **148**, 241–248.

152. Wild, P., Perdrix, A., Romazini, S., Moulin, J. J., and Pellet, F. Lung cancer mortality in a site producing hard metals. *Occup. Environ. Med.* **57**, 568–573.

153. Leonard, A. and Lauwerys, R. (1990) Mutagenicity, carcinogenicity and teratogenicity of cobalt metal and cobalt compounds. *Mutat. Res.* **239**, 17–27.

154. Anard, D., Kirsch-Volders, M., Elhajouji, A., Belpaeme, K., and Lison, D. (1997) In vitro genotoxic effects of hard metal particles assessed by alkaline single cell gel and elution assays. *Carcinogenesis* **18**, 177–184.

155. De Boeck, M., Lison, D., and Kirsch-Volders, M. (1998) Evaluation of the in vitro direct and indirect genotoxic effects of cobalt compounds using the alkaline comet assay. Influence of interdonor and interexperimental variability. *Carcinogenesis* **19**, 2021–2029.

156. De Boeck, M., Hoet, P., Lombaert, N., et al. (2003) In vivo genotoxicity of hard metal dust: induction of micronuclei in rat type II epithelial lung cells. *Carcinogenesis* **11**, 1793–1800.

157. International Agency for Research on Cancer (IARC). (2006). Cobalt in hard metals and cobalt sulfate, gallium arsenide, indium phosphide and vanadium pentoxide. IARC, Monogr Eval Carcinog Risks Hum, Vol. 86. Lyon, France: IARC.

158. Duffus, J. H. (1996) Epidemiology and the identification of metals as human carcinogens. *Sci. Prog.* **79**, 311–326.

159. Navarro Silvera, S. A., and Rohan, T. E. Trace elements and cancer risk: a review of the epidemiologic evidence. *Cancer Causes Control* **18**, 7–27.

160. Desoize, B. (2004) Metals and metal compounds in cancer treatment. *Anticancer Res.* **24**, 1529–1544.

Chapter 7

Breast Cancer and the Role of Exercise in Women

Beverly S. Reigle and Karen Wonders

Abstract

Cancer of the breast is a significant health problem for women from the time of diagnosis through the treatment and survivorship trajectory. The disease and treatments are an assault to a woman's body, resulting in sequelae that can be debilitating. Although women diagnosed with breast cancer are living longer, concerns about functional limitations, recurrence, and survival remain paramount. Physical activity and exercise are preventative and rehabilitative measures that can be employed at various points along the breast cancer trajectory. Current research supports the beneficial role that physical activity and exercise play in reducing the risk for developing breast cancer and preventing or attenuating disease and treatment-related impairments.

Key words: Breast cancer, exercise, prevention, recurrence.

1. Incidence and Mortality

Cancer of the breast is the most common cancer in US women and ranks second to lung cancer in cancer deaths (1). The American Cancer Society (1) estimates that in 2007 more than 182,460 women will develop invasive breast cancer, more than 67,770 will develop in situ carcinoma, and an estimated 40,480 women will die of the disease. Early detection is the primary method of combating the disease, which is underscored by the current 5-year survival rate of 98% for localized tumors, 84% for regionally metastasized tumors, and 27% for those involving distant metastasis (1).

M. Verma (ed.), *Methods of Molecular Biology, Cancer Epidemiology, vol. 472*
© 2009 Humana Press, a part of Springer Science+Business Media, Totowa, NJ
Book doi: 10.1007/978-1-60327-492-0

A noticeable decrease in the incidence rate of breast occurred in 2002. In the 1990s, the rate of breast cancer incidence increased steadily at about 0.5% per year *(2)*. However, between mid 2002 and 2004, the age-adjusted incidence rate dropped approximately 6.7%. A comparison of the incidence rates of 2001 and 2004 indicated a decrease of 8.6%, which was evident only in women 50 years of age and older and associated more with estrogen receptor-positive tumors *(2)*. The researchers suggested that this decrease in incidence could be attributed to a 38% drop in the use of hormone-replacement therapy (HRT), which began declining in mid 2002. This sharp decrease in the use of HRT among women of this age followed the highly publicized findings of the Women's Health Initiative *(3)*, in which an increase in the incidence of coronary heart disease and breast cancer was associated with the use of estrogen—progestin therapy *(2)*.

Breast cancer mortality rates decreased by 24% between the years 1990 and 2000 *(4)*. For women aged 49 years and younger, the drop in breast cancer mortality was greater than for women 50 years and older *(1)*. The drop in number of breast cancer deaths is attributed to early detection and adjuvant therapy *(2)*. Recent findings indicated that screening mammography accounted for 25 to 65% (median of 46%) of the drop in breast cancer mortality, and the remaining amount was attributed to adjuvant therapy *(5)*. As a result, over 2 million women in the USA are breast cancer survivors *(6)*.

Racially and ethnically, white women have the highest breast cancer incidence rate *(1)*. However, African American women have the highest mortality rate and, in comparison to Hispanic/Latino, Native American, and Asian women, they have the highest incidence rate. Hispanic/Latino women have the highest breast cancer incidence and mortality rates when compared with Asian and Native American women *(1)*. The higher incidence and mortality rates among some racial and ethnic populations may be attributed to inequities in socioeconomic status and cancer care as well as cultural and genetic factors *(1)*. In a descriptive study involving a multiracial cohort of 124,934 women who were listed in 1 of 11 population-based tumor registries, researchers *(7)* found that African American and Hispanic white women presented with a more advanced stage of breast cancer at the time of diagnosis than non-Hispanic white women. Findings also indicated that certain racial and ethnic groups did not receive the recommended standard of care for their primary treatment. The differences in disease management among certain race and ethnic populations may be attributed to "socioeconomic factors, patient—physician interactions, and knowledge" *(7*; p. 34).

1.1. Risk Factors

A woman's chances of developing breast cancer within her lifetime are one in eight or 12.5% *(8)*. Of the multiple risk factors, gender (being female), and age are the most significant. As a woman ages, her chances of developing the disease increases. Thus, women who are 50 to 59 years of age have a 2.63% chance of developing breast cancer compared with a 0.43% chance for women aged 30 to 39 *(8)*. Other risk factors include, but are not limited to, inherited genetic mutations (BRCA 1, 2), a personal or family history of the disease, atypical proliferative hyperplasia, reproductive factors (e.g., early menarche, late menopause, nulliparity, HRT), postmenopausal obesity, physical inactivity, and consumption of one or more alcoholic beverages per day *(2)*. Few of the known risk factors are modifiable. However, physical inactivity is a behavior that can be changed and, if women increase their level of physical activity, their chances for developing breast cancer may decrease *(9, 10)*.

In this chapter, the authors discuss the breast cancer trajectory and the role of physical activity and exercise. For clarity, differentiation between the two terms is warranted. According to the US Department of Health and Human Services *(11)*, physical activity is the "bodily movement that is produced by the contraction of skeletal muscle and that substantially increases energy expenditure" *(11*; p. 21). Exercise, a specific type of physical activity, is defined as "planned, structured, and repetitive bodily movements done to improve or maintain one or more components of physical fitness *(11*; p. 21).

2. Exercise Physiology

Knowledge of exercise physiology provides a backdrop for understanding the role of physical activity and exercise in the breast cancer population. Basically, all plants and animals rely on energy to support life. This energy originates from the sun in the form of light energy. Through the process of photosynthesis, plants use light energy from the sun to drive the chemical reactions necessary to form carbohydrates, fats, and proteins. Humans acquire these nutrients by eating plants and the animals who feed on these plants. In turn, the body uses the carbohydrates, fats, and proteins obtained from food to provide the necessary energy to maintain cellular activities both at rest and during exercise. The nutrients we obtain from eating plants and animals may be broken down through the process of metabolism to release the stored energy. Metabolism is the sum of the chemical reactions occurring in living organisms.

The energy within the molecular bonds of carbohydrates, fats, and proteins is chemically released in the form of the high-energy phosphate compound adenosine triphosphate (ATP). The formation of ATP occurs by combining adenosine diphosphate (ADP) and inorganic phosphate (Pi). Energy is stored within the chemical bond that joins ADP and Pi. Accordingly, if this bond breaks, energy that may be used for muscular contraction is released:

$$ATP \rightarrow ADP + Pi + energy.$$

A limited amount of ATP is stored within the body cells and serves as an immediate source of energy for muscular contraction. Since muscular exercise requires a constant supply of ATP to sustain muscular contraction, three metabolic pathways exist within muscle cells, giving them the capacity to produce ATP. The first pathway is called the phosphagen system, and involves the formation of ATP by the breakdown of phosphocreatine (PC). As ATP is broken down into ADP + Pi at the onset of exercise, PC donates a phosphate to the ADP molecule, thereby reforming ATP. Thus:

$$ADP + Pi \rightarrow ATP.$$

The phosphagen pathway is anaerobic (does not use oxygen) and can rapidly form ATP. However, just as with stores of ATP, the body only stores limited amounts of PC. Therefore, only a small amount of ATP can be formed through this system. Consequently, the phosphagen system supplies energy at the onset of exercise and during short-duration (i.e., less than 10 seconds), high-intensity exercise.

The second metabolic pathway used to make ATP is glycolysis. In the body, carbohydrates are ultimately converted to the simple sugar, glucose. Glucose is transported via the blood to body tissues. At rest, glucose is taken up by the muscles and liver and is stored as a more complex sugar molecule called glycogen. During exercise, glycogen is converted back to glucose and transported to active tissues where it is metabolized, via glycolysis. Glycolysis is an anaerobic pathway that involves a series of reactions, whereby glucose is ultimately degraded into two molecules of pyruvic acid. The presence of oxygen determines the fate of pyruvic acid. In the absence of oxygen, pyruvic acid is converted to lactic acid, and a net of two ATP molecules are formed.

In the presence of oxygen, pyruvic acid is converted to the compound acetyl coenzyme A (acetyl CoA), and the production of ATP continues via the third metabolic pathway, oxidative phosphorylation. This is the most complex of the three energy systems, and involves the interaction of two metabolic pathways: the Krebs cycle and the electron transport chain. Once formed, acetyl CoA enters the Krebs cycle. A series of complex reactions follows, leading to the complete oxidation of acetyl CoA. The end products of the Krebs cycle are two molecules of ATP, carbon dioxide, and hydrogen.

The hydrogen released during the Krebs cycle combines with two electron carriers, nicotinamide adenine dinucleotide (NAD) and flavin adenine dinucleotide (FAD). NAD and FAD carry the hydrogen atoms to the electron transport chain, whereby the hydrogen ultimately combines with oxygen to form water. During this process, electrons are split from the hydrogen, and pass through a series of reactions. These electrons provide energy needed for the phosphorylation of ADP, thus forming ATP.

The energy for muscular contraction comes from the breakdown of ATP. During maximal, short-duration exercise, ATP is generated primarily from the degradation of carbohydrates, while stored body fat is considered the ideal fuel for prolonged exercise, as it contains large quantities of energy per unit of weight. Proteins typically provide little energy for cellular function, and are instead used as the body's building blocks.

2.1. Cardiorespiratory Fitness

One of the most important factors determining an individual's ability to perform endurance exercise is his or her maximal oxygen uptake, or VO_{2max}. This is defined as the maximal rate at which oxygen can be taken up, distributed, and used by the body during physical activity. VO_{2max} is usually expressed in terms of milliliters of oxygen consumed per kilogram of body weight per minute ($mL \cdot kg^{-1} \cdot min^{-1}$) and typical values range from 20 to 70 $mL \cdot kg^{-1} \cdot min^{-1}$. Individuals with a higher VO_{2max} are better able to perform endurance exercise.

Direct measurement of VO_{2max} requires a computerized metabolic cart. This method offers the most valid and reliable marker of cardiorespiratory fitness. However, direct measurement of VO_{2max} is expensive, time-consuming, and requires highly trained personnel and is often not practical for most testing environments, particularly for large populations involved in epidemiological studies of exercise and disease. Therefore, several researchers have developed regression equations that predict VO_{2max} based on physiological responses (usually heart rate) to submaximal exercise. In these submaximal exercise tests, the workload is typically fixed and heart rate is measured during and at the completion of the test. Three assumptions allow for the prediction of VO_{2max} from submaximal exercise tests:

1. A linear relationship exists between heart rate, oxygen uptake, and workload.

2. The maximum heart rate at a given age is uniform.

3. The mechanical efficiency is the same for everyone.

Once an individual's VO_{2max} has been determined, it can be useful in prescribing exercise intensity. In order to make improvements to an individual's VO_{2max}, one must exercise at a percentage of his/her VO_{2max}. In healthy populations, this percentage is generally around 60 to 70%. A second way in which exercise intensity may be expressed is in terms of a metabolic equivalent, or a MET. One MET is equal to the resting oxygen consumption of the reference average human, approximately 3.5 mL · kg^{-1} · min^{-1}. The harder the body works during the activity, the higher the MET. In general, any activity that burns 3 to 6 METs is considered moderate-intensity physical activity. Any activity that burns > 6 METs is considered vigorous-intensity physical activity.

3. Breast Cancer Trajectory Framework

The Model of Disability and Prevention of Disability (MDPD) *(12, 13)* provides a framework for conceptualizing the breast cancer continuum from pathology to disability and the potential for introducing physical activity and exercise as preventative and rehabilitative measures *(14)*. Four of the MDPD's concepts are presented as a continuum: 1) pathology, 2) impairment, 3) functional limitation, and 4) disability (*see* **Fig. 7.1**). Two concepts are depicted as interacting in a reciprocal manner along the continuum: 1) risk factors (i.e., biological, environmental, and lifestyle) and 2) quality of life (QOL).

Application of the MDPD to breast cancer begins with pathology or the carcinogenesis that occurs in the breast. This abnormal cellular change leads to biochemical and physiological abnormalities called impairments. Impairments, prior to treatment, consist of changes in consistency and structure of the breast and possibly adjacent skin and lymph nodes. Following surgery and adjuvant therapies, impairments may consist of numbness, swelling, pain *(15)*, fatigue *(16)*, nausea and vomiting (17), muscle weakness, decreased joint range of motion *(18)*, and decreased cognitive abilities *(19)*. These impairments, whether disease or treatment related, may lead to functional limitations such as difficulty performing self-care (e.g., combing hair) ambulating, remembering, and difficulty performing household activities and occupational responsibilities, According to the MDPD, disability occurs when functional limitations exist and resources or accommodations are not available to assist the woman in performing her social and work-related roles *(12)*. Thus, disability is based on society's response to a woman's functional limitations.

Risk factors, as mentioned earlier, have a reciprocal interaction with the disablement continuum. Certain biological (e.g., nulliparity), environmental (e.g., radiation), and lifestyle (e.g., physical inactivity) factors may negatively impact points along the breast cancer trajectory and increase a woman's risk for developing the disease, incurring impairments, developing functional limitations,

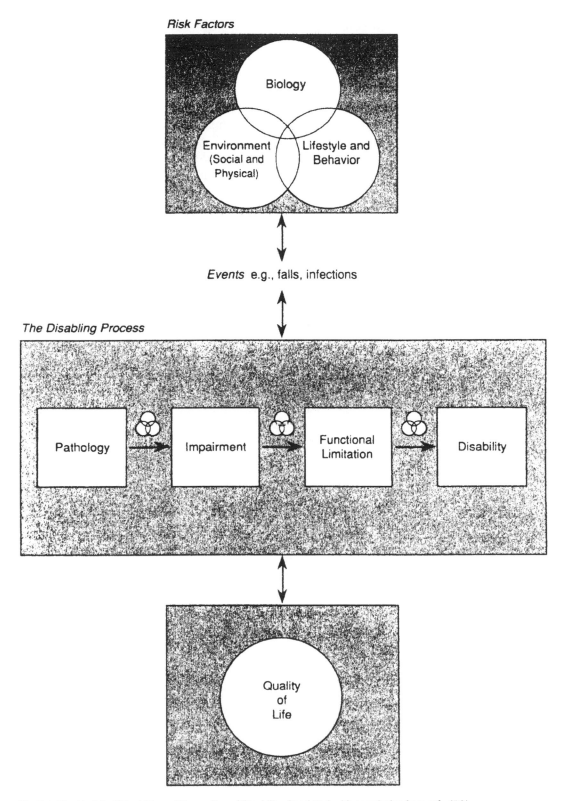

Fig. 7.1. The Model of Disability and Prevention of Disability. Reprinted with permission from ref. *(13)*

or becoming disabled. The reciprocal nature of the risk factor concept is supported in a study *(20)* in which researchers found that exercise improved immune function in breast cancer survivors following chemotherapy. Immunosuppression is a side effect of chemotherapeutic drugs which, in turn, places a woman at risk for infection *(21)*. Exercise is an intervention that can positively impact the immune system; thus, decreasing a woman's chances of infection *(20)*.

QOL, a multidimensional concept, represents a woman's perceptions of her emotional, physical, social, and functional well-being *(22)*. The impairments and functional abilities that develop following a diagnosis of breast cancer influence a woman's QOL *(23)*. The reciprocal nature of the QOL concept was demonstrated by Darga et al. *(24)* in a study that examined whether QOL in a sample of 39 breast cancer survivors with a body mass index (BMI) of 30 to 44 kg/m² predicted weight loss and whether weight loss had an effect on QOL at 12 months after intervention. Their findings indicated that, at baseline, physical and functional QOL scores were significantly associated with weight loss and at 12 months after intervention, weight loss was associated with significant improvement in several QOL subscales. Interestingly, women who reported impaired physical and functional QOL scores at baseline lost more weight, suggesting that such impairments may be a motivating factor to weight loss adherence and not inhibitory *(24)*. The intervention in this study consisted of both dietary counseling and a recommended moderate exercise regimen of 30 to 45 minutes per day. Thus, exercise, as an intervention, introduced at points along the MDPD continuum can have a positive effect on QOL *(23)*.

4. Prevention of Breast Cancer Occurrence

Physical activity and exercise are interventions that can be introduced at several points along the breast cancer continuum as depicted by the MDPD. The first intervention point is prior to pathology, which is the prevention of carcinoma of the breast. In a review of 44 studies that examined the association between physical activity and breast cancer, 32 studies supported a 30 to 40' reduction in breast cancer risk among women who were physically active *(25)*.

The specific amount of physical activity necessary to infer a risk reduction has yet to be fully elucidated; however, many studies suggest that a moderate level of physical activity plays a key role in primary prevention against breast cancer *(26–31)*. Friedenreich et al. *(29)* reviewed 21 studies on physical activity and breast cancer. Of these 21 cases, 15 cases (71%) suggested that physical activity reduces breast cancer risk. In addition, Gammon et al. *(30)* reviewed epidemiological studies published from 1966 to present and reported that 11 of 16 studies found a 12 to 60% risk reduction among premenopausal and postmenopausal women as their level of recreational exercise increased. Conversely, Gammon et al. *(32)* did not find any relationship between physical activity and breast cancer in 1,668 women aged 45 years and younger versus 1,505 controls. Likewise, a prospective study by Moore et al. *(33)* did not detect any relationship between breast cancer and physical activity in women between 55 and 69 years of age.

The inconsistencies observed among studies could be the assessment of physical activity at different time periods of a woman's life. Only a few case—control studies examined the relationship between lifetime physical activity and breast cancer *(34–36)*. Many studies do not include household chores or occupational activities, which may be an important component of physical activity in women. Friedenreich et al. *(35)*, however, examined breast cancer risk associated with lifetime recreational, household, and occupational activities separately and in combination. While no association was made between lifetime activity and breast cancer risk in premenopausal women, lifetime activity was found to reduce breast cancer risk in postmenopausal women. Interestingly, household and occupational activities were associated with the largest risk reductions in this group.

Currently, no scientific consensus exists on the appropriate intensity, duration, or frequency of physical activity needed to influence breast cancer risk. Bernstein et al. *(27)* reported a strong reduction in breast cancer risk in a case—control study of women younger than 40 years of age. In this investigation, subjects completed a detailed physical activity assessment instrument that quantified the average number of hours per week women spent doing recreational physical activity. It was determined that an average of 3.8 hours or more of physical activity per week was associated with the greatest reductions in breast cancer risk.

Rockhill and colleagues *(37)* analyzed data from a prospective study of women between the ages of 30 and 55 years, who reported on the average number of hours per week they spent in various moderate and vigorous recreational physical activity over the previous year. Women who were more physically active had a lower risk of breast cancer than those who were less physically active. In addition, women who reported engaging in moderate or vigorous physical activity for 7 hours or more each week had a relative risk of 0.82 compared with those who reported engaging in physical activity for less than 1 hour per week.

4.1. Mechanism for Reducing Breast Cancer Risk Through Physical Activity

Although physical activity may reduce a woman's risk of developing breast cancer, the underlying mechanism remains unclear. In some studies, physical activity has been associated with body size and fat stores (38–41). Regular physical activity is often accompanied by a reduction in body fat, which leads to reduced substrate for the production of estrogen from androstenedione in fat tissue (41). In addition, physical activity may also increase levels of sex hormone-binding globulin, thereby reducing the amount of estradiol (40). Thus, since breast cancer is an estrogen-dependent disease, it is possible that exercise reduces risk by lowering a woman's exposure to estrogen.

Another possible mechanism may involve lipid peroxidation and the production of reactive oxygen species (ROS). Numerous studies have shown that physical exercise is a strong inducer of lipid peroxidation. Aerobic metabolism is dependent on oxidative phosphorylation, a process whereby ATP is formed through mitochondrial electron transport. The mitochondrial electron transport system involves the sequential transfer of electrons through a series of oxidation/reduction reactions. Cytochrome c oxidase serves as the final electron acceptor for this system; and, under normal conditions, reduces oxygen to water. However, intermediate proteins in the mitochondrial electron transport system are not always entirely efficient in the transfer of electrons, and occasionally may release electrons directly to oxygen. This results in the formation of ROS, partially reduced and highly reactive metabolites of oxygen (42). Therefore, increases in oxygen consumption observed during exercise are accompanied by a concomitant increase in ROS. ROS cause damage by binding to proteins, lipids, and nucleic acids, thereby altering their conformation and function (43, 44).

The body is equipped with an antioxidant system to protect against, or minimize, damage caused by oxidative stress. Three enzymatic antioxidants in this system include superoxide dismutase (SOD), catalase (CAT), and glutathione peroxidase (GPx). SOD catalyzes the dismutation of O_2- to H_2O_2 and O_2 (45). Three types of SOD isoenzymes have been identified in mammals, and are characterized by prosthetic metal ions and their cellular location within the body. Manganese-containing SOD (Mn-SOD) is found in the mitochondria of the heart, kidney, and liver. Copper- and zinc-containing SOD (CuZn-SOD) is predominantly located in the cytoplasm of erythrocytes, heart, and liver. Lastly, copper- and zinc-containing extracellular SOD (EC-SOD) can be found in the extracellular space of the lung and kidney (46).

CAT catalyzes the reduction of H_2O_2 to water and ½ O_2. GPx is located in the cytoplasm and mitochondria of cardiomyocytes and uses glutathione (GSH) as a substrate to reduce H_2O_2 to water (20). GSH is primarily synthesized by the liver and is transported to tissues via blood circulation. GSH is thought to play a critical role in protecting against oxidative stress, in that it can neutralize free radicals by donating two electrons *(47)*.

If the amount of ROS exceeds the cell's antioxidant capacity, a state of oxidative stress results, initiating a cascade of events leading to lipid peroxidation, DNA damage, and apoptosis *(48, 49)*. Apoptosis is a highly regulated chemical form of programmed cell death. The complex process by which apoptosis induces cellular death involves four distinct phases; a stimulus phase, a signal transduction phase, a degradation phase, and a clearance phase. The stimulation phase involves a mechanism of stimulation to activate the relevant genetic machinery allowing the cell to begin apoptosis. These stimuli may originate from inside or outside of the cell *(50)*. Free radicals are one such stimulus that originates outside the cell and modulates apoptosis *(49)*. Various drugs and chemotherapy agents are other mechanisms that may advance apoptosis *(51)*. Finally, the tumor necrosis factor (TNF) family of ligands and receptors are known to trigger apoptosis directly through receptor-mediated apoptosis *(50)*.

The second phase of apoptosis involves intracellular signal transduction. Signal transduction occurs by two overlapping pathways: ligand-mediated activation following binding to a receptor and a mitochondrial-dependent pathway. The binding of a TNF ligand to its receptor activates the death domain within the cell and leads to the activation of caspases *(50)*. Caspases are proteases that cleave the carboxyl, C-terminal of aspartic acid resi-dues of proteins. They are expressed as procaspases, inactive precursors to caspases, in the cytosol of nearly every cell in the body. There are 13 known caspases that are responsible for mediating the biochemical degradation of approximately 70 cytosolic and nuclear targets that lead to the distinguishing morphological features of apoptosis. Different caspases have different roles in initiating apoptotic cell death. Caspases-1 and -11 cleave precursors to produce mature cytokines. Caspases-8 and -9 initiate the propagation of apoptotic cell death signals, and caspases-3, -6, and -7 execute apoptosis by cleaving several vital proteins *(52)*.

There are two ways by which mitochondria participate in apoptosis. First, they house cytochrome c and apoptosis-inducing factor (AIF), two pro-apoptotic proteins. The release of cytochrome c from the mitochondria leads to the activation of caspase-9 and caspase-3 *(53)*. AIF has the ability to act on the nucleus directly, without activation of caspases *(54)*. Second, mitochondria produce ROS, which is believed to be an early triggering event in the apoptotic pathway *(55)*. Researchers *(56)* hypothesize that ROS activates mitogen-activated protein kinases (MAPKs), which mediate cellular responses. Activation of MAPK and cross-talk between its family members determine if the cell will undergo proliferation, differentiation, or death.

The third stage of apoptosis includes the morphological and biochemical changes associated with apoptosis, involving cell dismantling, DNA fragmentation, and expression of phagocyte recognition molecules. The final stage of apoptosis is the recognition and ingestion of apoptotic bodies by phagocytes (50).

It is possible that exercise may induce oxidative stress and subsequent apoptosis of premalignant and malignant cells of the breast, and thus protect against breast cancer. This hypothesis was tested by Radak et al. (57), using an animal model. In this investigation, solid leukemia tumor cells were transplanted into three groups of mice: control, exercise trained with the exercise being terminated at the time of transplantation, and exercise trained with the animals continuing exercise throughout the experiment. At 18 days post-transplantation, tumors in the exercise trained animals who continued to exercise were 50% smaller than the tumors in the other two groups (p < 0.05). The decrease in tumor size was associated with an increase in levels of lipid peroxidation.

5. Exercise and Primary and Adjuvant Treatment Complications

Women diagnosed with breast cancer represent the largest cancer survivor group in the USA (58). Once diagnosed, most women undergo a multimodality approach to treating their disease (59). Typically, surgery is the primary treatment for Stage I, II, IIIA, and operable IIIC breast cancer (60), with irradiation, chemotherapy, hormone therapy, or a combination of the three used as adjuvant approaches (61, 62). The assault to their bodies, from both the disease and treatments, is frequently characterized by sequelae such as nausea and vomiting (63), hair loss (64), fatigue (65, 66), depression (67), poor body image (67–69), pain (70), decreased upper body flexibility and strength (23, 71, 72), lymphedema (73–75), weight gain (76), and osteoporosis (77). Breast cancer survivors also report difficulty sleeping and pulling in the arm or axilla (78). Exercise is an intervention that can prevent, alleviate, or reduce the severity of many of these problems. The following is a brief discussion about the role of exercise in women who are undergoing primary and adjuvant therapies.

5.1. Surgery and Exercise

The primary treatment of a malignant breast tumor is typically surgical excision. The most common types of breast cancer surgery are lumpectomy, total mastectomy, and modified radical mastectomy (62). The type of surgery is based on tumor and personal factors such as tumor size, axillary node involvement, tumor stage, and patient preference (1). Of the three surgical procedures, lumpectomy conserves as much breast tissue as possible, removing only the tumor and a margin of tissue surrounding the tumor. The total mastectomy removes the entire breast and a modified radical mastectomy removes the entire breast and a select number of axillary lymph nodes (e.g., 10 to 15 nodes) *(62)*. Axillary lymph node dissection (ALND) may also accompany a lumpectomy and total mastectomy based on the outcome of a less invasive lymph node sampling procedure called sentinel node biopsy (SNB) *(79)*. The sentinel node is the first node or nodes of the lymphatic system into which the breast tumor drains. If the node or nodes are positive for malignancy then further ALND is required *(62, 79)*. The SNB is less invasive; therefore, the expectation is that women will experience less postsurgical morbidity. However, Rietman and colleagues *(80)* found no significant difference in upper-limb morbidity (e.g., pain, decreased range of motion and muscle strength, and perceived activities of daily living (ADL) disability) between women who had SNB or ALND. Baron et al. *(81)* found that women reported sensations such as numbness and tenderness even 2 years after SNB or ALND; however, the severity of these sensations was less for those who had SNB. Even though the removal of axillary lymph nodes is associated with postsurgical morbidity; axillary lymph node status remains the primary determinant of a woman's breast cancer prognosis *(82)*.

The sequelae that follow surgical treatment can impact a woman's ability to perform her usual personal, household, and occupational activities. Two hundred and four patients with Stage I or II breast cancer were assessed preoperatively and 6 weeks postoperatively for shoulder range of motion, muscle strength, grip strength, pain, upper and forearm edema, shoulder disability and perceived ADL disability following breast cancer surgery with either ALND or SNB *(80)*. Findings indicated that, between baseline and 6 weeks following surgery, women experienced pain, decreased range of motion, numbness, loss of shoulder abductor and elbow flexor strength, and perceived ADL disability. In a study of 400 breast cancer survivors who had ALND as part of their surgery, researchers *(83)* found that pain, numbness, loss of strength, sensitive scar and shoulder, and neck and back discomfort were the most frequent complaints 5 months after completing primary and adjuvant therapies. Of the 400 women, 25 to 35% reported difficulty performing ADL, which included lifting heavy objects and completing household chores.

Lymphedema is often a late effect of ALND and radiation treatment *(66, 73)*. This effect occurs when the transport of lymph fluid is interrupted and collects in the tissues of the extremity *(73)*. To prevent lymphedema, women who have undergone ALND have been advised by health professionals to avoid "vigorous, repetitive, or excessive upper body exercise" *(84)*. However, such advice was not supported by research *(84)* and, in fact, current findings support the performance of vigorous exercise (i.e., dragon boat training) following treatment for breast cancer without the development of lymphedema *(85)*.

Exercises following breast cancer surgery have been recommended for many years by the ACS Reach to Recovery program *(86)*; however, these exercises were not research based. To the authors' knowledge, no national consensus exists regarding the type, intensity, duration, frequency, and time of initiation of postoperative exercises for breast cancer survivors. Some controversy *(87, 88)* exists regarding how soon after the surgical procedure (e.g., postoperative day 1 or following drain removal) upper arm exercises should be initiated, due to concern about seroma development and wound drainage. Na et al. *(88)* conducted a quasi-experimental study involving 33 subjects who had a modified radical mastectomy or partial mastectomy to determine whether those receiving early postmastectomy rehabilitation (40 minutes of physical therapy and 30 minutes of exercise four times per day) had greater improvement in range of shoulder motion and performance of functional activities than patients who received exercise instruction only. Additionally, they determined whether postoperative complications (e.g., seromas) were associated with early rehabilitation. Measurements occurred preoperatively and postoperatively at 3 days, discharge, and 1 month. Interestingly, the average hospital stay was 18 days for the experimental and 12 for the control group. Findings indicated that the experimental group had greater range of shoulder motion and less difficulty performing five activities of the functional assessment than the control group and that early rehabilitation did not increase postoperative complications. This supports the findings of a 1984 experimental study *(89)* in which 49 women who had modified radical mastectomies and received immediate postoperative physical therapy (30 minutes two times per day for about 10 days) were compared with 41 women who had modified radical mastectomies and no physical therapy. Women who performed exercises (active assistive shoulder progressing to active resistive and functional activities) demonstrated better shoulder range of motion and less difficulty with functional activities. In addition, no statistically significant difference in postoperative complications or hospital stay was found between the two groups.

Unfortunately, a paucity of studies exist that address postoperative exercises for women diagnosed with breast cancer (e.g., when to initiate, type, intensity, frequency, and duration of exercise). Based on a few studies, Harris *(79)* recommends a postoperative regimen that includes range of motion exercises, active-assisted movements, and hand and elbow isometric/concentric exercises beginning the day of surgery up to the day 14 postoperatively.

5.2. Adjuvant Therapy

Adjuvant therapy is treatment that is initiated after the primary treatment. As mentioned earlier, the primary treatment is often surgery and adjuvant therapies most commonly include chemotherapy, irradiation, and hormonal therapy. Adjuvant therapies impact the body systemically or locally. Chemotherapy is a systemic treatment involving medication that is usually administered orally or intravenously *(62)* to prevent micrometastasis *(79)*. Irradiation is a localized treatment that involves the use of external beam or interstitial radiation at the tumor or adjacent sites to reduce the risk of local or regional recurrence. Hormonal or endocrine therapy is also systemic and involves the use of antiestrogen medications (e.g., Tamoxifen and aromatase inhibitors) to prevent recurrence or the development of a new primary breast cancer *(79)*.

Most of the current studies that address the benefits of exercise in the breast cancer population involve breast cancer survivors who have completed primary treatment (i.e., surgery) and are either undergoing or have completed adjuvant therapy. Kirschbaum *(90)* conducted a critical review of the literature that addressed the benefits of whole body exercise during and after breast cancer treatment. Findings indicated support for all types of aerobic exercise administered during adjuvant therapy as compared with after treatment. In particular, she found strong evidence that aerobic exercises decrease cancer-related fatigue. Courneya and colleagues *(59)* also conducted an extensive literature review of studies that examined the effect of aerobic or resistance exercise regimens on cardiovascular function and muscle strength in breast cancer survivors. Based on the findings, they recommended that during and after treatment, breast cancer survivors engage in 20 to 60 minutes of an aerobic exercise of moderate intensity 3 to 5 days per week. Additionally, they recommended the inclusion of resistance training.

Kolden et al. *(23)* investigated the feasibility, safety, and benefits of a 16-week group exercise training (GET) for 40 sedentary women aged 46 years and older. Subjects had undergone a modified radical mastectomy or breast-conserving surgery and most were undergoing adjuvant therapies. Findings indicated a significant improvement at 16 weeks in resting systolic blood pressure, flexibility, aerobic capacity (estimated VO_{2max}), strength, as well as QOL (enhanced well-being, increased positive affect, decreased distress, and improved functioning). Based on the findings of this pilot study, a randomized controlled trial is recommended to determine the efficacy of this exercise intervention.

Headley and colleagues *(91)* conducted a unique quasi-experimental study to determine the effect of a seated exercise on fatigue and QOL in women with Stage IV breast cancer and undergoing outpatient chemotherapy. Of the 32 subjects, 16 were randomly assigned to the experimental group. The experimental group viewed an exercise videotape and performed seated exercises three times per week during four cycles of chemotherapy. Those in the control group did not engage in the seated exercises, but could continue their usual physical activities. Findings indicated that subjects performing the seated exercises experienced a slower decline in physical well-being and less fatigue starting with the third cycle of chemotherapy than the control group.

A recent study designed specifically for breast cancer patients undergoing radiotherapy examined the effect of stretching as a method of increasing range of motion in the upper quadrant *(92)*. Following breast cancer surgery and prior to radiotherapy, 64 women were recruited and randomized to a control group or stretch group. The experimental group received instruction on how to perform daily low-load, prolonged pectoral stretches and the control group received no exercise instruction. No difference in shoulder range of motion, arm circumference, and QOL was found between the two groups.

Two experimental studies *(93, 94)* evaluated exercise in breast cancer survivors following primary and adjuvant therapies. One study examined the benefits of walking *(93)* and the other examined weight training *(94)*. The findings of both studies supported the post-treatment exercise. The home-based walking intervention effectively increased short-term activity in sedentary breast cancer survivors *(93)*. Weight training performed two times per week improved physical and psychosocial QOL scores and were associated with increased muscle mass and upper body strength *(94)*.

Overall, the benefits of exercise during and following breast cancer treatment are supported. However, further randomized controlled trials are needed to determine the type, intensity, frequency, and duration of exercise as well as when to initiate each type.

6. Prevention of Recurrence

Evidence exists to suggest that physical activity will reduce the risk of breast cancer recurrence and mortality. The Nurses Health Study *(95)*, a long-term, prospective, cohort study, has yielded some promising statistics regarding the relationship between breast cancer recurrence and exercise. Based on the results of a sample of 2,987 women diagnosed with Stage I, II, or III breast cancer, researchers concluded that walking 3–5 hours at a moderate pace reduces the risk of death from breast cancer by 50%. In addition, it was found that walking even 1 hour per week was associated with a reduction in the risk of breast cancer recurrence, death from breast cancer, and death from all causes. Although the current evidence is promising, further research is needed to determine the impact of exercise on breast cancer prognosis and disease-free survival *(96)*. Initiating exercise is important; however, maintaining an exercise regimen long term is a significant challenge. Developing strategies that facilitate adherence to an exercise program is essential to adequately determine the survival benefits. Currently, studies *(97)* are underway that will hopefully provide information about the impact of lifestyle factors such as diet and physical activity on recurrence and survival.

7. Conclusion

This chapter introduced the reader to the influential role physical activity and exercise plays along the breast cancer continuum. Physical activity and exercise are preventive and rehabilitative measures that can be instituted at various points along the breast cancer trajectory. Clinicians are encouraged to assess the physical activity level of breast cancer patients and to educate them on the potential benefits of exercise both prior to, during, and following treatment. However, further research is needed to address the types, intensity, frequency, and duration of exercise that women should employ at different points along the breast cancer trajectory.

References

1. American Cancer Society. (2008) Cancer facts and figures 2008. Atlanta, GA.

2. Ravdin, P.M., Cronin, KA., Howlader, N., Berg, C.D. (2007) The decrease in breast-cancer incidence in 2003 in the United States. N Engl J Med **356**, 1670–1674.

3. Nelson, H. D., Humphrey, L.L., Nygren, P., Teutsch, S.M., Allan, J.D. (2002) Postmenopausal hormone replacement therapy. JAMA **288**, 872–891.

4. Ozols, R. F., Herbst, R.S., Colson, U.L., Gralow, J., Bonner, J., Curran, W.J. Jr., et al. (2007) Clinical cancer advances 2006: Major research advances in cancer treatment, prevention and screening—a report from the American Society of Clinical Oncology. J Clin Onc **25**, 146–162.

5. Berry, D.A., Cronin, K.A., Plevritis, S.K., et al. (2005) Effect of screening and adjuvant therapy on mortality from breast cancer. N Engl J Med **353**, 1784–1792.

6. National Cancer Institute. A snapshot of breast cancer. September, 2006. Retrieved July 23, 2007 from http://planning.cancer.gov/disease/Breast-Snapshot.pdf.

7. Li, C.I., Malone, K.E., Daling, J.R. (2003) Differences in breast cancer stage, treatment, and survival by race and ethnicity. Arch Intern Med **163**, 49–56.

8. National Cancer Institute. Fact sheet: Probability of breast cancer in American women. October 5, 2006 Retrieved July 23, 2007 from http://www.cancer.gov/images/Documents/bd21295f-31fa-419b-b249-54311ca969a1/fs5_6.pdf.

9. Kruk, J. (2007) Lifetime physical activity and the risk of breast cancer: A case-control study. Cancer Detect Prev **31**, 19–28.

10. McTiernan, A., Kooperberg, C., White, E., Wilcox, S., Coates, R., Adams-Campbell, L.L., Woods, N., Ockene, J. (2003) Recreational physical activity and the risk of breast cancer in postmenopausal women: The Women's Health Initiative cohort study. JAMA **290**, 1331–1336.

11. US Department of Health and Human Services. (1966) Physical activity and

health: a report of the Surgeon General. Atlanta: Centers for Disease Control and Prevention, National Center for Chronic Disease Prevention and Health Promotion.

12. Nagi, S.Z. (1965). Some conceptual issues in disability and rehabilitation. In M. B. Sussman (Ed.), Sociology and Rehabilitation (pp. 100–13). Washington, DC: American Sociological Association.

13. Pope, A.M., Tarlov, A.R. (Eds.) (1991) Disability in America: Toward a national agenda for prevention. Washington, DC: National Academy Press.

14. Reigle, B.S. (2006) The prevention of disablement: A framework for the breast cancer trajectory. Rehab Nurs 31, 174–179.

15. Bosompra, K., Ashikaga, T., O'Brien, P.J., Nelson, L., Skelly, J. (2002) Swelling, numbness, pain, and their relationship to arm function among breast cancer survivors: A disablement process model perspective. Breast J 8, 338–348.

16. Mock, V., Pickett, M., Ropka, M.E., Lin, E.M., Stewart, K.J., Rhodes, V.A., et al. (2001) Fatigue and quality of life outcomes of exercise during cancer treatment. Cancer Prac 9, 119–127.

17. Bender, C.M., McDaniel, R.W., Murphy-Ende, K., Pickett, M., Rittenberg, C.N., Rogeres, M.P., et al. (2002) Chemotherapy-induced nausea and vomiting. Clin J Oncol Nurs 6, 94–102.

18. Pinto, B.M., Clark, M.M., Maruyama, N.C., Feder, S.I. (2003) Psychological and fitness changes associated with exercise participation among women with breast cancer. Psychooncology 12, 118–126.

19. Silverman, D.H.S., Dy, C.J., Castellon, S.A., Lai, J., Pio, B., Abraham, L., et al. (2007) Altered frontocortical, cerebellar, and basal ganglia activity in adjuvant-treated breast cancer survivors 5–10 years after chemotherapy. Breast Cancer Res Treat 103, 303–311.

20. Hutnick, N. A., Williams, N.I., Kraemer, W.J., Orsega-Smith, E., Dixon, R.H., Bleznak, A.D., Mastro, A.M. (2005) Exercise and lymphocyte activation following chemotherapy for breast cancer. Med Sci Sports Exerc 37, 1827–1835.

21. Mizuno, T., Katsumata, N., Mukai, H., Shimizu, C., Ando, M., Watanabe, T. (2007) The outpatient management of low-risk febrile patients with neutropenia: risk assessment over the telephone. Support Care Cancer 15, 287–291.

22. Brady, M.J., Cella, D.F., Mo, F., Bonomi, A.E., Tulsky, D.S., Lloyd, S.R., et al. (1997) Reliability and validity of the functional assessment of cancer therapy-breast quality-of-life instrument. J Clin Oncol 15, 974–986.

23. Kolden, G.G., Strauman, T.J., Ward, A., et al. (2002) A pilot study of group exercise training (GET) for women with primary breast cancer: Feasibility and health benefits. Psychooncology 11, 447–456.

24. Darga, L.L., Megnan, M., Mood, D., Hryniuk, W.M., DiLaura, N.M., Djuric, Z. (2007) Quality of life as a predictor of weight loss in obese, early-stage breast cancer survivors. Oncol Nurs Forum 34, 86–92.

25. Freidenreich, C.M., Orenstein, M.R. (2002) Physical activity and cancer prevention: Etiologic evidence and biological mechanisms. J Nutr 132, 3456S–3464S.

26. Frisch, R.E., Wyshak, G., Albright, N.L., et al. (1985) Lower prevalence of breast cancer and cancers of reproductive system among former college athletes compared to non-athletes. Br J Cancer 52, 885–891.

27. Bernstein, L., Henderson, B.E., Hanisch, R., et al. (1994) Physical exercise and reduced risk of breast cancer in young women. J Natl Cancer Inst 86, 1403–1408.

28. Matthews, C.E., Fowke, J.H., Dai, Q., et al. (2004) Physical activity, body size, and estrogen metabolism in women. Cancer Causes Control 15, 473–481.

29. Friedenreich, C.M., Thune, I., Brinton, L.A., et al. (1998) Epidemiologic issues related to the association between physical activity and breast cancer. Cancer 83, 600–610.

30. Gammon, M.E., John, E.M., Britton, J.A. (1998) Recreational and occupational physical activities and risk of breast cancer. J Natl Cancer Inst 90, 100–117.

31. Friedenreich, C.M.. (2001) Physical activity and cancer prevention from observational to intervention research. Cancer Epidemiol Biomarkers Prev 10, 287–301.

32. Gammon, M.D., Schoenberg, J.B., Britton, J.A., et al. (1998) Recreational physical activity and breast cancer risk among women under 45 years. Am J Epidemiol 147, 273–280.

33. Moore, D.B., Folsom, A.R., Mink, P.J., et al. (2000) Physical activity and incidence of postmenopausal breast cancer. Epidemiol 2000 11, 292–296.

34. Carpenter, C.L., Ross, R.K., Panganini-Hill, A., et al. (1999) Lifetime exercise activity and breast cancer risk among post-menopausal women. Br J Cancer **80**, 1852–1858.

35. Friedenreich, C.M., Bryant, H.E., Courneya, K.S. (2001) Case-control study of lifetime physical activity and breast cancer risk. Am J Epidemiol **154**, 336–347.

36. Young, D., Bernstein, L., Wu, A.H. (2003) Physical activity and breast cancer. Cancer **97**, 2565–2575.

37. Rockhill B., Willett, W.C., Hunter, D.J., et al. (1999) A prospective study of recreational physical activity and breast cancer risk. Arch Intern Med **159**, 2290–2296.

38. Broocks, A., Pirke, K.M., Schweiger, U., et al. (1990) Cyclic ovarian function in recreational athletes. J Appl Physiol **68**, 2083–2086.

39. Russell, J.B., Mitchell, D., Musey, P.I., et al. (1984) The relationship of exercise to anovulatory cycles in female athletes: Hormonal and physical characteristics. Obstet Gynecol **63**, 452–456.

40. McTiernan, A., Kooperberg, C., White, E., et al. (2003) Is exercise effective in reducing the risk of breast cancer in postmenopausal women? JAMA **290**, 1331–1336.

41. Gauley, J.A., Gutai, J.P., Kuller, L.II., et al. (1989) The epidemiology of serum sex hormones in postmenopausal women. Am J Epidemiol **129**, 1120–1131.

42. Cadenas, E., Davies, K.J. (2000) Mitochondrial free radical generation, oxidative stress, and aging. Free Radic Biol Med **29**, 222–230.

43. Kanter, M.M., Hamlin, R.L., Unverferth, D.V., et al. (1985) Effect of exercise training on antioxidant enzymes and cardiotoxicity of doxorubicin. J Appl Physiol **59**, 1298–1303.

44. Minotti, G., Cairo, G., Monti, E. (1999) Role of iron in anthracycline cardiotoxicity: new tunes for an old song? FASEB J **13**, 199–212.

45. Yu, B.P. (1994) Cellular defenses against damage from reactive oxygen species. Physiol Rev **74**, 139–162.

46. Nakao, C., Ookawara, T., Kizaki, T., et al. (2000) Effects of swimming training on three superoxide dismutase isoenzymes in mouse tissues. J Appl Physiol **88**, 649–654.

47. Meister, A., Anderson, M. E. (1983) Glutathione. Annu Rev Biochem **52**, 711–760.

48. Abraham, R., Basser, R.L., Green, M.D. (1996) A risk-benefit assessment of anthracycline antibiotics in antineoplastic therapy. Drug Saf **15**, 406–429.

49. Wencker, D., Chandra, M., Nguyen, K., (2003) A mechanistic role for cardiac myocyte apoptosis in heart failure. J Clin Invest **111**, 1497–1504.

50. Afford, S., Randhawa, S. (2000) Apoptosis. Am J Clinical Pathol **53**, 55–63.

51. Kalyanaranam, B., Joseph, J., Kalivendi, S., et al. (2002) Doxorubicin-induced apoptosis implications in cardiotoxicity. Mol Cell Biochem **234**, 119–124.

52. Primeau, A.J., Adhihetty, P.J., Hood, D.A. (2002) Apoptosis in heart and skeletal muscle. Can J Appl Physiol **27**, 349–395.

53. Green, P.S., Leeuwenburg, C. (2002) Mitochondrial dysfunction is an early indicator of doxorubicin-induced apoptosis. Biochimica et Biophysica Acta **1588**, 94–101.

54. Li, P., Nijhawan, D., Budihardjo, I., et al. (1997) Cytochrome c and dATP-dependent formation of Apaf-1/caspase-9 complex initiates an apoptotic protease cascade. Cell **91**, 479–489.

55. Nomura, K. Imai, H., Koumura, T., et al. (1999) Mitochondrial phospholipids hydroperoxide glutathione peroxidase suppresses apoptosis mediated by a mitochondrial death pathway. J Biol Chem **274**, 29294–29302.

56. Wang, X., Martindale, J.L., Liu, Y., et al. (1998) The cellular response to oxidative stress: influences of mitogen-activiated protein kinase signaling pathways on cell survival. Biochem J **333**, 291–300.

57. Radak, Z,. Gaal, D., Taylor, A.W., et al. (2002) Attenuation of the development of murine solid leukemia tumor by physical exercise. Antioxid Redox Signal **4**, 213–219.

58. Ries, L.A.G., Eisner, M.P., Kosary, C. L., Hankey, B. F., Miller, B.A., Clegg, L., et al. (Eds.). (2004) SEER cancer statistics review, 1975–2001, Bethesda, MD, NCI http://seer.cancer.gov/csr/1975_2001/.

59. Courneya, K.S., Mackey, J.R., McKenzie, D.C. (2002) Exercise for breast cancer survivors. Physic Sportsmed **30**, 1–12.

60. National Cancer Institute Breast cancer (PDQ): Treatment health professional version. Retrieved July 22, 2007 from http://www.cancer.gov/cancertoics/pdq/treatment/breast/healthprofessional/.

61. American Cancer Society. (2003) Breast cancer facts and figures 2003–2004. Atlanta, GA: American Cancer Society.

62. National Comprehensive Cancer Network and American Cancer Society. (2006) Breast cancer: Treatment guidelines for patients. Atlanta, GA: American Cancer Society.

63. Bender, C.M., McDaniel, R.W., Murphy-Ende, K., Pickett, M., Rittenberg, C.N., Rogeres, M.P., et al. (2002). Chemotherapy-induced nausea and vomiting. Clin J Oncol Nurs 6, 94–102.

64. Batchelor, D. (2001) Hair and cancer chemotherapy: Consequences and nursing care—a literature study. Eur J Cancer Care 10, 147–163.

65. Dimeo, F.C. (2001) Effects of exercise on cancer-related fatigue. Cancer 92, 1689–1693.

66. Kattlove, H., Winn, R.J. (2003) Ongoing care of patients after primary treatment for cancer. Ca Cancer J Clin 54, 172–196.

67. Aziz, N.M. (2002) Cancer survivorship research: Challenge and opportunity. J Nutr 132, 3494S–3503S.

68. Winick, L., Robbins, G.F. (1977) Physical and psychologic readjustment after mastectomy. Cancer 39, 478–486.

69. Pinto, B.M., Clark, M.M., Maruyama, N.C., Feder, S.I. (2003) Psychological and fitness changes associated with exercise participation among women with breast cancer. Psychooncology 12, 118–126.

70. Lash, T.L., Silliman, R.A. (2000) Patient characteristics and treatments associated with a decline in upper-body function following breast cancer therapy. J Clinl Epidemiol 53, 615–622.

71. Satariano, W.A., Ragland, D.R., DeLorenze, G.N. (1996) Limitations in upper-body strength associated with breast cancer: A comparison of black and white women. J Clin Epidemiol 49, 535–544.

72. Box, R.C., Reul-Hirche, H.M., Bullock-Saxton, J.E., Furnival, C.M. (2002) Shoulder movement after breast cancer surgery: Results of a randomized controlled study of postoperative physiotherapy. Breast Cancer Res Treat 75, 35–50.

73. Brown, J.R. (2004) A clinically useful method for evaluating lymphedema. Clin J Oncol Nurs 8, 35–38.

74. Pasket, E.D., Stark, N. (2000) Lymphedema: Knowledge, treatment, and impact among breast cancer survivors. Breast J 6, 373–378.

75. Miller, L.T. (2002). Management of breast cancer-related edemas. In Macken, E.J., Callahan, A.D., Osterman, A.L., Skirven, T.M., Schneider, L.H., Hunter, J.M., eds. Rehablitiation of the Hand and Upper Extremity. St. Louis, MO: Mosby, 914–928.

76. Holmes, M.D., Kroenke, C.H. (2004) Beyond treatment: Lifestyle choices after breast cancer to enhance quality of life and survival. Women's Health Issues 14, 11–13.

77. Fogelman, I., Blake, G.M., Blamey, R., Palmer, M., Sauerbrei, W., Schumacher, M., et al. (2003) Bone mineral density in premenopausal women treated for node-positive early breast cancer with 2 years of goserelin or 6 months of cyclophosphamide, methotrexate and 5-fluorouracil (CMF). Osteoporos Int 14, 1001–1006.

78. Shimozuma, K., Ganz, P.A., Petersen, L., Hirji, K. (1999) Quality of life in the first year after breast cancer surgery: Rehabilitation needs and patterns of recovery. Breast Cancer Res Treat 56, 45057.

79. Harris, S.R., Campbell, K.L., McNeely, M.L. (2005) Upper extremity rehabilitation for women who have been treated for breast cancer. Physiother Can 56, 202–214.

80. Rietman, J.S., Kijkstra, P.U., Geertzen, J.H.B., Baas, P., de Vries, J., Dolsma, W., et al. (2003) Short-term morbidity of the upper limb after sentinel lymph node biopsy or axillary lymph node dissection for stage I or II breast carcinoma. Cancer 98, 690–696.

81. Baron, R.H, Fey, J.V., Borgen, P.I., et al. (2004) Eighteen sensations after breast cancer surgery: A two-year comparison of sentinel lymph node biopsy and axillary lymph node dissection. Oncol Nurs Forum 31, 691–698.

82. Luini, A., Galimberti, V., Gati, G., Arnone, P., et al. (2005) The sentinel node biopsy after previous breast surgery: Preliminary results on 543 patients treated at the European Institute of Oncology. Breast Cancer Res Treat 89, 159–163.

83. Ververs, J.M.M.A., Roumen, R.M.H., Vingerhoets, A.J.J.M., Vreugdenhil, G., Coebergh, J.W.W., Crommelin, M.A., et al. (2001) Risk, severity and predictors of physical and psychological morbidity after axillary lymph node dissection for breast cancer. Eur J Cancer 37, 991–999.

84. Harris, S.R., Niesen-Vertommen, S.L. (2000) Challenging the myth of exercise-induced lymphedema following breast cancer: A series of case reports. J Surg Oncol 74, 95–99.

85. Lane, K., Jespersen, D., McKenzie, D.C. (2005) The effect of a whole body exercise programme and dragon boat training on arm volume and arm circumference in women treated for breast cancer. Eur J Cancer Care 14, 353–358.

86. Holleb, A.I. (1990) Two decades of Reach to Recovery: A tribute to the volunteers. CA Cancer J Clin **40**, 5–7.

87. Shamley, D.R., Barker, K., Simonite, V., Beardshaw, A. (2005) Delayed versus immediate exercises following surgery for breast cancer: A systematic review. Breast Cancer Res Treat **90**, 263–271.

88. Na,Y.M., Lee, J.S., Park, J.S., Kang, S.W., Lee, H.D., Koo, J.Y. (1999) Early rehabilitation program in postmastectomy patients: A prospective clinical trial. Yonsei Med J **40**, 1–8.

89. Wingate, L. (1985) Efficacy of physical therapy for patients who have undergone mastectomies: A prospective study. Phys Ther **65**, 896–900.

90. Kirshbaum, M.N. (2006) A review of the benefits of whole body exercise during and after treatment for breast cancer. J Clin Nurs **16**, 104–121.

91. Headley, J.A, Ownby, K., John, L.D. (2004) The effect of seated exercise on fatigue and quality of life in women with advanced breast cancer. Oncol Nurs Forum **31**, 977–983.

92. Lee, T.S., Kilbreath, S.L., Refshauge, K.M., Pendlebury, S.C., Beith, J.M., Lee, M.J. (2007) Pectoral stretching program for women undergoing radiotherapy for breast cancer. Breast Cancer Res Treat **102**, 313–321.

93. Matthew, C.E., Wilcox, S., Hanby, C.L., Ananian, C.D., Heiney, S.P., Gebretsadik, T., et al. (2007) Evaluation of a 12-week home-based walking intervention for breast cancer survivors. Support Care Cancer **15**, 203–211.

94. Ohira, T., Schmitz, K.H, Ahmed, R.L., Ye, D. (2006) Effects of weight training on quality of life in recent breast cancer survivors. Cancer **106**, 2076–2083.

95. Holmes, M.D., Chen, W.Y., Feskanich, D., Kroenke, C.H., Colditz, G.A. (2005) Physical activity and survival after breast cancer diagnosis. JAMA **293**, 2479–2486.

96. Denmark-Wahnefried, W., Pinto, B.M., Gritz, E.R. (2006) Promoting health and physical function among cancer survivors: Potential for prevention and questions that remain. J Clin Oncol **24**, 5125–5131.

97. Kushi, L.H., Kwan, M.I., Lee, M.M., Ambrosone, C.B. (2007) Lifestyle factors and survival in women with breast cancer. J Nutr **137**, 236S–242S.

Chapter 8

Energy Intake, Physical Activity, Energy Balance, and Cancer: Epidemiologic Evidence

Sai Yi Pan and Marie DesMeules

Abstract

Energy intake, physical activity, and obesity are modifiable lifestyle factors. This chapter reviews and summarizes the epidemiologic evidence on the relation of energy intake, physical activity, and obesity to cancer. High energy intake may increase the risk of cancers of colon–rectum, prostate (especially advanced prostate cancer), and breast. However, because physical activity, body size, and metabolic efficiency are highly related to total energy intake and expenditure, it is difficult to assess the independent effect of energy intake on cancer risk. There are sufficient evidences to support a role of physical activity in preventing cancers of the colon and breast, whereas the association is stronger in men than in women for colon cancer and in postmenopausal than in premenopausal women for breast cancer. The evidence also suggests that physical activity likely reduces the risk of cancers of endometrium, lung, and prostate (to a lesser extent). On the other hand, there is little or no evidence that the risk of rectal cancer is related to physical activity, whereas the results have been inconsistent regarding the association between physical activity and the risks of cancers of pancreas, ovary and kidney. Epidemiologic studies provide sufficient evidence that obesity is a risk factor for both cancer incidence and mortality. The evidence supports strong links of obesity with the risk of cancers of the colon, rectum, breast (in postmenopausal women), endometrium, kidney (renal cell), and adenocarcinoma of the esophagus. Epidemiologic evidence also indicates that obesity is probably related to cancers of the pancreas, liver, and gallbladder, and aggressive prostate cancer, while it seems that obesity is not associated with lung cancer. The role of obesity in other cancer risks is unclear.

Key words: Energy intake/restriction, physical activity, energy balance, obesity, overweight, cancer, colon, rectum, breast, prostate, lung, endometrium, esophagus, pancreas, ovary, kidney, liver, gallbladder.

1. Introduction

Animal experiments have consistently shown that energy restriction can reduce the development of a variety of spontaneous, induced, and transplanted tumors in rats and mice as

M. Verma (ed.), *Methods of Molecular Biology, Cancer Epidemiology, vol. 472*
© 2009 Humana Press, a part of Springer Science+Business Media, Totowa, NJ
Book doi: 10.1007/978-1-60327-492-0

well as non-human primates *(1–6)*. Animal experimental studies have suggested that calorie restriction may reduce cancer risk by reducing levels of plasma insulin and insulin-like growth factor (IGF)-I, inhibiting cell proliferation, increasing cell death due to apoptosis, increasing activities of antioxidant enzymes, enhancing DNA repair, reducing oncogene expression, and influencing level of immunological responsiveness *(1, 7, 8)*. These studies suggested the importance of energy balance as a determinant for cancer risk.

Although animal models clearly demonstrated a protective effect of energy restriction on cancer risk, it is less clear and there is little direct evidence that such a protective effect exists in humans, e.g., a study on normal weight humans found that 20% energy restriction for 10 weeks did not reduce oxidative DNA damage *(9)*. In free-living populations it is difficult to answer the important question, i.e., whether such effect may also operate on humans within the range of energy intake by human. For human populations, energy intake is determined by physical activity (PA), body size, and metabolic efficiency, and all these factors might be related to cancer risk, which makes the relationship between energy intake and cancer in humans complicated.

This chapter reviews and summarizes the epidemiologic evidence of energy intake, PA, and energy imbalance resulting from excess energy intake relative to total energy expenditure as risk factors for cancer in humans.

2. Energy Intake/ Restriction and Cancer

Very few studies have assessed the relationship between energy restriction and the risk of various cancer sites because of the ethical issue. One study of the 1944–1945 Dutch famine and subsequent overall cancer incidence *(10)* found no evidence that the short famine has affected overall cancer risk. However, higher energy intake in childhood may increase the risk of developing cancer in adult life *(11, 12)*. Because PA and body size are highly related to total energy intake, it is difficult to assess the independent effect of energy intake on cancer risk, and energy intake is also difficult to assess in large-scale epidemiologic studies.

2.1. Breast Cancer

Direct examination of energy (calorie) restriction and breast cancer risk has been conducted in several studies. One study observed an increased risk of breast cancer in women who were exposed to a short but severe famine during World War II (1944–1945 Dutch Famine) *(13)*. However, four Norwegian studies suggested a decreased risk *(14–17)* and a Dutch study detected no decreased risk *(18)* of breast cancer in women who experienced short-term, transient energy restriction during World War II. A Swedish cohort study on 7,303 women hospitalized for anorexia nervosa prior to age 40 years (therefore with abnormal low energy intake) found that these women have a 53% lower incidence of breast cancer *(19)*. High energy intake has not been consistently associated with increased risk of breast cancer: most case–control studies *(20–29)* and prospective studies *(30–33)* demonstrated a positive association, whereas several case–control studies *(34–36)* and prospective studies *(37–39)* noticed no relationship.

2.2. Colorectal Cancer

Only one study assessed the association between energy restriction and colorectal cancer risk *(40)*. This study observed no significant relationship between energy restriction early in life and subsequent colon carcinoma risk for men and women who had lived in a western city in 1944–1945 (hunger winter) in the Netherlands. However, most case–control studies suggested an increased risk of colorectal cancer associated with high energy intake *(41–52)*. A combined analysis of 13 case–control studies demonstrated a positive association with total energy intake for 11 of the 13 studies, and the association was similar between men and women, between younger (<50 years old) and older (>50 years old) people, between colon and rectal cancer, and between right and left colon cancer sites *(47)*. Another case–control study published after the aforementioned combined analysis also noticed a similar association for colon and rectal cancer *(46)*. On the other hand, cohort studies have usually reported a weak or null association *(53–55)*.

2.3. Prostate Cancer

The only study that examined the relation of energy restriction with prostate cancer, The Netherlands Cohort Study on Diet and Cancer, demonstrated no evidence for the hypothesis that energy restriction in childhood and adolescence during the Hunger Winter (1944–1945) in the Netherlands for a short duration (7 months) led to a decrease in prostate cancer risk among adults *(56)*. Migrant studies and ecological studies suggest that energy intake is related to prostate cancer incidence and mortality *(57)*. A review of 23 analytic epidemiologic studies *(57)* and studies published later *(58–61)* show that total energy intake might be positively associated with prostate cancer, and the association is stronger for, or restricted to, advanced prostate cancer *(57, 58)*. However, a case–control study found that total energy intake was associated with an increased risk for both local and regional/distant stage of prostate cancer *(60)*. The review and meta-analysis of 23 studies *(57)* reported that the summary odds ratio (OR) of prostate cancer comparing the top with the bottom quartiles of energy intake was 1.3 (95% confidence interval [CI], 1.1–1.4) from case–control studies with no evidence of an association from four cohort studies; and the summary OR of advanced prostate cancer was 1.6 (95% CI, 1.2–2.0) from the four case–control studies that evaluated the advanced disease.

3. PA and Cancer Risk

3.1. Colon/Colorectal Cancer

The evidence for the inverse relationship between PA and colon cancer is convincing, with a dose–response effect *(43, 62–73)*. This association has been shown in various populations, including Europe, Asia, and North America. The magnitude of reduction in colon cancer risk is between 30 and 40% *(62, 73)*. It is estimated that 12–14% of colon cancer could be attributed to lack of regular vigorous PA *(63)*. It seems that higher intensity activities and PAs performed over a longer period of time provide greater protection against colon cancer *(62)*. It has been estimated that 30–60 minutes/day of more intense types of activity are required to have the greatest effect on colon cancer risk *(62, 63)*. Although a meta-analysis of 19 cohort studies and 28 case–control studies indicated an inverse association for both men and women *(73)*, a stronger relationship has been found in men than women, especially in the more recent studies *(64, 71)*, or no association in women in some studies *(74, 75)*.

For rectal cancer, the above-mentioned meta-analysis showed that PA offered no protection against rectal cancer in either sex *(73)*. In addition, other studies that examined rectal cancer and colon cancer separately observed a much weaker or no association between rectal cancer risk and PA *(44, 62, 64, 67, 70–72)*.

3.2. Breast Cancer

There is a compelling evidence for an inverse association between regular PA and breast cancer risk, with a dose–response relationship observed in most studies *(62, 76–78)*. The inverse association was shown for both premenopausal and postmenopausal women, both occupational and recreational PA, activity at different periods of life, and at different level of intensity of PA, and the association is independent of weight gain *(62)*. A recent systematic review of 19 cohort studies and 29 case–control studies *(76)* demonstrated a 15–20% reduction in breast cancer risk with PA and a 6% (95% CI, 3–8%) decrease in breast cancer risk for each additional hour of PA per week, assuming that the level of activity would be sustained. This review also suggests that the evidence for the inverse association with PA is strong for postmenopausal women, with a range of 20–80% risk reduction, but the evidence for premenopausal women is much weaker. The much weaker association in premenopausal women may partly explain the inconsistency of study results, because these studies did not analyze women by menopausal status. It also appears that 30–60 minutes/day of moderate to vigorous-intensity PA is required to decrease the risk of breast cancer *(62)*.

The timing of PA within lifespan may be important. A review of 19 case–control studies and 4 cohort studies on the effect of PA in adolescence/young adulthood on breast cancer risk *(79)* reported a summary relative risk (RR) of 0.81 (95% CI, 0.73–0.89) for those who were most active in adolescence/young adulthood compared with those who were least active, with a 3% (95% CI, 0–6%) risk reduction for each 1-hour increase of recreational PA/week during adolescence. However, PA in adolescence/young adulthood may be strongly correlated to PA later in adulthood, therefore, the observed association could be a reflection of lifetime PA rather than resulting from PA at a specific time point. In addition, the International Agency for Research on Cancer (IARC) review also suggested that PA sustained over a lifetime provides the strongest protection against breast cancer *(62)*.

3.3. Prostate Cancer

The IARC review *(62)* and the review by Torti and Matheson *(80)* concluded that there is a probable link between PA and prostate cancer risk. In the latter review, 9 of 13 cohort studies and 5 of 11 case–control studies published between 1988 and 2002 showed an inverse association, and a total of 9 studies reported a significant reduction in risk, with a reduction range being 10 to 30% Since 2002, six prospective studies and four case–control studies have been published. Five of the six cohort studies found no association between PA and overall risk of prostate cancer *(81–85)*, while one cohort study indicated an increased risk among men with sedentary jobs compared with men with high activity levels *(86)*. However, an inverse association was reported in subgroups of these five null cohorts. All three cohort studies that assessed advanced or aggressive prostate cancer suggested that PA may be associated with a reduced risk of advanced prostate cancer *(82, 84, 85)*. Littman's study observed a decreased risk of prostate cancer associated with higher level of PA among men who were at a normal weight, 65 years old at diagnosis, and who had not had a recent prostate-specific antigen (PSA) *(81)*. Of the two cohort studies that evaluated prostate cancer mortality, one study found an inverse association with recreational PA *(82)*, while the other study demonstrated no association with occupational PA *(86)*. In addition, two cohorts noticed that the association was restricted to older population (65 years at diagnosis) *(81, 84)*. Of the four case–control studies, two found a reduced risk associated with strenuous PA *(61, 87)*, with no association for total lifetime PA in the latter study *(87)*. The case–control study in Italy observed a significant association with occupational, but not with recreational, PA *(88)*, while the case–control study in China showed a reduced risk with moderate PA *(89)*.

Overall, the results between studies are inconsistent, and the possible reason could be that the association is restricted to some subgroups, such as advanced prostate cancer. Therefore, further research on the advanced stage of the disease is needed.

3.4. Endometrial Cancer

Most studies and reviews suggested that PA probably has a protective role in endometrial cancer development (62, 90, 91). At least 16 of 21 studies (8 cohort and 13 case–control studies) reported a risk decrease in the most active women, with an average reduction at 30–40% (91–106). A systematic review and meta-analysis of 7 cohort studies and 13 case–control studies (90) showed that PA is associated with a decreased risk of endometrial cancer, with a summary estimate of risk reduction of 27% from 7 high-quality cohort studies for the most active women compared with the least active women. A dose–response relationship was demonstrated in 9 (91, 92, 94, 95, 97–99, 103, 106) of 15 studies that examined a dose–response effect (91–99, 101, 103, 106–109). However, it is unclear whether total PA or specific types or intensities or time period of PA are important for prevention of endometrial cancer. Some studies found a stronger effect of PA in women with a high calorie intake (103) or a high body mass index (BMI) (94, 103, 105), whereas other studies observed no significant interaction with BMI (91–93, 96, 109) and total energy intake (91, 96). In addition, there is no strong evidence of effect modification by menopausal status (92, 93, 105) and age (93, 94, 96, 98, 103), although there is a suggestion of a stronger but statistically nonsignificant association with household activities among premenopausal women than among postmenopausal women (91, 92).

3.5. Lung Cancer

Overall, two reviews (62, 110) and four cohort studies and one case–control study published after the reviews (111–115) showed evidence of an inverse association between lung cancer and PA. The five cohorts identified by the IARC review (62) all found a decrease in lung cancer risk, with the reduction ranging between 20 and 60% for both occupational and non-occupational PA. A dose–response effect was also demonstrated in these studies. The meta-analysis of recreational PA and lung cancer risk of seven cohort studies and two case–control studies (110) reported a summary estimate of 0.87 (95% CI, 0.79–0.95) for moderate recreational PA and 0.70 (95% CI, 0.62–0.79) for high recreational PA with a statistically significant inverse dose–response relationship. Furthermore, this meta-analysis suggested that the inverse association occurred for both sexes, although it was somewhat stronger for women than for men.

Of the four cohort studies and one case–control study not included in the above two reviews, Bak et al. (113) and Steindorf et al. (112) reported no association between occupational and non-occupational PA and lung cancer risk, but suggested that more vigorous recreational PAs, such as sports and cycling, were associated with a decreased risk of lung cancer. The Iowa's Women's Health Study noted a decreased risk of lung cancer in physically active women with the RR of 0.72 (95% CI, 0.55–0.94) in current active smokers and 0.63 (95% CI, 0.43–0.92) in former active smokers, but the RR was not significantly decreased in active never-smokers *(111)*. Among current and former smokers in the Beta Carotene and Retinol Efficacy Trial, higher PA was also found to be associated with a decreased risk of lung cancer incidence for younger participants and lung cancer mortality for women *(114)*. Furthermore, the hospital-based case–control study observed a protective effect for physical exercise among smokers only *(115)*.

Although all above studies were adjusted for smoking, there is still some concern on residual confounding from smoking and other lung diseases.

3.6. Ovarian Cancer

The influence of PA on ovarian cancer risk was assessed in at least 16 studies with inconsistent results. Two cohort studies *(116, 117)* and six case–control studies *(104, 107, 118–123)* suggested a reduction in ovarian cancer risk with a high level of PA, three cohort studies *(124–126)* and two case–control studies *(127)* showed no association, and two cohort studies found a positive association *(128, 129)*.

The Netherlands cohort study *(116)* and a Canadian case–control study *(119)* observed a decreased risk of ovarian cancer associated with moderate PA with no association for vigorous activity. Two cohort studies indicated that frequent vigorous leisure-time PA may increase the risk of ovarian cancer *(128, 129)*; however, there was no association with vigorous recreational activity in one case–control study *(127)*.

Of the six studies that examined specifically occupational PA, high occupational PA was associated with a decreased ovarian cancer risk in five case–control studies *(104, 107, 118, 119, 122)*, and no association in one cohort study *(124)*. Of the studies that investigated recreational PA, a reduction of ovarian cancer risk associated with high recreational PA was reported in four case–control studies *(119–121, 123)* and one cohort study *(116)*, and no association in two case–control studies *(122, 127)* and three cohort studies *(125, 128, 129)*.

Overall, the majority of cohort studies do not support an association and there is inadequate evidence to support a role of PA on ovarian cancer etiology.

3.7. Pancreatic Cancer

At least 13 cohort studies and 3 case–control studies have evaluated the relationship between PA and pancreatic cancer risk. Of the cohort studies, nine observed no association *(130–138)*, three reported a lower risk of pancreatic cancer with high level of PA

(139–141), and one found an increased risk of pancreatic cancer with high occupational PA for women and men (142). Of the three case–control studies, two noted a reduction in pancreatic cancer risk associated with high recreational PA (143, 144) and one showed a non-significant decrease in risk with high recreational PA (145). Most of above cohort studies assessed recreational PA, whereas one cohort study assessed occupational PA only, with no association observed (138). Of the four cohort studies that examined both recreational and occupational PA, one demonstrated no association with both types of PA (133), one noticed no association with recreational PA but a positive association with occupational PA (142), and two reported an inverse association with both occupational and recreational PA (139, 141). The Health Professional Follow-up Study and the Nurses' Health Study (140) indicated that moderate PA and walking/hiking were associated with a decreased risk of pancreatic cancer for men and women, but vigorous PA was not associated with a decreased risk. In the American Society Cancer Prevention Study II Nutrition Cohort study, PA at baseline and at the age of 40 years was not associated with pancreatic cancer risk, however, moderate activity (but not vigorous activity) in 1982 was associated with a significantly decreased risk for both men and women (135).

Overall, the majority of the cohort studies do not support a prevention role of PA on pancreatic cancer.

3.8. Kidney Cancer

The results on the association between PA and kidney cancer (mostly renal cell cancer) risk are inconsistent. Of the studies that assessed the relationship, three cohort studies (146–148) and five case–control studies (138, 149–152) observed no association, while four cohort studies (124, 153–155) and three case–control studies (156–158) found a decreased risk of kidney cancer with high level of either recreational or occupational PA. Of the studies that assessed occupational PA, three cohort studies (146, 147, 154) and five case–control studies (138, 150, 151, 157) demonstrated no association, whereas two cohort studies (124, 155) and two case–control studies (156, 158) suggested a reduction in kidney cancer risk associated with higher level of occupational PA. While most studies noticed no association with recreational PA (147–151, 156, 158), a reduced risk of kidney cancer was noted in male smokers (154), in men only (not in women) (146), and in both sexes (for total PA) (157). One cohort study observed a nonsignificant decrease in risk associated with total PA (including occupational and recreational PA) in women only but not in men (153). The largest cohort study in Sweden also found that the risk reduction associated with occupational PA occurred only in men, not in women (155). An Italy case–control study suggested that occupational PAs at age 12, 15–19, 30–39, and 50–59 years were all associated with a risk reduction (156).

3.9. Secondary Prevention

The evidence is accumulating that PA is associated with improved quality of life *(159–161)*, and decreased recurrence and risk of death from cancer *(162–166)* after cancer diagnosis. The recent reviews of literature of both randomized clinical trials (RCT) and observational studies indicate that PA is beneficial in improving cardiopulmonary function, overall quality of life, global health, strength, sleep, and self-esteem, and in reducing weight gain, depression, anxiety, and fatigue *(167, 168)*.

4. Overweight / Obesity and Cancer Risk

4.1. Breast Cancer

Most case–control studies and cohort studies found no or an inverse association between obesity and breast cancer risk in premenopausal women *(62, 169–173)*. Nevertheless, there is convincing evidence for a positive association between obesity and postmenopausal breast cancer risk *(62, 169–172, 174, 175)*. The association remains after adjusting for various reproductive and lifestyle factors, including PA *(169, 171, 172)*, and becomes stronger with increasing age and years after menopause *(171)*. It seems that the association was stronger in women with a family history of breast cancer *(169)* and in women who never used hormone-replacement therapy (HRT) *(169, 171)*. Systematic reviews and meta-analyses indicate that the increased risk associated with overweight and obesity is in the range of 20–50% *(171–173)*, with a 2% increase in risk per unit increase in BMI *(172)*. It is estimated that 22.6% of postmenopausal breast cancer cases in the USA, 16.7% in Europe *(173)*, and 12.6% in Canada *(176)* could be attributed to overweight and obesity.

As with general obesity (BMI), central obesity (measured as waist and waist-to-hip ratio (WHR)) is also strongly associated with breast cancer risk among postmenopausal women, and the relationship may result from the high correlation of waist and WHR with BMI; however, central (not general) obesity may be specifically associated with an increased risk of breast cancer in premenopausal women *(177)*.

It is suggested that adult weight gain is the strongest and most consistent predictor of increased risk of breast cancer in postmenopausal women and the association is stronger in post-menopausal women who never used HRT *(169, 173)*.

In addition, literature suggests that great body size is associated with a more advanced stage of breast cancer at diagnosis and has a adverse effect on breast cancer prognosis in both premeno-pausal and postmenopausal women even after adjustment for other prognostic factors *(178)*; all aspects of breast cancer prognosis, that is, mortality, recurrence, contralateral breast cancer, and overall mortality, are found to be higher in obese women. This adverse effect of obesity on breast cancer prognosis is also observed in women of races with a relatively low incidence of breast cancer *(178)*.

4.2. Colorectal Cancer

It has been consistently demonstrated that obesity increases the risk of colorectal cancer in men and women *(62, 169, 171, 172, 174–176, 179–186)*. The observed association is generally more consistent and stronger for men than for women *(62, 171, 181, 185, 186)*, for colon cancer than for rectal cancer *(62, 181–184)*, and for cancer of the distal colon than the proximal colon *(171, 179, 187, 188)*. Age, menopausal status, and HRT use may modify the association between BMI and colorectal cancer because some studies reported that BMI is related to colorectal cancer risk in only relatively young women *(181, 189)*, premenopausal women *(188, 190)*, and postmenopausal women who used HRT *(190, 191)*. However, some studies found no modification by estrogen exposure on the association between BMI and colorectal cancer among postmenopausal women *(181, 192)*. Most studies reported a nearly twofold increase in colorectal cancer risk (RR = 1.5 for women) in people with a BMI ≥ 30 kg/m^2 compared with those with a BMI < 23 kg/m^2 *(62, 173)*, with a 3% increase in colon cancer risk per unit increase in BMI *(172)*. It is estimated that 35.4% and 20.8% of colorectal cancer cases in US men and women as well as 27.5% and 14.2% in European men and women could be attributed to overweight and obesity *(173)*.

It is also shown that waist circumference and WHR (indicators of abdominal obesity) are strong indicators of colorectal cancer risk in both sexes, especially for women *(180, 187, 193–195)*, suggesting that fat distribution is more important than BMI for colorectal cancer risk in women.

Furthermore, a positive relationship was observed between body fatness and colorectal adenomas, with similar magnitude of association to the association with colorectal cancer, implying that obesity may affect progression from adenoma to cancer *(52, 169, 196–200)*. Some studies also noticed a stronger effect of BMI, WHR, or waist circumference on large adenomas than on small ones, or an effect restricted to large adenomas *(52, 196, 200–202)*.

4.3. Endometrial Cancer

Convincing and consistent evidence exists that overweight and obesity is strongly associated with endometrial cancer risk *(62, 171, 172, 174, 182, 186, 203)*. Obesity has been found to be associated with a twofold to fivefold increase in endometrial cancer risk in both premenopausal and postmenopausal women in a majority of prospective and case–control studies of various populations worldwide *(62, 94, 95, 171, 172, 174, 175, 203–208)*. Most studies observed a linear increase in risk with increasing BMI *(62, 94, 95, 203, 206, 208)*, with a 10% increase in endometrial cancer risk per unit increase in BMI *(172)*. Overweight and obesity has been estimated to account for about 40–45% of endometrial cancer incidence in Europe *(172, 173)* and 57% in the USA *(173)*.

The association for older women is generally similar to the association for younger women *(94, 209, 210)* or somewhat stronger than the association for younger women *(203, 211–213)*. It is also shown that the association was stronger for postmenopausal than premenopausal women *(206)*, for oral contraceptives never-users than ever-users *(206, 207)*, among none-users of HRT than ever-users *(206)*, and for women with a history of diabetes mellitus than for those without the history *(207, 214)*. One recent large cohort study suggested that BMI-related risk increase was most pronounced for Type I tumors but also seen for Type II tumors, sarcomas, and mixed tumors *(203)*. It is also found that large body size increased the risk of hyperplasia of the endometrium *(215)*.

Studies that assessed the relationship of other measurements, such as waist circumference, WHR, waist-to-thigh circumference, and skinfold thickness to endometrial cancer risk also demonstrated positive associations *(206, 207, 216–219)*. However, whether the associations are independent of BMI remains uncertain.

Most studies that evaluated adult weight gain reported a substantial increase in endometrial cancer risk associated with weight gain during adult life *(95, 206, 208, 212, 217–219)*, with a linear dose-dependent pattern *(62)*.

4.4. Kidney Cancer

Renal cell cancer is one of the cancer sites that have been most consistently observed to be associated with obesity *(62, 146, 153, 171, 172, 176, 182–185, 204, 220–222)*. The risk of renal cell cancer is 1.5- to 2.5-fold higher in overweight and obese men and women than those of normal weight, with a dose–response relationship demonstrated in most studies. These studies covered populations worldwide, including North America, northern and southern Europe, Asia, and Australia. The summary RR estimate from 14 studies on each sex in a meta-analysis was 1.07 (95% CI, 1.04–1.09) for men and 1.07 (95% CI, 1.05–1.09) for women per unit increase of BMI *(220)*. It was estimated that 56.7% and 45.2% of the renal cell cancer cases among Americans and Europeans could be related to overweight and obesity *(173)*. Some studies suggested a stronger association in women than in men *(62, 153)*; however, the aforementioned meta-analysis found that BMI is equally strongly associated with renal cell cancer risk for both sexes *(220)*. This meta-analysis also showed comparable strengths of association between cohort and case–control studies, between small and large studies, between populations of the USA and other countries, and between studies adjusted for and not adjusted for smoking. In addition, the obesity-associated risk of renal cell cancer seems to be independent of blood pressure *(223, 224)*.

4.5. Adenocarcinoma of the Esophagus and Gastric Cardia

Three reviews *(62, 171, 225)* and three recently published cohort studies *(183, 226, 227)* and a recently published case–control study *(228)* have consistently linked obesity with increased risk of adenocarcinoma of the esophagus and gastric cardia, with a stronger association with esophageal adenocarcinoma than with cardia adenocarcinoma. The systematic review and meta-analysis of 2 cohort studies and 12 case–control studies *(225)* showed summary RRs of 1.9 (95% CI, 1.5–2.4) and 2.4 (95% CI, 2.0–2.8) associated with overweight and obesity for esophageal adenocarcinoma, and 1.2 (95% CI, 1.0–1.5) and 1.5 (95% CI, 1.2–1.9) for gastric cardia adenocarcinoma. It is estimated that 52.3% and 42.7% of esophageal adenocarcinoma cases among American and European populations could be attributed to overweight and obesity *(173)*.

An increased risk of adenocarcinoma of esophagus and gastric cardia was also observed to be positively associated with central obesity (waist circumference) *(227)* and change in BMI during adulthood *(226)*. Furthermore, a stronger association was seen in nonsmokers than in smokers *(204, 229)*. However, no association was reported between BMI and the risk of esophageal squamous cell carcinoma or noncardia gastric adenocarcinoma *(62, 183, 227, 229)*.

4.6. Prostate Cancer

The relationship of prostate cancer to obesity appears complex. Many studies have assessed the association between obesity and prostate cancer incidence in various populations with inconsistent results. A recent published systematic review and meta-analysis of 31 cohort studies and 25 case–control studies *(230)* indicates that obesity is weakly associated with an increased risk of prostate cancer, with a summary RR of 1.05 (95% CI, 1.01–1.08) per 5 kg/m^2 increment of BMI, with an increased risk for advanced disease only (summary RR of 1.12 per 5 kg/m^2 increase in BMI; 95% CI, 1.01–1.23) but not for localized diseases (summary RR of 0.96 per 5 kg/m^2 increase in BMI; 95% CI, 0.89–1.03). Recent published studies and reviews suggested that obesity seems to contribute to a greater risk of aggressive or advanced or fatal prostate cancer but perhaps to a lower risk of nonaggressive prostate cancer *(231–236)*. The differential effect of obesity by prostate cancer aggressiveness may in part be explained by an inherent bias in our ability to detect prostate cancer in obese men (lower PSA values and larger sized prostates, making biopsy less accurate for finding an existing cancer) *(236)*. The above-mentioned meta-analysis also showed that waist circumference and WHR were weakly associated with the risk of overall prostate cancer incidence, with the summary RRs being 1.03 (95% CI, 0.99–1.07) per 10-cm increment of waist circumference and 1.11 (95% CI, 0.95–1.30) per 0.1-unit increment of WHR, however, the summary RRs were based on small number of studies.

Although epidemiological studies have not consistently shown that obesity is a risk factor for prostate cancer incidence, studies on prostate cancer mortality have more clearly demonstrated a positive association *(204, 232, 237–240)*.

4.7. Ovarian Cancer

The evidence from both case–control studies and cohort studies has been inconsistent on the relationship between obesity and ovarian cancer *(62, 169, 182, 241–244)*. However, a recent published systematic review and meta-analysis of 28 studies *(245)* supported a positive association between obesity and ovarian cancer risk, with pooled effect estimates of 1.2 (95% CI, 1.0–1.3) for overweight and 1.3 (95% CI, 1.1–1.3) for obesity, with a stronger association among case–control studies (OR = 1.5) than cohort studies (OR = 1.1). This review also suggested an increased risk of ovarian cancer associated with overweight/obesity in early adulthood but found no evidence that the association with obesity varied by histological subtype of ovarian cancer.

The timing of overweight, menopausal status, and race may be risk modifiers and may account for some of the inconsistent results. Some studies found a positive association with higher BMI in early adulthood *(128, 244, 246–248)*, but not with recent or current BMI *(128, 244, 247)*. Among studies that examined BMI-related risk of ovarian cancer by menopausal status, some studies observed a positive association among premenopausal women only *(242, 247, 249)*. In addition, one studies noted that a higher BMI was associated with ovarian cancer risk among African American women only, not among white women *(243)*.

4.8. Pancreatic Cancer

Evidence from increasing number of published studies suggests that obesity is associated with higher risk of pancreatic cancer *(130, 145, 176, 184, 186, 250, 251)*, although there is some inconsistency with no association detected in some studies. A recent published meta-analysis of 21 prospective studies *(250)* demonstrated an association between BMI and risk of pancreatic cancer in both men and women, with estimated summary RR of 1.12 (95% CI, 1.06–1.17) per 5 kg/m² increase in BMI. This review also observed a stronger association in men than in women, in studies conducted in United States than in Europe (but no association found in studies done in Asia), among studies based on self-reported weight and height than those based on measured anthropometry, and among studies adjusted for diabetes than those did not. Furthermore, several cohort studies also reported statistically significant association of pancreatic cancer risk with weight gain *(135, 141)*, waist circumference, and WHR *(133, 252, 253)*.

4.9. Other Cancers

BMI has been observed to be inversely associated with lung cancer risk in some cohort and case–control studies *(62, 183–185)* or not associated with lung cancer risk *(175, 176, 186, 254, 255)*.

However, this inverse association may be explained by weight loss due to preclinical disease or a residual confounding effect of smoking *(62, 183)*.

There have only been a few studies on gallbladder cancer and obesity. Although most of these studies are relatively small, they consistently demonstrated an increased risk for women *(173, 175, 184)*. For the relationship between liver cancer and obesity, there is only limited number of studies. Most of these studies found an elevated risk *(183–185, 204, 254, 255)*, while three studies suggested no association *(175, 176, 186)*.

4.10. All Cancers Combined

The results from several studies indicate that overweight and obesity are associated with the risk of incidence *(175, 176, 182–186, 254)* and mortality *(204, 256)* from all types of cancer combined. It has been estimated that overweight and obesity may contribute to 7% of all cancer incidence in Canada *(176)* and 5% in Europe *(172)*, and in the USA, for 14% and 20% of all cancer-related mortality in men and women *(204)*.

5. Conclusion

This review presents the epidemiologic evidence on the relationship of energy intake, PA, and obesity with cancer. In summary, high energy intake may increase the risk of cancers of colon–rectum, prostate (especially advanced prostate cancer), and breast. However, because PA, body size, and metabolic efficiency are highly related to total energy intake and expenditure, it is difficult to assess the independent effect of energy intake on cancer risk. The reverse associations of PA with colon and breast cancer are well established, whereas the association is stronger in men than in women for colon cancer and in postmenopausal than in premenopausal women for breast cancer. The evidence also suggests that risks of cancers of endometrium, lung, and prostate (to a lesser extent) are likely decreased by PA. On the other hand, there is little or no evidence that physical activity is related to rectal cancer risk, while there are inconsistent results regarding the association between physical activity and the risks of cancers of pancreas, ovary and kidney. Epidemiologic studies provide sufficient evidence that obesity is a risk factor for both cancer incidence and mortality. The evidence supports strong associations of obesity with risks of cancers of the colon, rectum, breast (in postmenopausal women), endometrium, kidney (renal cell), and adenocarcinoma of the esophagus. Epidemiologic evidence also indicates that obesity is probably related to cancers of the pancreas, liver, and gallbladder, and aggressive prostate cancer, while it seems that obesity is not associated with lung cancer. Results have been inconsistent for other cancers regarding the association with obesity. Energy intake, PA, and obesity are modifiable lifestyle factors; therefore, adopting a healthy lifestyle by avoiding excess energy intake, increasing PA, and maintaining a healthy weight would be an important strategy to prevent cancer and reduce the burden of cancer.

References

1. Hursting SD, Lavigne JA, Berrigan D, Perkins SN, Barrett JC (2003) Calorie restriction, aging, and cancer prevention: mechanisms of action and applicability to humans. *Annu Rev Med* **54**: 131–152.

2. Patel AC, Nunez NP, Perkins SN, Barrett JC, Hursting SD (2004) Effects of energy balance on cancer in genetically altered mice. *J Nutr* **134**: 3394S–3398S.

3. Lane MA, Black A, Handy A, Tilmont EM, Ingram DK, Roth GS (2001) Caloric restriction in primates. *Ann N Y Acad Sci* **928**: 287–295.

4. Roth GS, Ingram DK, Lane MA (1999) Calorie restriction in primates: will it work and how will we know? *J Am Geriatr Soc* **47**: 896–903.

5. Dirx MJ, Zeegers MP, Dagnelie PC, van den Bogaard T, van den Brandt PA (2003) Energy restriction and the risk of spontaneous mammary tumors in mice: a meta-analysis. *Int J Cancer* **106**: 766–770.

6. Cleary MP, Hu X, Grossmann ME, et al. (2007) Prevention of mammary tumorigenesis by intermittent caloric restriction: does caloric intake during refeeding modulate the response? *Exp Biol Med (Maywood)* **232**: 70–80.

7. Kritchevsky D (1997) Caloric restriction and experimental mammary carcinogenesis. *Breast Cancer Res Treat* **46**: 161–167.

8. Thompson HJ, Jiang W, Zhu Z (1999) Mechanisms by which energy restriction inhibits carcinogenesis. *Adv Exp Med Biol* **470**: 77–84.

9. Loft S, Velthuis-te Wierik EJ, Van den BH, Poulsen HE (1995) Energy restriction and oxidative DNA damage in humans. *Cancer Epidemiol Biomarkers Prev* **4**: 515–519.

10. Elias SG, Peeters PH, Grobbee DE, Van Noord PA (2005) The 1944–1945 Dutch famine and subsequent overall cancer incidence. *Cancer Epidemiol Biomarkers Prev* **14**: 1981–1985.

11. Frankel S, Gunnell DJ, Peters TJ, Maynard M, Davey SG (1998) Childhood energy intake and adult mortality from cancer: the Boyd Orr Cohort Study. *BMJ* **316**: 499–504.

12. Uauy R, Solomons N (2005) Diet, nutrition, and the life-course approach to cancer prevention. *J Nutr* **135**: 2934S–2945S.

13. Elias SG, Peeters PH, Grobbee DE, Van Noord PA (2004) Breast cancer risk after caloric restriction during the 1944–1945 Dutch famine. *J Natl Cancer Inst* **96**: 539–546.

14. Robsahm TE, Tretli S (2002) Breast cancer incidence in food- vs non-food-producing areas in Norway: possible beneficial effects of World War II. *Br J Cancer* **86**: 362–366.

15. Nilsen TI, Vatten LJ (2001) Adult height and risk of breast cancer: a possible effect of early nutrition. *Br J Cancer* **85**: 959–961.

16. Tretli S, Gaard M (1996) Lifestyle changes during adolescence and risk of breast cancer: an ecologic study of the effect of World War II in Norway. *Cancer Causes Control* **7**: 507–512.

17. Vatten LJ, Kvinnsland S (1990) Body height and risk of breast cancer. A prospective study of 23,831 Norwegian women. *Br J Cancer* **61**: 881–885.

18. Dirx MJ, van den Brandt PA, Goldbohm RA, Lumey LH (1999) Diet in adolescence and the risk of breast cancer: results of the Netherlands Cohort Study. *Cancer Causes Control* **10**: 189–199.

19. Michels KB, Ekbom A (2004) Caloric restriction and incidence of breast cancer. *JAMA* **291**: 1226–1230.

20. Varela G, Carbajal A, Nunez C, Belmonte S, Moreiras O (1996) (Influence of energy intake and body mass index in the incidence of cancer of the breast. Case-control study in a sample from 3 Spanish hospital populations). *Nutr Hosp* **11**: 54–58.

21. Malin A, Matthews CE, Shu XO, et al. (2005) Energy balance and breast cancer risk. *Cancer Epidemiol Biomarkers Prev* **14**: 1496–1501.

22. Franceschi S, Favero A, Decarli A, et al. (1996) Intake of macronutrients and risk of breast cancer. *Lancet* **347**: 1351–1356.

23. Levi F, La VC, Gulie C, Negri E (1993) Dietary factors and breast cancer risk in Vaud, Switzerland. *Nutr Cancer* **19**: 327–335.

24. Toniolo P, Riboli E, Protta F, Charrel M, Cappa AP (1989) Calorie-providing nutrients and risk of breast cancer. *J Natl Cancer Inst* **81**: 278–286.

25. Yu SZ, Lu RF, Xu DD, Howe GR (1990) A case-control study of dietary and nondietary risk factors for breast cancer in Shanghai. *Cancer Res* **50**: 5017–5021.

26. Nkondjock A, Robidoux A, Paredes Y, Narod SA, Ghadirian P (2006) Diet, lifestyle and BRCA-related breast cancer risk among French-Canadians. *Breast Cancer Res Treat* **98**: 285–294.

27. Levi F, Pasche C, Lucchini F, La VC (2001) Dietary intake of selected micronutrients and breast-cancer risk. *Int J Cancer* **91**: 260–263.

28. Iscovich JM, Iscovich RB, Howe G, Shiboski S, Kaldor JM (1989) A case-control study of diet and breast cancer in Argentina. *Int J Cancer* **44**: 770–776.

29. Fioretti F, Tavani A, Bosetti C, et al. (1999) Risk factors for breast cancer in nulliparous women. *Br J Cancer* **79**: 1923–1928.

30. Chang SC, Ziegler RG, Dunn B, et al. (2006) Association of energy intake and energy balance with postmenopausal breast cancer in the prostate, lung, colorectal, and ovarian cancer screening trial. *Cancer Epidemiol Biomarkers Prev* **15**: 334–341.

31. Silvera SA, Jain M, Howe GR, Miller AB, Rohan TE (2006) Energy balance and breast cancer risk: a prospective cohort study. *Breast Cancer Res Treat* **97**: 97–106.

32. Barrett-Connor E, Friedlander NJ (1993) Dietary fat, calories, and the risk of breast cancer in postmenopausal women: a prospective population-based study. *J Am Coll Nutr* **12**: 390–399.

33. Gaard M, Tretli S, Loken EB (1995) Dietary fat and the risk of breast cancer: a prospective study of 25,892 Norwegian women. *Int J Cancer* **63**: 13–17.

34. Graham S, Hellmann R, Marshall J, et al. (1991) Nutritional epidemiology of postmenopausal breast cancer in western New York. *Am J Epidemiol* **134**: 552–566.

35. Holmberg L, Ohlander EM, Byers T, et al. (1994) Diet and breast cancer risk. Results from a population-based, case-control study in Sweden. *Arch Intern Med* **154**: 1805–1811.

36. Yuan JM, Wang QS, Ross RK, Henderson BE, Yu MC (1995) Diet and breast cancer in Shanghai and Tianjin, China. *Br J Cancer* **71**: 1353–1358.

37. Velie E, Kulldorff M, Schairer C, Block G, Albanes D, Schatzkin A (2000) Dietary fat, fat subtypes, and breast cancer in postmenopausal women: a prospective cohort study. *J Natl Cancer Inst* **92**: 833–839.

38. Byrne C, Rockett H, Holmes MD (2002) Dietary fat, fat subtypes, and breast cancer risk: lack of an association among postmenopausal women with no history of benign breast disease. *Cancer Epidemiol Biomarkers Prev* **11**: 261–265.

39. Kim EH, Willett WC, Colditz GA, et al. (2006) Dietary fat and risk of postmenopausal breast cancer in a 20-year follow-up. *Am J Epidemiol* **164**: 990–997.

40. Dirx MJ, van den Brandt PA, Goldbohm RA, Lumey LH (2003) Energy restriction early in life and colon carcinoma risk: results of The Netherlands Cohort Study after 7.3 years of follow-up. *Cancer* **97**: 46–55.

41. Satia-Abouta J, Galanko JA, Potter JD, Ammerman A, Martin CF, Sandler RS (2003) Associations of total energy and macronutrients with colon cancer risk in African Americans and Whites: results from the North Carolina colon cancer study. *Am J Epidemiol* **158**: 951–962.

42. Slattery ML, Potter J, Caan B, et al. (1997) Energy balance and colon cancer–beyond physical activity. *Cancer Res* **57**: 75–80.

43. Slattery ML, Caan BJ, Benson J, Murtaugh M (2003) Energy balance and rectal cancer: an evaluation of energy intake, energy expenditure, and body mass index. *Nutr Cancer* **46**: 166–171.

44. Mao Y, Pan S, Wen SW, Johnson KC (2003) Physical inactivity, energy intake, obesity and the risk of rectal cancer in Canada. *Int J Cancer* **105**: 831–837.

45. Levi F, Pasche C, Lucchini F, La VC (2002) Macronutrients and colorectal cancer: a Swiss case-control study. *Ann Oncol* **13**: 369–373.

46. Franceschi S, La VC, Russo A, et al. (1998) Macronutrient intake and risk of colorectal *cancer in Italy. Int J Cancer* **76: 321–324.**

47. Howe GR, Aronson KJ, Benito E, et al. (1997) The relationship between dietary fat intake and risk of colorectal cancer: evidence from the combined analysis of 13 case-control studies. *Cancer Causes Control* **8**: 215–228.

48. Le ML, Wilkens LR, Kolonel LN, Hankin JH, Lyu LC (1997) Associations of sedentary lifestyle, obesity, smoking, alcohol use, and diabetes with the risk of colorectal cancer. *Cancer Res* **57**: 4787–4794.

49. Gerhardsson d, V, Hagman U, Steineck G, Rieger A, Norell SE (1990) Diet, body mass

and colorectal cancer: a case-referent study in Stockholm. *Int J Cancer* **46**: 832–838.

50. Freudenheim JL, Graham S, Marshall JR, Haughey BP, Wilkinson G (1990) A case-control study of diet and rectal cancer in western New York. *Am J Epidemiol* **131**: 612–624.

51. Graham S, Marshall J, Haughey B, et al. (1988) Dietary epidemiology of cancer of the colon in western New York. *Am J Epidemiol* **128**: 490–503.

52. Boutron-Ruault MC, Senesse P, Meance S, Belghiti C, Faivre J (2001) Energy intake, body mass index, physical activity, and the colorectal adenoma-carcinoma sequence. *Nutr Cancer* **39**: 50–57.

53. Gaard M, Tretli S, Loken EB (1996) Dietary factors and risk of colon cancer: a prospective study of 50,535 young Norwegian men and women. *Eur J Cancer Prev* **5**: 445–454.

54. Stemmermann GN, Nomura AM, Heilbrun LK (1985) Cancer risk in relation to fat and energy intake among Hawaii Japanese: a prospective study. *Princess Takamatsu Symp* **16**: 265–274.

55. Kato I, Akhmedkhanov A, Koenig K, Toniolo PG, Shore RE, Riboli E (1997) Prospective study of diet and female colorectal cancer: the New York University Women's Health Study. *Nutr Cancer* **28**: 276–281.

56. Dirx MJ, van den Brandt PA, Goldbohm RA, Lumey LH (2001) Energy restriction in childhood and adolescence and risk of prostate cancer: results from the Netherlands Cohort Study. *Am J Epidemiol* **154**: 530–537.

57. Platz EA (2002) Energy imbalance and prostate cancer. *J Nutr* **132**: 3471S–3481S.

58. Platz EA, Leitzmann MF, Michaud DS, Willett WC, Giovannucci E (2003) Interrelation of energy intake, body size, and physical activity with prostate cancer in a large prospective cohort study. *Cancer Res* **63**: 8542–8548.

59. Hsieh LJ, Carter HB, Landis PK, et al. (2003) Association of energy intake with prostate cancer in a long-term aging study: Baltimore Longitudinal Study of Aging (United States). *Urology* **61**: 297–301.

60. Kristal AR, Cohen JH, Qu P, Stanford JL (2002) Associations of energy, fat, calcium, and vitamin D with prostate cancer risk. *Cancer Epidemiol Biomarkers Prev* **11**: 719–725.

61. Darlington GA, Kreiger N, Lightfoot N, Purdham J, Sass-Kortsak A (2007) Prostate cancer risk and diet, recreational physical activity and cigarette smoking. *Chronic Dis Can* **27**: 145–153.

62. IARC Handbooks of Cancer Prevention (2002) *Weight Control and Physical Activity*. Lyons, France: International Agency for Research on Cancer.

63. Slattery ML (2004) Physical activity and colorectal cancer. *Sports Med* **34**: 239–252.

64. Lee KJ, Inoue M, Otani T, Iwasaki M, Sasazuki S, Tsugane S (2007) Physical activity and risk of colorectal cancer in Japanese men and women: the Japan Public Health Center-based prospective study. *Cancer Causes Control* **18**: 199–209.

65. Isomura K, Kono S, Moore MA, et al. (2006) Physical activity and colorectal cancer: the Fukuoka Colorectal Cancer Study. *Cancer Sci* **97**: 1099–1104.

66. Mai PL, Sullivan-Halley J, Ursin G, et al. (2007) Physical activity and colon cancer risk among women in the California Teachers Study. *Cancer Epidemiol Biomarkers Prev* **16**: 517–525.

67. Friedenreich C, Norat T, Steindorf K, et al. (2006) Physical activity and risk of colon and rectal cancers: the European prospective investigation into cancer and nutrition. *Cancer Epidemiol Biomarkers Prev* **15**: 2398–2407

68. Larsson SC, Rutegard J, Bergkvist L, Wolk A (2006) Physical activity, obesity, and risk of colon and rectal cancer in a cohort of Swedish men. *Eur J Cancer* **42**: 2590–2597.

69. Zhang Y, Cantor KP, Dosemeci M, Lynch CF, Zhu Y, Zheng T (2006) Occupational and leisure-time physical activity and risk of colon cancer by subsite. *J Occup Environ Med* **48**: 236–243.

70. Steindorf K, Jedrychowski W, Schmidt M, et al. (2005) Case-control study of lifetime occupational and recreational physical activity and risks of colon and rectal cancer. *Eur J Cancer Prev* **14**: 363–371.

71. Chao A, Connell CJ, Jacobs EJ, et al. (2004) Amount, type, and timing of recreational physical activity in relation to colon and rectal cancer in older adults: the Cancer Prevention Study II Nutrition Cohort. *Cancer Epidemiol Biomarkers Prev* **13**: 2187–2195.

72. Wei EK, Giovannucci E, Wu K, et al. (2004) Comparison of risk factors for colon and rectal cancer. *Int J Cancer* **108**: 433–442.

73. Samad AK, Taylor RS, Marshall T, Chapman MA (2005) A meta-analysis of the association of physical activity with reduced risk of colorectal cancer. *Colorectal Dis* **7**: 204–213.

74. Calton BA, Lacey JV Jr, Schatzkin A, et al. (2006) Physical activity and the risk of colon cancer among women: a prospective cohort study (United States). *Int J Cancer* **119**: 385–391.

75. Lund Nilsen TI, Vatten LJ (2002) Colorectal cancer associated with BMI, physical activity, diabetes, and blood glucose. *IARC Sci Publ* **156**: 257–258.

76. Monninkhof EM, Elias SG, Vlems FA, et al. (2007) Physical activity and breast cancer: a systematic review. *Epidemiology* **18**: 137–157.

77. Vainio H, Kaaks R, Bianchini F (2002) Weight control and physical activity in cancer prevention: international evaluation of the evidence. *Eur J Cancer Prev* 11 Suppl 2: S94–100.

78. Friedenreich CM, Orenstein MR (2002) Physical activity and cancer prevention: etiologic evidence and biological mechanisms. *J Nutr* **132**: 3456S–3464S.

79. Lagerros YT, Hsieh SF, Hsieh CC (2004) Physical activity in adolescence and young adulthood and breast cancer risk: a quantitative review. *Eur J Cancer Prev* **13**: 5–12.

80. Torti DC, Matheson GO (2004) Exercise and prostate cancer. *Sports Med* **34**: 363–369.

81. Littman AJ, Kristal AR, White E (2006) Recreational physical activity and prostate cancer risk (United States). *Cancer Causes Control* **17**: 831–841.

82. Nilsen TI, Romundstad PR, Vatten LJ (2006) Recreational physical activity and risk of prostate cancer: A prospective population-based study in Norway (the HUNT study). *Int J Cancer* **119**: 2943–2947.

83. Zeegers MP, Dirx MJ, van den Brandt PA (2005) Physical activity and the risk of prostate cancer in the Netherlands cohort study, results after 9.3 years of follow-up. *Cancer Epidemiol Biomarkers Prev* **14**: 1490–1495.

84. Giovannucci EL, Liu Y, Leitzmann MF, Stampfer MJ, Willett WC (2005) A prospective study of physical activity and incident and fatal prostate cancer. *Arch Intern Med* **165**: 1005–1010.

85. Patel AV, Rodriguez C, Jacobs EJ, Solomon L, Thun MJ, Calle EE (2005) Recreational physical activity and risk of prostate cancer in a large cohort of U.S. men. *Cancer Epidemiol Biomarkers Prev* **14**: 275–279.

86. Norman A, Moradi T, Gridley G, et al. (2002) Occupational physical activity and risk for prostate cancer in a nationwide cohort study in Sweden. *Br J Cancer* **86**: 70–75.

87. Friedenreich CM, McGregor SE, Courneya KS, Angyalfi SJ, Elliott FG (2004) Case-control study of lifetime total physical activity and prostate cancer risk. *Am J Epidemiol* **159**: 740–749.

88. Pierotti B, Altieri A, Talamini R, et al. (2005) Lifetime physical activity and prostate cancer risk. *Int J Cancer* **114**: 639–642.

89. Jian L, Shen ZJ, Lee AH, Binns CW (2005) Moderate physical activity and prostate cancer risk: a case-control study in China. *Eur J Epidemiol* **20**: 155–160.

90. Voskuil DW, Monninkhof EM, Elias SG, Vlems FA, van Leeuwen FE (2007) Physical activity and endometrial cancer risk, a systematic review of current evidence. *Cancer Epidemiol Biomarkers Prev* **16**: 639–648.

91. Friedenreich C, Cust A, Lahmann PH, et al. (2007) Physical activity and risk of endometrial cancer: The European prospective investigation into cancer and nutrition. *Int J Cancer* **121**: 347–355.

92. Matthews CE, Xu WH, Zheng W, et al. (2005) Physical activity and risk of endometrial cancer: a report from the Shanghai endometrial cancer study. *Cancer Epidemiol Biomarkers Prev* **14**: 779–785.

93. Colbert LH, Lacey JV, Jr, Schairer C, Albert P, Schatzkin A, Albanes D (2003) Physical activity and risk of endometrial cancer in a prospective cohort study (United States). *Cancer Causes Control* **14**: 559–567.

94. Furberg AS, Thune I (2003) Metabolic abnormalities (hypertension, hyperglycemia and overweight), lifestyle (high energy intake and physical inactivity) and endometrial cancer risk in a Norwegian cohort. *Int J Cancer* **104**: 669–676.

95. Schouten LJ, Goldbohm RA, van den Brandt PA (2004) Anthropometry, physical activity, and endometrial cancer risk: results from the Netherlands Cohort Study. *J Natl Cancer Inst* **96**: 1635–1638.

96. Littman AJ, Voigt LF, Beresford SA, Weiss NS (2001) Recreational physical activity and endometrial cancer risk. *Am J Epidemiol* **154**: 924–933.

97. Salazar-Martinez E, Lazcano-Ponce EC, Lira-Lira GG, et al. (2000) Case-control study of diabetes, obesity, physical activity and risk of endometrial cancer among Mexican women. *Cancer Causes Control* **11**: 707–711.

98. Moradi T, Nyren O, Bergstrom R, et al. (1998) Risk for endometrial cancer in relation to occupational physical activity: a nationwide cohort study in Sweden. *Int J Cancer* **76**: 665–670.

99. Moradi T, Weiderpass E, Signorello LB, Persson I, Nyren O, Adami HO (2000) Physical activity and postmenopausal endometrial cancer risk (Sweden). *Cancer Causes Control* **11**: 829–837.

100. Goodman MT, Hankin JH, Wilkens LR, et al. (1997) Diet, body size, physical activity, and the risk of endometrial cancer. *Cancer Res* **57**: 5077–5085.

101. Hirose K, Tajima K, Hamajima N, et al. (1996) Subsite (cervix/endometrium)-specific risk and protective factors in uterus cancer. *Jpn J Cancer Res* **87**: 1001–1009.

102. Kalandidi A, Tzonou A, Lipworth L, Gamatsi I, Filippa D, Trichopoulos D (1996) A case-control study of endometrial cancer in relation to reproductive, somatometric, and life-style variables. *Oncology* **53**: 354–359.

103. Levi F, La VC, Negri E, Franceschi S (1993) Selected physical activities and the risk of endometrial cancer. *Br J Cancer* **67**: 846–851.

104. Zheng W, Shu XO, McLaughlin JK, Chow WH, Gao YT, Blot WJ (1993) Occupational physical activity and the incidence of cancer of the breast, corpus uteri, and ovary in Shanghai. *Cancer* **71**: 3620–3624.

105. Sturgeon SR, Brinton LA, Berman ML, et al. (1993) Past and present physical activity and endometrial cancer risk. *Br J Cancer* **68**: 584–589.

106. Terry P, Baron JA, Weiderpass E, Yuen J, Lichtenstein P, Nyren O (1999) Lifestyle and endometrial cancer risk: a cohort study from the Swedish Twin Registry. *Int J Cancer* **82**: 38–42.

107. Dosemeci M, Hayes RB, Vetter R, et al. (1993) Occupational physical activity, socioeconomic status, and risks of 15 cancer sites in Turkey. *Cancer Causes Control* **4**: 313–321.

108. Olson SH, Vena JE, Dorn JP, et al. (1997) Exercise, occupational activity, and risk of endometrial cancer. *Ann Epidemiol* **7**: 46–53.

109. Friberg E, Mantzoros CS, Wolk A (2006) Physical activity and risk of endometrial cancer: a population-based prospective cohort study. *Cancer Epidemiol Biomarkers Prev* **15**: 2136–2140.

110. Tardon A, Lee WJ, Delgado-Rodriguez M, et al. (2005) Leisure-time physical activity and lung cancer: a meta-analysis. *Cancer Causes Control* **16**: 389–397.

111. Sinner P, Folsom AR, Harnack L, Eberly LE, Schmitz KH (2006) The association of physical activity with lung cancer incidence in a cohort of older women: the Iowa Women's Health Study. *Cancer Epidemiol Biomarkers Prev* **15**: 2359–2363.

112. Steindorf K, Friedenreich C, Linseisen J, et al. (2006) Physical activity and lung cancer risk in the European Prospective Investigation into Cancer and Nutrition Cohort. *Int J Cancer* **119**: 2389–2397.

113. Bak H, Christensen J, Thomsen BL, et al. (2005) Physical activity and risk for lung cancer in a Danish cohort. *Int J Cancer* **116**: 439–444.

114. Alfano CM, Klesges RC, Murray DM, et al. (2004) Physical activity in relation to all-site and lung cancer incidence and mortality in current and former smokers. *Cancer Epidemiol Biomarkers Prev* **13**: 2233–2241.

115. Kubik A, Zatloukal P, Tomasek L, et al. (2007) Interactions between smoking and other exposures associated with lung cancer risk in women: diet and physical activity. *Neoplasma* **54**: 83–88.

116. Biesma RG, Schouten LJ, Dirx MJ, Goldbohm RA, van den Brandt PA (2006) Physical activity and risk of ovarian cancer: results from the Netherlands Cohort Study (The Netherlands). *Cancer Causes Control* **17**: 109–115.

117. Hannan LM, Leitzmann MF, Lacey JV, Jr, et al. (2004) Physical activity and risk of ovarian cancer: a prospective cohort study in the United States. *Cancer Epidemiol Biomarkers Prev* **13**: 765–770.

118. Chiaffarino F, Parazzini F, Bosetti C, et al. (2007) Risk factors for ovarian cancer histotypes. *Eur J Cancer* **43**: 1208–1213.

119. Pan SY, Ugnat AM, Mao Y (2005) Physical activity and the risk of ovarian cancer: a case-control study in Canada. *Int J Cancer* **117**: 300–307.

120. Riman T, Dickman PW, Nilsson S, Nordlinder H, Magnusson CM, Persson IR (2004) Some life-style factors and the risk of invasive epithelial ovarian cancer in Swedish women. *Eur J Epidemiol* **19**: 1011–1019.

121. Zhang M, Lee AH, Binns CW (2003) Physical activity and epithelial ovarian cancer risk: a case-control study in China. *Int J Cancer* **105**: 838–843.

122. Tavani A, Gallus S, La VC, et al. (2001) Physical activity and risk of ovarian cancer: an Italian case-control study. *Int J Cancer* **91**: 407–411.

123. Cottreau CM, Ness RB, Kriska AM (2000) Physical activity and reduced risk of ovarian cancer. *Obstet Gynecol* **96**: 609–614.

124. Pukkala E, Poskiparta M, Apter D, Vihko V (1993) Life-long physical activity and cancer risk among Finnish female teachers. *Eur J Cancer Prev* 2: 369–376.

125. Patel AV, Rodriguez C, Pavluck AL, Thun MJ, Calle EE (2006) Recreational physical activity and sedentary behavior in relation to ovarian cancer risk in a large cohort of US women. *Am J Epidemiol* 163: 709–716.

126. Weiderpass E, Margolis KL, Sandin S, et al. (2006) Prospective study of physical activity in different periods of life and the risk of ovarian cancer. *Int J Cancer* 118: 3153–3160.

127. Bertone ER, Newcomb PA, Willett WC, Stampfer MJ, Egan KM (2002) Recreational physical activity and ovarian cancer in a population-based case-control study. *Int J Cancer* 99: 431–436.

128. Anderson JP, Ross JA, Folsom AR (2004) Anthropometric variables, physical activity, and incidence of ovarian cancer: The Iowa Women's Health Study. *Cancer* 100: 1515–1521.

129. Bertone ER, Willett WC, Rosner BA, et al. (2001) Prospective study of recreational physical activity and ovarian cancer. *J Natl Cancer Inst* 93: 942–948.

130. Lin Y, Kikuchi S, Tamakoshi A, et al. (2007) Obesity, physical activity and the risk of pancreatic cancer in a large Japanese cohort. *Int J Cancer* 120: 2665–2671.

131. Nothlings U, Wilkens LR, Murphy SP, Hankin JH, Henderson BE, Kolonel LN (2007) Body mass index and physical activity as risk factors for pancreatic cancer: the Multiethnic Cohort Study. *Cancer Causes Control* 18: 165–175.

132. Luo J, Iwasaki M, Inoue M, et al. (2007) Body mass index, physical activity and the risk of pancreatic cancer in relation to smoking status and history of diabetes: a large-scale population-based cohort study in Japan–the JPHC study. *Cancer Causes Control* 18: 603–612.

133. Berrington de GA, Spencer EA, Bueno-de-Mesquita HB, et al. (2006) Anthropometry, physical activity, and the risk of pancreatic cancer in the European prospective investigation into cancer and nutrition. *Cancer Epidemiol Biomarkers Prev* 15: 879–885.

134. Sinner PJ, Schmitz KH, Anderson KE, Folsom AR (2005) Lack of association of physical activity and obesity with incident pancreatic cancer in elderly women. *Cancer Epidemiol Biomarkers Prev* 14: 1571–1573.

135. Patel AV, Rodriguez C, Bernstein L, Chao A, Thun MJ, Calle EE (2005) Obesity, recreational physical activity, and risk of pancreatic cancer in a large U.S. Cohort. *Cancer Epidemiol Biomarkers Prev* 14: 459–466.

136. Lee IM, Sesso HD, Oguma Y, Paffenbarger RS, Jr. (2003) Physical activity, body weight, and pancreatic cancer mortality. *Br J Cancer* 88: 679–683.

137. Lee IM, Paffenbarger RS, Jr (1994) Physical activity and its relation to cancer risk: a prospective study of college alumni. *Med Sci Sports Exerc* 26: 831–837.

138. Brownson RC, Chang JC, Davis JR, Smith CA (1991) Physical activity on the job and cancer in Missouri. *Am J Public Health* 81: 639–642.

139. Stolzenberg-Solomon RZ, Pietinen P, Taylor PR, Virtamo J, Albanes D (2002) A prospective study of medical conditions, anthropometry, physical activity, and pancreatic cancer in male smokers (Finland). *Cancer Causes Control* 13: 417–426.

140. Michaud DS, Giovannucci E, Willett WC, Colditz GA, Stampfer MJ, Fuchs CS (2001) Physical activity, obesity, height, and the risk of pancreatic cancer. *JAMA* 286: 921–929.

141. Isaksson B, Jonsson F, Pedersen NL, Larsson J, Feychting M, Permert J (2002) Lifestyle factors and pancreatic cancer risk: a cohort study from the Swedish Twin Registry. *Int J Cancer* 98: 480–482.

142. Nilsen TI, Vatten LJ (2000) A prospective study of lifestyle factors and the risk of pancreatic cancer in Nord-Trondelag, Norway. *Cancer Causes Control* 11: 645–652.

143. Hanley AJ, Johnson KC, Villeneuve PJ, Mao Y (2001) Physical activity, anthropometric factors and risk of pancreatic cancer: results from the Canadian enhanced cancer surveillance system. *Int J Cancer* 94: 140–147.

144. Inoue M, Tajima K, Takezaki T, et al. (2003) Epidemiology of pancreatic cancer in Japan: a nested case-control study from the Hospital-based Epidemiologic Research Program at Aichi Cancer Center (HERPACC). *Int J Epidemiol* 32: 257–262.

145. Eberle CA, Bracci PM, Holly EA (2005) Anthropometric factors and pancreatic cancer in a population-based case-control study in the San Francisco Bay area. *Cancer Causes Control* 16: 1235–1244.

146. van Dijk BA, Schouten LJ, Kiemeney LA, Goldbohm RA, van den Brandt PA (2004) Relation of height, body mass, energy intake, and physical activity to risk of renal cell carcinoma: results from the Netherlands Cohort Study. *Am J Epidemiol* 160: 1159–1167.

147. Bergstrom A, Terry P, Lindblad P, et al. (2001) Physical activity and risk of renal cell cancer. *Int J Cancer* **92**: 155–157.

148. Paffenbarger RS, Jr, Hyde RT, Wing AL (1987) Physical activity and incidence of cancer in diverse populations: a preliminary report. *Am J Clin Nutr* **45**: 312–317.

149. Pan SY, DesMeules M, Morrison H, Wen SW (2006) Obesity, high energy intake, lack of physical activity, and the risk of kidney cancer. *Cancer Epidemiol Biomarkers Prev* **15**: 2453–2460.

150. Mellemgaard A, Lindblad P, Schlehofer B, et al. (1995) International renal-cell cancer study. III. Role of weight, height, physical activity, and use of amphetamines. *Int J Cancer* **60**: 350–354.

151. Mellemgaard A, Engholm G, McLaughlin JK, Olsen JH (1994) Risk factors for renal-cell carcinoma in Denmark. III. Role of weight, physical activity and reproductive factors. *Int J Cancer* **56**: 66–71.

152. Goodman MT, Morgenstern H, Wynder EL (1986) A case-control study of factors affecting the development of renal cell cancer. *Am J Epidemiol* **124**: 926–941.

153. Wendy S, V, Stram DO, Nomura AM, Kolonel LN, Henderson BE (2007) Risk factors for renal cell cancer: The multiethnic cohort. *Am J Epidemiol*.

154. Mahabir S, Leitzmann MF, Pietinen P, Albanes D, Virtamo J, Taylor PR (2004) Physical activity and renal cell cancer risk in a cohort of male smokers. *Int J Cancer* **108**: 600–605.

155. Bergstrom A, Moradi T, Lindblad P, Nyren O, Adami HO, Wolk A (1999) Occupational physical activity and renal cell cancer: a nationwide cohort study in Sweden. *Int J Cancer* **83**: 186–191.

156. Tavani A, Zucchetto A, Dal ML, et al. (2007) Lifetime physical activity and the risk of renal cell cancer. *Int J Cancer* **120**: 1977–1980.

157. Menezes RJ, Tomlinson G, Kreiger N (2003) Physical activity and risk of renal cell carcinoma. *Int J Cancer* **107**: 642–646.

158. Lindblad P, Wolk A, Bergstrom R, Persson I, Adami HO (1994) The role of obesity and weight fluctuations in the etiology of renal cell cancer: a population-based case-control study. *Cancer Epidemiol Biomarkers Prev* **3**: 631–639.

159. Yeter K, Rock CL, Pakiz B, Bardwell WA, Nichols JF, Wilfley DE (2006) Depressive symptoms, eating psychopathology, and physical activity in obese breast cancer survivors. *Psychooncology* **15**: 453–462.

160. Milne HM, Gordon S, Guilfoyle A, Wallman KE, Courneya KS (2007) Association between physical activity and quality of life among Western Australian breast cancer survivors. *Psychooncology*.

161. Milne HM, Wallman KE, Gordon S, Courneya KS (2007) Effects of a combined aerobic and resistance exercise program in breast cancer survivors: a randomized controlled trial. *Breast Cancer Res Treat*.

162. Weitzen R, Tichler T, Kaufman B, Catane R, Shpatz Y (2006) [Body weight, nutritional factors and physical activity--their influence on prognosis after breast cancer diagnosis). *Harefuah* **145**: 820–825, 861.

163. Holmes MD, Chen WY, Feskanich D, Kroenke CH, Colditz GA (2005) Physical activity and survival after breast cancer diagnosis. *JAMA* **293**: 2479–2486.

164. Pierce JP, Stefanick ML, Flatt SW, et al. (2007) Greater survival after breast cancer in physically active women with high vegetable-fruit intake regardless of obesity. *J Clin Oncol* **25**: 2345–2351.

165. Meyerhardt JA, Giovannucci EL, Holmes MD, et al. (2006) Physical activity and survival after colorectal cancer diagnosis. *J Clin Oncol* **24**: 3527–3534.

166. Meyerhardt JA, Heseltine D, Niedzwiecki D, et al. (2006) Impact of physical activity on cancer recurrence and survival in patients with stage III colon cancer: findings from CALGB 89803. *J Clin Oncol* **24**: 3535–3541.

167. Kirshbaum MN (2007) A review of the benefits of whole body exercise during and after treatment for breast cancer. *J Clin Nurs* **16**: 104–121.

168. Schmitz KH, Holtzman J, Courneya KS, Masse LC, Duval S, Kane R (2005) Controlled physical activity trials in cancer survivors: a systematic review and meta-analysis. *Cancer Epidemiol Biomarkers Prev* **14**: 1588–1595.

169. Mao Y, Pan SY, Ugnat AM (2006) Obesity as a cancer risk factor: epidemiology. In: Awad AB, Bradford PG, eds. *Nutrition and Cancer Prevention*. Boca Raton: Taylor & Francis Group, pp. 541–563.

170. Carmichael AR, Bates T (2004) Obesity and breast cancer: a review of the literature. *Breast* **13**: 85–92.

171. Bianchini F, Kaaks R, Vainio H (2002) Overweight, obesity, and cancer risk. *Lancet ncol* **3**: 565–574.

172. Bergstrom A, Pisani P, Tenet V, Wolk A, Adami HO (2001) Overweight as an avoid-

able cause of cancer in Europe. *Int J Cancer* **91**: 421–430.

173. Calle EE, Kaaks R (2004) Overweight, obesity and cancer: epidemiological evidence and proposed mechanisms. *Nat Rev Cancer* **4**: 579–591.

174. Lundqvist E, Kaprio J, Verkasalo PK, et al. (2007) Co-twin control and cohort analyses of body mass index and height in relation to breast, prostate, ovarian, corpus uteri, colon and rectal cancer among Swedish and Finnish twins. *Int J Cancer* **121**: 810–818.

175. Kuriyama S, Tsubono Y, Hozawa A, et al. (2005) Obesity and risk of cancer in Japan. *Int J Cancer* **113**: 148–157.

176. Pan SY, Johnson KC, Ugnat AM, Wen SW, Mao Y (2004) Association of obesity and cancer risk in Canada. *Am J Epidemiol* **159**: 259–268.

177. Harvie M, Hooper L, Howell AH (2003) Central obesity and breast cancer risk: a systematic review. *Obes Rev* **4**: 157–173.

178. Carmichael AR (2006) Obesity and prognosis of breast cancer. *Obes Rev* **7**: 333–340.

179. Gunter MJ, Leitzmann MF (2006) Obesity and colorectal cancer: epidemiology, mechanisms and candidate genes. *J Nutr Biochem* **17**: 145–156.

180. Pischon T, Lahmann PH, Boeing H, et al. (2006) Body size and risk of colon and rectal cancer in the European Prospective Investigation Into Cancer and Nutrition (EPIC). *J Natl Cancer Inst* **98**: 920–931.

181. Adams KF, Leitzmann MF, Albanes D, et al. (2007) Body mass and colorectal cancer risk in the NIH-AARP cohort. *Am J Epidemiol* **166**: 36–45.

182. Lukanova A, Bjor O, Kaaks R, et al. (2006) Body mass index and cancer: results from the Northern Sweden Health and Disease Cohort. *Int J Cancer* **118**: 458–466.

183. Samanic C, Chow WH, Gridley G, Jarvholm B, Fraumeni JF, Jr (2006) Relation of body mass index to cancer risk in 362,552 Swedish men. *Cancer Causes Control* **17**: 901–909.

184. Samanic C, Gridley G, Chow WH, Lubin J, Hoover RN, Fraumeni JF, Jr (2004) Obesity and cancer risk among white and black United States veterans. *Cancer Causes Control* **15**: 35–43.

185. Oh SW, Yoon YS, Shin SA (2005) Effects of excess weight on cancer incidences depending on cancer sites and histologic findings among men: Korea National Health Insurance Corporation Study. *J Clin Oncol* **23**: 4742–4754.

186. Rapp K, Schroeder J, Klenk J, et al. (2005) Obesity and incidence of cancer: a large cohort study of over 145,000 adults in Austria. *Br J Cancer* **93**: 1062–1067.

187. MacInnis RJ, English DR, Hopper JL, Haydon AM, Gertig DM, Giles GG (2004) Body size and composition and colon cancer risk in men. *Cancer Epidemiol Biomarkers Prev* **13**: 553–559.

188. Terry PD, Miller AB, Rohan TE (2002) Obesity and colorectal cancer risk in women. *Gut* **51**: 191–194.

189. Terry P, Giovannucci E, Bergkvist L, Holmberg L, Wolk A (2001) Body weight and colorectal cancer risk in a cohort of Swedish women: relation varies by age and cancer site. *Br J Cancer* **85**: 346–349.

190. Slattery ML, Ballard-Barbash R, Edwards S, Caan BJ, Potter JD (2003) Body mass index and colon cancer: an evaluation of the modifying effects of estrogen (United States). *Cancer Causes Control* **14**: 75–84.

191. Hou L, Ji BT, Blair A, et al. (2006) Body mass index and colon cancer risk in Chinese people: menopause as an effect modifier. *Eur J Cancer* **42**: 84–90.

192. Lin J, Zhang SM, Cook NR, Rexrode KM, Lee IM, Buring JE (2004) Body mass index and risk of colorectal cancer in women (United States). *Cancer Causes Control* **15**: 581–589.

193. MacInnis RJ, English DR, Hopper JL, Gertig DM, Haydon AM, Giles GG (2006) Body size and composition and colon cancer risk in women. *Int J Cancer* **118**: 1496–1500.

194. MacInnis RJ, English DR, Haydon AM, Hopper JL, Gertig DM, Giles GG (2006) Body size and composition and risk of rectal cancer (Australia). *Cancer Causes Control* **17**: 1291–1297.

195. Moore LL, Bradlee ML, Singer MR, et al. (2004) BMI and waist circumference as predictors of lifetime colon cancer risk in Framingham Study adults. *Int J Obes Relat Metab Disord* **28**: 559–567.

196. Giovannucci E, Ascherio A, Rimm EB, Colditz GA, Stampfer MJ, Willett WC (1995) Physical activity, obesity, and risk for colon cancer and adenoma in men. *Ann Intern Med* **122**: 327–334.

197. Sedjo RL, Byers T, Levin TR, et al. (2007) Change in body size and the risk of colorectal adenomas. *Cancer Epidemiol Biomarkers Prev* **16**: 526–531.

198. Chung YW, Han DS, Park YK, et al. (2006) Association of obesity, serum glucose and lipids with the risk of advanced colorectal adenoma and cancer: a case-control study in Korea. *Dig Liver Dis* **38**: 668–672.

199. Guilera M, Connelly-Frost A, Keku TO, Martin CF, Galanko J, Sandler RS (2005) Does physical activity modify the association between body mass index and colorectal adenomas? *Nutr Cancer* **51**: 140–145.

200. Giovannucci E, Colditz GA, Stampfer MJ, Willett WC (1996) Physical activity, obesity, and risk of colorectal adenoma in women (United States). *Cancer Causes Control* **7**: 253–263.

201. Honjo S, Kono S, Shinchi K, et al. (1995) The relation of smoking, alcohol use and obesity to risk of sigmoid colon and rectal adenomas. *Jpn J Cancer Res* **86**: 1019–1026.

202. Shinchi K, Kono S, Honjo S, et al. (1994) Obesity and adenomatous polyps of the sigmoid colon. *Jpn J Cancer Res* **85**: 479–484.

203. Bjorge T, Engeland A, Tretli S, Weiderpass E (2007) Body size in relation to cancer of the uterine corpus in 1 million Norwegian women. *Int J Cancer* **120**: 378–383.

204. Calle EE, Rodriguez C, Walker-Thurmond K, Thun MJ (2003) Overweight, obesity, and mortality from cancer in a prospectively studied cohort of U.S. adults. *N Engl J Med* **348**: 1625–1638.

205. Chang SC, Lacey JV, Jr., Brinton LA, et al. (2007) Lifetime weight history and endometrial cancer risk by type of menopausal hormone use in the NIH AARP diet and health study. *Cancer Epidemiol Biomarkers Prev* **16**: 723–730.

206. Friedenreich C, Cust A, Lahmann PH, et al. (2007) Anthropometric factors and risk of endometrial cancer: the European prospective investigation into cancer and nutrition. *Cancer Causes Control* **18**: 399–413.

207. Xu WH, Matthews CE, Xiang YB, et al. (2005) Effect of adiposity and fat distribution on endometrial cancer risk in Shanghai women. *Am J Epidemiol* **161**: 939–947.

208. Trentham-Dietz A, Nichols HB, Hampton JM, Newcomb PA (2006) Weight change and risk of endometrial cancer. *Int J Epidemiol* **35**: 151–158.

209. La VC, Franceschi S, Decarli A, Gallus G, Tognoni G (1984) Risk factors for endometrial cancer at different ages. *J Natl Cancer Inst* **73**: 667–671.

210. Le ML, Wilkens LR, Mi MP (1991) Early-age body size, adult weight gain and endometrial cancer risk. *Int J Cancer* **48**: 807–811.

211. Tornberg SA, Carstensen JM (1994) Relationship between Quetelet's index and cancer of breast and female genital tract in 47,000 women followed for 25 years. *Br J Cancer* **69**: 358–361.

212. Xu W, Dai Q, Ruan Z, Cheng J, Jin F, Shu X (2002) Obesity at different ages and endometrial cancer risk factors in urban Shanghai, China. *Zhonghua Liu Xing Bing Xue Za Zhi* **23**: 347–351.

213. Levi F, La VC, Negri E, Parazzini F, Franceschi S (1992) Body mass at different ages and subsequent endometrial cancer risk. *Int J Cancer* **50**: 567–571.

214. Friberg E, Mantzoros CS, Wolk A (2007) Diabetes and risk of endometrial cancer: a population-based prospective cohort study. *Cancer Epidemiol Biomarkers Prev* **16**: 276–280.

215. Baanders-van Halewyn EA, Blankenstein MA, Thijssen JH, de Ridder CM, de Waard F (1996) A comparative study of risk factors for hyperplasia and cancer of the endometrium. *Eur J Cancer Prev* **5**: 105–112.

216. Swanson CA, Potischman N, Wilbanks GD, et al. (1993) Relation of endometrial cancer risk to past and contemporary body size and body fat distribution. *Cancer Epidemiol Biomarkers Prev* **2**: 321–327.

217. Shu XO, Brinton LA, Zheng W, et al. (1992) Relation of obesity and body fat distribution to endometrial cancer in Shanghai, China. *Cancer Res* **52**: 3865–3870.

218. Austin H, Austin JM, Jr, Partridge EE, Hatch KD, Shingleton HM (1991) Endometrial cancer, obesity, and body fat distribution. *Cancer Res* **51**: 568–572.

219. Olson SH, Trevisan M, Marshall JR, et al. (1995) Body mass index, weight gain, and risk of endometrial cancer. *Nutr Cancer* **23**: 141–149.

220. Bergstrom A, Hsieh CC, Lindblad P, Lu CM, Cook NR, Wolk A (2001) Obesity and renal cell cancer–a quantitative review. *Br J Cancer* **85**: 984–990.

221. Dal ML, Zucchetto A, Tavani A, et al. (2007) Renal cell cancer and body size at different ages: an Italian multicenter case-control study. *Am J Epidemiol* **166**: 582–591.

222. Bjorge T, Tretli S, Engeland A (2004) Relation of height and body mass index to renal cell carcinoma in two million Norwegian men and women. *Am J Epidemiol* **160**: 1168–1176.

223. Chow WH, Gridley G, Fraumeni JF, Jr, Jarvholm B (2000) Obesity, hypertension, and the risk of kidney cancer in men. *N Engl J Med* **343**: 1305–1311.

224. Yuan JM, Castelao JE, Gago-Dominguez M, Ross RK, Yu MC (1998) Hypertension, obesity and their medications in relation to renal cell carcinoma. *Br J Cancer* **77**: 1508–1513.

225. Kubo A, Corley DA (2006) Body mass index and adenocarcinomas of the esophagus or gastric cardia: a systematic review and meta-analysis. *Cancer Epidemiol Biomarkers Prev* **15**: 872–878.

226. Merry AH, Schouten LJ, Goldbohm RA, van den Brandt PA (2007) Body mass index, height and risk of adenocarcinoma of the oesophagus and gastric cardia: a prospective cohort study. *Gut* **56**: 1503–1511.

227. MacInnis RJ, English DR, Hopper JL, Giles GG (2006) Body size and composition and the risk of gastric and oesophageal adenocarcinoma. *Int J Cancer* **118**: 2628–2631.

228. Ryan AM, Rowley SP, Fitzgerald AP, Ravi N, Reynolds JV (2006) Adenocarcinoma of the oesophagus and gastric cardia: male preponderance in association with obesity. *Eur J Cancer* **42**: 1151–1158.

229. Chow WH, Blot WJ, Vaughan TL, et al. (1998) Body mass index and risk of adenocarcinomas of the esophagus and gastric cardia. *J Natl Cancer Inst* **90**: 150–155.

230. MacInnis RJ, English DR (2006) Body size and composition and prostate cancer risk: systematic review and meta-regression analysis. *Cancer Causes Control* **17**: 989–1003.

231. Giovannucci E, Liu Y, Platz EA, Stampfer MJ, Willett WC (2007) Risk factors for prostate cancer incidence and progression in the health professionals follow-up study. *Int J Cancer* **121**: 1571–1578.

232. Gong Z, Agalliu I, Lin DW, Stanford JL, Kristal AR (2007) Obesity is associated with increased risks of prostate cancer metastasis and death after initial cancer diagnosis in middle-aged men. *Cancer* **109**: 1192–1202.

233. Gong Z, Neuhouser ML, Goodman PJ, et al. (2006) Obesity, diabetes, and risk of prostate cancer: results from the prostate cancer prevention trial. *Cancer Epidemiol Biomarkers Prev* **15**: 1977–1983.

234. Littman AJ, White E, Kristal AR (2007) Anthropometrics and prostate cancer risk. *Am J Epidemiol* **165**: 1271–1279.

235. Rodriguez C, Freedland SJ, Deka A, et al. (2007) Body mass index, weight change, and risk of prostate cancer in the Cancer Prevention Study II Nutrition Cohort. *Cancer Epidemiol Biomarkers Prev* **16**: 63–69.

236. Freedland SJ, Platz EA (2007) Obesity and prostate cancer: making sense out of apparently conflicting data. *Epidemiol Rev* **29**: 88–97.

237. Andersson SO, Wolk A, Bergstrom R, et al. (1997) Body size and prostate cancer: a 20-year follow-up study among 135006 Swedish construction workers. *J Natl Cancer Inst* **89**: 385–389.

238. Rodriguez C, Patel AV, Calle EE, Jacobs EJ, Chao A, Thun MJ (2001) Body mass index, height, and prostate cancer mortality in two large cohorts of adult men in the United States. *Cancer Epidemiol Biomarkers Prev* **10**: 345–353.

239. Snowdon DA, Phillips RL, Choi W (1984) Diet, obesity, and risk of fatal prostate cancer. *Am J Epidemiol* **120**: 244–250.

240. Wright ME, Chang SC, Schatzkin A, et al. (2007) Prospective study of adiposity and weight change in relation to prostate cancer incidence and mortality. *Cancer* **109**: 675–684.

241. Lacey JV, Jr., Leitzmann M, Brinton LA, et al. (2006) Weight, height, and body mass index and risk for ovarian cancer in a cohort study. *Ann Epidemiol* **16**: 869–876.

242. Beehler GP, Sekhon M, Baker JA, et al. (2006) Risk of ovarian cancer associated with BMI varies by menopausal status. *J Nutr* **136**: 2881–286.

243. Hoyo C, Berchuck A, Halabi S, et al. (2005) Anthropometric measurements and epithelial ovarian cancer risk in African-American and White women. *Cancer Causes Control* **16**: 955–963.

244. Peterson NB, Trentham-Dietz A, Newcomb PA, et al. (2006) Relation of anthropometric measurements to ovarian cancer risk in a population-based case-control study (United States). *Cancer Causes Control* **17**: 459–467.

245. Olsen CM, Green AC, Whiteman DC, Sadeghi S, Kolahdooz F, Webb PM (2007) Obesity and the risk of epithelial ovarian cancer: a systematic review and meta-analysis. *Eur J Cancer* **43**: 690–709.

246. Engeland A, Tretli S, Bjorge T (2003) Height, body mass index, and ovarian cancer: a follow-up of 1.1 million Norwegian women. *J Natl Cancer Inst* **95**: 1244–1248.

247. Fairfield KM, Willett WC, Rosner BA, Manson JE, Speizer FE, Hankinson SE (2002) Obesity, weight gain, and ovarian cancer. *Obstet Gynecol* **100**: 288–296.

248. Lubin F, Chetrit A, Freedman LS, et al. (2003) Body mass index at age 18 years and during adult life and ovarian cancer risk. *Am J Epidemiol* **157**: 113–120.

249. Kuper H, Cramer DW, Titus-Ernstoff L (2002) Risk of ovarian cancer in the United States in relation to anthropometric measures: does the association depend on menopausal status? *Cancer Causes Control* **13**: 455–463.

250. Larsson SC, Orsini N, Wolk A (2007) Body mass index and pancreatic cancer risk:

A meta-analysis of prospective studies. *Int J Cancer* **120**: 1993–1998.

251. Fryzek JP, Schenk M, Kinnard M, Greenson JK, Garabrant DH (2005) The association of body mass index and pancreatic cancer in residents of southeastern Michigan, 1996–1999. *Am J Epidemiol* **162**: 222–228.

252. Larsson SC, Permert J, Hakansson N, Naslund I, Bergkvist L, Wolk A (2005) Overall obesity, abdominal adiposity, diabetes and cigarette smoking in relation to the risk of pancreatic cancer in two Swedish population-based cohorts. *Br J Cancer* **93**: 1310–1315.

253. Ansary-Moghaddam A, Huxley R, Barzi F, et al. (2006) The effect of modifiable risk factors on pancreatic cancer mortality in populations of the Asia-Pacific region. *Cancer Epidemiol Biomarkers Prev* **15**: 2435–2440.

254. Wolk A, Gridley G, Svensson M, et al. (2001) A prospective study of obesity and cancer risk (Sweden). *Cancer Causes Control* **12**: 13–21.

255. Moller H, Mellemgaard A, Lindvig K, Olsen JH (1994) Obesity and cancer risk: a Danish record-linkage study. *Eur J Cancer* **30A**: 344–350.

256. Okasha M, McCarron P, McEwen J, Smith GD (2002) Body mass index in young adulthood and cancer mortality: a retrospective cohort study. *J Epidemiol Community Health* **56**: 780–784.

Chapter 9

Contribution of Alcohol and Tobacco Use in Gastrointestinal Cancer Development

Helmut K. Seitz and Chin Hin Cho

Abstract

Tobacco smoke and alcohol are major risk factors for a variety of cancer sites, including those of the gastrointestinal tract. Tobacco smoke contains a great number of mutagenic and carcinogenic compounds, including polycyclic carbohydrates, nitrosamines, and nicotine, while ethanol per se has only weak carcinogenic potential, but its first metabolite, acetaldehyde, is a mutagen and carcinogen, since it forms stable adducts with DNA. The possibility of proto-oncogene mutation in gastrointestinal mucosa cells may be associated with tobacco smoking-induced cancers through the formation of unfavorable DNA adducts. Individuals with defective DNA repair mechanisms and unfavorable genetic make-up for carcinogen metabolism may be at increased risk for gastrointestinal cancers. Individuals with a high production rate of acetaldehyde from ethanol also have an increased cancer risk when they drink chronically. These include individuals with a genetically determined increased acetaldehyde production due to alcohol dehydrogenase polymorphism and those with a decreased detoxification of acetaldehyde due to acetaldehyde dehydrogenase mutation. In addition, oral bacterial overgrowth due to poor oral hygiene also increases salivary acetaldehyde. Dietary deficiencies such as a lack of folate, riboflavine, and zinc may also contribute to the increase cancer risk in the alcoholic patient. It is of considerable importance that smoking and drinking act synergistically. Smoking increases the acetaldehyde burden following alcohol consumption and drinking enhances the activation of various procarcinogens present in tobacco smoke due to increased metabolic activation by an induced cytochrome P450-2E1-dependent microsomal biotransformation system in the mucosa of the upper digestive tract and the liver.

Key words: Alcohol, acetaldehyde, tobacco, gastrointestinal cancer, tobacco carcinogens, alcohol dehydrogenase, acetaldehyde dehydrogenase, liver cancer, pancreatic cancer, gastrointestinal bacteria.

M. Verma (ed.), *Methods of Molecular Biology, Cancer Epidemiology, vol. 472*
© 2009 Humana Press, a part of Springer Science + Business Media, Totowa, NJ
Book doi: 10.1007/978-1-60327-492-0

1. Introduction

Smoking and alcohol consumption are major risk factors for a variety of cancers. However, in the present overview only the effect of alcohol and smoking on the risk of gastrointestinal cancers, including those of the pancreas and the liver, will be discussed. With respect to other types of cancer, especially those of the respiratory tract induced by smoking (1) and of the breast due to alcohol (2), the reader is referred to the most recent review articles.

One of five people who die is a smoker. Therefore, cigarette smoke is considered to be the most preventable cause of cancer mortality in the world. Smoking is associated with an increased risk for at least 15 different cancer types. The risk for development of cancer is 2.24 times greater for smokers than nonsmokers. Cigarette smoke is strongly associated with cancers of the esophagus, lung, pancreas, and bladder, and it has been included among the risk factors for colon and gastric cancers (3–6). Cigarette smoke comprises a combination of more than 4,700 components. About 60 of these are considered to be carcinogenic, namely polycyclic aromatic hydrocarbons, nitrosamines, aromatic amine, trace metals, as well as nicotine. Understanding the carcinogenic actions of tobacco smoke would put us in a better position to know how to treat and even prevent cancers.

With respect to alcohol, the most comprehensive estimates come from the World Health Organisation (WHO) global burden of disease project, which showed that more than 389,000 cases of cancer were attributable to alcohol drinking worldwide, representing 3.6% of all cancers (7, 8). A most recent analysis of a working group of experts at the International Agency for Research on Cancer (IARC) in Lyon, France came to the conclusion that alcohol is a risk factor for upper aerodigestive tract (UADT) cancer (oral cavity, pharynx, hypopharynx, larynx, and esophagus), liver cancer, colorectal cancer, and breast cancer (9). Some of these cancers are difficult to treat, including complex and high risk surgery as well as radiochemotherapy with poor response. In this context it is noteworthy that alcohol consumption and smoking has a synergistic effect on the risk of some of these cancers.

In the first part of this chapter, general mechanisms of tobacco and its active components, such as nicotine and its metabolite nitrosamines, and of ethanol with its major toxic metabolite acetaldehyde in carcinogenesis will be discussed. In the second part, however, the major emphasis will be on organ-specific formation and development of gastrointestinal cancers due to tobacco and alcohol, and will include the oropharynx, esophagus, stomach, pancreas, liver, and colorectum.

2. Carcinogenetic Mechanisms of Tobacco and Alcohol

2.1. The Carcinogenic Action of Nicotine and its Metabolite Nitrosamines

Nicotine is one of the active components in cigarette smoke, but its association with tumorigenesis is enigmatic *(10)*. Nicotine-replacement therapy (NRT) is increasingly used by many smokers quitting on their own, and people can access NRT, notwithstanding the socioeconomic and cultural barriers *(11)*. This has led to recent evaluations of their effectiveness and possible side-effects derived from this continuation of nicotine intake in the general population. Nicotine could act as a mutagen, a procarcinogen, and/or a mitogen. Several lines of evidence support the idea that nicotine is mutagenic. It induces sister-chromatid exchanges and increases chromosome aberration frequency in a time- and dose-dependent manner in Chinese hamster ovary cells at concentrations achievable in the saliva of tobacco chewers *(12, 13)*. It has also been reported that nicotine dose dependently forms adducts with liver DNA, lung DNA, histone H1/H3, hemoglobin, and albumin in mice *(14, 15)*.

Nicotine-derived tobacco-specific nitrosamines that are strong carcinogens play critical roles in the initiation and promotion of smoking-related malignancies in humans. Evolving evidence suggests that these carcinogenic compounds are only found in tobacco, but can also be endogenously metabolized from nicotine *(16)*. One of these compounds, 4-(methylnitrosamine)-1-(3-pyridyl)-1-butanone (NNK), has been reported to play a key role in the initiation and promotion of smoking-related malignancies *(17)*. It directly stimulates human colon cancer cell growth through the activation of β-adrenoceptors *(18)*. Importantly, it has also been shown that the amount of NNK in tobacco smoke is so high that the total estimated doses to smokers and long-term snuff-dippers are similar in magnitude to the total doses required to produce cancer in laboratory animals *(19)*. These exposures thus represent an unacceptable risk to cigarette smokers and nonsmokers exposed to years of environmental tobacco smoke.

The ability of nicotine to promote the growth of gastrointestinal tumors is widely studied. It stimulates gastric and colon cancer cell growth in vitro and the mitogenic effect is likely to be mediated through β-adrenoceptors and the downstream protein kinases, including protein kinase C (PKC) and extracellular signal-regulated kinase-1/2 (ERK 1/2), and the subsequent induction of the arachidonic acid cascade *(20)*. Moreover, nicotine in drinking water enhances the growth of gastric and colon cancers in the nude mouse xenograft model *(21, 22)*. With respect to smoking-associated cervical cancer, physiologically attainable concentrations of nicotine is shown to enhance the proliferation of human cervical cells in vitro *(23)*. Nicotine also has pro-angiogenic action. Cigarette smoke increases the formation of ulcerative colitis-associated colonic adenoma in mice, and is associated with increased angiogenesis through the upregulation of vascular endothelium growth factor (VEGF) and matrix metalloproteinase (MMP) in colon and gastric cancer xenografts in athymic mice *(21, 24, 25)*.

2.2. The Carcinogenicity of Acetaldehyde, the First Metabolite of Ethanol

Ethanol is only a weak carcinogen in animal experiments *(26)*. However, acetaldehyde, the first metabolite of ethanol has been classified as a carcinogen by the IARC *(27, 28)*, since in animal experiments the inhalation of acetaldehyde results in nasal tumours *(29)*. Acetaldehyde is highly toxic, mutagenic, and carcinogenic. It interferes with DNA synthesis and repair, injures the cellular antioxidative defense system, results in cellular hyperregeneration of the mucosa, and finally, most importantly, binds to DNA, forming stable adducts with mutagenic properties *(30–36)*. The generation of mutagenic adducts is especially enhanced in hyperregenerative tissues such as the upper and lower gastrointestinal mucosa (due to chronic ethanol consumption) due to the fact that biogenic amines present in hyperregenerative tissues favour the adduct formation *(36)*.

Acetaldehyde is generated from ethanol oxidation and the enzyme responsible for this reaction is alcohol dehydrogenase (ADH). Various ADH isozymes exist and two of them reveal polymorphism (ADH1B and ADH1C). While the ADH1B*2 allele encodes for an enzyme that is approximately 40 times more active than the enzyme encoded by the ADH1B*1 allele, ADH1C*1 transcription leads to an ADH isoenzyme 2.5 times more active than that from ADH1C*2 *(37)*. ADH1B*2 allele frequency is high in Asians but low in Caucasians. It protects Asians from alcoholism, because the high amounts of acetaldehyde produced are associated with severe side effects such as flush, tachycardia, nausea, and vomiting.

With respect to ADH1C, the allele frequency is almost equally distributed in the Caucasian population and some, but not all, studies, showed an increased risk for UADT cancer and for breast cancer in patients with ADH1C*1 homozygosity who consume considerable amounts of alcohol *(38–43)*. These individuals generate more acetaldehyde after alcohol consumption.

The concentration of acetaldehyde in tissues or in the blood does not only depend on the rate of generation but also on the rate of degradation. The most important enzyme responsible for acetaldehyde oxidation is acetaldehyde dehydrogenase (ALDH) 2 with a relatively low K_m for ethanol. In Asia up to 50% of the population carries a mutation of the ALDH2 gene that encodes for an enzyme with very low activity leading to elevated acetaldehyde concentrations after alcohol consumption in the blood and in the saliva. While homozygotes are completely protected against alcoholism and alcohol-associated diseases due to the fact that they cannot tolerate alcohol even at very small doses without developing severe side effects, heterozygotes (ALDH2*1,2) have an increased risk for gastrointestinal cancer *(44)*. Landmark studies from Japan have shown a strikingly increased risk for esophageal and colorectal cancer in these individuals, with a relative risk (RR) of more than 10 for esophageal cancer and up to more than 50 for a metachronic esophageal carcinoma *(44–46)*.

Acetaldehyde can also be generated by bacterial oxidation of ethanol. This can take place in the oral cavity and in the large intestine. In animal experiments it has been shown that acetaldehyde production in the colon was significantly reduced in germ-free mice as compared with conventional animals following ethanol administration. This was associated with mucosal injury and hyperregeneration *(47, 48)*. Furthermore salivary acetaldehyde concentrations are lower in humans after a mouthwash with an antiseptic *(49)*, emphasizing the role of oral bacteria in the production of acetaldehyde from ethanol.

Thus, in summary, in vitro data, animal experiments, and genetic linkage studies support strongly the carcinogenic role of acetaldehyde as a pathogenetic mechanisms in gastrointestinal cancer development following chronic ethanol ingestion. Most recently it was concluded from a working group of the IARC that strong mechanistic evidence exist in humans that endogenous acetaldehyde derived from the consumption of ethanol in alcoholic beverages plays a causal role in the development of malignant esophageal tumours in individuals who are deficient in aldehyde dehydrogenase *(9)*.

Besides acetaldehyde, other mechanisms may explain the carcinogenicity of ethanol including oxidative stress, altered methyl transfer, and deficiency of retinoic acid. These mechanisms may be primarily relevant for cancer of the liver, where acetaldehyde is of minor importance due to an efficient acetaldehyde oxidation capacity. With respect to these mechanisms, the reader is referred to recent review articles *(33, 50–52)*.

3. Interaction Between Alcohol and Tobacco

Alcohol consumption and smoking have a synergistic effect on the risk of UADT cancer. This synergistic effect has been shown in countless studies. For example, a case-control study of oral and pharyngeal cancer conducted in the USA regarding tobacco and alcohol use of 1,114 patients and 1,268 population-based control subjects demonstrated that the risk for these cancers among nondrinkers increased with the amount smoked, and conversely that the risks among nonsmokers increased with the level of alcohol intake. Among consumers of both products, risk of oropharyngeal cancer tended to combine more in a multiplicative than additive fashion and were increased more than 35-fold among those who consumed two or more packs of cigarettes and more than four alcoholic drinks per day. Cessation of smoking was also associated with a sharply reduced risk of this cancer *(53)*.

Various factors may contribute to this effect including the local permeabilizing effects of alcohol on the penetration of tobacco-specific carcinogens and other carcinogens across the oral mucosa *(54)*. Acetaldehyde is a known constituent of tobacco smoke. Smokers have been shown to have elevated breath acetaldehyde concentrations after acute cigarette smoking *(55)* and also endogenously after several weeks of smoking cessation. During ethanol ingestion, smokers have about two times higher acetaldehyde levels in their saliva as compared with non-smokers. This is due to a change in the capacity of oral bacteria to produce acetaldehyde from ethanol *(56, 57)*. Smokers have an increased incidence of yeast infections and occurrence of Gram-positive bacteria, which are known to have a high capacity for ethanol oxidation *(56, 57)*. Thus, smoking increases the acetaldehyde load in the saliva following alcohol consumption.

In addition, chronic alcohol consumption results in the induction of cytochrome P450-2E1 (CYP2E1) in various tissues including the mucosa of the UADT *(58, 59)*. CYP2E1 is part of the microsomal ethanol-oxidizing system (MEOS), which oxidizes ethanol to acetaldehyde by utilizing oxygen and NADPH (which is generated by the ADH reaction). In the chronic alcoholic patient, MEOS contributes up to 30% in ethanol oxidation, which is less than 10% in the normal state. CYP2E1 is induced by ethanol, but this induction varies interindividually and may occur as soon as 1 week after the ingestion of 40 g of ethanol daily *(60)*. The CYP2E1-dependent ethanol oxidation not only produces acetaldehyde, but also reactive oxygen species (ROS), such as O^{2-}, OH^-, or hydroxyethyl radicals. In addition, and this is of great importance, some procarcinogens require CYP2E1-dependent metabolism to become ultimate carcinogens. Among these are some present in tobacco smoke, such as polycyclic hydrocarbons and various nitrosamines. Due to the induction of CYP2E1 by ethanol, these procarcinogens have enhanced activation in the mucosal cells of the UADT, and this may be another mechanism by which chronic ethanol exerts its carcinogenicity, especially in smokers *(61)*.

4. Epidemiology and Pathogenesis of Alcohol and Tobacco in Gastrointestinal Carcinogenesis

4.1. Cancer of the Oropharynx and the Esophagus

Tobacco smoking is a major risk factor for oropharyngeal and esophageal cancer. A fourfold to sixfold increase in risk among subjects with medium or high tobacco consumption was observed, as well as a trend in increasing risk with duration and with earlier age at the start of smoking. Other findings include a sharp reduction in risk with cessation of smoking. In Italy, smokers of pipes and cigars showed a more elevated risk of cancer of the oral cavity and esophagus than did cigarette smokers (62). In another study from Cuba, 82% of oral cancer cases were attributed to tobacco smoking, and 19% to smoking cigars or a pipe only. Smoking more than 30 cigarettes per day showed an odds ratio (OR) of 20.8, similar to smoking more than four cigars daily (OR = 20.5). In comparison, drinking more than 70 drinks per week showed an OR of 5.7 (63).

Information on the role of the tar yield of cigarettes in upper digestive tract cancer was also important. Significant excess risk was observed even in the lower tar category (64).

The reason why only a particular group of patients who smoke would suffer from oropharyngeal cancer is still inconclusive. Jourenkova-Mironova and coworkers studied the involvement of microsomal epoxide hydrolase (mEH), encoded by the EPHX1 gene in the metabolism of tobacco carcinogens. They investigated the effect of exon 3 and 4 polymorphisms of the EPHX1 gene in 121 patients with oropharyngeal cancer, and 172 control subjects without cancer, all Caucasians regular smokers. They concluded that EPHX1 polymorphisms may be one factor of importance in the susceptibility to smoking-related cancers of the UADT (65).

To date, high-incidence areas for esophageal cancer include China (21 per 100,000), South America (13 per 100,000) and the former Soviet Union (8 per 100,000) (66). Globally, esophageal cancer is more common in men than in women, with decreasing sex ratios in higher-risk areas and vice versa for lower-risk areas. The incidence rate for esophageal cancer increases with age, the lowest incidence rate occurring at age 30 years and the highest at 70 years old. The highest mortality rates reported in China are 26.5% in men and 19.7% in women (67).

Esophageal cancer is a multifactor disease. Smoked food has a high content of nitrosamines and nitrites. Methyl alkyl nitrosamines appear to be specific inducers of carcinoma of the esophagus, regardless of their route of administration. Smoking is also believed to be a major etiological factor in esophageal cancer, as is alcohol consumption worldwide *(68)*. Smokers have four to ten times the risk of dying from esophageal cancer compared with nonsmokers. Squamous cell carcinomas associated with smoking and alcohol abuse have historically been the most common esophageal carcinomas in Western countries. Recently, a shift towards more adenocarcinomas commonly associated with Barrett's metaplasia has been noted *(69)*.

Despite improvements in the detection of premalignant pathology, and newer preventive strategies, the overall incidence of esophageal carcinomas has risen. Treatment modalities include surgery, chemotherapy, radiation therapy, or a combination of these. On the other hand, prevention strategies are also emphasized, including smoking and alcohol cessation *(70)*. However, searching for new mediators in the etiology of esophageal cancer remains the primary approach in the treatment of the disease in the future. Prostaglandins (PGs) are thought to be one of the important mediators that participate in the carcinogenesis of solid tumors, in particular, cancers of the gastrointestinal tract.

PG synthesis is initiated by the release of free arachidonate from cell membrane, a process catalyzed by membrane phospholipases. Free arachidonic acid is subsequently converted to PGG2 in a two-step enzymatic process catalyzed by the cyclooxygenase enzyme (COX). COX is a bifunctional enzyme that plays a key and rate-limiting role in the biosynthesis of PGs. The inducible form of COX is regulated by numerous factors, including growth factors, oncogenes, tumour-suppressor genes, and various tumour promoters such as tobacco smoke and bile acids *(71, 72)*. Benzo(a)pyrene, a constituent of tobacco smoke and char-broiled foods, induces COX-2 in cultured cells *(71)*. Similarly, both conjugated and unconjugated bile acids have been shown to induce COX-2 in esophageal cell lines *(72, 73)*. From these studies, both tobacco smoke and bile acids are heavily implicated in the pathogenesis of esophageal cancer, and COX-2 may play a significant role.

Indeed, increased levels of COX-2 are commonly found in adenocarcinoma as well as in squamous cell carcinoma of the esophagus *(74, 75)*. In addition, over-expression of COX-2 has been found in premalignant conditions of the esophagus, such as squamous dysplasia and Barrett's esophagus *(76, 77)*. Shirvani et al. *(78)* reported a progressive increase in COX-2 expression with increased histological severity from metaplasia to low- and high-grade dysplasia. Increased COX-2 expression is also associated with decreased survival in patients with esophageal adenocarcinoma *(79)*. COX-2 has both oxygenase and peroxidase functions. The peroxidase activity catalyzes the conversion of procarcinogens to carcinogens in extrahepatic tissues such as the upper digestive tract *(80, 81)*. COX-2 activity is responsible for the conversion of the procarcinogen benzo[a]pyrene, present in tobacco smoke, to the powerful mutagen benzo[a]pyrene diolepoxide. The enzyme is itself induced by procarcinogens, thereby amplifying the effect of a given dose of benzo[a]pyrene on tumour initiation *(71)*. Smoking is a known predisposing factor for the two common cell types of esophageal cancer, and the abrogation of COX-2 activity by COX-2 inhibitors may play an important role in cancer prevention by preventing tobacco smoke-related DNA damage. Furthermore, there is compelling epidemiological evidence that the regular or occasional use of aspirin or other nonsteroidal anti-inflammatory drugs (NSAIDs) is inversely related to the risk of esophageal cancer *(82, 83)*. These data suggest a potential role for aspirin and other NSAIDs in the prevention and possible treatment of esophageal cancer and perhaps also other types of cancers in the gastrointestinal tract.

Several genes are involved in both tobacco- and alcohol-related pathways that modulate the susceptibility to esophageal cancer. Results suggest that ALDH2, NQO1, and XRCC1 polymorphisms alter the susceptibility to esophageal cancer and they may also modulate the effects of cigarette smoking and alcohol consumption on esophageal cancer risk in the Chinese population. No clear association with the risk for esophageal cancer was found for polymorphisms of CYP2E1 and TP53 (alias p53) *(84)*. However, CYP1A1 Val/Val and glutathione-*S*-transferase (GST) M1 deletion genotypes are genetic susceptibility biomarkers for esophageal cancer. The risk increases for persons with the CYP1A1 Val/Val and GSTM1 deletion genotype. These two metabolic enzymes seem to have interactions with tobacco smoking, but the mechanism still needs further study *(85)*.

Regarding the GSTM1 gene polymorphisms, the GSTM1-null genotype is associated with an increased OR for esophageal cancer (OR = 2.17; 95% confidence interval [CI]: 1.34–3.50), but not for stomach cancer. A combined effect was also found between smoking and the GSTM1-null genotype with regard to esophageal cancer risk. Tea drinking is a protective factor for both cancers, its effect being independent of the GSTT1 and GSTM1 genotypes. These findings suggest that the GSTM1 polymorphism is involved in the susceptibility to esophageal cancer development, and tea consumption reduces the risk of esophageal and stomach cancers *(86)*.

p53, an apoptosis gene, is the most extensively studied gene in esophageal adenocarcinoma cancer. The reported mutation data show that ~50% of these tumours have p53 mutations, whereas in Barrett's esophagus and Barrett's esophagus with dysplasia, p53 mutation is less frequent *(87)*. Most of these mutations are located in exons 5, 7, and 8. p53 over-expression is significantly influenced by the presence of codon 72 polymorphisms. The incidence of p53 over-expression increases additively with environmental exposure to cigarette smoke, alcohol, and reca quid in Taiwan. When compared with individuals exposed to only one of these environmental risk factors, patients who had exposure to two or three risk factors have ORs of 6.11 (95% CI: 1.80–20.75) and 6.22 (95% CI: 1.81–21.34), for p53 over-expression, respectively. Elderly patients (>70 years old) are more likely to have p53 over-expression, with an OR of 5.63 (95% CI: 1.53–20.64) compared with over-expression among patients younger than 55 years old. It is concluded that the presence of p53 codon 72 variants can be a significant factor influencing p53 over-expression in esophageal cancer, with over-expression also influenced by combined or prolonged environmental exposures (88).

Chronic alcohol consumption is also a major risk factor for cancer of the oropharynx and esophagus (9). It has been estimated that 25–68% of UADT cancers are attributed to alcohol and up to 80% of these tumours can be prevented by abstaining from alcohol and smoking (89–91). In a meta-analysis including 235 studies, pooled RRs for alcohol 25, 50, or 100 g/day for oral cavity and pharyngeal cancer were 1.76, 2.87, and 6.10, respectively, and for esophageal cancer were 1.51, 2.21, and 4.23, respectively (92). In a carefully designed French study, Tuyns was able to demonstrate that alcohol consumption of more than 80 g/day (approximately one bottle of wine) increases the RR of esophageal cancer by a factor of 18, while smoking alone of more than 20 cigarettes leads to an increased RR of 5. Taken together, both factors act synergistically resulting in an increased RR of 44 (93). An epidemiologic study by Maier et al. showed that 90% of all patients with head and neck cancer consumed alcohol regularly in quantities twice the amount of a control group with a significant dose-response relationship (94). If the RR for an individual with a daily alcohol consumption of 25 g was assumed to be 1, the RR rose to 32 if alcohol consumption exceeded 100 g. Bruguere and coworkers found RR values of 13.5 for oral cancer, 15.2 for oropharyngeal cancer, and 28.6 for hypopharyngeal cancer when 100–159 g of alcohol was consumed daily (95). It is noteworthy that even with these high daily alcohol dosages, the alcohol-associated cancer risk is not saturable. Alcohol consumption of exceeding 1.5 bottles of wine daily results in a 100-fold increased RR for esophageal cancer (96). In an epidemiologic study of the American Cancer Society (ACS) on more than 750,000 individuals, Bofetta and Garfinkel found an increased RR for esophageal cancer already at a dose of 12 g alcohol daily (RR = 1.37) rising to an RR = 5.8 following 72 g of alcohol daily (97). A follow-up study of the ACS found the same results (98). Similar dose-dependent data have also been demonstrated in case-control studies involving non-smokers.

During the last decade, one mechanism of ethanol-associated upper digestive tract cancer has been elucidated. It has been shown that the accumulation of acetaldehyde after alcohol consumption due to genetic polymorphisms (*see* **above**) was found to be associated with increased levels of acetaldehyde-derived DNA adducts as well as an increase in sister chromatid exchanges and micronuclei of peripheral lymphocytes *(34, 99, 100)*, and that these individuals were at extreme high risk when they consume ethanol chronically *(44)*. High levels of acetaldehyde occur in saliva, and these levels are further increased in individuals with ADH1C*1 homozygosity *(40)* and ALDH2*1,2 heterozygosity *(101)*, in smokers (*see* **above**), and in individuals with poor oral hygiene and bacterial overgrowth *(102)*. Saliva rinses the mucosa and acetaldehyde may enter the cell and result in DNA adduct formation. In addition, continuous contact of the mucosa with acetaldehyde derived from saliva leads to mucosal hyperproliferation, a precancerous condition *(103, 104)*. Other factors such as nutritional deficiencies of folate, retinoic aid, riboflavine, iron, and zinc may also contribute to the increased cancer risk in the alcoholic patient *(50)*, but these factors have not been studied in detail.

4.2. Gastric Cancer

Gastric cancer is estimated to be second in frequency worldwide. *Helicobacter pylori* (*HP*) infection, salt intake, cigarette smoking, micronutrients, and family history are risk factors for stomach cancer in different countries. The familial aggregation of stomach cancer may be due to shared environments and genetic susceptibility. However, the major causes appear to be environmental rather than genetic. A relationship has been suggested between tobacco smoking and gastric cancer. All the cohort studies show a significantly increased risk of gastric cancer, on the order of 1.5–2.5. However, evidence from case-control studies is less consistent. A meta-analysis on 40 studies provided a quantitative estimate on the order of 1.5–1.6 as compared with non-smokers. The RR is higher in men (1.59) than in women (1.11). A dose-response relationship existed in four gastric cancer studies attributable to tobacco smoking occurring worldwide, in total over 80,000 cases of gastric cancer may be attributed to tobacco smoking each year. This figure is larger than that estimated for other cancers associated with tobacco smoking, such as pancreatic and renal cancers *(105)*.

With respect to GST polymorphism, only the GSTM1 homozygous-null genotype is associated with an increased risk of gastric cancer (OR = 1.73; 95% CI: 1.10–3.04). After grouping according to smoking status, the GSTM1-null genotype was associated with an increased gastric cancer risk for smokers (OR = 2.15; 95% CI: 1.02–4.54) *(106)*. Regarding the enzyme activity, cancer patients have significantly lower GST activity in tumour and tumour-adjacent tissues compared with normal tissues. Also, smokers have lower GST activity in both tumour and tumour-adjacent tissues than nonsmokers. In addition, GST is significantly lower in tissues positive for *HP* infection than in *HP*-negative tissues.

Another metabolizing enzyme is also affected by smoking. There is a significant reduction in total CYP activity in tumour and tumour-adjacent tissues versus normal stomach. In the case of smokers, CYP activity is 1.8-fold higher in tumour-adjacent than in corresponding tumour tissues, but no such difference occurs in nonsmokers. It is likely that alterations in the activities of CYP and GST may be in part associated with an increased risk of gastric cancer *(107)*, which could be modified by tobacco smoking.

People with a methylenetetrahydrofolate reductase (MTHFR) C677T variant genotype and a smoking habit are at a significantly higher risk of developing stomach cancer (OR = 7.72; 95% CI: 2.23–27.70) compared with those with a wild-type homozygous (C/C) genotype and no smoking habit. This also applied to frequent alcohol consumption (OR = 3.08; 95% CI: 1.30–7.23) when compared with those with the C/C genotype and low consumption of alcohol. Individuals with habits of frequent alcohol consumption and smoking have 12.96-fold (95% CI: 2.76–70.46) risk of developing stomach cancer. Polymorphism of MTHFR C677T is associated with risk of developing stomach cancer and there is a coordinating effect between habits of smoking and alcohol consumption on MTHFR genotype in the development of stomach cancer *(108)*. Another study shows that MTHFR C677T may interact with smoking, moldy food intake, wheat porridge intake, eating salty food, and *HP ca*gA infection to increase the risk of stomach cancer. No such interaction was found with alcohol consumption or green tea intake *(109)*. One report shows that thymidylate synthetase (TS) and MTHFR are major enzymes in the metabolism of folates, involved in DNA "break", instability, and hypomethylation. TS polymorphism may modify the risk of esophageal and stomach cancers in smokers *(110)*.

There is no convincing evidence that the risk of gastric cancer is modified by chronic alcohol consumption.

4.3. Pancreatic Cancer

The main risk factors for pancreatic cancer include tobacco smoking and dietary habits. Tobacco smoking is estimated to account for 25–29% of pancreatic cancer incidence, the RR of smokers being at least 1.5 times higher than the non-smoking population. The risk increases with the level of tobacco smoking. The highest risk ratio, tenfold, has been reported in men who consume more than 40 cigarettes daily and the excess risk levels off 10 to 15 years after smoking cessation *(5, 111, 112)*. Similar observations have been reported in the Asian countries *(113, 114)*. The second most important risk factor associated with pancreatic cancer seems to be diet, although it may not be as consistent as that of smoking *(5, 111, 112)*.

A number of environmental and lifestyle factors, such as smoking, alcohol use, coffee consumption, and exposure to organochlorine or hydrocarbon solvents are associated with the frequency and spectrum of k-ras mutation in pancreatic tumours. Dietary intake and serum levels of folate are associated with the risk of pancreatic cancer among male smokers. These findings demonstrate the potential of the molecular epidemiological approach in understanding the etiology of pancreatic cancer and further studies should be performed to understand the interactive relationship between genetic and environmental factors in the etiology of pancreatic cancer *(115)*.

DNA adducts derived from exposure to polycyclic aromatic hydrocarbons and aromatic amines from tobacco smoke have been detected in pancreatic tissues and related cancer risk. Oxidative DNA damage and lipid peroxidation-induced DNA adducts also occur in the pancreas. The level of aromatic DNA adducts is correlated with the spectrum of k-ras mutation in the tumour. The increase in k-ras mutation during pancreatic carcinogenesis that occurs in cigarette smokers is also found in alcohol users *(116–118)*. Pancreatic cancer has the highest frequency (>85%) of k-ras mutation among all human cancers, and this is associated with cigarette smoking or alcohol consumption. These observations support the notion that individuals with a deficiency in repairing DNA alkylation products seem to have an increased risk of pancreatic cancer.

Metabolic activation is another prerequisite for the carcinogenic effect of many carcinogens. Many studies of smoking-related cancers have shown that genetic variations in carcinogen metabolism affect individual susceptibility to carcinogen exposure and further increase cancer risk. Limited studies show an association between genetic polymorphisms of drug-metabolizing enzymes and the risk of pancreatic cancer. In a study of 45 cases and 53 healthy control subjects, no association was found between susceptibility to pancreatic cancer and genetic polymorphisms of CYP2E1 and CYP1A1, the enzymes that activate chemical carcinogens *(119)*. In another study with a larger population, again no association was found between the risk of pancreatic cancer and polymorphisms of GST1, GSTT1, and CYP1A1 *(120)*. However, significant over-expression of GSTM1 AB and B genotypes was found in all pancreatic disease cases *(121)*. Recently, in a large-scale population-based case-control study, a significant interaction was reported between the GSTT1-null genotype and cigarette smoking in pancreatic cancer *(122)*. Evidence in the same study also showed a significant interaction between heavy smoking and an Arg399Gln polymorphism of the DNA repair gene XRCG1 *(123)*. Polymorphisms of CYP1A2 and N-acetyltransferase (NAT) genes can modify the risk of pancreatic cancer. Heavy smokers with CYP1A2*1D (T-2467delT) delT, CYP1A2* 1F (A-163C) allele, and NAT1 "rapid" or NAT2 "slow„ alleles had ORs of 1.4 (95% CI: 0.7–2.3), 1.9 (95% CI: 1.1–3.4), 3.0 (95% CI: 1.6–5.4), and 1.5 (95% CI: 0.8–2.6), respectively, compared with people who had never smoked or carried the not-at-risk alleles *(124)*. All these data support the proposition that individuals who have deficient carcinogen detoxification and DNA repair capacities are at increased risk of pancreatic cancer.

Although chronic alcohol consumption is a risk factor for chronic pancreatitis, there is no convincing evidence that alcohol per se is carcinogenic for the pancreas *(125)*.

4.4. Colorectal Cancer

Tobacco smoking is consistently associated with a high risk for colon adenoma and hyperplastic polyp formation *(126, 127)* as well as increased incidence of colorectal carcinoma *(128–130)*. A large-scale clinical trial demonstrated a dose-dependency of smoking on colon adenoma and cancer formation *(131)*. Heavy and long-term cigarette smoking (>35 years) leads to a higher OR for colon cancer. Moreover, the risk of death from colorectal cancer is higher in current or former smokers than in non-smokers *(132)*.

Previous studies showed that passive cigarette smoking promotes the formation of inflammation-associated colonic adenoma in mice through an angiogenic pathway *(21, 24)*, and 5-lipoxygenase (5-LOX) plays a central role in this process *(133)*. In this regard, inhibition of 5-LOX not only decreases the expression of VEGF, MMP-2, and MMP-9 induced by a cigarette smoke extract but also suppresses cell proliferation of human umbilical vascular endothelial cells, a biological activity closely related to angiogenesis in tumour growth *(133)*. Indeed, suppression of 5-LOX is more effective than COX-2 inhibition in the prevention of colon cancer formation promoted by cigarette smoke, as inhibition of COX-2 may lead to a shunt of arachidonic acid metabolism towards the LOX pathway during tumourigenesis in these conditions *(134)*.

Breslow and Enstrom *(135)* were the first to consider the possibility of an association between beer drinking and the occurrence of rectal cancer. In 1992, a review on this issue was conducted by Kune and Vitetta *(136)* gathering the results of more than 50 major epidemiologic studies from 1957 to 1991. This review included 7 correlation studies, more than 40 case-control studies, and 17 prospective cohort studies on the role of alcohol on the development of colorectal cancer. An association was found in five of the seven correlation studies and in more than half of the case-control studies. In the majority of case-control studies in which community-based individuals were used as controls, a positive correlation between alcohol consumption and colorectal cancer was detected. However, this was not the case when hospital-based controls were used, possibly due to the high prevalence of alcohol consumption and alcohol-related diseases in hospital controls. Eleven of the seventeen cohort studies also demonstrated a positive association with alcohol. A positive trend with respect to dose-response was found in five of the ten case-control studies and in all prospective cohort studies in which a dose-response analysis has been taken into consideration.

Between 1992 and 1997 another 12 epidemiological studies were published *(137)*, and the data on alcohol consumption and the risk for colorectal cancer have not been consistent. A prospective cohort study in Japan reported a positive dose-response relationship between alcohol intake and colon cancer risk in both sexes *(138)*. On the other hand, a Danish population-based cohort study showed no association *(139)*.

Most recently, Cho et al. *(140)* pooled eight cohort studies from North America and Europe and showed a significant trend between an increased amount of alcohol intake and the risk for colorectal cancer. Consumption of more than 45 g alcohol per day increased the risk by 45%.

Five out of six studies of the effect of alcohol on the occurrence of adenomatous polyps in the large intestine showed a positive association with alcohol *(137)*. The same was true for hyperplastic polyps. When more than 30 g alcohol per day was consumed, the RR for men was 1.8 and for woman was 2.5 *(141)*.

Finally, alcohol may influence the adenoma-carcinoma sequence at different early steps as reported recently by Boutron et al. *(142)*. High alcohol intake favours high-risk polyps or colorectal cancer occurrence among patients with adenoma *(143)*. The authors reported that a reduction in ethanol intake for individuals with genetic predisposition for colorectal cancer had a large beneficial effect on tumour incidence *(144)*.

In 1999, epidemiological data on alcohol and colorectal cancer were reviewed by a panel of experts at the WHO Consensus Conference on Nutrition and colorectal cancer *(145)*. It was concluded that although the data are still somewhat controversial, chronic alcohol ingestion even at low daily intake (10–40 g), especially when consumed as beer, results in a 1.5- to 3.5-fold risk for rectal cancer and to a lesser extent for colonic cancer in both sexes, but predominantly in men. Epidemiologic studies also underline the importance of nutritional deficiencies such as methionine, folate, and vitamin B6, which may modulate the ethanol-associated colorectal cancer risk *(146, 147)*.

Subsequently, a recent prospective follow-up study of more than 10,000 US citizens concluded that the consumption of one ore more alcoholic beverages per day at baseline is associated with an approximately 70% greater risk of colon cancer with a strong positive dose-response relationship *(148)*. The most important factor for colorectal cancer appeared to be liquor consumption.

The mechanisms by which alcohol exerts its carcinogenic effect on the colorectal mucosa are not clear, but again acetaldehyde produced predominantly by fecal bacteria from ethanol may injure the mucosa leading to secondary hyperregeneration, a precancerous condition *(48, 149)*. Acetaldehyde may also interact with methyl transfer leading to DNA hypomethylation, which is associated with increased cancer risk *(150)*. For more detail, the reader is referred to the most recent review articles *(50, 51)*.

4.5. Hepatocellular Cancer

Alcohol use in common in the USA and Western Europe and is increasing in Asia. In the USA, 7% of the adult population meet the definition for alcohol misuse or dependence, thereby exceeding the prevalence of hepatitis C (HCV) by fivefold *(151)*. Similar data exist for some countries in Europe, including Germany, where 1.5 million individuals are alcohol-dependent and approximately 3 million people have alcohol-associated organ damage. Case–control studies in countries with a high prevalence of alcohol use and a moderate prevalence of viral hepatitis, as well as studies from countries with a high prevalence of chronic viral hepatitis and a lower prevalence of alcohol use, report that chronic ethanol consumption is associated with an approximately two-fold increased risk for hepatocellular cancer (HCC) *(152)*. The ORs increase further to fivefold to sevenfold when ethanol use exceeds 80 g/day for more than 10 years *(153, 154)*. In general, patients with alcoholic liver cirrhosis show HCC incidence of 1–2% per year.

Although alcohol itself leads to liver cirrhosis and promotes HCC, it is also a co-factor for the development of HCC in other chronic liver diseases. Thus, chronic alcohol misuse may enhance and/or accelerate hepatocarcinogenesis in patients with hepatitis B virus (HBV) and HCV infection, with hereditary hemochromatosis, or with non-alcoholic fatty liver disease (NAFLD). With respect to viral hepatitis, alcohol may stimulate oxidative stress and may, therefore, contribute to inflammation (*see* **below**). It has been shown that chronic alcohol consumption of more than 25 g/day leads to a 10-years earlier occurrence of HCC in a Japanese population *(155)*, indicating an accelerating effect of alcohol in HBV-driven hepatocarcinogenesis. Chronic alcohol misuse also increases the risk of HCV infection *(156)*. Whether this is due to impaired function of the immune system following alcohol ingestion or relates to the risky lifestyle of alcoholics is still unknown. In addition, alcohol may increase viral replication, possibly by immunosuppression. Finally, alcohol may stimulate inflammation and, thus, oxidative stress *(156)*.

In hereditary hemochromatosis, hepatic iron overload is a major factor in hepatocarcinogenesis *(157)* and alcohol enhances iron deposition in the liver, resulting in increases oxidative stress (*see* **below**).

With respect to NAFLD, it has become clear that type 2 diabetic patients are at increased risk for HCC *(158)*. The pathogenesis of NAFLD includes the accumulation of fat in the liver, which may be predominantly induced by hyperinsulinemia due to peripheral insulin resistance. Free fatty acids induce CYP2E1 and lead to ROS *(159)*. Alcohol also increases CYP2E1 and enhances this pathophysiological pathway. In addition, tumour necrosis factor (TNF)-α is elevated in NAFLD and alcoholic liver disease, resulting in further aggravation of peripheral insulin resistance and in oxidative stress. It has been shown that the RR for HCC in type 2 diabetic patients is approximately 4, and it increases to almost 10 for consumption of more than 80 g alcohol per day *(154, 158)*.

It should be pointed out that 30–50% of individuals with HCC show a loss of heterozygosity of the long arm of chromosome 4 *(160)*. In French patients with HCC, a loss of 4Q34-3 in particular was reported *(161)*. However, a large proportion of these patients were infected with HCV.

Various mechanisms may contribute to alcohol-associated carcinogenesis, including chronic inflammation resulting in increased oxidative stress, such as in alcoholic steatohepatitis *(33)*, acetaldehyde and its detrimental effect on proteins and DNA *(30–32)*, induction of CYP2E1 leading to increased ROS production, lipid peroxidation and DNA damage *(33)*, a decrease in antioxidant defense and DNA repair *(33)*, disturbed methyl transfer associated with DNA hypomethylation *(51)* decreased hepatic retinoic acid (RA) *(52)* iron overload *(157)*, and profound impairment of the immune system *(50)*.

5. Conclusion

The aim of the present review was to summarize the current evidence for the contributory role of smoking and chronic alcohol consumption to the cancer burden worldwide based on experimental and epidemiologic data demonstrating a causal relationship between these lifestyle factors and cancer of the gastrointestinal tract. Considering the high frequencies of these cancers especially in the Western World (colorectal cancer is the leading cancer in men and women in some countries), the link between smoking, drinking, and these tumours has important consequences for prevention and early detection. It is well established that no threshold and thus no safe smoking exists, far less is known about safe margins of alcohol consumption, especially when individual genetic or epigenetic risk factors may be considered. The combination of smoking and alcohol drinking is an extremely strong risk factor for some types of cancer, since smoking and drinking alcohol have a synergistic effect on cancer development in various tissues such as the mucosa of the UADT. Although difficult to implement, health authorities must introduce more effective measures in educating the public of potential hazards of smoking and of passive smoking (especially in the presence of small children) and regular and excessive alcohol consumption to avoid not only a variety of diseases associated with these behaviours, but also to prevent cancer development.

References

1. Fiore, M. C. (1992) Cigarette smoking: a clinical guide to assessment and treatment. *Med. Clin. North Am.* **76**, 289–303.
2. Singletary, K. W. and Gapstur, S. M. (2001) Alcohol and breast cancer: a review of epidemiologic and experimental evidence and potential mechanisms. *JAMA.* **286**, 2143–2151.
3. Shin, V. Y. and Cho, C. H. (2005) Nicotine and gastric cancer. *Alcohol.* **35**, 259–264
4. Das, S. K. (2003) Harmful health effects of cigarette smoking. *Mol. Cell. Biochem.* **253**, 159–165.
5. Muscat, J. E., Stellman, S. D., Hoffmann, D., and Wynder, E. L. (1997) Smoking and pancreatic cancer in men and women. *Cancer Epidemiol. Biomarkers Prev.* **6**, 15–19.
6. Zeegers, M. P. A., Goldbohm, R. A., and van den Brandt, P. A. (2002) A prospective study on active and environmental tobacco smoking and bladder cancer risk (The Netherlands). *Cancer Causes Control.* **13**, 83–90.
7. Boffeta, P. and Hashibe, M. (2006) Alcohol and cancer. *Lancet Oncol.* **7**, 149–156.
8. Boffetta, P., Hashibe, M., La Vecchia, C., Zatonski, W., and Rehm, J. (2006) The burden of cancer attributable to alcohol drinking. *Int. J. Cancer* **119**, 884–887.
9. Baan, R., Straif, K., Grosse, Y., Secretan, B., El Ghissassi, F., Bouvard, V., Altieri, A., and Cogliano, V., WHO International Agency for Research on Cancer Monograph Working Group. (2007) Carcinogenicity of alcoholic beverages. *Lancet Oncol.* **8**, 292–293.
10. Wu, W. K. K., Wong, H. P.S., Yu, L., and Cho, C. H. (2006) Nicotine and cancer, in *Alcohol Tobacco and Cancer* (Cho, C. H., and Purohit, V., eds.) Karger, Switzerland, pp. 253–267.
11. Levinson, A. H., Perez-Stable, E. J., Espinoza, P., Flores, E. T., and Byers, T. E. (2004) Latinos report less use of pharmaceutical aids when trying to quit smoking. *Am. J. Prev. Med.* **26**, 105–111.
12. Riebe M. and Westphal, K. (1983) Studies on the induction of sisterchromatid exchanges in Chinese hamster ovary cells by various tobacco alkaloids. *Mutat. Res.* **124**, 281–286.
13. Trivedi, A. H., Dave, B. J., and Adhvaryu, S. G. (1990) Assessment of genotoxicity of nicotine employing in vitro mammalian test system. *Cancer Lett.* **54**, 89–94.
14. Li, X. S., Wang, H. F., Shi, J. Y., Wang, X. Y., and Liu, Y. F. (1996) Genotoxicity

study on nicotine and nicotine-derived nitrosamine by accelerator mass spectrometry. *Radiocarbon* **38**, 347–353.
15. Wu, X. H., Wang, H. F., Liu, Y. F., Lu, X. Y., Wang, J. J., and Li, K. (1997) Histone adduction with nicotine: a bio-AMS study. *Radiocarbon* **39**, 293–297.
16. Hecht, S. S., Hochalter, J. B., Villalta, P. W., and Murphy, S. E. (2000) Hydroxylation of nicotine by cytochrome P450 2A6 and human liver microsomes: formation of a lung carcinogen precursor. *Proc. Natl. Acad. Sci. U.S.A.* **97**, 12493–12497.
17. Wu, W. K. and Cho, C. H. (2004) The pharmacological actions of nicotine on the gastrointestinal tract. *J. Pharmacol. Sci.* **94**, 348–358.
18. Wu, W. K. K., Wong, H. P.S., Luo, S. W., Chan, K., Huang, F. Y., Hui, M. K. C., Lam, E. K, Y., Shin, V. Y., Ye, Y. N., Yang, Y. H., and Cho, C. H. (2005) 4-(Methylnitrosamino)-1-(3-pyridyl)-1-butanone from cigarette smoke stimulates colon cancer growth via β-adrenoceptors. *Cancer Res.* **65**, 5272–5277.
19. Chepiga, T. A., Morton, M. J., Murphy, P. A., Avalos, J. T., Bombick, B. R., Doolittle, D. J., Borgerding, M. F., and Swauger, J. E. (2000) A comparison of the mainstream smoke chemistry and mutagenicity of a representative sample of the US cigarette market with tow Kentucky reference cigarettes (K1R4F and K1R5F). *Food Chem. Toxicol.* **38**, 949–962.
20. Shin, V. Y., Wu, W. K. K., Chu, K. M., Koo, M. W. L., Wong, H. P. S., Lam, E. K. Y., Tai, E. K. K., and Cho, C. H. (2007) Functional roles of β-adrenergic receptors in the mitogenic action of nicotine on gastric cancer cells. *Tox. Sci.* **96**, 21–29.
21. Ye, Y. N., Liu, E. S., Shin, V. Y., Wu, K. K., Luo, J. C., and Cho, C. H. (2004) Nicotine promoted colon cancer growth via epidermal growth factor receptor, c-Src and 5-lipoxygenase-mediated signal pathway. *J. Pharmacol. Exp. Ther.* **308**, 66–72.
22. Shin, V. Y., Wu, K. K., Ye, Y. N., So, W. H., Koo, M. W., Luo, E. S., Luo, J. C., and Cho, C. H. (2004) Nicotine promotes gastric tumour growth and neovascularization by activating extracellular signal-regulated kinase and cyclooxygenase-2. *Carcinogenesis* **25**, 2487–2495.
23. Waggoner, S. E. and Wang, X. (1994) Effect of nicotine on proliferation of normal, malignant and human papillomavirus-transformed

human cervical cells. *Gynecol. Oncol.* **55**, 91–95.

24. Liu, E. S., Ye, Y. N., Shin, V. Y., Yuen, S. T., Leung, S. Y., Wong, B. C., and Cho, C. H. (2003) Cigarette smoke exposure increases ulcerative colitis-associated colonic adenoma formation in mice. *Carcinogenesis* **24**, 1407–1413.

25. Shin, V. Y., Wu, K. K., Chu, K. M., Wong, H. P., Lam, K. Y., Tai, K. K., Koo, M. W., and Cho, C.H. (2005a) Nicotine induces cyclooxygenase-2 and vascular endothelial growth factor-2 in association with tumor-associated invasion and angiogenesis in gastric cancer. *Mol. Cancer Res.* **3**, 607–615.

26. Soffritti, M., Belpoggi, F., Lambertin, L., Lauriola, M., Padovani, M., and Maltoni, C. (2002) Results of long term experimental studies on the carcinogenicity of methyl alcohol and ethyl alcohol in rats. *Ann N.Y. Acad Sci.* **982**, 46–69.

27. International Agency for Research on Cancer. (1999) Re-evaluation of some organic chemicals, hydrazine and hydrogen peroxide. Acetaldehyde. IARC Monogr. Eval. Carcinog. Risks Chem. Hums. Vol 77, Lyon, pp. 319–335.

28. International Agency for Research on Cancer. (2007) Alcoholic beverage consumption and ethyl carbamate (urethane). IARC Monogr. Eval. Carcinog. Risks Hums. Vol. 96. Lyon (in press).

29. Woutersen, R. A., Appelman, L. M., van Garderen Hoetmer, A., and Feron, V. J. (1986) Inhalation toxicity of acetaldehyde in rats. III. Carcinogenicity study. *Toxicology* **41**, 213–231.

30. Seitz, H. K. and Meier, P. (2007) The role of acetaldehyde in upper digestive tract cancer in alcoholics. *Translational Med.* **149**, 293–297.

31. Seitz, H. K. (2007) The role of acetaldehyde in alcohol-associated cancer of the gastrointestinal tract, in *Acetaldehyde-Related Pathology: Bridging the Trans-disciplinary Divide* (Chadwick., D. J., ed.), Novartis Foundation Symposium No. 285, John Wiley and Son, London, U.K.

32. Salaspuro, M., Salaspuro, V., and Seitz, H. K. (2006) Alcohol and upper aerodigestive tract cancer, in *Alcohol, Tobacco and Cancer* (Cho C. H., Purohit, V., eds.), Karger, Basel, pp. 48–62.

33. Seitz, H. K. and Stickel, F. (2006) Risk factors and mechanisms of hepatocarcinogenesis with special emphasis on alcohol and oxidative stress. *Biol Chem.* **387**, 349–360.

34. Fang, J. L. and Vaca, C. E. (1997) Detection of DNA adducts of acetaldehyde in peripheral white blood cells of alcohol abusers. *Carcinogenesis.* **18**, 627–632.

35. Matsuda, T., Terashima, I., Matsumoto, Y., Yabushita, H., Matsui, S., and Shibutani, S. (1999) Effective utilization of N2-ethyl-2′-deoxyguanosine triphosphate during DNA synthesis catalyzed by mammalian replicative DNA polymerases. *Biochemistry* **38**, 929–935.

36. Theravathu, J. A., Jaruga, P., Nath, R. G., Dizdaroglu, M., and Brooks, P. J. (2005) Polyamines stimulate the formation of mutagenic 1, N2-propanodeoxyguanosine adducts from acetaldehyde. *Nucleic Acids Res.* **33**, 3513–3520.

37. Bosron, W. F. and Li, T. K. (1986) Genetic polymorphism of human liver alcohol and aldehyde dehydrogenase and their relationship to alcohol metabolism and alcoholism. *Hepatology* **6**, 502–510.

38. Harty, L. C., Caporaso, N. E., Hayes, R. B., Winn, D. M., Bravo-Otero, E., Blott, W. J., Kleinmen, D. V., Brown, L. M., Armenian, H. K., Fraumeni, J. F. Jr., and Shields, P. G. (1997) Alcohol dehydrogenase 3 genotype and risk of oral cavity and pharyngeal cancers. *J. Natl. Cancer Inst.* **89**, 1689–1705.

39. Homann, N., Stickel, F., König, I. R., Jacobs, A., Junghanns, K., Benesova, M., Schuppan, D., Himsel, S., Zuberjerger, I., Hellerbrand, C., Ludwig, D., Caselmann, W. H., and Seitz, H. K. (2005) Alcohol dehydrogenase 1C*1 allele is a genetic marker for alcohol-associated cancer in heavy drinkers. *Int. J. Cancer* **118**, 1998–2002.

40. Visapää, J-P., Götte, K., Benesova, M., Li, J., Homann, N., Conradt, C., Inoue, H., Tisch, M., Hörrmann, K., Väkeväinen, S., Salaspuro, M., and Seitz H. K. (2004) Increased cancer risk in heavy drinkers with the alcohol dehydrogenase 1C*1 allele, possibly due to salivary acetaldehyde. *Gut* **53**, 871–876.

41. Coutelle, C., Höhn, B., Benesova, M., Oneta, C. M., Quattrochi, P., Roth, H.-J., Schmidt-Gayk, H., Schneeweiss, A., Bastert, G., and Seitz, H. K. (2004) Risk factors in alcohol associated breast cancer: Alcohol dehydrogenase polymorphism and estrogens. *Int. J. Oncol.* **25**, 1127–1132.

42. Terry, M. B., Gammon, M. D., Zhang, F. F., Knight, J. A., Wang, Q., Britton, J. A., Teitelbaum, S. L., Neugut, A. I., and Santella, R. M. (2006) ADH3 genotype, alcohol intake and breast cancer risk. *Carcinogenesis* **27**, 840–847.

43. Freudenheim, J. L., Ambrosone, C. B., Moysich, K. B., Vena, J. E., Graham, S., Marshall, J. R., Multi, P., Laughlin, R., Nemoto, T., Harty, L. C., Crits, G. A., Chan, A. W. K., and Shields, P. G. (1999) Alcohol dehydrogenase 3 genotype modification of the association of alcohol consumption with breast cancer risk. *Cancer Causes Control* **10**, 369–377.

44. Yokoyama, A., Muramatsu, T., Ohmori, T., Yokoyama, T., Okoyama, K., Takahashi, H., Hasegawa, Y., Higuchi, S., Maruyama, K., Shirakura, K., and Ishii, H. (1998) Alcohol-related cancers and aldehyde dehydrogenase-2 in Japanese alcoholics. *Carcinogenesis* **19**, 1383–1387.

45. Yokoyama, A., Watanabe, H., Fukuda, H., Haneda, T., Kato, H., Yokoyama, T., Muramatsu, T., Igaki, H., and Tachimori, Y. (2002) Multiple cancers associated with esophageal and oropharyngolaryngeal squamous cell carcinoma and the aldehyde dehydrogenase-2 genotype in male Japanese drinkers. *Cancer Epidemiol. Biomarkers Prev.* **11**, 895–900.

46. Matsuo, K., Hamajima, N., Shinoda, M., Hatooka, S., Inoue, M., Takezaki, T., and Tajima, K. (2006) Gene-environment interaction between an aldehyde dehydrogenase-2 (ALDH2) polymorphism and alcohol consumption for the risk of esophageal cancer. *Carcinogenesis* **22**, 913–916.

47. Seitz, H. K., Simanowski, U. A., Garzon, F. T., Rideout, J. M., Peters, T. J., Koch, A., Berger, M. R, Einecke, H., and Maiwald, M. (1990) Possible role of acetaldehyde in ethanol-related rectal cocarcinogenesis in the rat. *Gastroenterology* **98**, 406–413.

48. Simanowski, U. A., Suter, P., Russell, R. M., Heller, M., Waldherr, R., Ward, R., Peters, T.J., Smith, D., and Seitz, H. K. (1994) Enhancement of ethanol-induced rectal hyperregeneration with age in F344 rats. *Gut* **35**, 1102–1106.

49. Homann, N., Jousimies-Somer, H., Jokelainen, K., Heine, R., and Salaspuro, M (1997) High acetaldehyde levels in saliva after ethanol consumption: methodological aspects and pathogenetic implications. *Carcinogenesis* **18**, 1739–1743.

50. Pöschl, G. and Seitz, H. K. (2004) Alcohol and cancer (review). *Alcohol Alcohol* **39**, 155–165.

51. Stickel, F., Herold, C., Seitz, H. K., and Schuppan, D. (2006) Alcohol and transmethylation: implication for hepatocarcinogenesis, in *Liver Diseases: Biochemical Mechanisms and New Therapeutic Insights* (Ali, S., Mann, D., and Friedman, S., eds). Plenum Press, New York, pp. 45–58.

52. Wang, X. D. (2005) Alcohol, vitamin A, and cancer. *Alcohol* **35**, 251–258.

53. Blot, W. J., McLaughlin, J. K., Winn, D. M., Austin, D. F., Greenberg, R. S., Preston-Martin, S., Bernstein, L., Schoenberg, J. B., Stemhagen, A., and Fraumeni, J. F. (1988) Smoking and drinking in relation to oral and pharyngeal cancer. *Cancer Res.* **48**, 3282–3287.

54. Du, X., Squier, C.A., Kremer, M. J., and Wertz, P. W. (2000) Penetration of N-nitrosonornicotine (NNN) across oral mucosa in the presence of ethanol and nicotine. *J. Oral Pathol. Med.* **29**, 80–85.

55. Salaspuro, M., Salaspuro, V., and Seitz, H. K. (2006) Interaction of alcohol and tobacco in upper aerodigestive tract and stomach cancer, in *Alcohol, Tobacco and Cancer* (Cho C. H., and Purohit, V., eds) Karger, Basel, pp. 48–62.

56. Salaspuro, M. (2003) Acetaldehyde, microbes, and cancer of the digestive tract. *Crit. Rev. Clin. Lab. Med.* **40**, 183–208.

57. Salaspuro, V. and Salaspuro, M. (2004) Synergistic effect of alcohol drinking and smoking on in vivo acetaldehyde concentration in saliva. *Int. J. Cancer* **111**, 480–483.

58. Lieber, C. S. (1994) Alcohol and the liver. *Update Gastroenterology* **106**, 1085–1105.

59. Shimizu, M., Lasker, J. M., Tsutsumi, M., and Lieber, C. S. (1990) Immunohistochemical localization of ethanol inducible cytochrome P4502E1 in the rat alimentary tract. *Gastroenterology* **93**, 1044–1050.

60. Oneta, C. M., Lieber, C. S., Li, J., Rüttimann, S., Schmid, B., Lattmann, J., Rosman, A. S., and Seitz, H. K. (2002) Dynamics of cytochrome P-4502E1 activity in man: induction by ethanol and disappearance during withdrawal phase. *J. Hepatol.* **36**, 47–52.

61. Seitz, H. K. and Osswald, B. R. (1992) Effect of ethanol on procarcinogen activation, in *Alcohol and Cancer* (Watson R. R., ed.) CRC Press, Boca Raton, pp. 55–72.

62. Franceschi, S., Falamini, R., Barra, S., Barón, A. E., negri, E., Bidoli, E., Serraino, D., and La Vecchia, C. (1990) Smoking and drinking in relation to cancers of the oral cavity, pharynx, larynx, and esophagus in northern Italy. *Cancer Res.* **50**, 6502–6507.

63. Garrote, L. F., Herrero, R., Reyes, R. M., Vaccarella, S., Anta, J. L., Ferbeye, L., Muñoz, N., and Franceschi, S. (2001) Risk factors for cancer of the oral cavity and oropharynx in Cuba. *Br. J. Cancer* **85**, 46–54.

64. Gallus, S., Altieri, A., Bosetti, C., Franceschi, S., Levi, F., Negri, E., Dal Maso, L., Conti, E., Zambon, P., and La Vecchia, C.

(2003) Cigarette tar yield and risk of upper digestive tract cancers: case-control studies from Italy and Switzerland. *Ann. Oncol.* **14**, 209–213.

65. Jourenkova-Mironova, N., Mitrunen, K., Bouchardy, C., Dayer, P., Benhbamou, S., and Hirvonen, A. (2000) High-activity microsomal epoxide hydrolase genotypes and the risk of oral, pharynx, and larynx cancers. *Cancer Res.* **60**, 534–536.

66. Pickens, A. and Orringer, M. (2003) Geographical distribution and the racial disparity in esophageal cancer. *Ann. Thorac. Surg.* **76**, S1367–S1369.

67. Li, J. Y. (1982) Epidemiology of esophageal cancer in China. *Natl. Cancer Inst. Monog.* **62**, 113–120.

68. McCabe, M. L. and Dlamini, Z. (2005) The molecular mechanisms of esophageal cancer. *Int. Immunopharmacol.* **5**, 1113–1130.

69. Blackstock, A.W. (2007) Esophageal cancer. *Semin. Radiat. Oncol.* **17**, 1.

70. Layke, J. C. and Lopez, P. P. (2006) Esophageal cancer: a review and update. *Am. Fam. Physician* **73**, 2187–2194.

71. Kelly, D. J., Mestre, J. R., Subbaramaiah, K., Sacks, P. G., Schantz, S. P., Tanabe, T., Inoue, H., Ramonetti, J. T., and Dannenberg, A. J. (1997) Benzo[a]pyrene upregulates cyclooxygenase-2 gene expression in oral epithelial cells. *Carcinogenesis* **18**, 795–799.

72. Zhang, F., Altorki, N. K., Wu, Y. C., Soslow, R. A., Subbaramaiah, K., and Dannenberg, A. J. (2001) Duodenal reflux induces cyclooxygenase-2 in the esophageal mucosa of rats: evidence for involvement of bile acids. *Gastroenterology* **121**, 1391–399.

73. Zhang, F., Subbaramaiah, K., Altorki, N., and Dannenberg, A. J. (1998) Dihydroxy bile acids activate the transcription of cyclooxygenase-2. *J. Biol. Chem.* **273**, 2424–2428.

74. Zimmermann, K. C., Sarbia, M., Weber, A. A., Borchard, F., Gabbert, H. E., and Schror, K. (1999) Cyclooxygenase-2 expression in human esophageal carcinoma. *Cancer Res.* **59**, 198–204.

75. Wilson, K. T., Fu, S., Ramanujam, K. S., and Meltzer, S. J. (1998) Increased expression of inducible nitric oxide synthase and cyclooxygenase-2 in Barrett's esophagus and associated adenocarcinomas. *Cancer Res.* **58**, 2929–934.

76. Shamma, A., Yamamoto, H., Doki, R., Okami, J., Kondo, M., Fujiwara, Y., Yano, M., Inoue, M., Matsuura, N., Shiozaki, H., and Monden, M. (2000) Up-regulation of cyclooxygenase-2 in squamous carcinogenesis of the esophagus. *Clin. Cancer Res.* **6**, 1229–1238.

77. Kaur, B. S., Khamnehei, N., Iravani, M., Namburu, S. S., Lin, O., and Triadafilopoulos, G. (2002) Rofecoxib inhibits cyclooxygenase-2 expression and activity and reduces cell proliferation in Barret's esophagus. *Gastroenterology* **123**, 60–67.

78. Shirvani V. N., Ouatu-Lasca R., Kaur B. S., Omary M. B., Triadafilopoulos G. (2000) Cyclooxygenase 2 expression in Barrett's esopagus and adenocarcinoma: Ex vivo induction by bile salts and acid exposure. *Gastroenterology* **118**, 487–196.

79. Risrimaki, A., Honkanen, N., Jankala, H., Sipponen, P., and Harkonen, M. (1997) Expression of cyclooxygenase-2 in human gastric carcinoma. *Cancer Res.* **57**, 1276–1286.

80. Marnett, L. J., Reed, G. A., and Dennison, D. J. (1978) Prostaglandin synthetase-dependent activation of 7, 8-dihydro-7, 8-dihydroxygeno[a] pyrene to mutagenic derivatives. *Biochem. Biophys. Res. Commun.* **82**, 210–216

81. Eling, T. E., Thompson, D. C., Fourman, G. L., Curtis, J. F., and Hughes, M. F. (1990) Prostaglandin H synthase and xenobiotic oxidation. *Annu. Rev. Pharmacol. Toxicol.* **30**, 1–45.

82. Thun, M. J., Namboodiri, M. M., Calle, E. E., Flanders, W. D., and Heath, C. W. Jr. (1993) Aspirin use and risk of fatal cancer. *Cancer Res.* **53**. 1322–1327.

83. Farrow, D. C., Vaughan, T. L., Hansten, P. D., Stanford, J. L., Risch, H. A., Gammon, M. D., Chow, W. H., Dubrow, R., Ahsan, H., Mayne, S. T., Schoenberg, J. B., West, A. B., Rotterdam, H., Fraumeni, J. R. Jr., and Blot, W. J. (1998) Use of aspirin and other nonsteroidal anti-inflammatory drugs and risk of esophageal and gastric cancer. *Cancer Epidemiol. Biomarkers Prev.* 7, 97–102.

84. You, N. C., Mu, L. N., Yu, S. Z., Jiang, Q. W., Cao, W., Zhou, X. F., Ding, B. G., Wang, R. H., Cai, L., and Zhang, Z. F. (2004) Polymorphisms of alcohol- and smoking-related susceptibility genes and risk of esophageal cancer. *Ann. Epidemiology* **14**, 595–596.

85. Wang, A. H., Sun, C. S., Li, L.S., Huang, J. Y., and Chen, Q. S. (2002) Relationship of tobacco smoking CYP1A1, GSTM1 gene polymorphism and esophageal cancer in Xi'an. *World J. Gastroenterol.* **8**, 49–53.

86. Gao, C. M., Takezaki, T., Wu, J. Z., Liu, Y. T., Li, S. P., Ding, J. H., Su, P., Hu, X., Xu, T. L., Sugimura, H., and Tajima, K. (2002) Glutathione-S-transferase M1 (GSTM1) and

GSTT1 genotype, smoking, consumption of alcohol and tea and risk of esophageal and stomach cancers: a case-control study of a high-incidence area in Jiangsu Province, China. *Cancer Lett.* **188**, 95–102.

87. Altorki, N. K., Oliveria, S., and Schump, D. S. (1997) Epidemiology and molecular biology of Barrett's adenocarcinoma. *Semin. Surg. Oncol.* **13**, 270–280.

88. Lee, J. M., Shun, C. T., Wu, M. T., Chen, Y. Y., Yang, S. Y., Hung, H. I., Chen, J. S., Hsu, H. H., Huang, P. M., Juo, S. W., and Lee, Y. C. (2006) The associations of p53 overexpression with p53 codon 72 genetic polymorphisms in esophageal cancer. *Mutation Res.* **594**, 181–188.

89. Tuyns, A. J., Esteve, J., Raymond, L., Berrino, F., Benhamou, E., Blanchet, F., Boffetta, P., Crosignani, P., Del Moral, A., Lehmann, W., Merletti, F., Pequignot, G., Riboli, E., Sancho-Garnier, H., Terracini, B., Zubiri, A., and Zubiri, L. (1988) Cancer of the larynx/hypopharynx, tobacco and alcohol: IARC international case-control study in Turin and Varese (Italy), Zaragoza and Navarra (Spain), Geneva (Switzerland) and Calvados (France). *Int. J. Cancer.* **41**, 483–491.

90. Franceschi, S., Talamini, R., Barra, S., Baron, A. E., Negri, E., Bidoli, E., Serraino, D., and La Vecchia, C. (1990) Smoking and drinking in relation to cancers of the oral cavity, pharynx, larynx, and esophagus in northern Italy. *Cancer Res.* **50**, 6502–6507.

91. Blot, W. J. (1992) Alcohol and cancer. *Cancer Res.* **52 Suppl**, 2119–2123.

92. Bagnardi, V., Blangiardo, M., La Veccia, C., and Corrao, G. (2001) A meta-analysis of alcohol drinking and cancer risk. *Br. J. Cancer* **85**, 1700–1705.

93. Tuyns, A. (1978) Alcohol and cancer. *Alcohol Health Res. World* **2**, 20–31.

94. Maier, H., Zöller, J., Herrmann, A., Kreiss, M., and Heller, W. D (1993) Dental status and oral hygiene in patients with head and neck cancer. *Otolaryngol. Head Neck Surg.* **1088**, 655–661.

95. Brugere, J., Guenel, P., Leclerc, A., and Rodriguez, J. (1986) Differential effects of tobacco and alcohol in cancer of the larynx, pharynx, and mouth. *Cancer* **57**, 391–395.

96. Tuyns, A. (1983) Esophageal cancer in non-smoking drinkers and in non-drinking smokers. *Int. J. Cancer* **32**, 443–444.

97. Boffetta, P. and Garfinkel, L. (1990) Alcohol drinking and mortality among men enrolled in an American Cancer Society prospective Study. *Epidemiology* **5**, 342–348.

98. Thun, M. J., Peto, R., Lopez, Ad., Monaco, J. H., Henley, S. J., Heath, C. W. Jr., and Doll, R. (1997) Alcohol consumption and mortality among middle-aged and elderly U. S. adults. *N. Engl. J. Med.* **337**, 1705–1714.

99. Morimoto, K. and Takeshita, T. (1996) Low Km aldehyde dehydrogenase (ALDH2) polymorphism, alcohol drinking behaviour, and chromosome alterations in peripheral lymphocytes. *Environ. Health Perspect.* **104** (Suppl 3), 563–567.

100. Ishikawa, H., Yamamoto, H., Tian, Y., Kawano, M., Yamauchi, T., and Yokoyama, K. (2003) Effect of ALDH2 gene polymorphism and alcohol drinking behaviour on micronuclei frequency in non-smokers. *Mut Res.* **541**, 71–80.

101. Väkeväinen, S., Tillonen, J., Agarwal, D. P., Svirastava, N., and Salaspuro, M. (2000) High salivary acetaldehyde after a moderate dose of alcohol in ALDH2-deficient subjects: strong evidence for the local carcinogenic action of acetaldehyde. *Alcohol Clin. Exp. Res.* **24**, 873–877.

102. Homann, N., Tillonen, J., Rintamäki, H., Salaspuro, M., Lindqvist, C., and Meurman, J. H. (2001) Poor dental status increases the acetaldehyde production from ethanol in saliva: a possible link to the higher risk of oral cancer among alcohol-consumers. *Oral Oncol.* **37**, 153–158.

103. Homann, N., Kärkkäinen, P., Koivisto, T., Nosova, T., Jokelainen, K., and Salspuro, M. (1997) Effects of acetaldehyde on cell regeneration and differentiation of the upper gastrointestinal tract mucosa. *J. Natl. Cancer Inst.* **89**, 1692–1697.

104. Simanowski, U. A., Suter, P., Stickel, F., Maier, H., Waldherr, R., Smith, D., Russell, R. M., and Seitz, H. K. (1993) Esophageal epithelial hyperproliferation following long term alcohol consumption in rats: effect of age and salivary function. *J. Natl. Cancer Inst.* **85**, 2030–2033.

105. Tredaniel, J., Boffetta, P., Buiatti, E., Saracci, R., and Hirsch, A. (1997) Tobacco smoking and gastric cancer: review and meta-analysis. *Int. J. Cancer* **72**, 565–573.

106. Tamer, L., Ates, N. A., Ates, C. Ercan, B. Elipek, T. Yildirim, H., Camdeviren, H. Atik, U., and Aydin, S. (2005) Glutathione S-transferase M1, T1 and P1 genetic polymorphisms, cigarette smoking and gastric cancer risk. *Cell Biochem. Funct.* **23**, 267–272.

107. Kim, H. S., Kwack, S. J., and Lee, B. M. (2005) Alternation of cytochrome P450

and glutathione S-transferase activity in normal and malignant human stomach. *J. Toxcol. Environ. Health* **68**, 1611–1620.

108. Gao, C., Wu, J., Ding, J., Liu, Y., Zang, Y., Li, S., Su, P., Hu, X., Xu, T., Toshiro, K., and Kazuo, T. (2002). Polymorphisms of methylenetetrahydrofolate reductase C677T and the risk of stomach cancer. *Zhoghua Liu Xing Bing Xue Za Zhi* **23**, 289–292.

109. Mu, L. N., Ding, B. G., Chen, C. W., Wei, G. R., Zhou, X. F., Wang, R. H., Cai, l., Zhang, Z. F., Jiang, Q. W., and Yu, S. Z. (2004) A case-control study on the relationship between methyl-tetrahydrofolic acid reductase 677 gene polymorphism and the risk of stomach cancer. *Zhonghua Liu Xing Bing Xue Za Zhi* **25**, 495–498.

110. Gao, C. M., Tekezaki, T., Wu, J. Z., Lui, Y. T., Ding, J. H., Li, S. P., Su, P. Hu, X., Kai, H. T., Lu, Z. Y., Matsuo, K., Hamajima, N., Sugimura, H., and Tajima, K. (2004) Polymorphisms in thymidylate synthase and methylenetetrahydrofolate reductase genes and the susceptibility to esophageal and stomach cancer with smoking. *Asian Pac. J. Cancer Prev.* **5**, 133–138.

111. Ahkgren, J. D. (1996) Epidemiology and risk factors in pancreatic cancer. *Semin. Oncol.* **23**, 241–250.

112. Silverman, D. T., Dunn, J. A., Hoover, R. N., Schiffman, M., Lillemoe, K. D., Schoenberg, J. B., Brown, L. M., Greenberg, R. S., Hayes, R. B., and Swanson G. M. (1994) Cigarette smoking and pancreas cancer: a case-control study based on direct interview. *J. Natl. Cancer Inst.* **86**, 1510–1516.

113. Wang, L., Miao, X., Tan, W., Lu, X., Zhao, P., Zhao, X., Shan, Y., Li, H., and Lin, D. (2005) Genetic polymorphisms in methylenetetrahydrofolate reductase and thymidylate synthase and risk of pancreatic cancer. *Clin. Gastroenterol. Hepatol.* **3**, 743–751.

114. Yun, J. E., Jo, I., Park, J., Kim, M. T., Ryu, H. G., Odongua, N., Kim, E., and Jee, S. H. (2006) Cigarette smoking elevated fasting serum glucose, and risk of pancreatic cancer in Korean men. *Int. J. Cancer* **119**, 208–212.

115. Li, D. H. and Jiao, L. (2003) Molecular epidemiology of pancreatic cancer. *Int. J. Gastrointest. Cancer* **33**, 3–14.

116. Berger, D. H., Chang, H., Wood, M., Huang, L. I., Heath, C. W., Lehman, T., and Ruggeri, B. A. (1999) Mutation activation of k-ras in non-neoplastic exocrine pancreatic lesions in relation to cigarette smoking status. Cancer **85**, 326–329.

117. Malats, N., Porra, M., Corominas, J. M., Pinol, J. L., Rifa, J., and Real, F. X. (1997) Ki-ras mutations in exocrine pancreatic cancer: association with clinico-pathological characteristics and with tobacco and alcohol consumption. *Int. J. Cancer* **70**, 661–667.

118. Li, D. H. (2001) Molecular epidemiology of pancreatic cancer. *Cancer J.* **7**, 259–265.

119. Lee, H. C., Yoon, Y. B., and Kim, C. Y. (1997) Association between genetic polymorphisms of the cytochrome P-450 (1A1, 2D6 and 2E1) and the susceptibility to pancreatic cancer. *Korean J. Intern. Med.* **12**, 128–136.

120. Bartch, H., Malaveille, C., and Lowenfels, A. B. (1998). Genetic polymorphism of N-acetyltransferases, glutathione S-transferase M1 and NAD (P)H: quinine oxidoreductase in relation to malignant and benign pancreatic disease risk. The International Pancreatic Disease Study Group. *Eur. J. Cancer Prev.* **7**, 215–223.

121. Liu, G., Ghadirian, P., Vesprini, D., Hamel, N., Paradis, A. J., Lal, G., Gallinger, S., Narod, S.A., and Foulkes, W. D. (2000) Polymorphism in GSTM1, GSTT1 and CYP1A1 and risk of pancreatic adenocarcinoma. *Br. J. Cancer* **82**, 1646–1649.

122. Duell, E. J., Holly, E. A., Bracci, P. M., Liu, M., Wiencke, J. K., and Kelsey, K. T. (2002) A population-based, case-control study of polymorphisms in carcinogen-metabolizing genes, smoking and pancreatic adenocarcinoma risk. *J. Natl. Cancer Inst.* **94**, 297–306.

123. Duell, E. J., Holly, E. A., Bracci, P. M., Wiencke, J. K., and Kelsey, K. T. (2002) A population-based study of the Arg399Gln polymorphism in X-ray repair cross-complementing group 1 (XRCC1) and risk of pancreatic adenocarcinoma. *Cancer Res.* **62**, 4630–4636.

124. Li, D. H., Jiao, L., Li, Y. N., Doll, M. A., Hein, D. W., Bondy, M. L., Evans, D. B., Wolff, R. A., Lenzi, R., Pisters, P. W., Abbruzzese, J. L., and Hassan, M. M. (2006) Polymorphisms of cytochrome P4501A2 and N-acetyltransferase genes, smoking, and risk of pancreatic cancer. *Carcinogenesis* **27**, 103–111.

125. Welsch, T., Kleeff, J., Seitz, H. K., Büchler, P., Friess, H., and Büchler, W. (2006) Update on pancreatic cancer and alcohol-associated risk. *J Gastroenterol. Hepatol.* **21**, 77–84.

126. Martinez, M. E., McPgerson, R. S., Levin, B., and Glober, G. A. (1997) A case-control study of dietary intake and other lifestyle risk factors for hyperplastic polyps. *Gastroenterology* **113**, 423–429.

127. Potter, J. D., Bigler, J., Fosdick, L., Bostick, R. M., Kampman, E., Chen, C., Louis, T. A.,

and Grambsch, P. (1999) Colorectal adenomatous and hyperplastic polyps: smoking and N-acetyltransferase 2 polymorphisms. *Cancer Epidemiol. Biomark Prev.* **8**, 69–75.

128. Newcomb, P. A., Storer, B. E., and Marcus, P. M., (1995) Cigarette smoking in relation to risk of large bowel cancer in women. *Cancer Res.* **55**, 4906–4909.

129. Terry, P., Ekbom, A., Lichtenstein, P., Feychting, M., and Wolk, A. (2001) Long-term tobacco smoking and colorectal cancer in a prospective cohort study. *Int. J. Cancer* **91**, 585–587.

130. Limburg, P. J., Vierkant, R. A., Cerhan, J. R., Yang, P., Lazovich, D., Potter, J. D., and Sellers, T. A. (2003) Cigarette smoking and colorectal cancer: long-term, subsite-specific risks in a cohort study of postmenopausal women. *Clin. Gastroenterol. Hepatol.* **1**, 202–210.

131. Giovannucci, E., Colditz, G. A., Stampfer, M. J., and Willett, W. C. (1996) Physical activity, obesity and risk colorectal adenoma in women (United States). *Cancer Causes Control* **6**, 253–263.

132. Heineman, E. F., Zahm, S. H., McLaughlin, J. K., and Vaught, J. B. (1994) Increased risk of colorectal cancer among smokers: results of a 26-year follow-up of US veterans and a review. *Int. J. Cancer* **59**, 728–738.

133. Ye, Y. N., Wu, W. K. K., Shin, V. Y., and Cho, C. H. (2005) A mechanistic study of colon cancer growth promoted by cigarette smoke extract. *Eur. J. Pharmacol.* **519**, 52–57.

134. Ye, Y. N., Wu, W. K. K., Shin, V. Y., Bruce, I. C., Wong, B. C. Y., and Cho, C. H. (2005a) Dual inhibition of 5-LOX and COX-2 suppresses colon cancer formation promoted by cigarette smoke. *Carcinogenesis* **26**, 827–834.

135. Breslow, N. E. and Enstrom, J. E. (1974) Geographic correlations between mortality rates and alcohol, tobacco consumption in the United States. *J. Natl. Cancer Inst.* **53**, 631–639.

136. Kune, G. A. and Viletta, L. (1992) Alcohol consumption and the etiology of colorectal cancer: a review of the scientific evidence from 1957 to 1991. *Nutr. Cancer* **18**, 97–111.

137. Seitz, H. K., Pöschl, G., and Stickel, F. (2002) Alcohol and colorectal cancer, in *Exogenous Factors in Colonic Carcinogenesis* (Scheppach, W., and Scheurlen, M., eds.) Falk Symposium 128, Kluwer Academic Publishers, Dordrecht, Boston, London, pp. 128–141.

138. Shimizu, N, Nagata, C., Shimizu H., Kametani, M. Takeyama, N., Ohnuma, T., and Matsushita S. (2003) Height weight, and alcohol consumption in relation to the risk of colorectal cancer in Japan: a prospective study. *Br. J. Cancer* **88**, 1038–1043.

139. Pedersen, A., Johansen, C., and Gronbaek, M. (2003) Relations between amount and type of alcohol and colon and rectal cancer in a Danish population based cohort study. *Gut* **52**, 861–867.

140. Cho, E., Smith-Warner, S. A., Ritz, J., van den Brandt, P. A., Colditz, G. A. Folsom, A. R., Freudenheim, J. L., Giovannucci, E. Goldbohm, R. A., Graham, S. Holmberg, L., Kim, D. H., Malila, N., Miller, A. B., Pietinen, P., Rohan, T. E., Sellers, T. A., Speizer, F. E., Willett, W. C. Wolk, A., and Hunter, D. J. (2004) Alcohol intake and colorectal cancer: a pooled analyses of 8 cohort studies. *Ann. Intern. Med.* **140**, 603–613.

141. Kearny, J., Giovannucci, E., Rimm, E. B., Stampfer, M. J., Colditz, G. A., Ascherio, A., Bleday, R., and Willett, W. C. (1995) Diet, alcohol, and smoking and the occurrence of hyperplastic polyps of the colon and rectum (United States). *Cancer Causes Control* **6**, 45–56.

142. Boutron, M. C., Faivre, J. Dop, M. C, Quipourt, V., and Senesse, P. (1995) Tobacco, alcohol, and colorectal tumors: a multistep process. *Am. J. Epidemiol.* **141**, 1038–1046.

143. Bardou, M., Montembault, S., Giraud, V., Balian, A., Borotto, E., Houdayer, C., Capron, F., Chaput, J. C., and Naveau, S. (2002) Excessive alcohol consumption favours high risk polyp or colorectal cancer occurrence among patients with adenomas: a case control study. *Gut* **50**, 38–42.

144. Le Marchand, L, Wilkens, L. R., Hankin, J. H., Kolonel, L. N., and Lyu, L. C. (1999) Independent and joint effects of family history and lifestyle on colorectal cancer risk: implications for prevention. *Cancer Epidemiol. Biomarkers Prev.* **8**, 845–851.

145. Scheppach, W., Bingham, S., Boutron-Ruault, M. C., Gerhardsson de Verdier, M., Moreno, V., Nagengast, F. M., Reifen, R., Riboli, E., Seitz, H. K, and Wahrendorf, J. (1999) WHO consensus statement on the role of nutrition in colorectal cancer. *Eur. J. Cancer Prev.* **8**, 57–62.

146. Larsson, S. C., Giovannucci, E., and Wolk, A. (2005) Vitamin B6 intake, alcohol consumption, and colorectal cancer: a longitudinal population-based cohort of women. *Gastroenterology* **128**, 1830–1837.

147. Giovannucci, E., Rimm, E. B., Ascherio, A., Stampfer, M. J., Colditz, G. A., and Willett, W. C. (1995) Alcohol, low methionine-low

folate diets, and risk of colon cancer in men. *J. Natl. Cancer Inst.* **87**, 265–273.

148. Su, L. J. and Arab, L (2004) Alcohol consumption and risk of colon cancer: evidence from the national health and nutrition examination survey I epidemiologic follow-up study. *Nutr. Cancer* **50**, 111–119.

149. Simanowski, U. A., Homann, N., Knühl, M., Arce, L., Waldherr, R., Conradt, C., Bosch, F. X., and Seitz, H. K. (2001) Increased rectal cell proliferation following alcohol abuse. *Gut* **49**, 418–422.

150. Choi, S. W., Stickel, F. Baik, W., Kim, Y. I., Seitz, H. K., and Mason, J. C. (1999) Chronic alcohol consumption induces genomic, but not p53-specific DNA hypomethylation in the colon of the rat. *J. Nutr.* **129**, 1945–1950.

151. Grant, B., Harfort, T., Dawson, D., Chou, P., DuFour, M., and Pickering, R. (1994) Prevalence of DSM-IV alcohol abuse and dependence: United States, 1992. *Alcohol Health Res. World* **18**, 243–248.

152. Morgan, T. R., Mandayam, S., and Jamal, M. M. (2004) Alcohol and hepatocellular carcinoma. *Gastroenterology* **127**, 87–96.

153. Tagger, A., Donato, F., Ribero, M. L., Chiesa, R., Portera, G., Gelatti, U., Alberini, A., Fasola, M., Moffetta, P., and Nardi, G. (1999) Case control study on hepatitis C virus (HCV) as a risk factor for hepatocellular carcinoma: the role of HCV genotypes and the synergism with hepatitis B virus and alcohol. Brescia HCC study. *Int. J. Cancer* **81**, 695–699.

154. Hassan, M. M., Hwang, L. Y., Hatten, C. J., Swaim, M., Li, D., Abbruzzese, J. L., Beasley, P., and Patt, Y. Z (2002) Risk factors for hepatocellular carcinoma: synergism of alcohol with viral hepatitis and diabetes mellitus. *Hepatology* **36**, 1206–1213.

155. Ohnishi, K. (1992) Alcohol and hepatocellular cancer, in *Alcohol and Cancer*, (Watson, R. R., ed.) CRC Press, Boca Raton, FL, USA, pp. 179–202.

156. Inoué, H. and Seitz, H. K. (2001) Viruses and alcohol in the pathogenesis of primary hepatic carcinoma. *Eur. J. Cancer Pres.* **10**, 1–4.

157. Kowdley, K. V. (2004) Iron, hemochromatosis, and hepatocellular carcinoma. *Gastroenterology* **127**, 79–86.

158. El-Serag, H. B. (2004) Hepatocellular carcinoma: recent trends in the United States. *Gastroenterology* **127**, 27–34.

159. Neuschwander-Tetri, B. A. and Caldwell, S. H. (2003) Nonalcoholic steatohepatitis: summary of an AASLD single topic conference. *Hepatology* **37**, 1202–1219.

160. Laurent-Puig, P., Legoix, P., Bluteau, O., Belghiti, J., Franco, D., Binot, F., Monges, G., Thomas, G., Bioulac-Sage, P., and Zucman-Rossi, J. (2001) Genetic alterations associated with hepatocellular carcinomas define distinct pathways of hepatocarcinogenesis. *Gastroenterology* **120**, 1763–1773.

161. Bluteau, O., Beaudoin, J. C. Pasturaus, P., Belghiti, J., Franco, D., Bioulac-Sage, P., Laurent-Puig, P., and Zacman-Rossi, J. (2002) Specific association between alcohol intake, high grade of differentiation and 4q34-q35 deletions in hepatocellular carcinomas identified by high resolution allelotyping. *Oncogene* **21**, 1225–1232.

Chapter 10

Role of Xenobiotic Metabolic Enzymes in Cancer Epidemiology

Madhu S. Singh and Michael Michael

Abstract

The cause of the majority of cancers is poorly understood albeit multifactorial. The ultimate consequence of etiological factors where defined is an alteration within the cellular genotype, which is manifested in the cells acquiring malignant phenotype. There are several environmental carcinogens that contribute to carcinogenesis. These carcinogens are metabolized by a large number of enzymes, including the cytochrome P 450 group, glutathione-S-transferase (GST), the uridine glucuronyl transferase (UGT) superfamily, alcohol-metabolizing enzymes, sulphatases, etc. These enzymes can either inactivate carcinogens or in some cases generate reactive moieties that lead to carcinogenesis.

This review summarises the available evidence regarding the role of xenobiotic metabolic enzymes and their role in cancer epidemiology. The available data and studies have identified correlates between expression of various metabolizing enzymes with risk of malignancies known to be induced by their substrates. The data may have relevance in one population but not for another for a specific malignancy and at times may be conflicting. We believe that with mature data in the future it may be possible to stratify patients by risk.

Key words: Xenobiotic, cancer epidemiology, P450, alcohol dehydrogenase, aldehyde dehydrogenase, glutathione-S-transferase, sulphatase, cancer risk.

1. Introduction

Cancer will most likely be the single largest cause of death worldwide between 2002 and 2030 (1). Despite this, the cause for the majority of cancers is poorly understood albeit multifactorial. The

M. Verma (ed.), *Methods of Molecular Biology, Cancer Epidemiology, vol. 472*
© 2009 Humana Press, a part of Springer Science + Business Media, Totowa, NJ
Book doi: 10.1007/978-1-60327-492-0

ultimate consequence of the etiological factors where defined is an alteration within the cellular genotype, which is then manifested in the cell acquiring the malignant phenotype: the ability to divide in an uncontrollable dysregulated fashion and the potential to metastasize. Aetiological factors include hereditable or acquired mutations in the DNA sequence leading to altered expression of proto-oncogenes and tumor suppressor genes that have been linked to several cancers; for example, chronic myeloid leukemia, where the pathognomic 9:22 chromosomal translocation results in the expression of bcr-abl tyrosine kinase. Similarly, in BRCA-associated breast cancer *(2)*, where cells with BRCA1 and BRCA2 loss-of-function mutations have abnormalities in DNA repair, which starts a cascade of events causing ultimately the initiation of carcinogenesis *(3)*.

There are also several environmental carcinogens that contribute to carcinogenesis. These include microbiological agents. For example, cancer of the cervix is associated with certain subtypes of human papilloma virus, hepatocellular cancer with chronic infection with hepatitis B and C, gastric cancer with chronic infection with *Helicobacter pylori*. A fifth of total cancers worldwide are related to chronic infections *(4)*. Environmental carcinogens include ultraviolet radiation exposure, which is associated with an increased incidence of melanoma, asbestos exposure with mesothelioma and lung adenocarcinoma and tobacco smoke with cancers of the lung and the upper aerodigestive tract.

In terms of environmental carcinogen exposure, these compounds are often dealt with by the body's own array of metabolic enzymes within the mucosal surfaces (lung, gastrointestinal tract, urogenital system, etc.) and the liver. These enzymes families include the cytochrome P450 *(5)*, glutathione-*S*-transferase (GST), and uridine glucuronyl transferases (UGTs) superfamilies, the alcohol-metabolizing enzymes, and sulphatases. The metabolic enzymes are categorized into two distinct groupings (**Table 10.1**): (a) Phase I, where the enzymes catalyse oxidation, reduction, hydroxylation, etc., includes the cytochromes, esterases, and alkoreductases; and (b) Phase II, where the enzymes catalyse conjugation of the Phase I enzyme metabolites with other moieties including glutathione and glucuronide, includes the UGTs and GSTs. These enzymes can either inactivate these compounds or in some cases generate reactive moieties that can lead to carcinogenesis. These metabolic enzymes systems are polymorphic and inducible and hence their activity can vary significantly between individuals. Hence it follows that effects of carcinogen exposures and hence the risk of cancer development may also potentially vary significantly based on these polymorphism distributions.

The role of these metabolic enzyme systems in carcinogenesis and hence their relevance in epidemiological studies identifying the

Table 10.1
The metabolic enzyme categories and their membership

Phase I enzymes	CYP, monoamine oxidase, peroxidases, oxidases, lipoxygenases, monooxygenases, dioxygenases, cyclooxygenases, hydroxylases, epoxygenases, esterases, carboxylesterases, reductases, aldoketoreductases, hydrolases, sulphatases, glycosylases, glucuronidases, aldoketoreductases, reductases, NAD-dependent enzymes
Phase II enzymes	Acetyltransferases, acyltransferases, methyltransferases, transaminases, epoxidases, uridine diphosphate glucuronostyltransferases, glutathione transferases

The classification of enzymes is not rigid and the same enzyme may act as a Phase I and Phase II enzyme under different circumstances

at-risk populations for specific malignancies is reviewed here. Their potential role in screening studies will also be summarised. This review focuses mainly on the cytochrome P450 and the GST systems as they represent the major focus of the reported literature.

2. The Cytochrome P450 System

The cytochrome P450 system is a group of primitive haeme-containing, mainly oxidative enzymes that have a very diverse range of functions. They were first discovered approximately 40 years ago and were temporarily named P function. It was observed by Garfinkel and Klingenberg in 1963 that pigment in liver microsomes had an unusual carbon monoxide-binding pigment with a maximum absorbance at 450 nM. This pigment was subsequently named P450 by Omura and Sato (International Society for the Study of Xenobiotics). The nomenclature of enzymes is based on the amino acid sequence and the reader is referred to a website *(6)* for more information regarding the same.

The CYP enzymes have the most significant role in the Phase I enzyme reaction, which consists of detoxification and metabolic activation through oxidation, reduction, hydroxylation, etc. They are involved in the metabolism of arachidonic acid and its derivatives including prostaglandins, prostacyclins, leukotrienes, thromboxanes (Eicosanoids), cholecalciferol, etc. Many enzymes from the P450 group are involved in epoxidation, reduction, and oxidation of more than 100 eicosanoid moieties involved in maintaining homeostasis. These are involved in several crucial chemical reactions in inflammation, bronchoconstriction, smooth muscle contraction, cell adherence and mitogenesis, renal vaso-constriction, etc. *(7)*.

Approximately 70–80% of the Phase I xenobiotic metabo-lizing enzymes are from the P450 group *(8)*. Xenobiotics are a generic term representing any foreign chemicals including drugs and food that normally exists outside the organism but to which an organism can be exposed *(9)*. Xenobiotics also have a role in drug metabolism/activation and inactivation, drug resistance, and drug interactions. The P450 family of enzymes metabolises over 50% of the therapeutic agents used clinically and their substrates include many of the agents used in oncology *(10)* **(Table 10.2)**.

The P450 groups of enzymes have a key role in carcinogen-esis because of their role in either the activation or deactivation of carcinogens *(5, 11)*. They are involved in the detoxification of potential carcinogens such as chemicals within cigarette smoke including polycyclic aromatic hydrocarbons, N-nitrosamine, aro-matic amines, 1,3-butadiene, and ethylene oxide *(12)*. They may also convert pro-carcinogens to carcinogens *(5, 11)*. Studying the relevant metabolic enzymes therefore may help to risk-strat-ify the population based on genetic and environmental factors (occupational and non-occupational) in terms of development of screening programs for specific cancers as well as to better tailor the pharmacological treatment when a malignancy develops. The latter aspect will not be discussed in this chapter. We first consider the genetic variability of these enzymes and the evidence relating them to the causality of specific malignances, and then focus on specific P450 families and subfamilies.

2.1. The Polymorphic Nature of the CYP P450 System

Humans have 57 CYP genes and 59 pseudo genes divided among 18 families and 43 subfamilies, with variable distribution within organs and tissues, corresponding to their role as first line of defense through xenobiotics metabolism in mucosal surfaces and viscera following oral or inhalational absorption or cellular meta-bolic processes.

In addition to their variable tissue distribution, the genes encoding for them are polymorphic to differing extents. There have been more than 400 alleles documented across the whole family and within the subfamilies. For example, within the CYP2 family, the CYP2B6 subfamily has 48 alleles, the CYP2C9 subfamily has 32, the CYP2D6 subfamily has 92, and within the CYP3A4 subfamily there are 34 alleles. As with any polymorphic enzyme system, the impact of various alleles varies significantly ranging from production of abbreviated proteins or proteins with variable or no catalytic activity i.e. non-functional proteins.

Table 10.2
Substrates (and medications) metabolized by Phase I and II enzymes

Enzyme classes and subclasses	Cytotoxic agent substrates	Pro-carcinogen substrates
Phase I cytochrome P450s		
1A1 Inducible, polymorphic; mainly extrahepatic (lung, GIT, kidney, lymphocytes)	Tamoxifen, toremifene, imatinib, flutamide	Polycyclic aromatic hydrocarbons, benzo(a)pyrene, dimethylbenzanthracene, PhIP
1A2 13% total hepatic CYP, polymorphic, inducible	Tamoxifen, toremifene, flutamide	Aryl and heterocyclic amine activation, N-nitrosodimethylamine, 4-aminobiphenyl, 2-aceto amino fluorene, N-nitrosodiethylamine, PhIP, IQ, aflatoxin B1
1B1 <1% total hepatic CYP, polymorphic, mainly extrahepatic (kidney, skin, breast, prostate, uterus)	Tegafur, docetaxel, flutamide	Polycyclic aromatic hydrocarbons, benzopyrene, dimethylbenz(a) anthracene, benz(a)anthracene, 3-methylcholanthrene, DMBA, estradiol
2A6 4% total hepatic CYP, polymorphic, extrahepatic sites: lung, nasal mucosa, others	Cyclophosphamide, ifosfamide	N-Nitrosamines: NNK, NNAL, NDEA, NNN, NATB, aflatoxin B1, 1,3-butadiene, 2,6-dichlorobenzonitrile
2B6 <1% total hepatic CYP, mainly extrahepatic (lung, GIT)	Tamoxifen Cyclophosphamide, ifosfamide	Low activity Aflatoxin B1 and NNK
2C8[a] Polymorphic Extrahepatic sites: breast Ovary, GIT, kidney	Paclitaxel, all-trans retinoic acid Cyclophosphamide, ifosfamide Tegafur	
2C9 Polymorphic	Tamoxifen Toremifene Imatinib Cyclophosphamide, ifosfamide, Targretin, 9-cis retinoic acid	
2C19 Polymorphic, Mainly extrahepatic (GIT especially duodenum, lower hepatic levels than 2C9)	Tamoxifen Cyclophosphamide, ifosfamide, thalidomide, imatinib	

(continued)

Table 10.2
(continued) Substrates (and medications) metabolized by Phase I and II enzymes

Enzyme classes and subclasses	Cytotoxic agent substrates	Pro-carcinogen substrates
2D6 Mainly hepatic, <2.5% of total hepatic CYP Polymorphic	Vinorelbine, tamoxifen, imatinib	
2E1	Vinorelbine	Low molecular weight toxicants; benzene, carbon tetrachloride, chloroform, vinyl chloride, vinyl bromide, NDEA, NNK
Polymorphic <7% of total hepatic CYP Also lung and others		
CYP 3A4/5/7 3A4: 30% total hepatic CYP 70% total small bowel CYP, also lung, kidney, uterus Inducible	Paclitaxel, docetaxel, vinca alkaloids, etoposide, teniposide, irinotecan, topotecan, gefitinib, imatinib, medroxy-progesterone acetate, tamoxifen, Targretin, 9-cis-retinoic acid, cyclophosphamide, ifosfamide	Aflatoxin B1, aflatoxin G1, benzo(a)pyrene, naphthalene, NNN, 1 nitro pyrene, 6 amino chrysene, estradiol, senecionine, stergmato cysteine
CYP3A5[b] Polymorphic, variable amounts In the liver, also GIT and kidney	Ifosfamide Tamoxifen Paclitaxel	
Non-cytochrome Phase I, II enzymes		
Dihydropyrimidine dehydrogenase Polymorphic Mainly liver and peripheral blood leucocytes, less other tissues	5FU	
Uridine diphospho-glucuronosyltransferases (UGTs) [4, 5] Polymorphic Liver, mucosal surfaces, breast, gonads, prostate	Irinotecan, topotecan, doxorubicin, epirubicin, etoposide, all-trans retinoic acid tamoxifen, flutamide	
Glutathione-S-transferase (GST) [6] Polymorphic Widespread	Substrates that are catalytically conjugated to GSH: chlorambucil, melphalan, nitrosourea, nitrogen mustards, ifosfamide, cyclophosphamide and their active metabolites (phosphoramide mustard and acrolein)	

(continued)

Table 10.2

(continued) Substrates (and medications) metabolized by Phase I and II enzymes

Enzyme classes and subclasses	Cytotoxic agent substrates	Pro-carcinogen substrates
NAD[P] quinone oxidoreduct- ase 1 (NQO1 or DT-Dia- phorase) Polymorphic	Mitomycin C	

GIT, gastrointestinal tract; *PhIP*, 2-amino-1-methyl-6-phenyl imidazo-[4,5-b]pyridine; *CYP*, cyto-chrome; *IQ*, 2-amino-3-methylimidazo[4,5-f]quinoline; *DMBA*, 7,12,-dimethylbenz[a]anthracene; *NNK*, 4-(methylnitrosoamino)-1-(3-pyridyl)-1-butanone; *NNAL*, 4-(methylnitrosoamino)-1-(3-pyridyl)-1-butanol; *NDEA*, N-nitrosodiethylamine; *NNN*, N9-nitrosonornicotine; *NATB*, N-nitrosoanatabine; *5FU*, 5-fluorouracil; *GSH*, glutathione

[a]The cytochrome 2C family contributes 18% of the total hepatic CYP

[b]Cytochrome 3A5 shares most substrates of CYP3A4, referred to here are examples in which 3A5 specifically has been studied

Their distribution and penetrance may also vary within a specific ethnic population.

2.2. The Link Between Cytochrome Expression and Cancer Incidence

Several diseases are epidemiologically linked to defects in specific CYP phenotypes, for example, CYP2D6 and lung cancer *(13)*. There is also data to suggest that some of the enzymes may have protective effect e.g. the GSTP1*C variant possibly has a protective effect in the elderly against pancreatic cancer and imparts a survival advantage in those treated with 5-fluorouracil relative to the wild type; multivariate hazard ratio, 0.45; 95% confidence interval (CI), 0.22–0.94 *(14)*. The relationships between specific CYP families/subfamilies and cancer risk is detailed below.

It must be emphasized that the interaction between pro-carcinogenic and protective or "anti-cancer" effects of these enzymes along with the exact nature and level of exposure of the known relevant carcinogen(s) is quite complex and hence the pathway to cancer induction is also complex. There is obvious substantial variation in enzyme activity within an individual but also variation in the level of exposure to single but often multiple carcinogens. Similarly, the enzyme kinetics may also vary with the level of carcinogen exposure and the effects of concurrent exposure to other xenobiotics on enzyme activity are usually not at all defined.

2.3. CYP1A1 and CYP1A2

CYP1A1 is involved in the metabolism of several hydrophobic aromatic hydrocarbons, including those that are commonly found in cigarette smoke (*see* **Table 10.2**) *(15)*. The enzyme is predominantly expressed extrahepatically *(15)*. Structurally it is very similar to CYP1A2, and CYP1A1 and CYP1A2 have a similar aryl hydrocarbon receptor. CYP1A2 is expressed in the liver.

Both of these enzymes have a role in metabolism of polycyclic aromatic hydrocarbons and polyhalogenated hydrocarbons *(16)*. Both CYP1A1 and CYP1A2 have an aryl hydrocarbon receptor that can bind to estrogen receptors *(17)*, retinoblastoma protein-1 *(18)*, and nuclear factor-κB *(19)*, all of which have a role in carcinogenesis *(20–24)*. Therefore CYP1A1 and CYP1A2 have effects on the cell cycle and can contribute to carcinogenesis. The CYP1A enzyme along with the CYP1B enzyme also catalyses the hydroxylation reaction of estrogen. One particular variant (CYP1A1) has been shown to have been associated with decreased capacity to metabolize estradiol *(25)*.

In a meta-analysis of literature evaluating Phase I/II enzyme polymorphisms and esophageal cancer risk, it was found that individuals with the Ile-Val substitution in the CYP1A1 exon 7 had increased esophageal cancer risk. The odds ratio (OR) for the increased incidence for Ile-Val, Val/Val, and the combined group (Ile-Val, Val/Val) compared with Ile/Ile (wild type) was 1.37 (95% CI: 1.09–1.71), 2.52 (95% CI: 1.62–3.91), and 1.44 (95% CI: 1.17–1.78), respectively *(26)*.

There is data to suggest that the CYP1A1 genotype was not associated with colon or rectal cancer. The presence of GST-M1, a CYP1A1 variant allele, and the *N*-acetyltransferase rapid-acetylator, NAT2, imputed phenotype was associated with increased risk of colon cancer (OR = 1.7; 95% CI: 1.2–2.3). Among men, the greatest colon cancer risk was observed for having any CYP1A1 variant allele and currently smoking (OR = 2.5; 95% CI: 1.3=4.8; Wald χ^2 test: P <0.01) *(27)*.

Landi et al. (2005) genotyped various metabolic enzymes in 377 patients with sporadic colorectal cancer (CRC) and in 326 control subjects *(28)*. They investigated the role of single nucleotide polymorphisms (SNPs) within genes of Phase I (CYP1A1, CYP1A2, CYP1B1, CYP2A6, CYP2D6, CYP2E1, CYP2C9, CYP2C19, CYP3A4, ADH2, and EPHX1) and Phase II (ALDH2, COMT, GSTA2, GSTA4, GSTM1, GSTM3, GSTP1, GSTT2, MTHFR, NAT1, NAT2, NQO1, MnSOD2, SULT1A1, and TPMT) enzymes of xenobiotic metabolism *(28)*. They used oligonucleotide microarray and the arrayed primer extension technique (APEX). *N*-acetyl-transferase 1 "rapid" phenotype and CYP1A2 —164C>A carriers were associated with increased risk of CRC. Also patients homozygous for the allele 48G within CYP1B1, a variant with an increased activity towards several substrates including sex hormones, were at increased risk of developing cancer relative to the wild type (OR = 2.81; 95% CI: 1.32–5.99). Moreover, CYP1A1 SNPs T461N and –1738A>C were associated with a reduced risk of cancer (OR = 0.52; 95% CI: 0.31–0.88; and OR = 0.69; 95% CI: 0.50–0.94 for carriers, respectively) (28).

Another factor in the equation is that these enzymes may be induced by substrates e.g. CYP1A2 has been shown to be induced by cigarette smoking (29). Smoking is associated with an increased risk of CRC. Therefore there may be a complex interaction between the carcinogen (cigarette smoke) the high risk genotype (e.g. CYP1A2 –164C>A) and CYP1A2 induction along with a large number of other factors, many of which are not yet well defined, which determines a person's chance of developing CRC.

2.4. CYP1B1

This extrahepatic enzyme has a role in metabolism in the aromatic hydrocarbons and steroids including estrogens (**Table 10.2**). Several metabolites of estrogen are produced, including 4-hydroxy estrogen (4-OH-E), which is thought to increase risk of breast cancer, and 2OH-E, which is protective (30, 31). Because of these metabolites, CYP1B1 has been implicated in the pathogenesis of both breast (32) and prostrate cancers (33). Estrogen metabolites have also been shown to be associated with an increased risk of carcinogenesis in the kidney (31).

There is some epidemiological correlation between certain CYP1B1 genotypes and ovarian cancer. There is data to suggest that the high-activity Val432 allele of the CYP1B1 gene, which may be linked to oxidative stress through elevated 4-hydroxylated catecholestrogen formation, is associated with an increased risk of ovarian cancer (34). The Val/Leu genotype for CYP1B1 was associated with an OR of 1.8 (95% CI: 1.0–3.3) and the Val/Val genotype with an OR of 3.8 (95% CI: 1.2–11.4) of increased risk of ovarian cancer compared with the wild type Leu/Leu genotype (P = 0.005) (34). Patients who were tobacco smokers with at least one CYP1A1 (MspI) m2 allele were at significantly increased risk of ovarian cancer compared with never-smoking women with an m1/m1 genotype (OR = 2.6; CI: 1.2–6.0). Cancer risk in smokers with one CYP1B1 Val allele was also increased (OR = 3.8; 95% CI: 1.6–9.8) compared with non-smokers and the wild Leu/Leu genotype. Subjects with the catechol-O-methyl transferase (COMT) Met allele or the CYP1A2 A/A alleles were also at significantly increased risk of ovarian cancer (OR = 2.2; 95% CI: 1.0–4.7; OR = 2.6; 95% CI: 1.1–5.9, respectively) compared with the reference population (34).

Certain genotypes may be associated with renal cell cancer. Sasaki et al. (2004) demonstrated that the frequencies of CYP1B1 119T/T and 432G/G genotype were significantly higher in renal cell cancer patients compared with healthy control subjects.

The relative risks were calculated as 3.01 and 2.17 for genotypes 119T/T and 432G/G, respectively, in renal cell carcinoma patients relative to the healthy control subjects (35).

Sasaki (2003) also demonstrated that the distributions of CYP1B1 genotypes at codons 119 and 432 were significantly different between endometrial cancer patients and healthy control subjects. The relative risks of 119T/T and 432G/G in endometrial cancer were calculated as 3.32 and 2.49 compared with wild types (36).

There is also some data to suggest that certain CYP1B1 genotypes may have increased expression in patients with prostate cancer. In an analysis of allelic, genotypic, and haplotype frequencies of 13 SNPs of CYP1B1 among 159 hereditary prostate cancer (HPC) and 245 sporadic prostate cancer patients and 222 unaffected men (33). When each of the SNPs was analysed separately, marginally significant differences were observed for allele frequencies between sporadic cases and controls for three consecutive SNPs (–1001C/T, –263G/A, and –13C/T; P = 0.04–0.07). Similarly, marginally significant differences between sporadic cases and controls in the frequency of variant allele carriers were observed for five consecutive SNPs (–1001C/T, –263G/A, –13C/T, +142C/G, and +355G/T; P = 0.02–0.08) (33).

There is data regarding the role of certain CYP1B1 genotypes with breast and squamous cell lung cancers. The Ala-Ser polymorphism at codon 119, in the presumed substrate recognition site 1, has been associated with the incidence of breast cancer and lung cancer (37). The frequency distribution of the genotypes of Ala-Ser polymorphism in patients with breast cancer was found to be slightly but statistically significantly different from that in 361 healthy control subjects (χ^2 = 8.32; degrees of freedom (d.f.) = 2; P = 0.016) and from that in 238 healthy control women (χ^2 = 6.17; d.f. = 2; P = 0.044). The frequency of CYP1B1 genotype Ser/Ser among lung cancer patients was 2.8-fold higher than that among the healthy control subjects. A positive association was found between the Ala-Ser polymorphism and increased risk to squamous cell carcinoma (SCC) of the lung, a cancer which is most closely associated with cigarette smoking (χ^2 = 7.02; d.f. = 2; P = 0.03) (37).

2.5. The CYP2 Family

The CYP2 family is a large family comprising the subfamilies 2A, 2B, 2C, 2D, and 2E, which will each be considered separately.

2.5.1. CYP2A6

The CYP2A6 enzyme has a role in metabolism of a large number of products of tobacco consumption (**Table 10.2**). In a Japanese study (38), it was found that a particular genotype of this enzyme, CYP2A6*4, has a protective role in smokers against lung cancer. A markedly reduced adjusted OR for lung cancer risk, 0.23 (95% CI: 0.08–0.67), was seen in the group with homozygous deletion (*4/*4) when the OR for a group with homozygous wild type (*1A/*1A) was defined to be 1.00 by logistic regression *(38)*. The (*4/*4) genotype was not found in patients with SCC (0 of 105) or small cell carcinoma (0 of 44), indicating that subjects with the (*4/*4) genotype have low risk for lung cancers, particularly those caused by tobacco smoke *(38)*. A significant reduction of daily cigarette consumption was observed in smokers with the (*4/*4) genotype, suggesting a possibility that complete lack of CYP2A6 affected smoking behavior *(38)*. The CYP2A6 has a role in nicotine metabolism *(39)*, hence individuals with deficiency of this enzyme have reduced nicotine tolerance and thus smoke fewer cigarettes, which may contribute to the lower incidence *(40)*. The other deduction that may be derived from this data is that perhaps due to reduced activity the pro-carcinogens are not converted to more potent metabolites that induce carcinogenesis.

2.5.2. CYP2B6

The CYP2B6 enzyme is found mainly in liver, although it has been found in extrahepatic organs including the skin, kidneys, brain, and lung. CYP2B6 has a major role in the metabolism of several drugs (Table 10.2). CYP2B6 also has a role in testosterone metabolism.

In terms of carcinogenesis, it was observed that a reduced CYP2B6 immunoreactivity in prostate cancer tissue was inversely correlated with a higher Gleason score ($P < 0.001$) and a poorer prognosis ($P < 0.0001$) *(41)*. CYP2B6 has a role in testosterone inactivation in liver *(42)*. It thus appears that reduced CYP2B6 activity contributes to development and progression of prostate cancer through the decreased metabolism of testosterone. Hence the decreased expression of CYP2B6 may be a useful prognostic marker for prostate cancer *(41)*.

2.5.3. CYP2C

The mainly hepatic CYP2C enzyme is involved in the metabolism of a large number of chemotherapeutic drugs **(Table 10.2)**. It has been reported that CYP2C and CYP3A4 messenger RNA (mRNA) expression was significantly reduced in malignant tissue of esophageal SCC in comparison with tissue taken from surrounding areas *(43)*. In a further study where CYP2 profiling was performed on ten breast cancer specimens, it was found that none of specimens had CYP2C18 and CYP2C19, while CYP2C8 and CYP2C9 were found in 100% of the samples *(44)*. However it appears at this juncture that as yet there is no data relating the expression of CYP2C enzymes or genotypic variation within this group and the risk of malignancy.

2.5.4. CYP2D6

The CYP2D6 enzyme has immense importance in the metabolism of several drugs, including anti-cancer drugs (Table 10.2) and carcinogens. Individuals who were extensive metabolisers of debrisoquine, a marker of CYP2D6 activity, were found to have a fourfold increased risk of lung cancer compared with people with slow metabolism (OR = 6.1; 95% CI: 2.2–17.1) *(45)*. This difference was found irrespective of differences in age, gender, smoking history, and occupation *(45)*. Both black and white individuals who were extensive metabolisers of debrisoquine were at significantly increased risk after similar adjustment: for blacks, OR = 4.5; 95% CI: 1.1–18.1; and for whites, OR = 10.2; 95% CI: 2.0–51.4 *(45)*.

Subsequently a few studies were published that have contradicted the findings of Caporaso et al. *(45)*. Certain mutations have been identified at the CYP2D6 locus (CYP2D6*3, CYP2D6*4, CYP2D6*5, and CYP2D6*6A), as well as those mutations that impair but do not abolish enzyme activity (CYP2D6*9 and CYP2D6*10A). Compared with subjects with homozygous inactivating mutations, no association with lung cancer was observed for those with homozygous or heterozygous functional alleles (OR were 0.4 and 0.7, respectively) *(46)*. The risk of lung cancer associated with the CYP2D6 poor-metaboliser genotype (OR = 1.5; 95% CI: 0.5–4.3) did not differ from that in the reference category of extensive-metaboliser and ultra-rapid-metaboliser genotypes combined. Lung cancer risks for the CYP2D6 poor-metaboliser genotype amongst light smokers (tobacco consumption 20 g/day) or heavy smokers (>20 g/day) were not significantly different *(47)*.

There is some data to suggest that there is a protective effect of certain CYP2D6 genotypes in hematological malignancies *(48)*. The CYP2D6*3 variant allele frequency was lower in the overall acute leukemia patients (0.6%) compared with control subjects ($P = 0.03$). The CYP2D6*1/*3 genotype frequency also showed a protective association in incidence of acute myeloid leukemia (AML) (OR = 0.09; 95% CI: 0.01–1.7; $P = 0.04$) *(48)*.

2.5.5. CYP2E1

CYP2E1 has role in metabolism of a large number of aromatic hydrocarbons as well as a role in metabolism of several drugs (Table 10.2). A Turkish group observed a risk association for the presence of the CYP2E1*5 genotype and an increased risk of acute lymphoblastic leukemia (ALL) and AML (OR = 3.6; 95% CI: 1.4–9.4; and OR = 3.9; 95% CI: 1.4–10.5, respectively), relative to the wild type *(48)*. Certain genotypes may also have a protective effect in gastric cancer. The variant allele PstI had been associated with a reduced risk of having gastric cancer (OR = 0.09; 95% CI: 0.01–0.83) *(49)*.

There is some evidence to point a role of CYP2E in women with heavy alcohol consumption and breast cancer. No statistically significant overall differences were seen in the genotype frequencies between breast cancer cases and controls. However, the "ever"-drinking women with the CYP2E1 c2 allele-containing genotypes had a 1.9-fold risk (95% CI: 0.99–3.83) for developing breast cancer compared with non-drinkers with the CYP2E1 c1/c1 genotype ($P = 0.043$) (50).

2.6. CYP3A

The mainly hepatic CYP3A enzyme is single most important enzyme for drug metabolism, accounting for the metabolism of over 50% of currently utilised drugs. CYP3A also metabolizes a large number of carcinogens and thus may have a role in carcinogenesis (**Table 10.2**).

Early menarche is a known breast cancer risk factor (51). The CYP3A4*1B/1B genotype has been found to be associated with early menarche. This variant, which primarily metabolizes testosterone catalyzing its 6-Beta, 2-Beta, and 15-Beta hydroxylation (52), showed a striking association with the onset of puberty (adjusted OR = 3.21; 95% CI: 1.62–6.89) for the homozygotes of the variant relative to the wild-type patients (53). It is hypothesized that this may be due to alteration in ratio of estrogen and testosterone.

There is also some data linking this same genotype to prostate cancer in men with benign prostatic hypertrophy (54). Another study has also reported that this CYP3A4*3 genotype was associated with family history positive prostate cancer (age and race adjusted OR = 5.86; 95% CI: 1.10–31.16) (55).

Cytochrome 3A5 expression is the result of genetic polymorphism and is limited to those individuals who bear the wild-type allele CYP3A5*1. It ranges from 10 to 20% in Caucasians and 40% in the Japanese to 55% in African Americans. CYP3A5 can account for 50% of the total CYP3A protein in these individuals and hence may have a major role in the variation in the CYP3A-mediated drug metabolism (56, 57). From a South African study, there is some evidence to suggest that individuals homozygous for defective CYP3A5 have a reduced risk of developing esophageal cancer ($P = 0.032$) (58). People who are homozygous with a particular genotype of CYP3A5 A6986G have a 0.23-fold decreased chance of developing low-grade prostate cancer ($P = 0.23$) and a 0.31-fold decreased risk of developing localized (Stage A—C) prostrate cancer ($P = 0.044$). The CYP3A5 A6986G polymorphism may be specifically associated with decreased risk of low-grade and early stage prostate cancer (59).

The relationship between CYP3A5 genotypes and prostate cancer is, however, not consistent. The association between CYP3A4 and five gene variants has been evaluated in a study of 622 incident prostate cancer patients and 396 control subjects (55). No association of CYP3A5 genotypes with prostate cancer and disease severity was found in this study. CYP3A43*3 was associated with family history-positive prostate cancer (age- and race-adjusted OR = 5.86; 95% CI: 1.10–31.16). CYP3A4*1B was associated inversely with the probability of having prostate cancer in Caucasians (age-adjusted OR = 0.54; 95% CI: 0.32–0.94) *(55)*.

3. The GST Family

The GST family is a family of Phase II detoxification enzymes that have a role in the conjugation of glutathione to a number of xenobiotics (**Table 10.2**). This has a role in protecting the cell from environment and oxidative stress. Unfortunately this can also manifest as accelerated detoxification of a drug from the cell leading to acquired resistance to the chemotherapeutic agents. The GST family is divided into three families: cytosolic, mitochondrial, and membrane-bound microsomal *(60)*. Five subclasses of GST enzymes have also been described (α, π, μ, θ, and ζ) and three polymorphisms (in the GSTπ-1, GSTθ-1, and GSTμ-1 genes) have been reported to decrease or abolish GST activity, i.e. the null genotypes. GST levels, in particular the GSTπ1 isozyme, have been found to be overexpressed in many tumor types relative to normal tissue, including ovarian, colonic, lung, and gastric cancers *(56)*.

There is some emerging evidence of the role of this family of enzymes with several cancers. The GSTμ-1 polymorphism was associated with an increased risk of developing CRC (OR = 1.62; 95% CI: 1.06–2.46) *(61)*. The risk of CRC associated with the GSTT1-null genotype was increased by a factor of 1.64 (95% CI: 1.10–2.59). There was no difference observed for the GSTπ-1 genotype *(61)*. Another study *(62)* has reconfirmed these results and also reported that patients with simultaneous GSTμ-1 and GSTθ-1 null genotypes had an even greater relative risk of developing this malignancy (OR = 4.98; 95% CI: 2.77–9.00) *(62)*. This group also reported an increased incidence of gastric cancer with the GSTθ-1-null genotype (OR = 2.58; 95% CI: 1.53–4.36) and for patients with simultaneous carriage with GSTM1- and GSTT1-null (OR = 3.32; 95% CI: 1.62–6.77). Carriers of GSTπ-1 104Val/Val had reduced risk of gastric cancer (OR = 0.20; 95% CI: 0.02–0.86). The GSTπ-1 Ile/Val genotype and Val allele had also been associated with gall bladder cancer risk (P = 0.013; OR = 1.9; 95% CI: 1.3–3.1; P = 0.027; OR =1.5; 95% CI: 1.0–2.1, respectively) *(63)*.

There is also evidence regarding the role of GST mutations in the risk of lung cancer in smokers. Schneider et al. showed that the GSTπ-1-null genotype expression was associated with a 34% increased risk of lung cancer (OR = 1.34; 95% CI: 0.99–1.81) that the GSTθ-1-null genotype was associated with a reduced risk (OR = 0.88; 95% CI: 0.59–1.32) relative to the wild-type patients *(64)*. Stratified analysis between tobacco smoking and variant genotypes revealed that heavy smokers (>60 pack years) had an increasing risk for the presence of at least one copy of the GSTπ-1 variant allele (OR = 50.56; 95% CI: 15.52–164.79). The corresponding risk for the GSTμ-1-null genotype was OR = 112.08 (95% CI: 23.02–545.71) and for the GSTθ-1-null genotype was OR = 158.49 (95% CI: 17.75–1,415.06) in smokers with greater than 60 pack years (64).

4. Alcohol Dehydrogenase and Aldehyde Dehydrogenase

Alcohol (ethanol) consumption has been implicated as a risk factor for oral cavity, pharynx, hypopharynx, larynx, and esophageal cancers (65). It has a role in development of primary liver cancer (66), as well as in colorectal and breast cancers (65). Alcohol is a known mutagen and carcinogen (67, 68).

There are several enzymes involves in the metabolism of alcohol, key enzymes include alcohol dehydrogenase (ALD), which converts alcohol to acetaldehyde (65). Aldehyde dehydrogenase (ALDH) is involved in the metabolism of acetaldehyde. ALDH polymorphisms and expression have been extensively studied in terms of cancer risk and carcinogenesis in relation to alcohol-related malignancies. There is some evidence to suggest that acetaldehyde has a greater role in causing alcohol-related cancers. Acetaldehyde causes mutation by formation of DNA—DNA and/or DNA—protein cross-links (68).

The ADH1B histidine allele at codon 48 has been associated with a decreased risk of upper aerodigestive tract cancer; OR = 0.36 (95% CI: 0.17–0.77) for medium/heavy drinkers and 0.57 (95% CI: 0.36–0.91) for never/light drinkers, respectively (69). Medium/heavy drinkers who were heterozygous or homozygous at the ALDH2 nucleotide position 248 were at a significantly increased risk of upper aerodigestive tract cancer (OR = 1.76; 95% CI: 1.13–2.75; and OR = 5.79; 95% CI: 1.49–22.5, respectively), with a significant dose response for carrying variant alleles ($P = 0.0007$) (69).

There is also early data to associate alcohol consumption with the risk of lung cancer, partially mediated by ADH and ALDH. In a case—control study, a significant association was noted between alcohol consumption and the risk of lung cancer (70). The ORs for light and heavy drinkers were 1.76 and 1.95, respectively ($P = 0.12$). The risk of lung cancer in alcohol consumers who also had the ALDH2 variant allele was increased ($P < 0.0001$) relative to patients with the wild-type allele. The adjusted OR for heavy drinkers bearing this variant allele was 6.15 compared with non-drinkers with this allele (70).

It was observed that compared with non-drinkers with the ADH3(1—1) genotype, consumers of at least 57 alcoholic drinks per week with the ADH3(1-1), ADH3(1-2), and ADH3(2-2) genotypes had 40.1-fold (95% CI: 5.4–296.0), 7.0-fold (95% CI: 1.4–35.0), and 4.4-fold (95% CI: 0.6–33.0) increased risk of oral cancer, respectively *(71)*. The risk associated with the ADH3(1-1) genotype, compared with the ADH3(1-2) and ADH3(2-2) genotypes combined, was 5.3 (95% CI: 1.0–28.8) among such drinkers *(71)*.

Individuals with ADH1B*1/*1 genotype have also been found to have a 3.99-fold increased risk (95% CI: 2.13–7.48) of developing esophageal cancer compared with those with the ADH1B*2/*2 genotype, after adjusting for the appropriate covariates. Individuals with ALDH2*1/*2 and ALDH2*2/*2 had a 4.99-fold risk (95% CI: 3.11–7.99) and 4.24-fold risk (95% CI: 1.52–11.84), respectively, of developing esophageal cancer compared with those with ALDH2*1/*1 after adjusting for the appropriate covariates *(72)*.

In another study, people with the combined genotypes ADH2(1)/ADH2(1) and ALDH2(1)/ALDH2(2) were at extraordinarily high risk for esophageal SCC, with an OR of 17.9 ($P < 0.001$) *(73)*.

5. Sulphatase

This group of enzymes has a role in the metabolism of estrogen. Sulphatase (STS) hydrolyzes steroid sulfates, such as estrone sulfate and dehydroepiandrosterone sulfate (DHEAS), to estrone and DHEA, which can be converted to steroids with potent estrogenic properties, that is, estradiol and androstenediol, respectively *(74)*. They may have a role in aetiology of breast cancer. Certain genotypes in the genes coding for the sulfatases have been associated with higher risk of breast cancer. The genetic polymorphisms of the estrogen-related genes SULT1A1 (OR = 2.5; 95% CI: 1.28–4.98) and CYP17 (OR = 4.1; 95% CI: 1.78–9.63) were associated with an increased risk of breast cancer among postmenopausal women compared with the wild type *(75)*.

These may also have a role in the pathological characteristics of the tumor at the time of presentation. The SULT1A1*1/*1 high-activity genotype was associated with tumor size ≤2 cm (OR = 2.63; 95% CI: 1.25–5.56; $P = 0.02$), possibly due to estrogen inactivation *(76)*.

These may have some role of development of endometrial cancer in women who take estrogen. A statistically significant interaction has been observed between estrogen-replacement therapy use in patients bearing the SULT1A1*2 genotype *(77)*. Patients with the SULT1A1*2 allele who had long-term use of estrogen-replacement therapy were associated with statistically significantly higher risk of endometrial cancer (adjusted OR = 3.85; 95% CI: 1.48 to 10.00) than those patients bearing the SULT1A1*2 allele but with no estrogen-replacement therapy use *(77)*.

SULT1A1 has also been implicated in the risk of lung cancer *(78)*. A cohort of 463 Caucasian patients and 485 matched controls were assessed for the SULT1A1*2 variant allele, which has been associated with decreased activity and thermal stability of the SULT1A1 enzyme. There was an overall significant increase in difference between cases and controls when adjusted by sex and smoking status (adjusted OR = 1.41; 95% CI: 1.04–1.91). The adjusted OR was higher for women (OR = 1.64; 95% CI: 1.06–2.56) than for men (OR = 1.23; 95% CI: 0.80–1.88). Furthermore, the risk was significantly higher in current smokers (OR = 1.74; 95% CI: 1.08–2.29) and heavy smokers (OR = 1.45; 95% CI: 1.05–2.00) *(78)*.

A particular allele, SULT1 His 213, has been associated with esophageal cancer in non-smokers, non-drinker, and Areca non-chewers *(79)*. The study conduced in Taiwan comprised of a cohort of 188 patients and 308 controls. After adjusting for substance use and other covariates, individuals with the Arg/His variant had a 3.53-fold higher risk (95% CI: 2.12–5.87) of developing esophageal cancer than those with the wild-type Arg/Arg. Unexpectedly, this positive association was found to be even stronger (adjusted OR = 4.04–4.80) among non-smokers, non-drinkers, or Areca non-chewers *(79)*.

6. Discussion

The data and studies summarized in this chapter have identified correlates between the expression of various xenobiotics-metabolizing enzymes, whether the native enzyme or genetic variants, with the risk of various malignancies known to be induced by their substrates. The studies have varied substantially in terms of the populations assessed and in particular their relative exposures and types of environmental carcinogens, the interaction of other concurrent risk factors for specific malignancy. Similarly the detection techniques and genetic variants of the enzymes assessed have also varied from study to study. The correlations can be conflicting and may be relevant for one population but not for another for a specific malignancy.

The question remains whether the expression of these enzymes or their polymorphic variants can be used to identify at-risk populations and that may then lead to an increase in surveillance, or a reduction of environmental exposure or at-risk behavior, leading to a decrease in cancer incidence. At this current stage to the best of our knowledge, there have been no reported studies that have achieved these aims.

To achieve this aim, specific factors must be incorporated within future well-powered prospective trials. The at-risk population must be identified from observational and populations studies where the risk of cancer has been related to the possible exposure of specific environmental or endogenous xenobiotics. The relevant carcinogen or pro-carcinogen must be well characterized, and these will obviously differ for each population, whether derived from specific industries or geographical regions or ethnic groups or those with at-risk social behaviors. Similarly the relevant enzymes as well their related genetic variants (inactivating or high activity alleles) must also be well characterized and demonstrate a reasonable frequency and penetrance within the specific population. The malignancy itself must represent a major health problem within the populations assessed in order to make any preventative measures economically feasible.

Other additional risk factors related to an increased malignancy risk must be considered simultaneously. These may include family history, social history, additional xenobiotics exposure (drug, tobacco, alcohol, industrial compounds, etc.). Their interaction with the xenobiotic metabolizing enzyme expression in relation to cancer risk must be fully evaluated. The impact of the enzyme expression may be independent of these other risk factors or codependent, reducing or amplifying their importance. Germline microarray genetic and serum proteomic analysis may also be relevant here. The studies finally must be appropriately powered to demonstrate a meaningful correlation of these factors with the cancer risk.

Hence, the at-risk population needs to well characterized and the relevant etiological factors for the specific malignancy fully defined. Once these have been achieved, the efficacy of screening programs or changes in work social or practices in economically reducing cancer incidence can be properly assessed through prospective trials.

References

1. Mathers CD. Projection of Global Mortality and Burden of Disease from 2002 to 2030. WHO 2006.
2. Key TJ, Verkasalo PK, Banks E. Epidemiology of breast cancer. Lancet Oncology 2001; 2:133.
3. Boulton SJ. Cellular functions of the BRCA tumour-suppressor proteins. Biochem Soc Trans. 2006; 34(Pt 5):633–645.
4. www.who.int/mediacentre/factsheets/fs297/en/index.html.
5. Gonzalez FJ, Gelboin HV. Role of human cytochromes 450 in the metabolic activation of chemical carcinogens and toxins. Drug Metab Rev 1994; 26:165–183.
6. www.drnelson.utmem.edu.
7. Capdevila Harris RC, Falck JR: Microsomal P450 function and Eicosanoid metabolism: Cell Mol Life Science 2002; 59(5):780–789.
8. Evans WE, Relling MV. Pharmacogenomics: translating functional genomics into rational therapeutics. Science 1999; 286:487–491.

9. Nebert DW, Dalton TD. The role of cytochrome P450 enzymes in endogenous signaling pathways and environmental carcinogenesis. Nat Rev Cancer 2006; 6:947–960.

10. Rendic S, DiCarlo FJ. Human cytochrome P 450 enzymes: Status report summarizing their reactions, substrates, inducers and inhibitors. Drug Metab Rev 1997; 29:413–580.

11. Windmill KF, McKinnon RA, Zhu X, Gaedigk A, Grant DM, McManus ME. The role of xenobiotic metabolizing enzymes in arylamine toxicity and carcinogenesis: functional and localization studies. Mutat Res 1997 May 12; 376(1–2):153–160.

12. Hecht SS . Biochemistry, biology and carcinogenicities of Tobacco Specific N-Nitrosamines Chem Res Toxicology 1998; June, Vol 11 No. 6, 560–603.

13. Caporaso N, Hayes RB, Dosemeci M, Hoover R, Ayesh R, Hetzel M, Idle J. Lung cancer risk, occupational exposure, and the Debrisoquine metabolic phenotype. Cancer Res 1989; 49:3675–3679.

14. Jiao L, Bondy ML, Hassan MM, Chang DZ, Abbruzzese JL, Evans DB, Smolensky MH, Li D: Glutathione S-transferase gene polymorphisms and risk and survival of pancreatic cancer. Cancer 2007; 109(5):840–848.

15. Rodriguez-Antona C, Ingelman-Sundberg M. Cytochrome P450 pharmacogenetics and cancer. Oncogene 2006; 25:1679–1691.

16. Nebert DW, Dalton TP, Okey AB, Gonzalez FJ. Role of aryl hydrocarbon receptor-mediated induction of the CYP1 enzymes in environmental toxicity and cancer. J Biol Chem 2004; 279(23):23847–23850.

17. Ohtake F, Takeyama K, Matsumoto T, Kitagawa H, Yamamoto Y, Nohara K, Tohyama C, Krust A, Mimura J, Chambon P, Yanagisawa J, Fujii-Kuriyama Y, Kato S. Modulation of oestrogen receptor signaling by association with the activated dioxin receptor. Nature 2003; 423:545–550.

18. Puga A Barnes SJ, Dalton TP, Chang C, Knudsen ES, Maier MA. Aromatic hydrocarbon receptor interaction with retinoblastoma protein potentiates repression of E2F dependent transcription and cell cycle arrest. J Biol Chem 2000; 275:2943–2950.

19. Currier N, Solomon SE, Demicco EG, Chang DL, Farago M, Ying H, Dominguez I, Sonenshein GE, Cardiff RD, Xiao ZX, Sherr DH, Seldin DC. Oncogenic signaling pathways activated in DMBA-induced mouse mammary tumors. Toxicol Pathol 2005; 33:726–737.

20. Momand J Wu HH, Dasgupta G. MDM2—master regulator of the p53 tumor suppressor protein. Gene 2000; 242 (1–2): 15–29.

21. Liehr JG. Dual role of oestrogens as hormones and pro-carcinogens: tumour initiation by metabolic activation of oestrogens. Eur J Cancer Prev 1997; 6:3–10.

22. Zumoff B. Does postmenopausal estrogen administration increase the risk of breast cancer? Contributions of animal, biochemical, and clinical investigative studies to a resolution of the controversy. Proc Soc Exp Biol Med 1998; 217:30–7.

23. Russo J, Hasan Lareef M, Balogh G, Guo S, Russo IH. Estrogen and its metabolites are carcinogenic agents in human breast epithelial cells. J Steroid Biochem Mol Biol 2003; 87:1–25.

24. Basseres D, Baldwin Jr AS. Nuclear factor- B and inhibitor of B kinase pathways in oncogenic initiation and progression. Oncogene 2006; 25:6817–6830.

25. Aklillu E, Oscarson M, Hidestrand M, Leidvik B, Otter C, Ingelman-Sundberg M, et al. Functional analysis of six different polymorphic CYP1B1 enzyme variants found in an Ethiopian population. Mol Pharmacol 2002; 61(3):586–594.

26. Yang CX, Matsuo K, Wang ZM, Tajima K, et al. Phase I/II enzyme gene polymorphisms and esophageal cancer: a meta-analysis of the literature. World J Gastroenterol 2005; 11:2531–2538.

27. Slattery ML, Samowtiz W, Ma K, Murtaugh M, Sweeney C, Levin TR, Neuhausen S. CYP1A1, cigarette smoking, and colon and rectal cancer. Am J Epidemiol 2004; 160;842–852.

28. Landi S, Gemignani F, Moreno V, Gioia-Patricola L, Chabrier A, Guino E, Navarro M, de Oca J, Capellà G, Canzian F; Bellvitge Colorectal Cancer Study Group. Comprehensive analysis of phase I and phase II metabolism gene polymorphisms and risk of colorectal cancer. Pharmacogenet Genomics 2005; 15(8):535–546.

29. Rasmussen BB, Brix TH, Kyvik KO, Brøsen K. The Interindividual differences in the 3-demethylation of caffeine alias CYP1A2 is determined by both genetic and environmental factors. Pharmacogenetics. 2002; 12(6):473–478.

30. Van Ashwegen CH, Purdy RH, Wittliff JL. Binding of 2-hydroxyestradiol and 4-hydroxyestradiol to estrogen receptors from human breast cancers. J Steroid Biochem 1989; 32(4):485–492.

31. Zhu BT, Conney AH. Is 2-methoxyestradiol an endogenous estrogen metabolite that inhibits mammary carcinogenesis? Cancer Res 1998; 58(11):2269–2277.

32. Hanna IH, Dawling S, Roodi N, Guengerich FP, Parl FF. Cytochrome P450 1B1 (CYP1B1) pharmacogenetics: association of polymorphism with functional differences in estrogen hydroxylation activity. Cancer Res 2000; 60:3440–3444.

33. Chang BL, Zheng SL, Isaacs SD, Turner A, Hawkins GA, Wiley KE, Bleecker ER, Walsh PC, Meyers DA, Isaacs WB, Xu J. Polymorphisms in the CYP1B1 gene are associated with increased risk of prostate cancer. Br J Cancer 2003; 89(8):1524–1529.

34. Goodman MT, McDuffie K, Kolonel LN, Terada K, Donlon TA, Wilkens LR, Guo C, Le Marchand L. Case-control study of ovarian cancer and polymorphisms in genes involved in catecholestrogen formation and metabolism. Cancer Epidemiol Biomarkers Prev 2001; 10(3):209–216.

35. Sasaki M, Tanaka Y, Okino ST, Nomoto M, Yonezawa S, Nakagawa M, Fujimoto S, Sakuragi N, Dahiya R. et al. Polymorphisms of the CYP1B1 gene as risk factors for human renal cell cancer. Clin Cancer Res 2004; 10(6):2015–2019.

36. Sasaki M, Tanaka Y, Kaneuchi M, Sakuragi N, Dahiya R. CYP1B1 gene polymorphisms have higher risk for endometrial cancer, and positive correlations with estrogen receptor and estrogen receptor β expressions. Cancer Res 2003; 63(14):3913–3918.

37. Watanabe J, Shimada T, Gillam EM, Ikuta T, Suemasu K, Higashi Y, Gotoh O, Kawajiri K, et al. Association of CYP1B1 genetic polymorphism with incidence to breast and lung cancer. Pharmacogenetics 2000; 10(1):25–33.

38. Ariyoshi N, Miyamoto M, Umetsu Y, Kunitoh H, Dosaka-Akita H, Sawamura Y, Yokota J, Nemoto N, Sato K, Kamataki T, et al. Genetic polymorphism of CYP2A6 gene and tobacco-induced lung cancer risk in male smokers. Cancer Epidemiol Biomarkers Prev 2002; 11(9):890–894.

39. Nakajima M, Yamamoto T, Nunoya K, Yokoi T, Nagashima K, Inoue K, Funae Y, Shimada N, Kamataki T, Kuroiwa Y. Role of human cytochrome P4502A6 in C-oxidation of nicotine. Drug Metab Dispos 1996; 24(11):1212–1217.

40. Benowitz NL, Pérez-Stable EJ, Herrera B, Jacob P 3rd. Slower metabolism and reduced intake of nicotine from cigarette smoking in Chinese-Americans J Natl Cancer Inst 2002; 94(2):108–115.

41. Kumagai J, Fujimura T, Takahashi S, Urano T, Ogushi T, Horie-Inoue K, Ouchi Y, Kitamura T, Muramatsu M, Blumberg B, Inoue S. Cytochrome P450 2B6 is a growth-inhibitory and prognostic factor for prostate cancer. Prostate 2007; 67(10):1029–1037.

42. Waxman DJ, Attisano C, Guengerich FP, Lapenson DP. Human liver microsomal steroid metabolism: identification of the major microsomal steroid hormone 6 beta-hydroxylase cytochrome P-450 enzyme. Arch Biochem Biophys 1988; 263(2):424–436.

43. Bergheim I, Wolfgarten E, Bollschweiler E, Hölscher AH, Bode C, Parlesak A. Cytochrome P450 levels are altered in patients with esophageal squamous-cell carcinoma. World J Gastroenterol 2007; 13(7):997–1002.

44. Knupfer H, Schmidt R, Stanitz D, et al. CYP2C and IL-6 expression in breast cancer. Breast 2004; 343(44):28–34.

45. Caporaso NE, Tucker MA, Hoover RN, Hayes RB, Pickle LW, Issaq HJ, Muschik GM, Green-Gallo L, Buivys D, Aisner S, et al. Lung cancer and the debrisoquine metabolic phenotype: J Natl Cancer Inst 1990; 82(15):1264–1272.

46. Shaw GL, Falk RT, Frame JN, Weiffenbach B, Nesbitt JC, Pass HI, Caporaso NE, Moir DT, Tucker MA. Genetic polymorphism of CYP2D6 and lung cancer risk. Cancer Epidemiol Biomarkers Prev 1998; 7(3):215–219.

47. Laforest. L, Wikman H, Benhamou S, Saarikoski ST, Bouchardy C, Hirvonen A, Dayer P, Husgafvel-Pursiainen K. CYP2D6 gene polymorphism in Caucasian smokers: lung cancer susceptibility and phenotype-genotype relationships. Eur J Cancer 2000; 36(14):1825–1832.

48. Aydin-Sayitoglu M, Hatirnaz O, Erensoy N, Ozbek U, et al. Role of CYP2D6, CYP1A1, CYP2E1, GSTT1, and GSTM1 genes in the susceptibility to acute leukemias. Am J Hematol 2006; 81(3):162–170.

49. Gonzalez A, Ramírez V, Cuenca P, Sierra R. Polymorphisms in detoxification genes CYP1A1, CYP2E1, GSTT1 and GSTM1 in gastric cancer susceptibility Rev Biol Trop 2004; 52(3):591–600.

50. Choi JY, Abel J, Neuhaus T, Ko Y, Harth V, Hamajima N, Tajima K, Yoo KY, Park SK, Noh DY, Han W, Choe KJ, Ahn SH, Kim SU, Hirvonen A, Kang D. Role of alcohol and genetic polymorphisms of CYP2E1 and ALDH2 in breast cancer development. Pharmacogenetics 2003; 13(2):67–72.

51. Petridou E, Syrigou E, Toupadaki N, Zavitsanos X, Willett W, Trichopoulos D. Determinants of age at menarche as early life predictors of breast cancer risk. Int J Cancer 1996; 68:193–198.

52. Waxman DJ, Attisano C, Guengerich FP, Lapenson DP. Human liver microsomal steroid metabolism: identification of the major microsomal steroid hormone 6 beta-hydroxylase cytochrome P-450 enzyme. Arch Biochem Biophys 1988; 263(2):424–436.

53. Kadlubar FF, Berkowitz GS, Delongchamp RR, Wang C, Green BL, Tang G, Lamba J, Schuetz E, Wolff MS, et al. The CYP3A4*1B variant is related to the onset of puberty, a known risk factor for the development of breast cancer. Cancer Epidemiol Biomarkers Prev 2003; 12(4):327–331.

54. Keshava C, McCanlies EC, Weston A, et al. CYP3A4 polymorphisms—potential risk factors for breast and prostate cancer: a HuGE review. Am J Epidemiol 2004; 160(9):825–841.

55. Zeigler-Johnson C, Friebel T, Walker AH, Wang Y, Spangler E, Panossian S, Patacsil M, Aplenc R, Wein AJ, Malkowicz SB, Rebbeck TR. CYP3A4, CYP3A5, and CYP3A43 genotypes and haplotypes in the etiology and severity of prostate cancer. Cancer Res 2004; 64(22):8461 8467.

56. Michael M, Doherty MM. Tumoral drug metabolism: overview and its implications for cancer therapy. J Clin Oncol 2005; 23:205–229.

57. Lamba JK, Lin YS, Schuetz EG, Thummel KE. Genetic contribution to variable human CYP3A-mediated metabolism. Adv Drug Deliv Rev 2002; 54:1271–1294.

58. Dandara C, Ballo R, Parker MI, et al. CYP3A5 genotypes and risk of oesophageal cancer in two South African populations. Cancer Lett. 2005; 225(2):275–282.

59. Zhenhua L, Tsuchiya N, Narita S, Inoue T, Horikawa Y, Kakinuma H, Kato T, Ogawa O, Habuchi T. CYP3A5 gene polymorphism and risk of prostate cancer in a Japanese population. Cancer Letters 2005; 225(2):237–243.

60. McIlwain CC, Townsend DM, Tew KD, et al. Glutathione S-transferase polymorphisms: cancer incidence and therapy. Oncogene 2006; 25:1639–1648.

61. Ates NA, Tamer L, Ates C, Ercan B, Elipek T, cal K, Camdeviren H, et al. Glutathione S-transferase M1, T1, P1 genotypes and risk for development of colorectal cancer. Biochem Genet 2005; 43(3–4):149–163.

62. Martinez C, Martín F, Fernández JM, García-Martín E, Sastre J, Díaz-Rubio M, Agúndez JA, Ladero JM, et al. Glutathione S-transferases mu 1, theta 1, pi 1, alpha 1 and mu 3 genetic polymorphisms and the risk of colorectal and gastric cancers in humans. Pharmacogenomics 2006; 7(5):711–718.

63. Pandey SN, Jain M, Nigam P, Choudhuri G, Mittal B, et al. Genetic polymorphisms in GSTM1, GSTT1, GSTP1, GSTM3 and the susceptibility to gallbladder cancer in North India. Biomarkers 2006; 11(3):250–261.

64. Schneider J, Bernges U, Philipp M, Woitowitz HJ. GSTM1, GSTT1, and GSTP1 polymorphism and lung cancer risk in relation to tobacco smoking. Cancer Lett 2004; 208(1):65–74.

65. Seitz HK, Pöschl G, Simanowski UA. Alcohol and cancer. Recent Dev Alcohol 1998; 14:67–95.

66. Stickel F, Schuppan D, Hahn EG, Seitz HK. Cocarcinogenic effects of alcohol in hepatocarcinogenesis. Gut 2002; 51(1):132–139.

67. Obe G, Ristow H. Mutagenic, cancerogenic and teratogenic effects of alcohol. Mutat Res 1979; 65(4):229–259.

68. Dellarco VL, et al. A mutagenicity assessment of acetaldehyde. Mutat Res 1988; 195:1–20.

69. Hashibe M, Boffetta P, Zaridze D, Shangina O, Szeszenia-Dabrowska N, Mates D, Janout V, Fabiánová E, Bencko V, Moullan N, Chabrier A, Hung R, Hall J, Canzian F, Brennan P. Evidence for an important role of alcohol- and aldehyde-metabolizing genes in cancers of the upper aerodigestive tract. Cancer Epidemiol Biomarkers Prev 2006; 15(4).

70. Minegishi Y, Tsukino H, Muto M, Goto K, Gemma A, Tsugane S, Kudoh S, Nishiwaki Y, Esumi H, et al. Susceptibility to lung cancer and genetic polymorphisms in the alcohol metabolite-related enzymes alcohol dehydrogenase 3, aldehyde dehydrogenase 2, and cytochrome P450 2E1 in the Japanese population. Cancer 2007; 110(2):353–362.

71. Harty LC, Caporaso NE, Hayes RB, Winn DM, Bravo-Otero E, Blot WJ, Kleinman DV, Brown LM, Armenian HK, Fraumeni JF Jr, Shields PG, et al. Alcohol dehydrogenase 3 genotype and risk of oral cavity and pharyngeal cancers. J Natl Cancer Inst 1997; 89:1698–1705.

72. Chen YJ, Chen C, Wu DC, Lee CH, Wu CI, Lee JM, Goan YG, Huang SP, Lin CC, Li TC, Chou YP, Wu MT. Interactive effects of lifetime alcohol consumption and alcohol and aldehyde dehydrogenase polymorphisms

on esophageal cancer risks. Int J Cancer 2006; 119(12):2827–2831.

73. Hori H, Kawano T, Endo M, Yuasa Y. Genetic polymorphisms of tobacco- and alcohol-related metabolizing enzymes and human esophageal squamous cell carcinoma susceptibility. J Clin Gastroenterol 1997; 25(4):568–575.

74. Stanway SJ, Delavault P, Purohit A, Woo LW, Thurieau C, Potter BV, Reed MJ, et al. Steroid sulfatase: a new target for the endocrine therapy of breast cancer. Oncologist 2007; 12:370–374.

75. Chacko P, Rajan B, Mathew BS, Joseph T, Pillai MR. CYP17 and SULT1A1 gene polymorphisms in Indian breast cancer. Breast Cancer 2004; 11(4):380–388.

76. Shatalova EG, Walther SE, Favorova OO, Rebbeck TR, Blanchard RL. Genetic polymorphisms in human SULT1A1 and UGT1A1 genes associate with breast tumor characteristics: a case-series study. Breast Cancer Res 2005; 7(6):R909–921.

77. Rebbeck TR, Troxel AB, Wang Y, Walker AH, Panossian S, Gallagher S, Shatalova EG, Blanchard R, Bunin G, DeMichele A, Rubin SC, Baumgarten M, Berlin M, Schinnar R, Berlin JA, Strom BL, et al. Estrogen sulfation genes, hormone replacement therapy, and endometrial cancer risk. J Natl Cancer Inst 2006; 98(18):1311–1320.

78. Wang Y Y, Spitz MR, Tsou AM, Zhang K, Makan N, Wu X. Sulfotransferase (SULT) 1A1 polymorphism as a predisposition factor for lung cancer: a case-control analysis. Lung Cancer 2002; 35(2):137–142.

79. Wu MT, Wang YT, Ho CK, Wu DC, Lee YC, Hsu HK, Kao EL, Lee JM. SULT1A1 polymorphism and esophageal cancer in males. Int J Cancer 2003; 103(1):101–104.

Chapter 11

Genetic Polymorphisms in the Transforming Growth Factor-β Signaling Pathways and Breast Cancer Risk and Survival

Wei Zheng

Abstract

The transforming growth factor (TGF)-β signaling pathway plays a critical role in breast cancer development and progression. Limited data from human studies, however, are currently available to link biomarkers in this pathway directly to the risk and survival of breast cancer. Most of the previous epidemiologic studies have focused on evaluating polymorphisms in the *TGFB1* gene (*T+29C*, rs1982073) and the *TGFBR1* gene (*9A/6A*), and the results have been inconsistent. The present review summarizes epidemiologic evidence regarding the association of genetic polymorphisms in the TGFβ pathway genes with breast cancer risk and survival and provides rationale and new approaches to continuing the research in this area.

Key words: Breast cancer, genetic factors, genetic polymorphisms, survival, susceptibility, transforming growth factor-β, TGFβ.

1. Introduction

The transforming growth factor (TGF)-β signaling pathway has been the focus of extensive research over the past two decades since it was first discovered in 1981 *(1, 2)*. It has now been well established that this signaling pathway plays a critical role in the development and progression of a large number of human cancers, including cancers of the breast, colon, lung, prostate, and pancreas, as described in several recent reviews *(3–6)*. In human tissues, three TGFβ ligands have been identified and characterized; they are TGFβ1, TGFβ2, and TGFβ3. Each is encoded by a unique gene (*TGFB1*, *TGFB2*, or *TGFB3*). TGFβ1 is the most abundant and universally expressed isoform and, thus, has been the focus of

M. Verma (ed.), *Methods of Molecular Biology, Cancer Epidemiology, vol. 472*
© 2009 Humana Press, a part of Springer Science + Business Media, Totowa, NJ
Book doi: 10.1007/978-1-60327-492-0

many previous studies, including the majority of epidemiological studies conducted thus far to evaluate the association of genetic polymorphisms in the TGFβ pathway genes with breast cancer risk.

TGFβs are cytokines that have been shown to regulate a number of cell functions involved in cell growth, differentiation, and survival (3–6). The signaling of TGFβs is mediated through interaction with their receptors (TβRI, TβRII, and TβRIII) and commences with the binding of TGFβ ligands to the type II TGFβ receptor (TβRII), a transmembrane receptor Ser/Thr protein kinase. In some cells, the binding of ligands to TβRII is accomplished through their interaction with TβRIII. In particular, the presentation of TGFβ2 by TβRIII is critical for its binding to TβRII and the initiation of TGFβ2 signaling. The ligand-bound TβRII complex has a high affinity for binding to and transactivating the type I receptor (TβRI), which in turn activates the transcription regulators mothers against decapentaplegic homolog (SMAD)-2 and SMAD3 through phosphorylation. Phosphorylated SMAD2 and SMAD3, in association with SMAD4, are translocated into the cell nucleus to modulate the transcription of target genes involved in many cell functions. SMAD7 blocks SMAD2 and SMAD3 from interacting with the receptor and being phosphorylated. SMAD7 thus inhibits TGFβ signaling, while Smad anchor for activation (SARA) stabilizes the SMAD-TβRI interaction, facilitating TGFβ signaling. The molecules described above form the core group of molecules involved in TGFβ signaling, and changes in the expression and function of these molecules affect TGFβ signaling, leading to tumor growth and progression. Although the Smad-mediated pathway is by far the best characterized mechanism of TGFβ signaling, many studies have also shown that TGFβs can exert their effects through Smad-independent pathways, such as the activation of Ras, phosphoinositide-3 kinase (PI3K); mitogen-activated protein kinases (MAPK), such as MAP3K1; protein phosphatase 2A (PP2A); RhoA and AKT/protein kinase (PKB); extracellular signal-regulated kinase (ERK); and p38 and C-Jun N-terminal kinase (JNK). It is believed that these Smad-independent pathways also play a significant role in tumorigenesis.

2. Role of TGFβs in Mammary Gland Tumorigenesis

A large body of evidence has clearly demonstrated that TGFβs may be the most potent naturally occurring inhibitors of cell growth, as reviewed recently by Benson, Elliott, Bierie, and Galliher (3–6). TGFβs have been shown to have strong inhibitory effects on the growth of normal, premalignant, and early transformed cells through inhibition of cell proliferation, induction of apoptosis, and promotion of cell differentiation and genomic stability. The inhibitory effect has been clearly demonstrated in transgenic mice, in which the risk of mammary gland tumors is reduced with elevated TGFβ expression in mammary tissues (7). Yet the risk increases in mice with reduced TGFβ signaling, due to the expression of a dominant-negative mutant TβRII (8). In breast cancer tissue, the *TGFBR2* gene is substantially downregulated, particularly in tissue from advanced cancers, resulting in reduced sensitivity to TGFβ-mediated growth inhibitory signaling. Decreased nuclear levels of phosphorylated SMAD2 and SMAD3 have been correlated with the development and progression of various cancers, including cancers of the breast (9, 10), colorectum (11), skin (12), prostate (13), and endometrium (14). Specifically for breast cancer, reduced nuclear levels of phosphorylated SMAD2/3 have been associated with high tumor grade, high architectural grade, larger tumor size, and hormone receptor negativity (10).

Although TGFβs are potent inhibitors of cell growth in the early stages of carcinogenesis, virtually all epithelial-derived human cancers become resistant to these growth-inhibitory effects (4). The mechanisms behind this resistance are well described for some cancers, such as cancers of the colon and pancreas, in which a large percentage of cancers are found to have mutations in the genes encoding the SMAD proteins (predominantly SMAD4) and TGFβ receptors. For breast cancer, inactivating mutations or loss of expression in members of the TGFβ signaling pathway, such as TβRI and TβRII, has also been reported in some cases (15, 16). For many breast cancer cases, the expression levels of TGFβ receptors are reduced, resulting in insensitivity to TGFβ-mediated inhibitory effects. Furthermore, during the later stages of carcinogenesis, TGFβs switch from acting as a tumor suppressor to acting as a tumor promoter and function like an oncogene, promoting tumor growth and inducing cancer cell survival. It has been reported fairly consistently that TGFβ levels are elevated in breast cancer tissues, particularly in late stage cancers. Numerous *in vitro* and *in vivo* studies have shown that TGFβs enhance the epithelial-to-mesenchymal transition, downregulate cellular adhesion molecules, augment the expression of metalloproteases, increase tumor cell motility and tumor angiogenesis, and cause local and systemic immunosuppression, leading tumors to an invasive metastatic status (3–6).

Despite strong evidence from *in vitro* and *in vivo* experiments that support a critical role of the TGFβ signaling pathway in the development and progression of breast and other cancers, limited data from human studies are currently available to link biomarkers in the TGFβ pathway directly to the risk and survival of breast cancer. Several studies using biological samples from breast cancer patients have shown that elevated TGFβs in tumor tissues or peripheral blood may be associated with an advanced cancer and/or a poor disease outcome *(3, 17, 18)*. The results from these studies, however, have been inconsistent. Over the past few years, an increasing number of epidemiological studies have evaluated the hypothesis that genetic variants that affect TGFβ production and/or signaling may be related to the risk and survival of breast cancer.

3. *TGFB1* Gene Variants and Breast Cancer Risk

Although several genetic polymorphisms in the TGFβ pathway genes have been investigated in relation to breast cancer risk, most studies conducted thus far have focused on the evaluation of a nonsynonymous single nucleotide polymorphism (SNP) (rs1982073) located at exon 1 of the *TGFB1* gene *(19–32)*. This SNP, a *T*-to-*C* transition at the 29th nucleotide in the coding sequence, results in a leucine-to-proline substitution at codon 10 (L10P) and has been associated with an elevated blood level of TGFβ1 *(33)*. Given the inhibitory effect of TGFβ1 in breast carcinogenesis, it is hypothesized that women carrying the *C* allele may be at a lower risk of breast cancer.

The first report that evaluated this hypothesis was from a cohort of 3,075 older women who were recruited initially for a study of osteoporotic fractures *(19)*. After an average of 9.3 years of follow-up, 146 breast cancer cases were identified in the cohort. Women who had the *CC* genotype were found to have a 64% reduced risk of developing breast cancer (relative risk [RR] = 0.36; 95% confidence interval [CI] = 0.17–0.75). This finding is consistent with the inhibitory effect of TGFβ1 in breast carcinogenesis demonstrated in *in vitro* and *in vivo* experiments and suggests that genetic polymorphisms in TGFβ pathway genes may contribute to the susceptibility of developing breast cancer in humans.

Over a dozen epidemiological studies have been conducted since 2001 to further evaluate the promising association reported in the initial study described above *(19)* (**Table 11.1**). In a pooling analysis of three European case-control studies, including a total of 3,987 cases and 3,867 controls, an elevated risk of 1.24 (95% CI = 1.06–1.44) was found to be associated with the *CC* genotype *(20)*. This finding is in direct contrast to the result reported in the initial study *(19)*. In another large study, a case-control study nested in the Multiethnic Cohort Study conducted in the United States, Le Marchand *(24)* reported no apparent association of the *T+29C* polymorphism with breast cancer. The point estimates of risk associated with the *CC* genotype ranged from 0.81 to 1.46 across the five ethnic groups evaluated in the study

Table 11.1

Epidemiological studies of TGFB1 (*T+29C*) polymorphism and breast cancer risk

Author, year [reference]; study population	Study design	No. of cases/controls	C allele in controls (%)	Risk of T+29C genotype TT	CT	CC
Ziv et al., 2001 [19]; USA	Cohort	146/3,075[a]	39	1.00	1.04	0.36*
Dunning et al., 2003 [20]; Europe	Population-based case-control	3,987/3,867	38	1.00	1.05	1.24*
Hishida et al., 2003 [21]; Japan	Hospital-based case-control	232/172	52	1.00	0.81	0.77
Krippl et al., 2003 [22]; Austria	Hospital-based	495/499	41	1.00	0.88	0.84
Jin et al., 2004 [23]; Europe	Mixed case-control	223/240 (Finnish)	28	1.00	1.06	0.57
		415/205 (Polish)	42	1.00	0.79	0.96
Le Marchand et al., 2004 [24]; USA	Nested case-control	233/1,612 (Black)	43	1.00	1.11	1.15
		225/647 (Latina)	49	1.00	1.04	0.81
		299/402 (White)	42	1.00	1.00	0.82
		303/385 (Asian)	53	1.00	1.25	0.95
		63/268 (Hawaiian)		1.00	0.88	1.46
Saha et al., 2004 [25]; India	Hospital-based case-control	26/97	29	1.00	1.64	0.67
Sigurdson et al., 2004 [26]; USA	Kin-cohort	190/2,430	38	1.00[b]	0.51	
				1.00	0.80	
Kaklamani et al., 2005 [27]; USA	Hospital-based case-control	658/841	34	1.00	1.02	0.89
Lee et al., 2005 [28]; Korea	Hospital-based case-control	560/509	46	1.00	1.40*	1.30
Shin et al., 2005 [29]; China	Population-based case-control	1,114/1,228	53	1.00	0.88	0.92
Skerrett et al., 2005 [30]; USA	Hospital-based case-control	88/102	N/S	N/S[b]		
Feigelson et al., 2006 [31]; USA	Nested case-control	502/505	37	1.00	1.05	0.89
González-Zuluéta Ladd et al., 2007 [32]; Netherlands	Cohort	143/3,646[a]	36	1.00	1.40*[c]	

*p <0.05 [a]Number of at-risk subjects at baseline. [b]No association was found to be statistically significant. [c]TC/CC combined and none of them were statistically significant. In the Shanghai Breast Cancer Study, a large population-based case-control study conducted among Chinese women, again, no significant association was found between the *T+29C* polymorphism and breast cancer risk *(29)*. However, in a stratified analysis by cancer stage, the *CC* genotype was found to be associated with a reduced risk of early-stage cancer (odds ratio [OR] = 0.66; 95% CI = 0.45–0.96) but an elevated, although not statistically significant, risk of late-stage cancer (OR = 1.34; 95% CI = 0.76–2.36). Several other studies have also provided some evidence for a potential protective effect of the *CC* genotype in early-stage breast cancer but not in late-stage cancer *(22, 31)*. The results from these studies are consistent with data from *in vitro* and *in vivo* experiments and suggest that *TGFB1* gene variants may play a dual role in the development of breast cancer in humans.

Table 11.1 summarizes the major findings of epidemiological studies conducted to date that have evaluated the association between the *TGFB1 T+29C* polymorphism and breast cancer risk. With a few exceptions, most studies failed to find an association that was statistically significant at $p \le 0.05$. Several studies reported a significant association for a subset of women, such as premenopausal women in a Japanese study *(21)*, or for a subgroup of cases, such as cases diagnosed at an early stage *(29)*. It is notable that the majority of these studies reported a slightly, although mostly not statistically significant, reduced risk associated with the *C* allele. The summary OR of these studies, after excluding three studies that provided insufficient data for the meta-analysis *(26, 30, 32)*, was 0.92 (95% CI = 0.81–1.05) (homogeneity test, $p = 0.06$) for the *CC* genotype compared with the *TT* genotype. The heterogeneity of this summary OR was mainly due to the study by Dunning *(20)*, which has the largest sample size of all studies reported to date and showed a significantly elevated OR. Excluding data from this study resulted in a summary OR of 0.89 (95% CI = 0.80–0.99; homogeneity test, $p = 0.48$). Overall these previous studies provide some evidence for a potential role of *TGFB1* gene polymorphisms in the risk of human breast cancer.

Several previous studies also investigated the association of breast cancer risk with several other *TGFB1* gene variants *(20, 23, 25, 29, 30)*, including rs1800469 (C-509T) and rs1800468 (G-800A) in the promoter region, rs1800471 (Arg25Pro) in exon 1, and rs1800472 (Thr263Ile) in exon 5. Similar to the finding for the *T+29C* polymorphism, no consistent association has been found for these SNPs. The *C-509T* polymorphism is in strong linkage disequilibrium with the *T+29C* polymorphism and has been shown to modify *TGFB1* expression in several studies *(34, 35)*. It was reported that this SNP may affect the binding of transcription factor Yin Yang 1, and the *T* allele may enhance *TGFB1* promoter activity and increase *TGFB1* gene expression *(35)*.

There are some data suggesting that the *T+29C* polymorphism may also be functionally significant. Hoffmann et al. *(36)* reported that *in vitro* production of TGFβ1 may be decreased by the variant *C* allele, while Yokota et al. *(33)* showed elevated serum levels of TGFβ1 in association with the *C* allele. In a recent study using Hela cells transfected with *TGFB1 T+29C* gene variants, Dunning et al. *(20)* reported increased TGFβ1 production by the variant *C* allele. Given the strong linkage disequilibrium of the *T+29C* and *C-509T* polymorphisms, it is difficult to distinguish the effect of these two SNPs in epidemiological studies.

4. Genetic Polymorphisms in Other TGFβ Pathway Genes and Breast Cancer Risk

Several studies have investigated the association of breast cancer risk with the *9A/6A* polymorphism in the *TGFBR1* gene that encodes the TGFβ type I receptor *(23, 31, 37–39)*. The *TGFBR1*6* allele results from the deletion of three alanines within a nine-alanine (**9A*) stretch in exon 1. In vitro experiments have shown that the **6A* allele has reduced efficiency in mediating TGFβ growth inhibitory signals *(37, 40)*. Compared with the wild-type **9A* allele, carrying the **6A* allele was associated with an elevated risk of breast cancer in several studies, although the association was not statistically significant in all studies *(23, 37–39)*. Two other studies, however, reported no significant association with this polymorphism *(23, 31)*. **Table 11.2** summarizes the results of epidemiological studies investigating the association of the *TGFBR2 9A/6A* polymorphisms with breast cancer risk. The frequency of the **6A* allele ranges from 5 to 10% in the Caucasian population. However, this variant can be acquired somatically in a sizable number of colorectal cancers that metastasize to the liver. It was reported that approximately 29.5% of liver metastases from colorectal cancer acquired the **6A* allele *(40)*. Somatic acquisition of this allele, however, is uncommon in breast cancer cells. The cancer-specific acquisition of this functional variant is interesting and warrants further investigation.

In addition to the **6A* allele, an intronic SNP (*Int7G24A*, rs334354) in the *TGFBR1* gene has also been investigated in relation to breast cancer risk *(39)*. In a small case-control study including 223 patients and 153 non-cancer control subjects, the *A* allele was found to be associated with a 2.4-fold (95% CI = 1.6–3.8) elevated risk of breast cancer *(39)*. This finding is interesting and warrants further investigation.

Genetic polymorphisms in several other TGFβ pathway genes have also been reported in relation to breast cancer risk. Recently, a functional variant (-246ins), a 4-bp insertion at nucleotide

Table 11.2
Epidemiological studies of *TGFBR1* (9A/6A) polymorphism and breast cancer risk

Author, year [reference]; study population	Study design	No. of cases/ controls	TGFBR1 polymorphism	
			*9A/*9A	*6A/*9A or *6A/*6A
Pasche et al., *1999 [37]*; USA	Hospital-based case-control	152/735	1.00	1.57[a]
Baxter et al., *2002 [38]*; UK	Hospital-based case-control	355/248	1.00	1.6*
Jin et al., *2004 [23]*; Europe	Mixed case-control	221/234 (Finnish) 170/202 (Polish)	1.00 1.00	0.67[a] 1.45[a]
Kaklamani et al., *2005 [27]*; USA	Hospital-based case-control	611/690	1.00	1.50*
Chen et al., *2006 [39]*; USA	Hospital-based case-control	115/130	1.00	1.67
Feigelson et al., *2006 [31]*; USA	Nested case-control	481/484	1.00	0.95

*$p \leq 0.05$ [a]Calculated based on the data provided in the paper

position –246 relative to the transcriptional start site, has been reported in the *TGFB2* gene, which increases the promoter activity of this gene *(41)*. In a small case-control study of 78 cases and 143 controls, this polymorphism was not found to be associated with breast cancer risk. Analyses conducted among cases, however, showed that the presence of the –246ins was associated with lymph node metastasis in breast cancer. In a case-control study conducted in Finland and Poland, Jin et al. evaluated a SNP in the TGFBR2 gene (G-875A, rs3087465) that has been shown to affect the transcriptional activity of this gene *(23)*. No apparent association of this SNP with breast cancer risk, however, was found in the study.

Because overall TGFβ signaling may be determined by multiple genetic polymorphisms in several TGFβ pathway genes, several studies have assessed the combined effects of multiple TGFβ pathway gene variants in relation to breast cancer risk. Based on genotyping data of the *TGFB1* (*T+29C*) and *TGFBR1* (*9A/6A*) polymorphisms, Kaklamani et al. *(27)* classified study participants (660 cases and 880 controls) into low, intermediate, and high signalers and found that the risk of breast cancer increased (from 1.0 to 1.3 [CI = 0.9–1.7] and 1.7 [CI = 1.1–2.7]) with reductions in TGFβ signaling. This finding, however, was not replicated in a subsequent study *(31)*. In the study conducted by Jin et al. *(23)*, data from three polymorphisms in the *TGFB1* (*C-509T*), *TGFBR1* (*9A/6A*), and *TGFBR2* (*G-875A*) genes were used to estimate the level of TGFβ signaling. However, no apparent association was found. The sample size in these previous studies, however, was not large, which may have affected their ability to evaluate the combined effect of multiple genetic factors.

5. Genetic Polymorphisms in TGFβ Pathways Genes and Breast Cancer Survival

As discussed earlier, during carcinogenesis, TGFβ can switch from a tumor suppressor to a tumor promoter in the late stage of cancer. Therefore, it has been hypothesized that genetic polymorphisms that enhance TGFβ signaling may be associated with a poor disease outcome after cancer diagnosis. The Shanghai Breast Cancer Study provided one of the first pieces of evidence in support of this hypothesis. Based on the data from an average of 5.17 years of follow-up of 1,111 breast cancer patients recruited in the initial phase of the Shanghai Breast Cancer Study from 1996 to 1998, Shu et al. *(43)* reported that patients who carried the variant *C* allele in the *T+29C* polymorphism had a lower disease-free survival rate (hazard ratio [HR] = 1.4; 95% CI = 1.0–1.9) than those homozygous for the *T* allele. The risk of cancer recurrence and death was further increased among patients who also carried risk genotypes in the *VEGF* and *PAI-1* genes *(44, 45)*. The findings for the *TGFB1* gene variant were supported by a small study, in which an HR of 1.4 (95% CI = 1.1–2.0) was found for carriers of the *+29C* allele *(32)*. In a large follow-up study of UK patients, the *CC* genotype was also found to be associated with an elevated, although not statistically significant, risk of total death (HR = 1.3; 95% CI = 0.8–1.9), supporting a possible role of *TGFB1* gene variants in breast cancer survival *(46)*.

Several studies have evaluated genetic polymorphisms in other TGFβ pathway genes in relation to tumor progression in breast cancer patients. Beisner et al. *(41)* reported that the −246ins allele in the *TGFB2* gene was associated with lymph node metastasis in a study of 223 patients. Chen et al. *(39)* showed that the *Int7G24A* variant in the *TGFBR1* gene was more common in invasive breast cancer patients than control subjects or patients with a pre-invasive tumor. Although these studies did not directly investigate the association of genetic polymorphisms with breast cancer survival, they have shown that these genetic polymorphisms may be associated with certain tumor characteristics that are in turn associated with poor disease outcome.

6. Conclusion

The TGFβ signaling pathway plays a critical role in breast cancer development and progression. Numerous *in vitro* and *in vivo* experiments have clearly demonstrated the potent cancer-inhibitory effects of TGFβ signaling in normal and premalignant cells. As cancer develops, however, cancer cells become resistant to the growth-inhibitory effects of TGFβs, and the production of TGFβs by both cancer cells and cancer stromal cells often escalates, which promotes the growth of tumors and leads to tumors with an invasive metastatic status.

Although the dual role of TGFβ signaling has been clearly demonstrated in many studies based on cell cultures and animal models, limited data from human studies are currently available to link biomarkers in this pathway directly to the risk and survival of breast cancer. An increasing number of epidemiological studies have evaluated common genetic polymorphisms in TGFβ pathway genes in relation to breast cancer risk and survival. Most of these studies have focused on evaluating polymorphisms in the *TGFB1* gene (*T+29C*, rs1982073) and the *TGFBR1* gene (*9A/6A*), and the results have been inconsistent. Many previous studies are limited by a small sample size, suboptimal sampling frame, and/or potential bias in case and control selection. In addition, virtually all previous studies evaluated only a few polymorphisms in the TGFβ signaling pathway, which is inadequate to quantify the overall level of TGFβ signaling in study subjects. Given the critical role of TGFβ signaling in breast carcinogenesis, it is likely that genetic polymorphisms that alter TGFβ signaling affect breast cancer development and progression. Further studies are needed to comprehensively evaluate genetic variants in this pathway in relation to breast cancer risk and survival.

References

1. Moses HL, Branum EL, Proper JA, Robinson RA. (1981) Transforming growth factor production by chemically transformed cells. *Cancer Res* **41**, 2842–2848.

2. Roberts AB, Anzano MA, Lamb LC, Smith JM, Sporn MB. (1981) New class of transforming growth factors potentiated by epidermal growth factor: isolation from non-neoplastic tissues. *Proc Natl Acad Sci USA* **78**, 5339–5343.

3. Benson JR. (2004) Role of transforming growth factor β in breast carcinogenesis. *Lancet Oncol* **5**, 229–239.

4. Elliott RL, Blobe GC. (2005) Role of transforming growth factor beta in human cancer. *J Clin Oncol* **23**, 2078–2093.

5. Bierie B, Moses HL. (2006) TGFβ: the molecular Jekyll and Hyde of cancer. *Nat Rev Cancer* **6**, 506–520.

6. Galliher AJ, Neil JR, Scheimann WP. (2006) Role of transforming growth factor-β in cancer progression. *Future Oncology* **2**, 743–763.

7. Pierce Jr DF, Gorska AE, Chytil A, et al. (1995) Mammary tumour suppression by transforming growth factor-1 transgene expression. *Proc Natl Acad Sci USA* **92**, 4254–4258.

8. Gorska AE, Jensen RA, Shyr Y, Aakre ME, Bhowmick NA, Moses HL. (2003) Transgenic mice expressing a dominant-negative mutant type II transforming growth factor-beta receptor exhibit impaired mammary

development and enhanced mammary tumor formation. *Am J Pathol* **163**, 1539–1549.

9. Xie W, Mertens JC, Reiss DJ, Rimm DL, Camp RL, Haffty BG, Reiss M. (2002) Alterations of Smad signaling in human breast carcinoma are associated with poor outcome: a tissue microarray study. *Cancer Res* **62**, 497–505.

10. Jeruss JS, Sturgis CD, Rademaker AW, Woodruff TK. (2003) Down-regulation of activin, activin receptors, and Smads in high-grade breast cancer. *Cancer Res* **63**, 3783–3790.

11. Xie W, Rimm DL, Lin Y, Shih WJ, Reiss M. (2003) Loss of Smad signaling in human colorectal cancer is associated with advanced disease and poor prognosis. *Cancer J.***9**, 302–312.

12. Tannehill-Gregg SH, Kusewitt DF, Rosol TJ, Weinstein M. (2004) The roles of Smad2 and Smad3 in the development of chemically induced skin tumors in mice. *Vet Pathol* **41**, 278–282.

13. Perttu MC, Martikainen PM, Huhtala HS, Blauer M, Tammela TL, Tuohimaa PJ, Syvala H. (2006) Altered levels of Smad2 and Smad4 are associated with human prostate carcinogenesis. *Prostate Cancer Prostatic Dis* **9**, 185–189.

14. Piestrzeniewicz-Ulanska D, Brys M, Semczuk A, Jakowicki JA, Krajewska WM. (2003) Expression and intracellular localization of Smad proteins in human endometrial cancer. *Oncol Rep.***10**, 1539–1544.

15. Chen T, Carter D, Garrigue-Antar L, Reiss M. (1998) Transforming growth factor beta type I receptor kinase mutant associated with metastatic breast cancer. *Cancer Res* **58**, 4805–4810.

16. Lucke CD, Philpott A, Metcalfe JC, Thompson AM, Hughes-Davies L, Kemp PR, Hesketh R. (2001) Inhibiting mutations in the transforming growth factor beta type 2 receptor in recurrent human breast cancer. *Cancer Res* **61**, 482–485.

17. Desruisseau S, Palmari J, Giusti C, Romain S, Martin P-M, Berthois Y. (2006) Determination of TGFbeta1 protein level in human primary breast cancers and its relationship with survival. *Br J Cancer* **94**, 239–246.

18. Grau AM, Wen W, Ramroopsignh D, Gao YT, Zi J, Cai Q, Shu XO, Zheng W. (2007) Circulating transforming growth factor-beta 1 and breast cancer prognosis: Results from the Shanghai Breast Cancer Study. *Cancer Epidemiol Biomarker Prev* (Submitted).

19. Ziv E, Cauley J, Morin PA, Saiz R, Browner WS. (2001) Association between the T29→C polymorphism in the transforming growth

factor β1 gene and breast cancer among elderly white women: The Study of Osteoporotic Fractures. *JAMA* **285**, 2859–2863.

20. Dunning AM, Ellis PD, McBride S, Kirschenlohr HL, Healey CS, Kemp PR, Luben RN, Chang-Claude J, Mannermaa A, Kataja V, Pharoah PD, Easton DF, Ponder BA, Metcalfe JC. (2003) A transforming growth factor β1 signal peptide variant increases secretion in vitro and is associated with increased incidence of invasive breast cancer. *Cancer Res* **63**, 2610–2615.

21. Hishida A, Iwata H, Hamajima N, Matsuo K, Mizutani M, Iwase T, Miura S, Emi N, Hirose K, Tajima K. (2003) Transforming growth factor β1 T29C polymorphism and breast cancer risk in Japanese women. *Breast Cancer* (Tokyo, Japan) **10**, 63–69.

22. Krippl P, Langsenlehner U, Renner W, Yazdani-Biuki B, Wolf G, Wascher TC, Paulweber B, Bahadori B, Samonigg H. (2003) The L10P polymorphism of the transforming growth factor-beta 1 gene is not associated with breast cancer risk. *Cancer Lett* **201**, 181–184.

23. Jin Q, Hemminki K, Grzybowska E, Klaes R, Soderberg M, Zientek H, Rogozinska-Szczepka J, Utracka-Hutka B, Pamula J, Pekala W, Forsti A. (2004) Polymorphisms and haplotype structures in genes for transforming growth factor beta1 and its receptors in familial and unselected breast cancers. *Int J Cancer* **112**, 94–99.

24. Le Marchand L, Haiman CA, van den Berg D, Wilkens LR, Kolonel LN, Henderson BE. (2004) T29C polymorphism in the transforming growth factor β1 gene and postmenopausal breast cancer risk: the Multiethnic Cohort Study. *Cancer Epidemiol Biomarkers Prev* **13**, 412–415.

25. Saha A, Gupta V, Bairwa NK, Malhotra D, Bamezai R. (2004) Transforming growth factor- β1 genotype in sporadic breast cancer patients from India: status of enhancer, promoter, 5′-untranslated-region and exon-1 polymorphisms. *Eur J Immunogenet* **31**, 37–342.

26. Sigurdson AJ, Hauptmann M, Chatterjee N, et al. (2004) Kin-cohort estimates for familial breast cancer risk in relation to variants in DNA base excision repair, BRCA1 interacting and growth factor genes. *BMC Cancer* **4**, 9.

27. Kaklamani VG, Baddi L, Liu J, Rosman D, Phukan S, Bradley C, Hegarty C, McDaniel B, Rademaker A, Oddoux C, Ostrer H, Michel LS, Huang H, Chen Y, Ahsan H, Offit K, Pasche B. (2005) Combined

genetic assessment of transforming growth factor-β signaling pathway variants may predict breast cancer risk. *Cancer Res* **65**, 3454–3461.

28. Lee KM, Park SK, Hamajima N, Tajima K, Yoo KY, Shin A, Noh DY, Ahn SH, Hirvonen A, Kang D. (2005) Genetic polymorphisms of TGF-β1 & TNF-β and breast cancer risk. *Breast Cancer Res Treat* **90**, 149–155.

29. Shin A, Shu XO, Cai Q, Gao YT, Zheng W. (2005) Genetic polymorphisms of the *Transforming Growth Factor-β1* gene and breast cancer risk: A possible dual role at different cancer stages. *Cancer Epidemiol Biomarkers Prev* **14**, 1567–1570.

30. Skerrett DL, Moore EM, Bernstein DS. (2005) Cytokine genotype polymorphisms in breast carcinoma: associations of TGF- β1 with relapse. *Cancer Invest* **23**, 208–214.

31. Feigelson HS, Patel AV, Diver WR, Stevens VL, Thun MJ, Calle EE. (2006) Transforming growth factor β receptor type I and transforming growth factor β1 polymorphisms are not associated with postmenopausal breast cancer. *Cancer Epidemiol Biomarkers Prev* **15**, 1236–1237.

32. Gonzalez-Zuloeta Ladd AM, Arias-Vasquez A, Siemes C, Coebergh JW, Hofman A, Witteman J, Uitterlinden A, Stricker BH, van Duijn CM. (2007) Transforming-growth factor β1 Leu10Pro polymorphism and breast cancer morbidity. *Eur J Cancer* **43**, 371–374.

33. Yokota M, Ichihara S, Lin TL, Nakashima N, Yamada Y. (2000) Association of a T29→C polymorphism of the transforming growth factor- β1 gene with genetic susceptibility to myocardial infarction in Japanese. *Circulation* **101**, 2783–2787.

34. Grainger DJ, Heathcote K, Chiano M, Snieder H, Kemp PR, Metcalfe JC, Carter ND, Spector TD. (1999) Genetic control of the circulating concentration of transforming growth factor type beta1. *Hum Mol Genet* **8**, 93–97.

35. Silverman ES, Palmer LJ, Subramaniam V, Hallock A, Mathew S, Vallone J, Faffe DS, Shikanai T, Raby BA, Weiss ST, Shore SA. (2004) Transforming growth factor-β1 promoter polymorphism C-509T is associated with asthma. *Am J Respir Crit Care Med* **169**, 214–219.

36. Hoffman SC, Stanley EM, Darrin Cox E, Craighead N, DiMercurio BS, Koziol DE, Harlan DM, Kirk AD, Blair PJ. (2001) Association of cytokine polymorphic inheritance and in vitro cytokine production in anti-CD3/CD28-stimulated peripheral blood lymphocytes. *Transplantation* **72**, 1444–1450.

37. Pasche B, Kolachana P, Nafa K, Satagopan J, Chen YG, Lo RS, Brener D, Yang D, Kirstein L, Oddoux C, Ostrer H, Vineis P, Varesco L, Jhanwar S, Luzzatto L, Massague J, Offit K. (1999) *TβR-I(6A)* is a candidate tumor susceptibility allele. *Cancer Res* **59**, 5678–5682.

38. Baxter SW, Choong DY, Eccles DM, Campbell IG. (2002) Transforming growth factor β receptor 1 polyalanine polymorphism and exon 5 mutation analysis in breast and ovarian cancer. *Cancer Epidemiol Biomarkers Prev* **11**, 211–214.

39. Chen T, Jackson CR, Link A, Markey MP, Colligan BM, Douglass LE, Pemberton JO, Deddens JA, Graff JR, Carter JH. (2006) *Int7G24A* variant of transforming growth factor-β receptor type I is associated with invasive breast cancer. *Clin Cancer Res* **12**, 392–397.

40. Pasche B, Knobloch TJ, Bian Y, Liu J, Phukan S, Rosman D, Kaklamani V, Baddi L, Siddiqui FS, Frankel W, Prior TW, Schuller DE, Agrawal A, Lang J, Dolan ME, Vokes EE, Lane WS, Huang CC, Caldes T, Di Cristofano A, Hampel H, Nilsson I, von Heijne G, Fodde R, Murty VV, de la Chapelle A, Weghorst CM. (2005) Somatic acquisition and signaling of TGFBR1*6A in cancer. *JAMA* **294**, 1634–1646.

41. Beisner J, Buck MB, Fritz P, Dippon J, Schwab M, Brauch H, Zugmaier G, Pfizenmaier K, Knabbe C. (2006) A novel functional polymorphism in the transforming growth factor-β2 gene promoter and tumor progression in breast cancer. *Cancer Res* **66**, 7554–7561.

42. Seijo ER, Song H, Lynch MA, Jennings R, Qong X, Lazaridis E, Muro-Cacho C, Weghorst CM, Munoz-Antonia T. (2001) Identification of genetic alterations in the *TGF-beta type II receptor* gene promoter. *Mutat Res* **483**, 19–26.

43. Shu XO, Gao YT, Cai Q, Pierce L, Cai H, Ruan ZX, Yang G, Jin F, Zheng W. (2004) Genetic polymorphisms in the TGF-beta 1 gene and breast cancer survival: a report from the Shanghai Breast Cancer Study. *Cancer Res* **64**, 836–839.

44. Lu H, Shu XO, Cui Y, Kataoka N, Cai QY, Gao YT, Zheng W. (2005) Association of genetic polymorphisms in the *VEGF* gene with breast cancer survival. *Cancer Res* **65**, 5015–5019.

45. Zhang X, Shu XO, Cai Q, Ruan Z, Gao YT, Zheng W. (2006) Functional plasminogen activator inhibitor-1 gene variants and breast cancer survival. *Clin Cancer Res* **12**, 6037–6042.

46. Goode EL, Dunning AM, Kuschel B, Healey CS, Day NE, Ponder BA, Easton DF, Pharoah PP. (2002) Effect of germ-line genetic variation on breast cancer survival in a population-based study. *Cancer Res* **62**, 3052–3057.

Part II

Epidemiology of Organ Specific Cancer

Chapter 12

Molecular Epidemiology of DNA Repair Genes in Bladder Cancer

Anne E. Kiltie

Abstract

Bladder cancer is a common disease, whose major risk factors include smoking and occupational exposure to chemicals. Superficial bladder cancer has significant healthcare cost implications due to the need for repeated cystoscopic surveillance. Chemical carcinogens can undergo metabolic activation and detoxification in the liver and polymorphisms in the relevant genes have been shown to be associated with bladder cancer risk. In addition, DNA repair enzymes are required to repair the DNA damage associated with carcinogen exposure. The main pathways involved are nucleotide excision repair, base excision repair, and double strand break repair.

Investigation of individual polymorphisms in DNA repair genes in bladder cancer has yielded few robust positive findings, which is not surprising given the multifactorial nature of the disease. Pathway approaches using novel genotyping technologies will allow more comprehensive studies of multiple polymorphisms in multiple genes. It will also be possible to investigate gene–environment interaction more rigorously than heretofore, using novel statistical methodology, in larger studies and through collaborative efforts within consortia. The results of the genome-wide association studies in bladder cancer are awaited with interest. In the future, genetic tests might be used in the prevention of bladder cancer to encourage lifestyle changes in those at highest risk of developing the disease, and in the treatment of bladder cancer to optimise cure rates whilst minimising morbidity in a cost-effective manner.

Key words: Bladder cancer, consortia, DNA repair genes, polymorphism, surveillance.

1. Introduction

Bladder cancer is a common disease. Smoking and occupational exposure to chemicals are two major risk factors. The need for repeated cystoscopic surveillance of patients with superficial bladder cancer means that this disease has significant healthcare cost implications. An individual's genetic make-up appears to contribute

M. Verma (ed.), *Methods of Molecular Biology, Cancer Epidemiology, vol. 472*
© 2009 Humana Press, a part of Springer Science+Business Media, Totowa, NJ
Book doi: 10.1007/978-1-60327-492-0

to their risk of developing bladder cancer, possibly by modifying the effect of environmental exposures, but may also influence their risk of developing recurrent or progressive disease and their response to various treatments. In the future, genetic tests might be used in the prevention of bladder cancer to encourage lifestyle changes in those at highest risk of developing the disease and in treatment of bladder cancer, to optimise cure rates whilst minimising morbidity in a cost-effective manner.

2. Bladder Cancer

Bladder cancer is the fifth commonest cancer in the United Kingdom (*1*), but only the 8th commonest cause of cancer death (*2*). Ninety-five percent of cases are transitional cell carcinomas, but rarer forms include squamous cell carcinoma (most commonly seen in regions of the world where schistosomiasis is endemic), adenocarcinoma, small cell carcinoma, sarcoma, carcinosarcoma, and lymphoma. Bladder cancer is more prevalent in men than women, with men accounting for around 70% of cases. It is a disease of the elderly, with few patients diagnosed below 50 years of age. Up to half of bladder cancer cases in men and a third in women are caused by cigarette smoking (*3, 4*) and around 5–10% of male bladder cancer in Europe is caused by occupational exposure to various chemical carcinogens (*5*). These include occupations in the paint, plastics, rubber, leather, and chemical industries, textile, metal, and electrical workers, and transport operators, hairdressers, and machinists. Exposure to carcinogens results in their ingestion, inhalation, and skin absorption, followed by metabolism (activation or detoxification) in the liver and excretion in the urine. Rarer risk factors include exposure of the bladder to ionising radiation and cyclophosphamide chemotherapy. A positive family history is seen in 1.4–6% of bladder cancer cases (*6–8*), with clustering at an early age of onset, arguing in favour of a genetic component to familial bladder cancer rather than merely shared environmental exposures.

The urinary bladder is composed of a muscle wall, the muscularis propria, which contracts during urinary voiding, encased by a layer of fat and fibrous tissue. Inside the bladder wall is the lamina propria, a thin layer of connective tissue. This separates the muscularis from the transitional urothelium, which lines the bladder cavity and is exposed to urine (*see* **Fig. 12.1**). DNA in urothelial cells is therefore constantly under attack from urinary carcinogenic metabolites. Approximately 70% of patients present with superficial bladder cancer, that is, a tumour or tumours involving only the urothelium or lamina propria. Histologically,

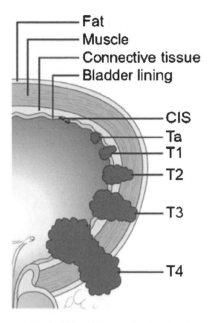

Fig. 12.1. T stages of bladder cancer. See text for details. From CancerHelp UK, the patient information website of Cancer Research UK: www.cancerhelp.org.uk, with permission.

these can be frond-like papillary tumours (pTa) or flat and solid (carcinoma in situ (CIS)). pTa tumours are generally well or moderately well differentiated (grade 1–2). Stage T1 tumours invade the lamina propria and are classified as superficial disease, but when poorly differentiated (grade 3), are likely to progress to invade muscle. T2 and T3 tumours invade the muscularis propria, with T3 disease extending outside the muscle wall either microscopically or macroscopically. T4 tumours invade adjacent structures such as the rectum, prostate, vagina, or uterus, or extend to the pelvic side wall. Transitional cell carcinomas can spread further to involve pelvic and distant lymph nodes, the bones, lungs, liver, or brain.

Superficial bladder cancer is managed by regular cystoscopic surveillance of the bladder, which may need to be life-long. Superficial disease has a propensity to recur, but may be stratified for risk (9). Although the risk of progression of superficial disease to muscle invasive disease is low overall, up to 50% of T1G3 tumours progress (about 10% of superficial disease) and early cystectomy (removal of the bladder) is often advocated. Treatment aims to prevent recurrence and progression, including intravesical installations of chemotherapy agents such as mitomycin C, which reduces the recurrence rate by around 50%, and Bacillus Calmette Guérin (BCG) installations for high-risk disease or CIS. BCG with maintenance treatment doubles the recurrence-free survival time compared with no maintenance (10). Muscle-invasive bladder tumours may be treated by cystectomy or radical radiotherapy to the bladder, with similar 5-year cause-specific survival rates of around 55% (*11*). Fitter patients usually also receive cisplatin-based neoadjuvant chemotherapy, which increases cure rates by 5% (*12*). When disease spreads beyond the bladder, chemotherapy and radiotherapy can be given as palliation.

3. Carcinogens Associated with Development of Bladder Cancer

The two major risk factors for transitional cell carcinoma of the bladder are cigarette smoking and occupational exposure to chemical carcinogens. Chemical carcinogens found in cigarette smoke include polyaromatic hydrocarbons (including benzo[a]pyrene), aromatic amines (including 4-aminobiphenyl, beta-naphthylamine, and benzidine), *N*-nitrosamines, and aldehydes (*13*). Individuals may also be exposed to these carcinogens through occupational exposure, e.g., aromatic amines in the dye industry, beta-naphthylamine in rubber workers, polyaromatic hydrocarbons in transport workers, and aromatic solvents and dyes in leather workers (*14*).

These carcinogens can undergo metabolic activation and detoxification in the liver. The Phase I enzymes of the cytochrome p450 family oxidise carcinogens such as polyaromatic hydrocarbons, aromatic amines, and *N*-nitrosamines to form carcinogenic metabolites, which can form adducts with DNA and also crosslink DNA. Phase II enzymes, including glutathione-S-transferases, can detoxify these metabolites. *N*-acetyltransferase (NAT)-2 inactivates aromatic amines, but can also activate certain arylamine metabolites. Polymorphisms in *NAT2* can result in slow acetylation and deletion of *GSTM1* results in a null phenotype characterised by deficient enzyme activity. As the balance between Phase I and Phase II enzymes determines the accumulation of DNA-damaging reactive intermediates and hence cancer development, polymorphisms in these genes have been investigated for association with cancer risk. Garcia-Closas et al. (*15*) undertook a meta-analysis of over 5,000 cases and controls and found NAT2 slow acetylators to have an increased risk of bladder cancer (odds ratio [OR], 1.4; 95% confidence interval [CI], 1.2–1.6) as did individuals with the *GSTM1* null phenotype (OR, 1.5; 95% CI, 1.3–1.6).

In addition to the chemical carcinogens that can form bulky adducts with DNA, oxidative byproducts are found in cigarette smoke. These include free radicals, such as superoxide and hydroxyl radicals, and hydrogen peroxide. Accumulation of these reactive oxygen species results in oxidative stress, which is a risk factor for cancer development.

4. DNA Repair Pathways

Modification or loss of DNA bases (mutations) can alter coding specificity leading ultimately to cancer (*16*). Such damage may be due to endogenous hydrolysis and oxidation reactions, or arise from exogenous insults including ionising radiation, drugs, and oxidative byproducts of cigarette smoke. The base excision repair (BER) pathway repairs this damage, which includes base modifications, abasic sites, and single strand breaks. The repair process involves lesion recognition and excision, followed by gap filling and ligation to repair the DNA backbone (*see* **Fig. 12.2** for details). Bulky DNA adducts, such as those from carcinogen exposure and cisplatin chemotherapy, are repaired by the nucleotide excision repair (NER) pathway, which involves the same principal steps as BER, namely lesion recognition, excision, gap filling, and ligation, but here the excision involves cleavage of a 24- to 32-base oligonucleotide containing the lesion (*17*) and a different set of proteins (*see* **Fig. 12.3** for details).

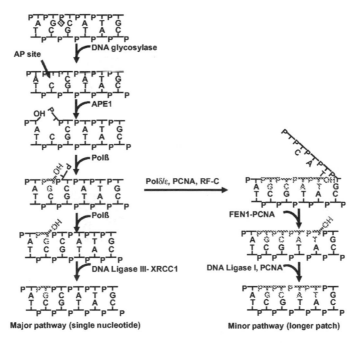

Fig. 12.2. Base excision repair (BER) pathways. The damaged base (G♦) is recognised and cleaved from the DNA backbone to generate an apurinic/apyrimidinic (*AP*) site, then apurinic/apyrimidinic endonuclease (*APE1*) cleaves the sugar-phosphate chain 5′ to the abasic site and recruits polymerase β (*polβ*) which adds one nucleotide to the 3′ end of the nick. In the major (short patch) pathway, the 5′ terminal deoxyribose-phosphate residue is excised by polβ, which interacts with the XRCC1-DNA Ligase III heterodimer, which completes the repair process. The longer patch pathway is required for more complex terminal sugar-phosphate residues. Polymerase δ/ε (*Polδ/ε*) adds a few more nucleotides to the 3′ end to create a flap, which is removed by flap endonuclease I (*FEN1*), stimulated by proliferating cell nuclear antigen (*PCNA*), then ligase I completes the repair. From ref. [50], by permission of The John Hopkins Bloomberg School of Public Health.

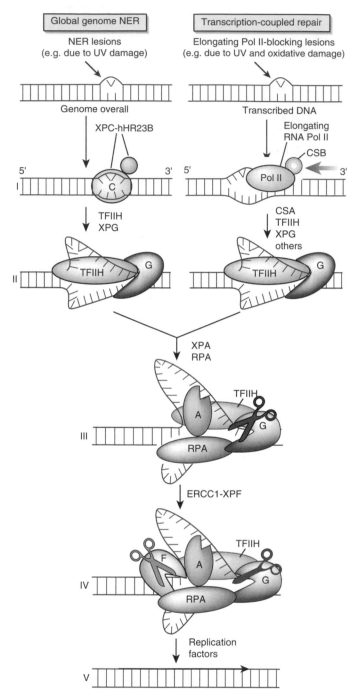

Fig. 12.3. Nucleotide excision repair (NER) pathways. NEP comprises two converging pathways, namely global genome repair (GGR) and transcription-coupled repair (TCR). GGR requires disrupted base pairing for activation, whilst TCR depends on the ability of the lesion to block RNA polymerase. In GGR, XPC and its cofactor hHR23B or XPE/DDB2 (not shown) recognise the lesion, whilst in TCR, CSA and CSB displace the stalled polymerase. Then in both pathways, the XPB and XPD subunits of TFIIH open approximately 30 base pairs of DNA around the damage, XPA confirms the presence of damage and RPA stabilises the open intermediate. XPG and ERCC1/XPF then cleave 3′ and 5′, respectively, and the gap is filled by the DNA replication machinery. GGR deficiency results in cancer development but not neurodegeneration, whilst the reverse is true for TCR deficiency. Reprinted from ref. [17], with permission from Macmillan Publishers Ltd.

The main double strand break (DSB) repair pathways are non-homologous end-joining, and homologous recombination (HR). DSB repair is more complex than BER and NER as there is no opposing DNA strand available to act as a template for repair. The key genes involved in non-homologous end-joining are *Ku70*, *Ku80*, *DNA PKcs*, Artemis, *Lig IV*, *XRCC4*, and Cernunnos (*17–19*); and in HR, are *RAD51*, *RAD51B*, *RAD51C*, *RAD51D*, *XRCC2*, *XRCC3*, *BRCA1*, *BRCA2*, *RAD52*, *RAD54*, and *RPA* (*17, 18*). DSB are formed from closely spaced single strand breaks on opposing DNA strands, and may arise during BER when the backbone is excised (*20*).

5. Single Nucleotide Polymorphisms in DNA Repair Genes

It is hypothesised that patients with a common, complex disease such as bladder cancer are likely to share some common, low penetrance alleles that increase their disease susceptibility (*21*). This is the basis on which association studies of single nucleotide polymorphisms (SNPs) have been undertaken. It appears that this is a valid starting point as common, low-penetrance variants are being found in genome-wide association studies (see below). SNPs are the most frequent form of genetic variants, involving the alteration of a single DNA base at polymorphic frequency, defined as >1%. Such variants in the coding region can be synonymous, where no amino acid substitution is observed, or non-synonymous, where the base substitution results in an alteration to the amino acid code that could affect protein structure and function. SNPs in the 3′ and 5′ untranslated regions of genes can alter messenger RNA (mRNA) stability and SNPs in intronic splice sites can result in alternative splicing and hence altered protein function. Rarely, SNP variants deep within introns can also have functional significance, as is the case for the *CDKN2A* gene (*22*).

Reduced protein function due to polymorphic variants in DNA repair genes can result in reduced DNA repair capacity (DRC) for carcinogenic adducts and oxidative lesions, resulting in mutations and hence cancer formation. DNA repair gene SNPs have been studied extensively in other tumour sites associated with cigarette smoking, including lung cancer and head and neck cancer, as well as in breast and prostate cancer. A few DNA repair polymorphisms are consistently associated with cancer risk across studies (see reviews in refs. (*23–25*)).

6. Case–Control Studies of DNA Repair Gene SNPs and Bladder Cancer Risk

6.1. Studies of Individual Polymorphisms

6.1.1. Overview of Results

Data regarding DNA repair SNPs in bladder cancer started to emerge in 2001, but early case–control studies were relatively small (**Tables 12.1–12.3**). Several studies found positive associations for single SNP variants with increased bladder cancer risk, but these results were not confirmed in subsequent studies. Due to the ascertainment bias known as the "winner's curse" (*26*), small, low-powered initial studies overestimated the actual genetic effect. For example, in 124 cases and 85 controls, Matullo et al. (*27*) found the *XRCC3* Thr241Met variant allele to be associated with an increased risk of bladder cancer, but this was not confirmed in eight subsequent larger studies (**Table 12.3**). Unless the prior probability of an association is high, a large proportion of genetic associations with marginal statistical significance ($p < 0.05$) in studies of low to moderate power will be false-positive results (*28*). Power is based on sample size, the frequency of the at-risk genetic variant, and the OR for a presumed association. In meta-analyses of common SNPs, the magnitude of effects were lower (ORs <1.5) than originally expected (*29*). In terms of prior probability, the relevance of the gene and the functional significance of the SNP are important. Only main effects are presented in Tables 12.1 to 12.3, as many subgroup analyses in smaller studies are likely to be spurious findings (*30*).

More recently, larger studies of at least 500 cases and/or controls have been published from four groups: The Spanish Bladder Cancer Study (*31–33*), the MD Anderson Bladder Cancer Study (*34–37*), the Leeds Bladder Cancer Study (*38–40*), and the New Hampshire Bladder Cancer Study (*41*). The most striking feature of Tables 12.1 to 12.3 is that the positive associations are seen in smaller studies and subsequently not confirmed in the larger studies or are seen as isolated findings in the larger studies. The latter may also be false positives, so the Spanish bladder cancer group used the false discovery rate (FDR) method (*32*) to determine the likelihood of false-positive results, and concluded that there was a substantial chance that their BER findings were false positives but three of six positive DSB repair polymorphism results were robust (*33*). They concluded that these results needed to be confirmed in future independent studies.

6.1.2. Functional Studies

Although case–control studies have shown associations with increased bladder cancer risk, they do not establish whether the variants result in altered DNA repair phenotypes. Several groups have performed assays by transfecting viable lymphocytes from patients

Table 12.1
The association between NER SNPs and bladder cancer

NER gene	SNP	Reference	Cases: controls	Comparison groups	OR (95% CI)
CSB/ERCC6	Arg1230Pro (G to C)	Garcia-Closas et al. (2006) [31][a]	1,055:978	GC/CC vs GG	1.0 (0.8–1.2)
		Wu et al. (2006) [35][b]	606:595	GC/CC vs GG	0.88 (0.65–1.19)
ERCC1	IVS5+33 (A to C)	Garcia-Closas et al. (2006) [31][a]	1,130:1,128	CA/AA vs CC	**1.2 (1.0–1.5)**
ERCC1	Asn118Asn (T to C)	Matullo et al. (2005) [54]	229:249	TC/CC vs TT	**0.62 (0.41– 0.95)**
hHR23B	IVS5-15 (A to G)	Garcia-Closas et al. (2006) [31][a]	1,124:1,119	GA/AA vs GG	**1.3 (1.1–1.5)**
hHR23B	Ala249Val (C to T)	Garcia-Closas et al. (2006) [31][a]	1,137:1,127	GA/AA vs GG	1.1 (0.9–1.4)
		Wu et al. (2006) [35][b]	607:595	GA/AA vs GG	1.08 (0.84–1.38)
XPC	Lys939Gln (A to C)	Sanyal et al. (2004) [72]	305:246	AC/CC vs AA	**1.49 (1.16– 1.92)**
		Sak et al. (2005) [38][c]	544:577	CC vs AC/AA	0.98 (0.68–1.42)
		Garcia-Closas et al. (2006) [31][a]	1,137:1,138	AC/CC vs AA	**1.2 (1.0–1.4)**
		Wu et al. (2006) [35][b]	606:596	AC/CC vs AA	0.99 (0.78–1.27)
		Zhu et al. (2007) [37][b]	550:554	AC/CC vs AA	0.99 (0.76–1.28)
XPC	PolyAT(– to +)	Broberg et al. (2005) [73]	61:155	+/ + vs –/ –	0.72 (0.28–1.9)
		Sak et al. (2005) [38][c]	532:561	+/ + vs –/ –	0.99 (0.69–1.43)
		Wu et al. (2006) [35][b]	617:604	–/ +, +/ + vs –/ –	1.19 (0.94–1.51)
		Andrew et al. (2006) [41][d]	348:435	+/ + vs –/ –	0.9 (0.6–1.4)
		Zhu et al. (2007) [37][b]	561:562	–/ +, +/ + vs –/ –	1.01 (0.78–1.30)
XPC	IVS11-6 (C to A)	Sak et al. (2005) [38][c]	536:566	AA vs CC	1.01 (0.70–1.46)

(continued)

Table 12.1
(continued)

NER gene	SNP	Reference	Cases: controls	Comparison groups	OR (95% CI)
		Garcia-Closas et al. (2006) [31][a]	982:994	AA vs CC	1.1 (0.8–1.4)
XPC	Arg492His (G to A)	Sak et al. (2006) [39][c]	535:567	GA/AA vs GG	1.05 (0.71–1.55)
		Garcia-Closas et al. (2006) [31][a]	1,111:1,118	GA/AA vs GG	1.1 (0.9–1.5)
XPC	Ala499Val (C to T)	Broberg et al. (2005) [73]	61:155	TT vs CC	3.1 (0.94–11)
		Sak et al. (2006) [39][c]	538:565	TT vs CT/CC	**1.70 (1.10–2.65)**
		Garcia-Closas et al. (2006) [31][a]	1,108:1,109	TT vs CC	1.2 (0.8–1.7)
		Wu et al. (2006) [35][b]	603:590	TT vs CC	1.09 (0.61–1.93)
		Zhu et al. (2007) [37][b]	546:549	CT/TT vs CC	0.91 (0.71–1.17)
XPC	3′ UTR (T to A) Ex15–184	Sak et al. (2006) [39][c]	520:560	AA vs TA/TT	**1.91 (1.19–3.09)**
XPC	3′ UTR (A to G) Ex15–177	Sak et al. (2006) [39][c]	528:560	GG vs AG/AA	**1.91 (1.19–3.07)**
XPD/ERCC2	Asp312Asn (G to A)	Schabath et al. (2005) [34][b]	497:477	GA/AA vs GG	1.19 (0.98–1.45)
		Broberg et al. (2005) [73]	57:145	AA v GG	3.6 (1.3–9.5)
		Matullo et al. (2005) [54]	292:305	AA v GG	1.14 (0.65–1.98)
		Garcia-Closas et al. (2006) [31][a]	1,129:1,122	GA/AA vs GG	1.1 (0.9–1.3)
		Wu et al. (2006) [35][b]	625:591	GA/AA vs GG	**1.28 (1.01–1.62)**
		Andrew et al. (2006) [41][d]	296:507	AA vs GG	1.2 (0.7–2.0)
XPD/ERCC2	Lys751Gln (A to C)	Matullo et al. (2001) [27]	124:47	AC/CC vs AA	0.71 (0.32–1.58)

(continued)

**Table 12.1
(continued)**

NER gene	SNP	Reference	Cases: controls	Comparison groups	OR (95% CI)
		Stern et al. (2002) [74]	229:210	CC vs AC/AA	0.8 (0.4–1.3)
		Shen et al. (2003) [75]	201:214	AC/CC vs AA	0.92 (0.62–1.37)
		Sanyal et al. (2004) [72]	307:246	AC/CC vs AA	1.13 (0.88–1.46)
		Schabath et al. (2005) [34][b]	480:461	AC/CC vs AA	1.11 (0.92–1.36)
		Broberg et al. (2005) [73]	61:154	CC vs AA	1.80 (0.77–4.4)
		Matullo et al. (2005) [54]	316:314	AC/CC vs AA	1.11 (0.76–1.60)
		Garcia-Closas et al. (2006) [31][a]	1,136:1,125	AC/CC vs AA	1.1 (0.9–1.3)
		Wu et al. (2006) [35][b]	614:599	AC/CC vs AA	1.03 (0.82–1.31)
		Andrew et al. (2006) [41][d]	317:544	CC vs AA	1.0 (0.6–1.6)
XPD/ERCC2	Arg156Arg (A to C)	Garcia-Closas et al. (2006) [31][a]	1,133:1,125	AC/CC vs AA	**1.3 (1.1–1.6)**
XPF/ERCC4	Ser835Ser (C to T)	Matullo et al. (2005) [54]	204:213	CC vs TT	1.06 (0.52–2.16)
		Garcia-Closas et al. (2006) [31][a]	1,091:1,019	CC vs TT	0.9 (0.7–1.3)
XPF/ERCC4	Ser662Pro (T to C)	Garcia-Closas et al. (2006) [31][a]	1,066:1,001	CT vs CC	1.2 (0.6–2.5)
		Wu et al. (2006) [35][b]	607:597	CT vs CC	2.19 (0.53–9.12)
XPG/ERCC5	Asp1104His (G to C)	Sanyal et al. (2004) [72]	299:284	CC vs GG	**0.38 (0.15–0.94)**
		Garcia-Closas et al. (2006) [31][a]	1,141:1,136	GC/CC vs GG	0.9 (0.8–1.1)
		Wu et al. (2006) [35][b]	615:600	GC/CC vs GG	1.10 (0.87–1.40)

(continued)

Table 12.1
(continued)

NER gene	SNP	Reference	Cases: controls	Comparison groups	OR (95% CI)
XPG/ERCC5	Met254Val (A to G)	Garcia-Closas et al. (2006) [31][a]	1,077:1,068	AG/GG vs AA	**1.4 (1.0–2.0)**
XPG/ERCC5	His46His (C to T)	Garcia-Closas et al. (2006) [31][a]	1,103:1,094	TT vs CC	**0.8 (0.6–1.0)**

Data presented for positive findings and for SNPs where more than one group have published. Negative findings reported in one study only: Matullo et al. (2005) [54] also studied XPF: Glu875Gly. Garcia-Closas et al. (2006) [31] also studied hHR23B: IVS5-66, IVS5-57; XPD: IVS19-70; ERCC1: Gln504Lys; XPF: Arg-415Gln, IVS9-35; XPG: Cys529Ser. Wu et al. (2006) [35] also studied ERCC1: 3′ UTR (rs3212986); XPA: 5′ UTR (ex1-176/+62, rs1800975), ERCC6: Met1097Val. Sak et al. (2006) [39] also studied XPC: Ex1-434, Ex1-356, Ex1-12, Ex1-7, Leu16Val, IVS3+73, IVS6-22, IVS6-70, Asp454Asp, Arg687Arg, IVS11-37, IVS14-51, IVS14-40, Ex15-111, Ex15-699. Bold face represents CI's not crossing 1.0. [a]Study reported from the Spanish Bladder Cancer Study. [b]Study reported from the MD Anderson Bladder Cancer Study. [c]Study reported from the Leeds Bladder Cancer Study. [d]Study reported from the New Hampshire Bladder Cancer Study. Published case–control studies only are presented so no account is taken for negative studies published in abstract form.

of varying SNP genotypes with a damaged plasmid (UV irradiated or benzo[a]pyrene diol epoxide [BPDE] treated), before testing the cells' ability to reactivate a luciferase reporter gene (host cell reactivation [HCR] assay). In lung cancer, *XPA* and *XPD* SNPs have been tested and an inverse association between DRC and lung cancer risk found (*42, 43*). Lin et al. (*44*) have established a HCR assay in bladder cancer using 4-aminobiphenyl as the damaging agent, but SNP genotypes have not yet been tested. This approach has been criticised because the lymphocytes tested are not isogenic, so as well as differing in the genotype of the SNP of interest, the lymphocytes may be variant for other SNPs in the same gene or pathway (*45*). A more direct approach is to clone the SNP of interest into deficient cells to look for restoration of function (*46–48*). SNPs showing no reduction in DRC in this assay may either lack functional significance or the assay may be insufficiently sensitive to detect small differences in DRC. Clarkson and Wood (*49*) have argued that, in contrast to the current approach, it is necessary to establish a functional effect for DNA repair gene polymorphisms, using SIFT (http://blocks.fhcrc.org/sift/SIFT.html) and Polyphen (http://www.bork.embl-heidelberg.de/PolyPhen/) prediction tools and functional in vitro assays, *before* undertaking association studies.

6.1.3. Meta-analyses

Several commonly investigated individual DNA repair SNPs in bladder cancer have been studied in meta-analyses: Hung et al. (*50*), analysed four studies comprising 991 cases and 1,088 controls and found an OR of 1.12 (95% CI, 0.95–1.33) for carriage of

Table 12.2
The association between BER SNPs and bladder cancer

BER geneSNP		Reference	Cases/ Controls	Comparison groups	OR (95% CI)
APEX1	Asp148Glu (T to G)	Broberg et al. (2005) [73]	61:155	GG vs TT	1.70 (0.64–4.3)
		Wu et al. (2006) [35][b]	596:590	GG vs TT	0.85 (0.61–1.19)
		Andrew et al. (2006) [41][d]	354:557	GG vs TT	0.80 (0.5–1.2)
		Terry et al. (2006) [76]	230:207	GG vs TT	1.4 (0.8–2.6)
		Figueroa et al. (2007) [32][a]	1,094:1,013	GG vs TT	0.89 (0.69–1.14)
		[Huang et al. (2007) [36][b]	596:590	GT/GG vs TT	0.91 (0.7–1.18)]
OGG1	5′ UTR (G to A) −1492	Figueroa et al. (2007) [32][a]	1,038:968	GA vs GG	**0.78 (0.63– 0.97)**
OGG1	Ser326Cys (C to G)	Karahalil et al. (2006) [77]	99:100	CG/GG vs CC	**2.41 (1.36– 4.25)**
		Wu et al. (2006) [35][b]	613:600	CG/GG vs CC	0.89 (0.70–1.12)
		[Huang et al. (2007) [36][b]	603:608	CG/GG vs CC	0.82 (0.65– 1.05)]
		Figueroa et al. (2007) [32][a]	1,088:1,018	GG vs CC	0.84 (0.57–1.26)
PARP1	Val762Ala (T to C)	Figueroa et al. (2007) [32][a]	1,138:1,131	TC/CC vs TT	**1.24 (1.02– 1.51)**
		Wu et al. (2006) [35][b]	606:595	TC/CC vs TT	0.89 (0.66–1.15)
		[Huang et al. (2007) [36][b]	606:595	TC/CC vs TT	0.89 (0.66– 1.15)]
PCNA	3′ UTR (G to C)	Matullo et al. (2005) [54]	284:293	CG/CC vs GG	**1.61 (1.00– 2.61)**
PolB	IVS1-89 (T to C)	Figueroa et al. (2007) [32][a]	1,086:1,033	TC/CC vs TT	**1.30 (1.04– 1.62)**
XRCC1	Val72Ala (T to C)	Figueroa et al. (2007) [32][a]		MAF <0.01	Not reported
		Sak et al. (2007) [40][c]		No variants	Not reported

(continued)

Table 12.2
(continued)

BER geneSNP	Reference	Cases/ Controls	Comparison groups	OR (95% CI)
XRCC1 Arg280His (G to A)	Stern et al. (2001) [78]	214:195	GA vs GG	1.2 (0.6–2.6)
	Figueroa et al. (2007) [32][a]	1,081:1,016	GA/AA vs GG	1.07 (0.81–1.43)
	Sak et al. (2007) [40][c]	513:560	GA/AA vs GG	1.50 (0.98–2.28)
XRCC1 Arg194Trp (C to T)	Stern et al. (2001) [78]	213:197	CT vs CC	0.6 (0.3–1.0)
	Matullo et al. (2005) [54]	315:313	CT vs CC	**0.69 (0.47–1.14)**
	Wu et al. (2006) [35][b]	614:600	CT/TT vs CC	0.94 (0.66–1.34)
	Andrew et al. (2006) [41][d]	299:512	CT/TT vs CC	0.80 (0.5–1.3)
	Figueroa et al. (2007) [32][a]	1,096:1,022	CT vs CC	0.98 (0.74–1.29)
	Sak et al. (2007) [40][c]	535:562	CT/TT vs CC	0.95 (0.65–1.40)
	Huang et al. (2007) [36][b]	614:600	CT/TT vs CC	0.94 (0.66–1.34)]
XRCC1 Arg399Gln (G to A)	Stern et al. (2001) [78]	214:197	AA vs GA/GG	0.70 (0.4–1.3)
	Matullo et al. (2001) [27]	124:47	GA/AA vs GG	0.8 (0.28–2.25)
	Shen et al. (2003) [75]	201:214	GA/AA vs GG	0.86 (0.59–1.28)
	Kelsey et al. (2004) [79][d]	355:544	AA vs GA/GG	**0.6 (0.4–1.0)**
	Sanyal et al. (2004) [72]	311:246	AA vs GG	1.27 (0.67–2.39)
	Matullo et al. (2005) [54]	311:312	GA/AA vs GG	0.77 (0.53–1.10)
	Broberg et al. (2005) [73]	61:155	AA vs GG	0.95 (0.27–3.3)
	Wu et al. (2006) [35][b]	613:596	GA/AA vs GG	1.05 (0.83–1.33)

(continued)

**Table 12.2
(continued)**

BER geneSNP	Reference	Cases/ Controls	Comparison groups	OR (95% CI)
	Andrew et al. (2006) [41][d]	306:538	AA vs GA/GG	0.6 (0.4–1.0)
	Karahalil et al. (2006) [77]	100:100	GA/AA vs GG	0.72 (0.41–1.26)
	Figueroa et al. (2007) [32][a]	1,061:996	AA vs GG	1.15 (0.86–1.56)
	Sak et al. (2007) [40][c]	532:560	AA vs GG	0.94 (0.64–1.39)
	[Huang et al. (2007) [36][b]	613:596	GA/AA vs GG	1.05 (0.83–1.33)]
	Hung et al. (2005) [50]	*991:1,088*	*GA/AA vs GG*	*1.12 (0.95–1.33)*
	Figueroa et al. (2007) [32][a]	*2,862:2,894*	*AA vs GG*	*0.99 (0.83–1.19)*
XRCC1 Pro206Pro (G to A)	Matullo et al. (2005) [54]	286:290	AG/GG vs AA	**1.73 (1.17–2.56)**
	Sak et al. (2007) [40][c]	515:545	AA vs GG	0.91 (0.64–1.31)

Data presented for positive findings and for SNPs where more than one group have published. Negative findings reported in one study only: Wu et al. (2006) [35] and Huang et al. (2007) [36] [same study group] also studied *MBD4*: Glu346Lys; *MUTYH*: Gln335His, *POLD1*: Arg119His. Figueroa et al. (2007) [32] also studied *APE1*: 5′ UTR (−655), Ex1+8;*MUTYH*: 5′ UTR (Ex1+8); *OGG1*: IVS7+110; *PARP1*: IVS2+82, Ex7+18, Ex8+45, IVS20-63, IVS21+59; *PARP3*: Q269R; *PARP4*: Ex3-89, IVS15-995, IVS17-110, Ex20-19, G1265A, G1280R, P1328T, A1331T, A1656P; *PolB*: IVS2-2264, IVS7+171; LIG1: Ex2-24, Ex7+44, IVS19-131, IVS25+19, Ex26+3; *LIG3*: Arg780His, IVS18-148, IVS18-39, 3′ UTR (Ex21-250); *POLD1*: IVS2+21; *PCNA*: IVS2-124, IVS2-4, IVS5+140. Sak et al. (2007) [40] also studied XRCC1: Ex1-1139, Ex1-1128, Ex1-900, Ex1-128, Ex1-52, IVS7-33, Gln632Gln, Ex17-123, Ex17-127. Studies in bold italics represent meta-analyses. Bold face represents CI's not crossing 1.0. [a]Study reported from the Spanish Bladder Cancer Study. [b]Study reported from the MD Anderson Bladder Cancer Study. [c]Study reported from the Leeds Bladder Cancer Study. [d]Study reported from the New Hampshire Bladder Cancer Study. Published case–control studies only are presented so no account is taken for negative studies published in abstract form.

the minor allele of *XRCC1* Arg399Gln, and subsequently Figueroa et al. (*32*) found an OR of 0.99 (95% CI, 0.83–1.19) for the homozygous variant versus wild-type genotype in 2,862 cases and 2,894 controls, suggesting no effect. Han et al. (*51*) studied *XRCC3* Thr241Met and found an OR of 1.11 (95% CI, 0.83–1.49) in six studies and the larger meta-analysis from Figueroa et al. (*33*) of 3,086 cases and 3,150 controls from seven studies found an OR of 1.17 (95% CI, 1.00–1.36) for homozygous variants versus homozygous wild-type individuals.

Table 12.3
The association between DSB repair SNPs and bladder cancer

DSB repair gene	SNP	Reference	Cases: controls	Comparison groups	OR (95% CI)
NBS1	Glu185Gln (G to C)	Sanyal et al. (2004) [72]	299:278	CC vs CG/GG	1.64 (0.92–2.90)
		Broberg et al. (2005) [72]	61:154	CC vs GG	0.53 (0.16–1.8)
		Wu et al. (2006) [35][b]	604:595	CC vs GG	1.28 (0.84–1.93)
		Figueroa et al. (2007) [33][a]	1,086:1,020	CC vs GG	1.19 (0.88–1.61)
XRCC2	Promoter (C to A) –73599	Figueroa et al. (2007) [33][a]	886:846	AA vs CC	**0.50 (0.31–0.81)**
XRCC2	Promoter (T to C) –53442	Figueroa et al. (2007) [33][a]	897:869	CC vs TT	**0.40 (0.19–0.84)**
XRCC2	Promoter (G to T) –998	Figueroa et al. (2007) [33][a]	906:875	TT vs GG	**0.36 (0.13–0.96)**
XRCC2	Arg188His (G to A)	Matullo et al. (2005) [54]	156:109	GA vs GG	1.78 (0.77–4.12)
		Wu et al. (2006) [35][b]	605:595	GA/AA vs GG	0.93 (0.67–1.28)
		Figueroa et al. (2007) [33][a]	1,138:1,1 29	AA vs GG	**0.36 (0.13–1.00)**
XRCC3	Thr241Met (C to T)	Matullo et al. (2001) [27]	124:85	CT/TT vs CC	**2.77 (1.55–4.93)**
		Stern et al. (2002) [80]	233:209	CT/TT vs CC	1.3 (0.9–1.9)
		Shen et al. (2003) [75]	201:214	CT/TT vs CC	0.63 (0.20–1.93)
		Sanyal et al. (2004) [72]	311:246	CT/TT vs CC	1.13 (0.88–1.46)
		Matullo et al. (2005) [54]	317:317	CT/TT vs CC	1.40 (0.97–2.03)
		Broberg et al. (2005) [73]	61:153	TT vs CC	0.62 (0.20–1.9)
		Andrew et al. (2006) [41][d]	355:557	TT vs CC	0.9 (0.6–1.4)
		Wu et al. (2006) [35][b]	612:596	CT/TT vs CC	1.20 (0.95–1.53)
		Figueroa et al. (2007) [33][a]	1,083:1,010	CT/TT vs CC	1.13 (0.94–1.36)

(continued)

Table 12.3
(continued)

DSB repair gene	SNP	Reference	Cases: controls	Comparison groups	OR (95% CI)
		Han et al. (2006) *[51]*	*1,310:2,118*	*CT/TT vs CC*	*1.11 (0.83–1.49)*
		Figueroa et al. (2007) [33][a]	*3,086:3,150*	*TT vs CC*	*1.17 (1.00–1.36)*
XRCC3	IVS7-14 (A to G)	Broberg et al. (2005) [73]	58:152	GG vs AA	0.30 (0.08–1.10)
		Matullo et al. (2005) [54]	309:311	GG vs AA	0.90 (0.44–1.84)
		Wu et al. (2006) [35][b]	600:592	GG vs AA	0.82 (0.55–1.22)
		Figueroa et al. (2007) [33][a]	1,085:1,032	GG vs AA	1.02 (0.69–1.50)
XRCC3	5' UTR (A to G) Ex 2+2	Matullo et al. (2005) [54]	316:315	GG vs AA	0.71 (0.27–1.85)
		Wu et al. (2006) [35][b]	599:595	AG/GG vs AA	0.97 (0.75–1.25)
		Figueroa et al. (2007) [33][a]	1,085:1,033	AG/GG vs AA	0.93 (0.77–1.11)
XRCC4	Asn298Ser (G to A)	Broberg et al. (2005) [73]	54:127	GA vs GG	1.1 (0.44–2.6)
XRCC4	IVS7-1 (G to A)	Wu et al. (2006) [35][b]	605:595	GA vs GG	1.20 (0.84–1.48)
		Figueroa et al. (2007) [33][a]	1,086:1,032	GA vs GG	**1.43 (1.14–1.80)**
ZNF350	Arg501Ser (A to T)	Figueroa et al. (2007) [33][a]	1,084:1,031	TT vs AA	**0.30 (0.11–0.83)**

Data presented for positive findings and for SNPs where more than one group have published. Negative findings reported in one study only: Broberg et al. (2005) [73] also studied *XRCC4*: Asn298Ser. Wu et al. (2006) [35] also studied *XRCC2*: 3′ UTR at nt41657; *BRCA2*: Asn372His; *RAG1*: Lys820Arg; *Ku70*: Gly593Gly; *Ku80*: 3′ UTR (rs10511685); *LIGIV* Thr9Ile; *ATM*: Asp1853Asn. Figueroa et al. (2007) [33] also studied *BRIP*: –1918, IVS1+12, IVS14+1, Glu879Glu, Ser919Pro,Tyr1137Tyr; *NBS1*: Leu34Leu, IVS8+1488, 3′ UTR (ex16+304); *RAD51*: –4719, IVS2+100, Ex1-96, IVS1+1398, IVS3+1932, IVS5-4480, IVS5-4016, IVS6+1598, 3′ UTR 1131bp 3′ of STP; *XRCC2*: –4644, –969, Ala16Ser, IVS2+5647, 3′ UTR Ex3+1443; *XRCC4*: –28073, IVS4-64, IVS7-6281, IVS7-61; *ZNF350*: Cys236Cys, 3′ UTR Ex5-229. Studies in bold italics depict meta-analyses. Bold represents CI's not crossing 1.0. [a]Study reported from the Spanish Bladder Cancer Study. [b]Study reported from the MD Anderson Bladder Cancer Study. [c]Study reported from the Leeds Bladder Cancer Study. [d]Study reported from the New Hampshire Bladder Cancer Study. Published case–control studies only are presented so no account is taken for negative studies published in abstract form.

6.2. Gene Dosage Effects: Haplotypes and Pathways

In a multistep, multigenic process such as carcinogenesis, single polymorphisms in single genes are unlikely to alter the expression or function of specific proteins to the extent of producing a pathological phenotype (*52*). However the combined effect of several SNPs in a gene could have more impact. Various studies have shown groups of SNPs within an individual gene to be associated with bladder cancer risk (*33*, *37*, *39*, *41*), although often the association is less strong than for an individual SNP. Due to linkage disequilibrium, SNPs are not inherited independently. Rather, sets of adjacent SNPs are usually inherited in blocks (*13*), resulting in different haplotypes (defined as the set of variants occurring together on a chromosome) in individuals. Each block has only a few haplotypes, so only a few SNPs are required to uniquely identify ("tag") each haplotype.

The HapMap Project (www.hapmap.org), which provides a public genome-wide database of common human sequence variation, has identified tagging SNPs, which capture groups of SNPs across the genome. Whilst Taqman is the commonest genotyping method for investigating single SNPs, this has been largely superseded by high-throughput multiplex genotyping platforms (*53*) for the study of multiple SNPs in multiple genes. The combined effect of multiple SNPs in several genes in one or more relevant DNA repair pathways could have a greater impact on pathological phenotype, i.e. DRC. Matullo et al. (*54*) found an increased risk for patients carrying more than five risk alleles (6–8 versus 0–4; OR, 1.76; 95% CI, 1.12–2.76) for SNPs in seven HR and NER genes, and Wu et al. (*35*) found a significant gene-dosage effect for increasing numbers of potential high-risk alleles in their study of DNA repair and cell cycle SNPs. In NER each additional allele was associated with a 1.21-fold increased risk (95% CI, 1.12–1.29). Garcia-Closas et al. (*31*) also found that genetic variation in 22 NER SNPs significantly predicted bladder cancer risk. Figueroa et al. (*33*) found a significant global association between 29 DSB repair variants and bladder cancer risk.

6.3. Gene–Environment Interaction

Cigarette smoking is associated with a twofold to threefold increased risk of developing bladder cancer (*3*). The effect of DNA repair polymorphisms on bladder cancer risk may only be apparent in the presence of DNA damaging agents, such as those in cigarette smoke, so groups have attempted to look at gene–smoking interactions. Studies have been hampered by small sample sizes and the influence of multiple testing on p values (*30*). However, novel computational algorithms have improved statistical power to detect interactions (gene–gene or gene–environment) over traditional logistic regression approaches. For example, multifactor dimensionality reduction (MDR) analysis (*55*) seeks to identify combinations of multilocus genotypes and discrete environmental factors that are associated with either high or low risk of disease (*41*). Classification tree analysis (CART) uses a binary recursive partitioning method that identifies a sub-group of high-risk subjects and detects higher-order interactions among a large number of variables (*35*). Splitting rules are used to stratify data into groups with homogeneous risk, which could be substantial (*31*). Using CART, the MD Anderson group found that smoking was the most important risk factor for bladder cancer, not unexpectedly in view of the ORs observed, and that NER gene polymorphisms were only relevant in smokers. They found an indication of a biologically meaningful interaction between NER and smoking and observed that smoking and three BER SNPs were a high-risk combination of factors (*35*, *36*). Although CART has identified potential gene–smoking interactions, this is a post-data mining tool, so findings require external validation in independent studies.

7. Genome-wide Association Studies

Genome-wide association studies have been undertaken using platforms of up to 550,000 tagging SNPs in a number of diseases. Such studies result in many null results and only a few SNPs across the genome are found to be of statistical significance, as critical p values are very low due to multiple testing. This approach detects variants in unstudied genes and SNPs of greater than 10% minor allele frequencies (MAF) but it is poor for MAFs of less than 5%. A major issues is the ability to achieve an adequate density of coverage of common sequence variation. Studies have recently been published on prostate cancer (*56–58*) and colorectal cancer (*59*), where variants were found in 8q24, a region with no known genes, and breast cancer (*60*). Whole genome association (WGA) studies in bladder cancer are underway.

8. DNA Repair SNPs and Response of Bladder Cancer to Therapies

Polymorphisms may be prognostic for events such as recurrence or progression of superficial bladder cancer, or predictive for response to radiotherapy and/or chemotherapy for muscle invasive disease. Knowledge of an individual's genetic risk profile could allow the intensity of cystoscopic surveillance to be modified based on risk of progression and for treatment of muscle invasive disease to be tailored to the individual. These studies lag behind

Table 12.4
Positive associations for DNA repair SNPs with prognostic factors and treatment outcomes in bladder cancer

Gene of interest	SNP	Reference	Outcome measured	Number of individuals affected	Comparison groups	HR/RR/OR (95% CI)
XPC	Ala499Val	Sak et al. (2006) [39]	Stage (Ta/T1 vs T2–T4)	469:87	CT/TT vs CC	$p = 0.01$ (χ^2)
			Grade (G1, 2, 3)	75:244:228	CT/TT vs CC	NS
XPD	Lys751Gln (A to C)	Sanyal et al. (2007) [63]	Progression	Not stated	AC/CC vs AA	0.4 (0.2–1.0)[c]
	XRCC1 Arg-399Gln	Sakano et al (2006) [71]	Cause specific survival after chemoradiation	Not stated	AC/CC vs AA and GA/AA vs GG	0.5 (0.19–0.97)[c]
XPG	Asp1104His (G to C)	Sakano et al. (2005) [62]	Stage (pT1 vs pTa)	53:171	GC/CC vs GG	1.9 (1.0–3.5)[d]
ERCC6 (CSB)	Met1097Val (A to G)	Gu et al. (2005) [61]	Recurrence vs no recurrence	77:120	AG/GG vs AA	1.54 (1.02–2.33)[a]
MSH6	Gly39Glu (G to A)	Sanyal et al. (2007) [63]	Grade (high vs low)	150:110	GA/AA vs GG	1.2 (1.0–1.5)[b]
		Sanyal et al. (2007) [63]	Stage (high vs low)	106:146	GA/AA vs GG	1.4 (1.0–2.0)[b]
	Lys751Gln with XRCC1 Arg399Gln (G to A)	Sanyal et al. (2007) [63]	Death	Not stated	AC/CC vs AA	0.6 (0.4–1.0)[c]
		Sanyal et al. (2007) [63]	Recurrence following installation treatment for TaG2	22 installations	GA/AA vs GG	0.4 (0.2–1.0)[c]
		Sanyal et al. (2007) [63]	Death following radiotherapy	11 treated	GA/AA vs GG	0.1 (0.0–0.8)[c]
OGG1	Ser326Cys (C to G)	Sanyal et al. (2007) [63]	Death following radiotherapy	10 treated	CG/GG vs CC	10.8 (1.2—99.5)[c]

NS, not significant.

[a]HR for recurrence versus no recurrence. [b]Relative risk (RR) for stage/grade. [c]HR for outcomes including death, recurrence, treatment response. [d]Odds ratio. [e]Risk ratio.

the case–control studies, hampered partly by small number of cases and by investigation of only relatively common variants whose functional significance is debatable.

8.1. SNPs as Prognostic Factors in Bladder Cancer

Table 12.4 shows the positive associations for DNA repair SNPs with prognostic factors and treatment outcomes. Gu et al. (*61*), in 261 superficial bladder tumour patients, found that increased numbers of high-risk variant alleles in NER genes were associated with higher recurrence rates for superficial disease and also shorter recurrence-free survival times (median 6.9 months versus 16.6 months), but there were no associations with progression. Sakano et al. (*62*), in 233 patients with superficial bladder cancer, found an association between the *XPG* Asp1104His variant allele with higher tumour stage (pT1 versus pTa), although there was no difference in terms of overall and cancer-specific survivals, but only 15 patients died from bladder cancer and cancer-specific survivals were 92.7% and 91.4%, respectively. Sanyal et al. (*63*), in 311 bladder cancer patients, 79% of whom had superficial tumours, found the variant allele of *MSH6* Gly39Glu to be associated with increased stage and grade of disease, whilst the *XPD* Lys-751Gln variant was associated with reduced risk of death and lower risk of progression. When the joint effect of the *XPD* Lys751Gln and *XPC* Lys939Gln variant alleles was determined, there was a significantly longer survival than for the rest of the patient population ($p < 0.001$).

8.2. Influence of DNA Repair SNPs on Somatic p53 Mutations

Alteration of the *TP53* gene is a crucial event in the development of muscle invasive bladder cancer. Carcinogens in cigarette smoke can cause *TP53* mutations and decreased DRC due to functional SNPs in DNA repair genes could result in somatic mutations in *TP53* and other important regulatory genes. Three groups have investigated the association between DNA repair SNPs and *TP53* mutations (*64, 65*) or p53 protein expression by immunohistochemistry (*66*). The two studies of both superficial and muscle-invasive disease found no statistically significant associations (*64, 65*), except that Stern et al. (*65*), in 139 patients, found 5 of 15 *TP53* G:C to A:T transitions to be associated with the *XRCC1* codon 751 homozygous variant genotype (OR, 3.7; 95% CI, 1.1–13). Sakano et al. (*66*), in 57 Japanese patients with muscle-invasive tumours, found the positive p53 expression rate by immunohistochemistry to be significantly lower in individuals homozygous for the variant allele of *XPC* codon 939 (OR < 0.01; $p = 0.005$) and heterozygous for the variant allele (OR, 0.36; 95% CI, 0.16–0.82). However, this finding was counter to the original hypothesis, and controversy exists regarding the relationship between *TP53* mutations status and protein expression by immunohistochemistry.

8.3. SNPs as Predictive Factors of Treatment Responses

In lung and colorectal cancer, individuals carrying the variant alleles in *XPC*, *ERCC1*, and *XRCC1* did worse after platinum-based treatment than individuals with wild-type alleles (*67–70*), contrary to the hypothesis that reduced DRC would increase sensitivity to cisplatin due to failure of adduct repair. Gu et al. (*61*) found that bladder cancer patients with *XPA* 5'-UTR or *ERCC6* Arg1230Pro variant alleles had shorter recurrence-free survivals following BCG treatment. Sanyal et al. (*63*) found the *XRCC1* Arg399Gln variant was associated with reduced recurrence rate following installation treatment for TaG2 disease (n = 22) and also with a reduced risk of death following radiotherapy (n = 11 patients treated). In contrast, the *OGG1* Ser326Cys variant allele was associated with an increased risk of death after radiotherapy (n = 10) but had no influence on survival in those who did not receive radiotherapy (n = 48).

Sakano et al. (*71*) studied NER, BER, and HR SNPs in 78 patients, looking at the effect on response and prognosis following platinum-based chemoradiotherapy. They found the recurrence rate to be significantly lower in patients with greater numbers of total variant alleles in all DNA repair genes and in NER genes ($p = 0.03$), and the total number of variant alleles were significantly associated with improved cancer-specific survival, in univariate analysis. On subgroup analysis for T3/4 patients (n = 38), the *XRCC1* genotypes and combined *XPD* and *XRCC1* genotypes were independently associated with cancer-specific survival in multivariate analysis. These data would fit with the hypothesis that SNP variants associated with reduced DRC result in improved response to chemotherapy and hence improved prognosis. Much larger series, investigating larger numbers of SNPs, are required to be able to make definitive conclusions about the role of DNA repair variants and treatment outcome.

9. Concluding Remarks

Investigation of individual DNA repair SNPs in bladder cancer has yielded few robust positive findings, which is not surprising given the multifactorial nature of the disease. Pathway approaches using novel genotyping technologies will allow more comprehensive studies of multiple SNPs in multiple genes, and it will be possible to investigate gene–environment interaction more rigorously than heretofore, using novel statistical methodology, in larger studies and through collaborative efforts within consortia. The results of the genome-wide association studies in bladder cancer are awaited with interest. Ultimately, genetic variation may be used to predict outcome from treatments in bladder cancer with a view to improving patient care in this disease.

Acknowledgments

I thank Tim Bishop and Jenny Barrett for critical reading of the manuscript and Anita Chatwin for her secretarial support.

References

1. Cancer Research UK. 2006. CancerStats Incidence-UK.
2. Cancer Research UK. 2007. CancerStats Mortality-UK.
3. Zeegers, M. P., Tan, F. E., Dorant, E., and van Den Brandt, P. A. (2000) The impact of characteristics of cigarette smoking on urinary tract cancer risk: a meta-analysis of epidemiologic studies. *Cancer Causes Control* 89, 630–639.
4. Puente, D., Hartge, P., Greiser, E., Cantor, K. P., King, W. D., González, C. A., et al. (2006) A pooled analysis of bladder cancer case-control studies evaluating smoking in men and women. *Cancer Causes Control* 17, 71–79.
5. Kogevinas, M., 't Mannetje, A., Cordier, S., Ranft, U., González, C. A., Vineis, P., et al. (2003) Occupation and bladder cancer among men in Western Europe. *Cancer Causes Control* 14, 907–914.
6. Kiemeney, L. A. and Schoenberg, M. (1996) Familial transitional cell carcinoma. *J Urol* 156, 867–872.
7. Lin, J., Spitz, M., R., Dinney, C., P., Etzel, C., J., Grossman, H., B., and Wu, X. (2006) Bladder cancer risk as modified by family history and smoking. *Cancer* 107, 705–711.
8. Murta-Nascimento, C., Silverman, D., T., Kogevinas, M., García-Closas, M., Rothman, N., Tardón, A., et al. (2007) Risk of bladder cancer associated with family history of cancer: do low-penetrance polymorphisms account for the increase in risk? *Cancer Epidemiol Biomarkers Prev* 16, 1595–600.
9. Guidelines on TaT1 (Non-Muscle Invasive) Bladder Cancer [http://www.uroweb.org/nc/professional-resources/guidelines/online].
10. Lamm, D. L., Blumenstein, B. A., Crissman, J. D., Montie, J. E., Gottesman, J. E., Lowe, B. A., et al. (2000) Maintenance bacillus Calmette-Guerin immunotherapy for recurrent TA, T1 and carcinoma in situ transitional cell carcinoma of the bladder: a randomized Southwest Oncology Group Study. *J Urol* 163, 1634–1124.
11. Kotwal, S., Choudhury, A., Johnston, C., Paul, A., B., Whelan, P., and Kiltie, A. (2008) Similar treatment outcomes for radical cystectomy and radical radiotherapy in invasive bladder cancer treated at a United Kingdom specialist treatment center. *Int J Radiat Oncol Biol Phys* 70, 456–463.
12. Advanced Bladder Cancer (ABC) Meta-analysis collaboration. (2005) Neoadjuvant chemotherapy in invasive bladder cancer: Update of a systematic review and meta-analysis of individual patient data. *Eur Urol* 48, 202–206.
13. Wu, X., Zhao, H., Suk, R., and Christiani, D. C. (2004) Genetic susceptibility to tobacco-related cancer. *Oncogene* 23, 6500–6523.
14. Engel, L. S., Taioli, E., Pfeiffer, R., Garcia-Closas, M., Marcus, P. M., Lan, Q., et al. (2002) Pooled analysis and meta-analysis of glutathione S-transferase M1 and bladder cancer: a HuGE review. *Am J Epidemiol* 156, 95–109.
15. García-Closas, M., Malats, N., Silverman, D., Dosemeci, M., Kogevinas, M., Hein, D. W., et al. (2005) NAT2 slow acetylation, GSTM1 null genotype, and risk of bladder cancer: results from the Spanish Bladder Cancer Study and meta-analyses. *Lancet* 366, 649–659.
16. Barnes, D. E. and Lindahl, T. (2004) Repair and genetic consequences of endogenous DNA base damage in mammalian cells. *Annu Rev Genet* 38, 445–476.
17. Hoeijmakers, J. H. (2001) Genome maintenance mechanisms for preventing cancer. *Nature* 411, 366–374.
18. O'Driscoll, M. and Jeggo, P. A. (2006) The role of double-strand break repair—insights from human genetics. Nature Reviews. *Genetics* 7, 45–54.
19. Buck, D., Malivert, L., de Chasseval, R., Barraud, A., Fondanèche, M. C., Sanal, O., et al. (2006) Cernunnos, a novel nonhomologous end-joining factor, is mutated in human immunodeficiency with microcephaly. *Cell* 124, 287–299.

20. Wallace, S. S. (1998) Enzymatic processing of radiation-induced free radical damage in DNA. *Radiat Res* **150**, 60–79.

21. Baynes, C., Healey, C. S., Pooley, K. A., Scollen, S., Luben, R. N., Thompson, D. J., et al. (2007) Common variants in the ATM, BRCA1, BRCA2, CHEK2 and TP53 cancer susceptibility genes are unlikely to increase breast cancer risk. *Breast Cancer Res* **9**, R27.

22. Harland, M., Taylor, C. F., Bass, S., Churchman, M., Randerson-Moor, J. A., Holland, E. A., et al. (2005) Intronic sequence variants of the CDKN2A gene in melanoma pedigrees. *Genes Chromosomes Cancer* **43**, 128–136.

23. Goode, E.L., Ulrich, C.M., and Potter, J.D. (2002) Polymorphisms in DNA repair genes and associations with cancer risk. *Cancer Epidemiol Biomarkers Prev* **11**, 1513–1530.

24. Kuschel, B., Auranen, A., McBride, S., Novik, K. L., Antoniou, A., Lipscombe, J. M., et al. (2002) Variants in DNA double-strand break repair genes and breast cancer susceptibility. *Hum Mol Genet* **11**, 1399–1407.

25. Kiyohara, C., Takayama, K., and Nakanishi, Y. (2006) Association of genetic polymorphisms in the base excision repair pathway with lung cancer risk: a meta-analysis. *Lung Cancer* **54**, 267–283.

26. Zollner, S. and Pritchard, J. K. (2007) Overcoming the winner's curse: estimating penetrance parameters from case-control data. *Am J Hum Genet* **80**, 605–615.

27. Matullo, G., Guarrera, S., Carturan, S., Peluso, M., Malaveille, C., Davico, L., et al. (2001) DNA repair gene polymorphisms, bulky DNA adducts in white blood cells and bladder cancer in a case-control study. *Int J Cancer* **92**, 562–567.

28. Wacholder, S., Chanock, S., Garcia-Closas, M., El Ghormli, L., and Rothman, N. (2004) Assessing the probability that a positive report is false: an approach for molecular epidemiology studies. *J Natl Cancer Inst* **96**, 434–442.

29. Bourgain, C., Génin, E., Cox, N., and Clerget-Darpoux, F. (2007) Are genome-wide association studies all that we need to dissect the genetic component of complex human diseases? *Eur J Hum Genet* **15**, 260–263.

30. Brennan, P. (2002) Gene-environment interaction and aetiology of cancer: what does it mean and how can we measure it? *Carcinogenesis* **23**, 381–387.

31. Garcia-Closas, M., Malats, N., Real, F. X., Welch, R., Kogevinas, M., Chatterjee, N., et al. (2006) Genetic Variation in the nucleotide excision repair pathway and bladder cancer risk. *Cancer Epidemiol Biomarkers Prev* **15**, 536–542.

32. Figueroa, J. D., Malats, N., Real, F. X., Silverman, D., Kogevinas, M., Chanock, S., et al. (2007) Genetic variation in the base excision repair pathway and bladder cancer risk. *Hum Genet* **121**, 233–242.

33. Figueroa, J. D., Malats, N., Rothman, N., Real, F. X., Silverman, D., Kogevinas, M., et al. (2007) Evaluation of genetic variation in the double-strand break repair pathway and bladder cancer risk. *Carcinogenesis* **28**, 1788–1793.

34. Schabath, M. B., Delclos, G. L., Grossman, H. B., Wang, Y., Lerner, S. P., Chamberlain, R. M., et al. (2005) Polymorphisms in XPD exons 10 and 23 and bladder cancer risk. *Cancer Epidemiol Biomarkers Prev* **14**, 878–884.

35. Wu, X., Gu, J., Grossman, H.B., et al. (2006) Bladder cancer predisposition: a multigenic approach to DNA-repair and cell-cycle-control genes. *Am J Hum Genet* **78**, 464–479.

36. Huang, M., Dinney, C. P., Lin, X., Lin, J., Grossman, H. B., and Wu, X. (2007) High-order interactions among genetic variants in DNA base excision repair pathway genes and smoking in bladder cancer susceptibility. *Cancer Epidemiol Biomarkers Prev* **16**, 84–91.

37. Zhu, Y., Lai, M., Yang, H., Lin, J., Huang, M., Grossman, H. B., et al. (2007) Genotypes, haplotypes and diplotypes of XPC and risk of bladder cancer. *Carcinogenesis* **28**, 698–703.

38. Sak, S. C., Barrett, J. H., Paul, A. B., Bishop, D. T, and Kiltie, A. E. (2005) The polyAT, intronic IVS11-6 and Lys939Gln XPC polymorphisms are not associated with transitional cell carcinoma of the bladder. *Br J Cancer* **92**, 2262–2265.

39. Sak, S. C., Barrett, J. H., Paul, A. B., Bishop, D. T., and Kiltie, A. E. (2006) Comprehensive analysis of 22 XPC polymorphisms and bladder cancer risk. *Cancer Epidemiol Biomarkers Prev* **15**, 2537–2541.

40. Sak, S. C., Barrett, J. H., Paul, A. B., Bishop, D. T., Kiltie, A. E. (2007) DNA repair gene XRCC1 polymorphisms and bladder cancer risk. *BMC Genet* **10**, 13.

41. Andrew, A. S., Nelson, H. H., Kelsey, K. T., Moore, J. H., Meng, A. C., Casella, D. P., et al. (2006) Concordance of multiple analytical approaches demonstrates a complex relationship between DNA repair gene SNPs, smoking and bladder cancer susceptibility. *Carcinogenesis* **27**, 1030–1037.

42. Spitz, M. R., Wu, X., Wang, Y., Wang, L. E., Shete, S., Amos, C. I., et al. (2001) Modulation of nucleotide excision repair capacity by XPD polymorphisms in lung cancer patients. *Cancer Res* **61**, 1354–1357.

43. Wu, X., Zhao, H., Wei, Q., Amos, C. I., Zhang, K., Guo, Z., et al. (2003) XPA polymorphism associated with reduced lung cancer risk and a modulating effect on nucleotide excision repair capacity. *Carcinogenesis* **24**, 505–509.

44. Lin, J., Kadlubar, F. F., Spitz, M. R., Zhao, H., and Wu, X. (2005) A modified host cell reactivation assay to measure DNA repair capacity for removing 4-aminobiphenyl adducts: a pilot study of bladder cancer. *Cancer Epidemiol Biomarkers Prev* **14**, 1832–1836.

45. Mohrenweiser, H. W., Wilson, D. M., and Jones, I. M. (2003) Challenges and complexities in estimating both the functional impact and the disease risk associated with the extensive genetic variation in human DNA repair genes. *Mutat Res* **526**, 93–125.

46. Khan, S. G., Metter, E. J., Tarone, R. E., Bohr, V. A., Grossman, L., Hedayati, M., et al. (2000) A new xeroderma pigmentosum group C poly(AT) insertion/deletion polymorphism. *Carcinogenesis* **21**, 1821–1825.

47. Seker, H., Butkiewicz, D., Bowman, E. D., Rusin, M., Hedayati, M., Grossman, L., et al. (2001) Functional significance of XPD polymorphic variants: attenuated apoptosis in human lymphoblastoid cells with the XPD 312 Asp/Asp genotype. *Cancer Res* **61**, 7430–7434.

48. Porter, P. C., Mellon, I., and States, J. C. (2005) XP-A cells complemented with Arg-228Gln and Val234Leu polymorphic XPA alleles repair BPDE-induced DNA damage better than cells complemented with the wild type allele. *DNA Repair* **2**, 341–349.

49. Clarkson, S. G. and Wood, R. D. (2005) Polymorphisms in the human XPD (ERCC2) gene, DNA repair capacity and cancer susceptibility: an appraisal. *DNA Repair* **4**, 1068–1074.

50. Hung, R. J., Hall, J., Brennan, P., and Boffetta, P. (2005) Genetic polymorphisms in the base excision repair pathway and cancer risk: a HuGE review. *Am J Epidemiol* **162**, 925–942.

51. Han, S., Zhang, H. T., Wang, Z., Xie, Y., Tang, R., Mao, Y., et al. (2006) DNA repair gene XRCC3 polymorphisms and cancer risk: a meta-analysis of 48 case-control studies. *Eur J Hum Genet* **14**, 1136–1144.

52. Matullo, G., Dunning, A. M., Guarrera, S., Baynes, C., Polidoro, S., Garte, S., et al. (2006) DNA repair polymorphisms and cancer risk in non-smokers in a cohort study. *Carcinogenesis* **27**, 997–1007.

53. Fan, J. B., Chee, M. S., and Gunderson, K. L. (2006) Highly parallel genomic assays. Nature reviews. *Genetics* **7**, 632–644.

54. Matullo, G., Guarrera, S., Sacerdote, C., Polidoro, S., Davico, L., Gamberini, S., et al. (2005) Polymorphisms/haplotypes in DNA repair genes and smoking: a bladder cancer case-control study. *Cancer Epidemiol Biomarkers Prev* **14**, 2569–2578.

55. Hahn, L. W., Ritchie, M. D., and Moore, J. H. (2003) Multifactor dimensionality reduction software for detecting gene-gene and gene-environment interactions. *Bioinformatics* **19**, 376–382.

56. Gudmundsson, J., Sulem, P., Manolescu, A., Amundadottir, L. T., Gudbjartsson, D., Helgason, A., et al. (2007) Genome-wide association study identifies a second prostate cancer susceptibility variant at 8q24. *Nat Genet* **39**, 631–637.

57. Haiman, C. A., Patterson, N., Freedman, M. L., Myers, S. R., Pike, M. C., Waliszewska, A., et al. (2007) Multiple regions within 8q24 independently affect risk for prostate cancer. *Nat Genet* **39**, 638–644.

58. Yeager, M., Orr, N., Hayes, R. B., Jacobs, K. B., Kraft, P., Wacholder, S., et al. (2007) Genome-wide association study of prostate cancer identifies a second risk locus at 8q24. *Nat Genet* **39**, 645–649.

59. Tomlinson, I., Webb, E., Carvajal-Carmona, L., Broderick, P., Kemp, Z., Spain, S., et al. (2007) A genome-wide association scan of tag SNPs identifies a susceptibility variant for colorectal cancer at 8q24.21. *Nat Genet* **39**, 984–988.

60. Easton, D. F., Pooley, K. A., Dunning, A. M., Pharoah, P. D., Thompson, D., Ballinger, D. G., et al. (2007) Genome-wide association study identifies novel breast cancer susceptibility loci. *Nature* **447**, 1087–1093.

61. Gu, J., Zhao, H., Dinney, C. P., Zhu, Y., Leibovici, D., Bermejo, C. E., et al. (2005) Nucleotide excision repair gene polymorphisms and recurrence after treatment for superficial bladder cancer. *Clin Cancer Res* **11**, 1408–1415.

62. Sakano, S., Kumar, R., Larsson, P., Onelöv, E., Adolfsson, J., Steineck, G., et al. (2005) A single-nucleotide polymorphism in the XPG gene, and tumour stage, grade, and clinical course in patients with non muscle-invasive neoplasms of the urinary bladder. *BJU Int* **97**, 847–851.

63. Sanyal, S., De Verdier, P. J., Steineck, G., Larsson, P., Onelöv, E., Hemminki, K., et al. (2007) Polymorphisms in XPD, XPC and the risk of death in patients with urinary bladder neoplasms. *Acta Oncologica* **46**, 31–41.

64. Ryk, C., Kumar, R., Sanyal, S., de Verdier, P. J., Hemminki, K., Larsson, P., et al. (2006) Influence of polymorphism in DNA repair and defence genes on p53 mutations in bladder tumours. *Cancer Lett* **241**, 142–149.

65. Stern, M. C., Conway, K., Li, Y., Mistry, K., and Taylor, J. A. (2006) DNA repair gene polymorphisms and probability of p53 mutation in bladder cancer. *Mol Carcinog* **45**, 715–719.

66. Sakano, S., Matsumoto, H., Yamamoto, Y., Kawai, Y., Eguchi, S., Ohmi, C., et al. (2006) Association between DNA repair gene polymorphisms and p53 alterations in Japanese patients with muscle-invasive bladder cancer. *Pathobiology* **73**, 295–303.

67. Park, D.J., Stoehlmacher J., Zhang, W., Tsao-Wei, D. D., Groshen, S., and Lenz, H. J. (2001) A Xeroderma pigmentosum group D gene polymorphism predicts clinical outcome to platinum-based chemotherapy in patients with advanced colorectal cancer. *Cancer Res* **61**, 8654–8658.

68. Stoehlmacher, J., Park, D. J., Zhang, W., Yang, D., Groshen, S., Zahedy, S., et al. (2004) A multivariate analysis of genomic polymorphisms: prediction of clinical outcome to 5-FU/oxaliplatin combination chemotherapy in refractory colorectal cancer. *Br J Cancer* **91**, 344–354.

69. Zhou, W., Gurubhagavatula, S., Liu, G., Park, S., Neuberg, D. S., Wain, J. C., et al. (2004) Excision repair cross-complementation group 1 polymorphism predicts overall survival in advanced non-small cell lung cancer patients treated with platinum-based chemotherapy. *Clin Cancer Res* **10**, 4939–4943.

70. Gurubhagavatula, S., Liu, G., Park, S., Zhou, W., Su, L., Wain, J. C., et al. (2004) XPD and XRCC1 genetic polymorphisms are prognostic factors in advanced non-small-cell lung cancer patients treated with platinum chemotherapy. *J Clin Oncol* **22**, 2594–2601.

71. Sakano, S., Wada, T., Matsumoto, H., Sugiyama, S., Inoue, R., Eguchi, S., et al. (2006) Single nucleotide polymorphisms in DNA repair genes might be prognostic factors in muscle-invasive bladder cancer patients treated with chemoradiotherapy. *Br J Cancer* **95**, 561–570.

72. Sanyal, S., Festa, F., Sakano, S., Zhang, Z., Steineck, G., Norming, U., et al. (2004) Polymorphisms in DNA repair and metabolic genes in bladder cancer. *Carcinogenesis* **25**, 729–734.

73. Broberg, K., Bjork, J., Paulsson, K., Hoglund, M., and Albin, M. (2005) Constitutional short telomeres are strong genetic susceptibility markers for bladder cancer. *Carcinogenesis* **26**, 1263–1271.

74. Stern, M. C., Johnson, L. R., Bell, D. A., and Taylor, J. A. (2002) XPD codon 751 polymorphism, metabolism genes, smoking, and bladder cancer risk. *Cancer Epidemiol Biomarkers Prev* **11**, 1004–1011.

75. Shen, M., Hung, R. J., Brennan, P., Malaveille, C., Donato, F., Placidi, D., et al. (2003) Polymorphisms of the DNA repair genes XRCC1, XRCC3, XPD, interaction with environmental exposures, and bladder cancer risk in a case-control study in northern Italy. *Cancer Epidemiol Biomarkers Prev* **12**, 1234–1240.

76. Terry, P. D., Umbach, D. M., and Taylor, J. A. (2006) APE1 genotype and risk of bladder cancer: evidence for effect modification by smoking. *Int J Cancer* **118**, 3170–3173.

77. Karahalil, B., Kocabas, N. A., and Ozçelik, T. (2006) DNA repair gene polymorphisms and bladder cancer susceptibility in a Turkish population. *Anticancer Res* **26**, 4955–4958.

78. Stern, M.C., Umbach, D. M., van Gils, C.H., Lunn, R.M., and Taylor, J. A. (2001) DNA repair gene XRCC1 polymorphisms, smoking, and bladder cancer risk. *Cancer Epidemiol Biomarkers Prev* **10**, 125–131.

79. Kelsey, K. T., Park, S., Nelson, H. H., and Karagas, M. R. (2004) A population-based case-control study of the XRCC1 Arg-399Gln polymorphism and susceptibility to bladder cancer. *Cancer Epidemiol Biomarkers Prev* **13**, 1337–1341.

80. Stern, M. C., Umbach, D. M., Lunn, R. M., and Taylor, J. A. (2002) DNA repair gene XRCC3 codon 241 polymorphism, its interaction with smoking and XRCC1 polymorphisms, and bladder cancer risk. *Cancer Epidemiol Biomarkers Prev* **11**, 939–943.

Chapter 13

Breast Cancer Screening and Biomarkers

Mai Brooks

Abstract

Annual screening mammograms have been shown to be cost-effective and are credited for the decline in mortality of breast cancer. New technologies including breast magnetic resonance imaging (MRI) may further improve early breast cancer detection in asymptomatic women. Serum tumor markers such as CA 15-3, carcinoembyonic antigen (CEA), and CA 27–29 are ordered in the clinic mainly for disease surveillance, and not useful for detection of localized cancer. This review will discuss blood-based markers and breast-based markers, such as nipple/ductal fluid, with an emphasis on biomarkers for early detection of breast cancer. In the future, it is likely that a combination approach to simultaneously measure multiple markers would be most successful in detecting early breast cancer. Ideally, such a biomarker panel should be able to detect breast cancer in asymptomatic patients, even in the setting of normal mammogram and physical examination results.

Key words: Breast cancer, mammogram, magnetic resonance imaging, MRI, tumor marker, nipple fluid.

1. Introduction

Breast cancer is the most common form of cancer and the second leading cause of cancer deaths in American women. In 2007, approximately 180,510 patients are estimated to be diagnosed with invasive breast cancer, and an estimated 40,910 will die of this disease in the USA *(1)*. Furthermore, about 62,030 female ductal carcinoma in situ (DCIS) breast cases will be newly diagnosed. For a woman of average risk, the lifetime incidence of breast cancer is one in eight.

M. Verma (ed.), *Methods of Molecular Biology, Cancer Epidemiology, vol. 472*
© 2009 Humana Press, a part of Springer Science + Business Media, Totowa, NJ
Book doi: 10.1007/978-1-60327-492-0

2. Screening

Screening of asymptomatic women has been accredited for the decline in mortality of breast cancer (2). The current recommendations from the American Cancer Society for normal-risk women are as follows: 1) Yearly mammogram starting at age 40 years. The age at which screening should be stopped should be individualized by considering the potential risks and benefits of screening in the context of overall health status and longevity. 2) Clinical breast exam every 3 years for women in their 20s and 30s, and every year for women 40 years and older (3). The evidence to justify mammography for population-based screening is derived from both randomized and several nonrandomized clinical trials. Eight randomized trials totaling hundreds of thousands of patients include the Health Insurance Plan of New York (4), four studies from Sweden (5–8), one study from the United Kingdom (9), and two studies from Canada (10, 11). The US Breast Cancer Detection Demonstration Project (BCDDP), the largest study of mammography and clinical breast exam, also demonstrated that screening decreases breast cancer mortality (12).

During the past decade, advances in mammography include digital techniques and computer-aided detection. Film (nondigital) mammography has been estimated to have an approximately 65–80% sensitivity at the desired specificity of 90% (13). The investigators from the Digital Mammographic Imaging Screening Trial (DMIST) reported that the overall diagnostic accuracy of digital and film mammography is similar (14). However, digital mammograms are more accurate in women under the age of 50 years, premenopausal or perimenopausal women, and those with radiographically dense breasts. Two years later, another large study compared film mammography with digital mammograms read with computer-aided detection software (15). The authors found that diagnostic specificity significantly decreases from 90.2% to 87.2% with computer-aided detection, whereas sensitivity does not change. The rate of biopsy increases by 19.7%. Thus, more expensive technology does not necessarily translate into better outcome (16).

In women at high risk for developing breast cancer, screening may also involve breast ultrasound and/or magnetic resonance imaging (MRI). High-risk factors include BRCA gene carriers, personal or strong family history of breast cancer, prior atypia such as atypical ductal hyperplasia (ADH) or lobular carcinoma in situ (LCIS), and prior chest irradiation. Sonography may be useful in dense breasts. Screening ultrasound can lead to biopsy in 2–4% of women, of which carcinoma was found in 10–16% of these biopsies *(17)*. The American College of Radiology (ACR) Imaging Network trial 6666 is evaluating screening sonography in high-risk women *(18)*. Breast MRI has also recently been used by clinicians in many high-risk patients. In previous reports, MRI resulted in biopsy in 7–18% of women; breast cancer was detected in 24–88% of these biopsies *(19)*. We do not know yet whether ultrasound or MRI decreases breast cancer mortality in the high-risk population beyond that achieved by screening mammography. Currently, breast MRI is also indicated in women with newly diagnosed unilateral breast cancer. A recent publication showed that MRI can detect cancer in the contralateral breast that is missed by mammography and clinical examination in 3.1% of cases *(20)*. The sensitivity of contralateral breast MRI is 91%, the specificity is 88%, and the negative predictive value is 99%.

Despite the proven success of breast cancer screening with mammography, many investigators in the US have noted a decline in its use. The National Health Interview Survey (NHIS) estimates from 2005 demonstrated a decline in mammogram screening to 66%, from 70% in 2000 *(21)*. This coincides with a reported decrease in the incidence of breast cancer *(22)*.

3. Biomarkers in Clinical Use

Serum tumor markers for breast cancer used in the clinic include CA 15-3, carcinoembyonic antigen (CEA), and CA 27-29. All have low sensitivity and specificity, and thus are not helpful in detecting early breast cancer. CA 15-3 levels are increased in approximately 5–30% of patients with stage 1 disease, 15–50% with stage 2, 60–70% with stage 3, and 65–90% with stage 4. CA 15-3 levels are also elevated in 15–20% of women with benign breast conditions, 50–60% with liver disease, 20–70% with pulmonary malignancies, 15–60% with gastrointestinal/colonic malignancies, and 40–60% with ovarian cancer *(23)*. CEA is more prevalent in colorectal cancer, whereas CA 27–29 is more specific for breast cancer. These three tumor markers have, however, been validated for monitoring treatment in patients with advanced disease, particularly if the cancer cannot be evaluated with conventional imaging *(24)*. The American Society of Clinical Oncology recommends the use of CEA, CA 15-3, and CA 27–29 only in metastatic settings *(25)*, whereas the European Group on Tumor Markers recommends their use in disease surveillance in general *(26)*.

4. Biomarkers Under Research

This discussion emphasizes biomarkers that are under investigation for early detection of breast cancer. Blood-based markers will be reviewed first, followed by a separate section at the end on breast-based markers, such as nipple/ductal fluid and breast fine needle aspiration (FNA).

4.1. Criteria

Guidelines have been proposed to clarify the development of new biomarkers for cancer detection (27). In Phase 1, preclinical exploratory studies are carried out to identify leads that may distinguish cancerous from benign cases. This phase also includes the use of various statistical algorithms for selecting promising markers from a large pool of potential leads. Phase 2 includes clinical assay development for clinical disease to optimize the procedures for performing the assay in a reproducible manner. The true-positive rate and the false-positive rate are calculated, and a receiver operating characteristic (ROC) curve is constructed. Phase 3 evaluates the biomarker with retrospective longitudinal repository studies. In Phase 4, prospective screening trials are performed to determine whether tumors can be detected early before standard clinical diagnosis. In the case of breast cancer, the biomarker would be compared with standard mammography. Finally, phase 5 addresses whether screening with the biomarker of interest reduces the burden of cancer on the population. The primary aim is to estimate the reduction in cancer mortality. Using these stringent criteria, it should be noted that none of the markers under investigation discussed below has reached Phase 4.

4.2. Cancer Cells

With the current technology, circulating tumor cells have been found in very few cases of early stage breast cancer (28). Circulating tumor cells detected in both localized and metastatic breast cancer patients have been associated with worse outcome (29, 30). Circulating tumor cells may also predict response to therapy (31). Of interest, circulating endothelial cells have also been reported to decrease with treatment (32).

4.3. DNA and RNA

Cell-free DNA can be detected in the blood of healthy controls at approximately 10 ng/mL (33). DNA levels can fluctuate up to 50-fold throughout the day, making this method of cancer detection unreliable (34). In general, breast cancer patients have elevated free DNA levels (35). This plasma DNA may result from active cell destruction, via apoptosis or necrosis (36). Circulating DNA has been reported to detect tumor progression and lymph node involvement (37), or predict prognosis (38). Cell-free RNA has been found in cancer patients. However, no RNA marker so far has shown any usefulness (39).

Genetic analysis of circulating DNA as a detection tool has received much interest. However, known mutations in genes associated with breast malignant transformation including p53, BRCA1 and BRCA2, and various kinases and phosphatases account for a minority of cases. Microsatellite instability and loss of heterozygosity have been found in serum DNA of breast cancer patients *(40)*, with unclear significance.

Recently, epigenetic analysis of abnormal DNA methylation has been promising in the detection of breast cancer. Hypermethylation of a gene is associated with loss of expression, and can inactivate tumor suppressor genes or other cancer genes *(41)*. Multiple methods are available to assess methylation, and ongoing efforts are made to standardize the assays *(42)*. Certain genes methylated in cancer cells have been found to also be methylated in benign cells. In general, tumor suppressor genes are more specific for malignant cells. The list of methylated DNA candidates include cyclin D2, RAR-β, and Twist promoters *(43)*; RASSF1A *(44)*; CDH1, GSTP1, and BRCA1 *(45)*; p16INK4a *(46)*; and DAPK *(47)*. In serum, promoter hypermethylation of APC, RASSF1A, and DAP-kinase was detected in DCIS and LCIS, as well as in invasive breast cancer *(48)*. Methylation of at least one gene out of four (APC, GSTP1, RASSF1A, and RAR-β2) in plasma identified breast cancer with a sensitivity of 62% and specificity of 87%, and detected 33% of early-stage cases *(49)*. Hypermethylation of one or more genes (BRCA1, p16, and 14-3-3σ) was found in 95% of sporadic breast cancers *(50)*. Concordance was reported between the gene methylation pattern detected in the primary tumor and matched patient samples from serum *(51)*. Another group found concordance between primary cancer, serum as well as bone marrow and sentinel node *(52)*. DNA methylation of APC and RASSF1A out of 39 genes was reported to be independently associated with poor outcome *(53)*. The combination of free DNA and promoter methylation status in plasma identified 54% of breast cancer patients *(54)*.

4.4. Proteins

Numerous peptides associated with breast malignant transformation have been extensively investigated in the blood of patients and compared with those found in control healthy women. Individually, none thus far has been sensitive or specific enough to detect early breast cancer. However, it is possible that future combinations of certain protein levels in the blood may be useful.

Members of the MUC family, other than CA 15.3 and CA 27.29, have been evaluated but found to have lower sensitivity. These include the glycoprotein CA 549 *(55)*. Other mucins, such as MUC2, MUC3, MUC4, MUC5, and MUC6 are under investigation *(56)*. Cytokeratins 8, 18, and 19 have been proposed as tumor markers. Tests for measuring levels of fragment of cytokeratin 19 (CYFRA 21.1) *(57)*, cytokeratin 18 fragment (TPS), and combined fragments of all three cytokeratins (TPA) have reported low sensitivity *(58)*.

With the successful introduction of Herceptin in the treatment of breast cancer *(59)*, serum HER2 has emerged as a biomarker candidate. In localized breast cancer, HER2 levels are too low to distinguish patients with cancer from those without *(60)*. Furthermore, circulating HER2 status does not correlate with tissue HER2 expression *(61)*. However, in HER2-positive breast cancer cases, HER2 levels in the blood may have a role in monitoring for tumor recurrence *(62)* and in predicting response to targeted therapy in metastatic cancer *(63, 64)*.

Other proteins have been proposed as possible breast tumor markers, such as mammoglobin *(65)*, kallikrein 14 *(66)*, osteopontin *(67)*, mutant p53 protein *(68)*, and crypto-1 *(69)*. Plasma prolactin concentrations are reported to associate with an increased risk of postmenopausal breast cancer *(70)*. Also, circulating insulin-like growth factor (IGF)-1 and IGF binding protein (IGFBP)-3 are positively associated with breast cancer risk in older women, not in younger women *(71)*.

As the process of angiogenesis plays a critical role in breast tumor growth, there has been much interest in the possible use of several angiogenic factors or inhibitors as biomarkers. In population studies, angiogenic factors are significantly elevated in cancer patients, in comparison with healthy controls. However, we observed that overlap values between cancer and healthy groups has made it difficult to diagnose breast tumor early at an individual basis *(72)*, although basic fibroblast growth factor (bFGF) may have the best sensitivity and specificity *(73)*. The same may apply to cytokines, such as interleukin (IL)-6 and tumor necrosis factor (TNF)-α *(74)*, hepatocyte growth factor *(75)*, and others *(76)*. It is possible that the level of angiogenic factor(s) may be useful for prognostic purpose or for monitoring therapeutic response. Treatment of breast cancer has resulted in decreasing plasma vascular endothelial growth factor (VEGF), Tie-2, and angiopoietin-1 *(77)*. bFGF has been reported to increase the predictive value of the conventional marker CA 15-3 in response to chemotherapy of advanced breast cancer *(78)*. High levels of plasma tissue inhibitor of metalloproteinase (TIMP)-1 predicts survival in women with metastatic breast cancer *(79)*, whereas low serum levels of pro-matrix metalloproteinase 2 correlates with aggressive behavior in operable breast cancer *(80)*. Preoperative E-selectin levels also correlate with advanced stage *(81)*.

4.5. Autoantibodies

Antibodies may reflect the immune response to the earliest cancer cells, or alternatively a robust antitumor defense associated with reduced risk of developing cancer. The utility of autoantibodies in the blood for diagnosing early breast cancer remains to be determined. The list of autoantibodies include those to

HER2 *(82)*; MUC1 *(83)*; endostatin *(84)*; p53 *(85)*; p80, S6, RPA32, NY-ESO-1, and annexin XI-A *(86)*; malignin *(87)*; and others *(88)*.

4.6. Genomics and Proteomics

Genomic studies have produced a number of useful tissue-based gene signatures that can predict prognosis. Two of these are already in clinical use for a subset of breast cancer patients, the Oncotype DX test *(89)* and the Mammaprint assay *(90)*. Different gene sets were tested, and found to be reliably prognostic for individual patients *(91)*.

Blood-based proteomics have identified several potential biomarkers, including heat shock protein (HSP)-27 *(92)*, transcriptional regulator 14-3-3σ *(93, 94)*, derivatives of the complement component C3a *(95)*, and a fragment of fibrinogen-α *(96)*. However, many complex technical issues need to be resolved before proteomics may make any progress *(97, 98)*. As many cancer proteins are heavily glycosylated, a glycomics approach has also been used to find glycan biomarkers in breast cancer serum *(99)*.

4.7. Nipple/Ductal Fluid

Breast cancer arises from the epithelial cells that line the ductal/lobular systems of the milk ducts. Therefore, it makes sense that examination of this ductal system or analysis of its secretions may reveal signs of early cancer *(100)*. It appears that many breast-related molecules exist at a higher concentration in nipple fluid than in blood. Although it is not universally available like blood, nipple fluid can be elicited in nearly all premenopausal women and in the majority of older women. Potential areas of usefulness include early detection of breast cancer risk or breast cancer, as well as monitor and/or predictor of preventive therapies *(101)*.

Certain peptides have emerged as potential tumor markers in nipple aspirate fluid. bFGF was found by our group to be significantly elevated in nipple fluid from cancerous breasts *(102, 103)*. This finding was confirmed by others to have a sensitivity of 90% and a specificity of 69% *(104)*. Other candidates include human glandular kallikrein *(105, 106)*, HER2 *(107)*, IGFBP-3 *(108)*, and urokinase-type plasminogen activator *(109)*. Recent work with proteomics technologies has produced varying nipple fluid proteome signatures by different researchers. Osteopontin, cathepsin D, gross cystic disease fluid protein-15, apolipoprotein D, and α1-acid glycoprotein *(110)*; human neutrophil peptides 1–3 *(111)*; 8-iso-prostaglandin F2α *(112)*; and others *(113–116)* were identified. Thus far, the best breast cancer predictive model included bFGF *(117)*.

4.8. Breast Cells

A few breast cells may be obtained from nipple aspirate fluid and many-fold more by ductal lavage with a microcatheter *(118)*. Some publications have disputed the usefulness of ductal lavage in the detection of new breast cancer *(119)*. It is clear that cancer cells may not be found even from known breast cancer, partly because the ducts are obstructed by the cancer itself or by biopsy-related swelling. However, there is a high likelihood of new breast cancer when malignant cells are discovered in the nipple fluid. Furthermore, there is much interest in the potential utility of nipple fluid or lavage-derived cells as a risk assessment tool (120). The evidence is mostly derived from long-term studies of nipple aspiration fluid or random FNA. Wrensch et al. showed a relative risk for breast cancer of 4.9 with atypical hyperplasia (121) and 2.4 associated with atypia on nipple aspiration fluids (122). In an FNA study, atypical hyperplasia was predictive of later breast cancer (123).

Molecular analysis of ductal cells has been promising. The HER2 gene has been detected by polymerase chain reaction (PCR) in cancer cells in spontaneous discharge (124). The Sukumar group tested ductal lavage cells by methylation-specific PCR to detect methylated alleles of cyclin D2, RAR-β, and Twist genes in 17/20 invasive carcinoma, 2/7 DCIS, and only in 5/45 control cases (43). A panel of six genes (GSTP1, RAR-β2, ONK4a, p14, RASSF1A, and DAP-kinase) showed hypermethylation in 82% of nipple fluids from cancerous breasts, and none from normal breasts (47). Interphase fluorescence in situ hybridization (FISH) analysis was used to show numeric changes on chromosomes 1, 8, 11, and/or 17 for a sensitivity of 71% and a specificity of 89% (125). DNA has been isolated successfully from nipple fluid and amplified with PCR for 11 microsatellite markers from seven chromosomes (126).

FNA-derived breast cells have been studied by PCR to detect c-myc amplification (127), and by FISH probes specific for chromosome arm 1q, c-myc, Her-2, and p53 (128). p53 and Her-2 protein content has been measured with accuracy from FNA specimens of the breast (129, 130). Using a 21-gene methylation panel, CCND2, RASSF1A, APC, and HIN1 were found to be 100% specific in FNA samples (45).

5. Conclusions

In the future, it is likely that a combination approach to measure simultaneously multiple markers would be most successful in detecting early breast cancer. Ideally, such a biomarker panel should be able to detect breast cancer in asymptomatic patients, and improve the accuracy of screening mammograms. A reliable biomarker signature may also signify new breast cancer, even in the setting of normal mammogram and physical examination results, and would indicate further more intensive diagnostic workup and/or preventive treatment.

References

1. Jemal, A., Siegel, R., Ward, E., Murray, T., Xu, J., and Thun, M.J. (2007) Cancer statistics, 2007. *CA Cancer J. Clin.* **57**, 43–66.

2. Rimer, B.K., Schildkraut, J.M., and Hiatt, R.A. (2005) Cancer screening. In: DeVita, V.T., Hellman, S., and Rosenberg, S.A., eds. Cancer: principles and practice of oncology. Philadelphia, PA: Lippincott-Raven, 567–579.

3. American Cancer Society. (2007) Cancer facts & figures 2007. Atlanta: American Cancer Society.

4. Shapiro, S. (1997) Periodic screening for breast cancer: the HIP Randomized Controlled Trial. Health Insurance Plan. *J. Natl. Cancer Inst. Monogr.* **22**, 27–30.

5. Hendrick, R.E., Smith, R.A., Rutledge, J.H., and Smart, C.R. (1997) Benefit of screening mammography in women aged 40–49: a new meta-analysis of randomized controlled trials. *J. Natl. Cancer Inst. Monogr.* **22**, 87–92.

6. Andersson, I., Aspegren, K., Janzon, L., Landberg, T., Lindholm, K., Linell, F., Ljungberg, O., Ranstam, J., and Sigfússon, B. (1998) Mammographic screening and mortality from breast cancer: the Malmö mammographic screening trial. *BMJ* **297**, 943–948.

7. Tabér, L., Vitak, B., Chen, H.H., Duffy, S.W., Yen, M.F., Chiang, C.F., Krusemo, U.B., Tot, T., and Smith, R.A. (2000) The Swedish Two-County Trial twenty years later. Updated mortality results and new insights from long-term follow-up. *Radiol. Clin. North Am.* **38**, 625–651.

8. Humphrey, L.L., Helfand, M., Chan, B.K., and Woolf, S.H. (2002) Breast cancer screening: a summary of the evidence for the U.S. Preventive Services Task Force. *Ann. Intern. Med.* **137**, 347–360.

9. Alexander, F.E., Anderson, T.J., Brown, H.K., Forrest, A.P., Hepburn, W., Kirkpatrick, A.E., Muir, B.B., Prescott, R.J., and Smith, A. (1999) 14 years of follow-up from the Edinburgh randomised trial of breast-cancer screening. *Lancet* **353**, 1903–1908.

10. Miller, A.B., To, T., Baines, C.J., and Wall, C. (2000) Canadian National Breast Screening Study-2: 13-year results of a randomized trial in women aged 50–59 years. *J. Natl. Cancer Inst.* **92**, 1490–1499.

11. Miller, A.B., To, T., Baines, C.J., and Wall, C. (2002) The Canadian National Breast Screening Study-1: breast cancer mortality after 11 to 16 years of follow-up. A randomized screening trial of mammography in women age 40 to 49 years. *Ann. Intern. Med.* **137**, 305–312.

12. Smart, C.R., Hendrick, R.E., Rutledge, J.H., and Smith, R.A. (1995) Benefit of mammography screening in women ages 40 to 49 years. Current evidence from randomized controlled trials. *Cancer* **75**, 1619–1626.

13. Esserman, L., Cowley, H., Eberle, C., Kirkpatrick, A., Chang, S., Berbaum, K., and Gale, A. (2002) Improving the accuracy of mammography: volume and outcome relationships. *J. Natl. Cancer Inst.* **94**, 369–375.

14. Pisano, E.D., Gatsonis, C., Hendrick, E., Yaffe, M., Baum, J.K., Acharyya, S., Conant, E.F., Fajardo, L.L., Bassett, L., D'Orsi, C., Jong, R., Rebner, M., and Digital Mammographic Imaging Screening Trial (DMIST) Investigators Group. (2005) Diagnostic performance of digital versus film mammography for breast-cancer screening. *N. Engl. J. Med.* **353**, 1773–1783.

15. Fenton, J.J., Taplin, S.H., Carney, P.A., Abraham, L., Sickles, E.A., D'Orsi, C., Berns, E.A., Cutter, G., Hendrick, R.E., Barlow, W.E., and Elmore, J.G. (2007) Influence of computer-aided detection on performance of screening mammography. *N. Engl. J. Med.* **356**, 1399–1409.

16. Hall, F.M. (2007) Breast imaging and computer-aided detection. *Engl. J. Med.* **356**, 1464–1466.

17. Berg, W.A. (2003) Rationale for a trial of screening breast ultrasound: American College of Radiology Imaging Network (ACRIN) 6666. *Am. J. Roentgenol.* **180**, 1225–1228.

18. Berg, W.A., Blume, J.D., Cormack, J.B., Mendelson, E.B., Madsen, E.L., and ACRIN 6666 Investigators. (2006) Lesion detection and characterization in a breast US phantom: results of the ACRIN 6666 Investigators. *Radiology* **239**, 693–702.

19. Morris, E.A., Liberman, L., Ballon, D.J., Robson, M., Abramson, A.F., Heerdt, A., and Dershaw, D.D. (2003) MRI of occult breast carcinoma in a high-risk population. *Am. J. Roentgenol.* **181**, 619–626.

20. Lehman, C.D., Gatsonis, C., Kuhl, C.K., Hendrick, R.E., Pisano, E.D., Hanna, L., Peacock, S., Smazal, S.F., Maki, D.D., Julian, T.B., DePeri, E.R., Bluemke, D.A., Schnall, M.D., and ACRIN Trial 6667 Investigators Group. (2007) MRI evaluation of the contralateral breast in women with recently diagnosed breast cancer. *N. Engl. J. Med.* **356**, 1295–1303.

21. Breen, N., Cronin, K., Meissner, H.I., Taplin, S.H., Tangka, F.K., Tiro, J.A., and McNeel, T.S. (2007) Reported drop in mammography: is this cause for concern? *Cancer* **109**, 2405–2409.

22. Ravdin, P.M., Cronin, K.A., Howlader, N., Berg, C.D., Chlebowski, R.T., Feuer, E.J., Edwards, B.K., and Berry, D.A. (2007) The decrease in breast-cancer incidence in 2003 in the United States. *N. Engl. J. Med.* **356**, 1670–1674.

23. Stearns, V., Yamauchi, H., and Hayes, D.F. (1998) Circulating tumor markers in breast cancer: accepted utilities and novel prospects. *Breast Cancer Res. Treat.* **52**, 239–259.

24. Duffy, M.J. (2006) Serum tumor markers in breast cancer: are they of clinical value? *Clin. Chem.* **52**, 345–351.

25. Bast, R.C., Ravdin, P., Hayes, D.F., Bates, S., Fritsche, H., Jessup, J.M., Kemeny, N., Locker, G.Y., Mennel, R.G., Somerfield, M.R., and American Society of Clinical Oncology Tumor Markers Expert Panel. (2001) 2000 update of recommendations for the use of tumor markers in breast and colorectal cancer: clinical practice guidelines of the American Society of Clinical Oncology. *J. Clin. Oncol.* **19**, 1865–1878.

26. Molina, R., Barak, V., van Dalen, A., Duffy, M.J., Einarsson, R., Gion, M., Goike, H., Lamerz, R., Nap, M., Sölétormos, G., and Stieber, P. (2005) Tumor markers in breast cancer—European Group on Tumor Markers recommendations. *Tumour Biol.* **26**, 281–293.

27. Pepe, M.S., Etzioni, R., Feng, Z., Potter, J.D., Thompson, M.L., Thornquist, M., Winget, M., and Yasui, Y. (2001) Phases of biomarker development for early detection of cancer. *J. Natl. Cancer Inst.* **93**, 1054–1061.

28. Ntoulia, M., Stathopoulou, A., Ignatiadis, M., Malamos, N., Mavroudis, D., Georgoulias, V., and Lianidou, E.S. (2006) Detection of Mammaglobin A-mRNA-positive circulating tumor cells in peripheral blood of patients with operable breast cancer with nested RT-PCR. *Clin. Biochem.* **39**, 879–887.

29. Cristofanilli, M., Budd, G.T., Ellis, M.J., Stopeck, A., Matera, J., Miller, M.C., Reuben, J.M., Doyle, G.V., Allard, W.J., Terstappen, L.W., and Hayes, D.F. (2004) Circulating tumor cells, disease progression, and survival in metastatic breast cancer. *N. Engl. J. Med.* **351**, 781–791.

30. Müller, V., Hayes, D.F., and Pantel, K. (2006) Recent translational research: circulating tumor cells in breast cancer patients. *Breast Cancer Res.* **8**, 110.

31. Lacroix, M. (2006) Significance, detection and markers of disseminated breast cancer cells. *Endocr. Relat. Cancer* **13**, 1033–1067.

32. Fürstenberger, G., von Moos, R., Lucas, R., Thürlimann, B., Senn, H.J., Hamacher, J., and Boneberg, E.M. (2006) Circulating endothelial cells and angiogenic serum factors during neoadjuvant chemotherapy of primary breast cancer. *Br. J. Cancer* **94**, 524–531.

33. Fournié, G.J., Gayral-Taminh, M., Bouché, J.P., and Conté, J.J. (1986) Recovery of nanogram quantities of DNA from plasma and quantitative measurement using labeling by nick translation. *Anal. Biochem.* **158**, 250–256.

34. Zhong, X.Y., Bürk, M.R., Troeger, C., Kang, A., Holzgreve, W., and Hahn, S. (2000) Fluctuation of maternal and fetal free extracellular circulatory DNA in maternal plasma. *Obstet. Gynecol.* **96**, 991–996.

35. Zanetti-Dallenbach, R.A., Schmid, S., Wight, E., Holzgreve, W., Ladewing, A., Hahn, S., and Zhong, X.Y. (2007) Levels of circulating cell-free serum DNA in benign and malignant breast lesions. *Int. J. Biol. Markers* **22**, 95–99.

36. Levenson, V.V. (2007) Biomarkers for early detection of breast cancer: what, when, and where? *Biochim. Biophys. Acta.* **1770**, 847–856.

37. Umetani, N., Giuliano, A.E., Hiramatsu, S.H., Amersi, F., Nakagawa, T., Martino, S., and Hoon, D.S. (2006) Prediction of breast tumor progression by integrity of free circulating DNA in serum. *J. Clin. Oncol.* **24**, 4270–4276.

38. Silva, J.M., Silva, J., Sanchez, A., Garcia, J.M., Dominguez, G., Provencio, M., Sanfrutos, L., Jareño, E., Colas, A., España, P., and Bonilla, F. (2002) Tumor DNA in plasma at diagnosis of breast cancer patients is a valuable predictor of disease-freesurvival. *Clin. Cancer Res.* **8**, 3761–3766.

39. Rykova, E.Y., Wunsche, W., Brizgunova, O.E., Skvortsova, T.E., Tamkovich, S.N., Senin, I.S., Laktionov, P.P., Sczakiel, G., and Vlassov, V.V. (2006) Concentrations of circulating RNA from healthy donors and cancer patients estimated by different methods. *Ann. N.Y. Acad. Sci.* **1075**, 328–333.

40. Schwarzenbach, H., Müller, V., Stahmann, N., and Pantel, K. (2004) Detection and characterization of circulating microsatellite-DNA in

blood of patients with breast cancer. *Ann. N.Y. Acad. Sci.* **1022**, 25–32.

41. Herman, J.G. and Baylin, S.B. (2003) Gene silencing in cancer in association with promoter hypermethylation. *N. Engl. J. Med.* **349**, 2042–2054.

42. Kagan, J., Srivastava, S., Barker, P.E., Belinsky, S.A., and Cairns, P. (2007) Towards clinical application of methylated DNA sequences as cancer biomarkers: a joint NCI's EDRN and NIST workshop on standards, methods, assays, reagents and tools. *Cancer Res.* **67**, 4545–4549.

43. Evron, E., Dooley, W.C., Umbricht, C.B., Rosenthal, D., Sacchi, N., Gabrielson, E., Soito, A.B., Hung, D.T., Ljung, B.M., Davidson, N.E., and Sukumar, S. (2001) Detection of breast cancer cells in ductal lavage fluid by methylation-specific PCR. *Lancet* **357**, 1335–1336.

44. Honorio, S., Agathanggelou, A., Schuermann, M., Pankow, W., Viacava, P., Maher, E.R., and Latif, F. (2003) Detection of RASSF1A aberrant promoter hypermethylation in sputum from chronic smokers and ductal carcinoma in situ from breast cancer patients. *Oncogene* **22**, 147–150.

45. Jeronimo, C., Monteiro, P., Henrique, R., Dinis-Ribeiro, M., Costa, I., Costa, V.L., Filipe, L., Carvalho, A.L., Hoque, M.O., Pais, I., Leal, C., Teixeira, M.R., and Sidransky, D. (2008) Quantitative hypermethylation of a small panel of genes augments the diagnostic accuracy in fine-needle aspirate washings of breast lesions. *Breast Cancer Res. Treat.* **109**, 27–34.

46. Silva, J.M., Dominguez, G., Villanueva, M.J., Gonzalez, R., Garcia, J.M., Corbacho, C., Provencio, M., España, P., and Bonilla, F. (1999) Aberrant DNA methylation of the p16INK4a gene in plasma DNA of breast cancer patients. *Br. J. Cancer* **80**, 1262–1264.

47. Krassenstein, R., Sauter, E., Dulaimi, E., Battagli, C., Ehya, H., Klein-Szanto, A., and Cairns, P. (2004) Detection of breast cancer in nipple aspirate fluid by CpG island hypermethylation. *Clin. Cancer Res.* **10**, 28–32.

48. Dulaimi, E., Hillinck, J., Ibanez de Caceres, I., Al-Saleem, T., and Cairns, P. (2004) Tumor suppressor gene promoter hypermethylation in serum of breast cancer patients. *Clin. Cancer Res.* **10**, 6189–6193.

49. Hoque, M.O., Feng, Q., Toure, P., Dem, A., Critchlow, C.W., Hawes, S.E., Wood, T., Jeronimo, C., Rosenbaum, E., Stern, J., Yu, M., Trink, B., Kiviat, N.B., and Sidransky, D. (2006) Detection of aberrant methylation of four genes in plasma DNA for the detection of breast cancer. *J. Clin. Onc.* **24**, 4262–4269.

50. Jing, F., Zhang, J., Tao, J., Zhou, Y., Jun, L., Tang, X., Wang, Y., and Hai, H. (2007) Hypermethylation of tumor suppressor genes BRCA1, p16 and 14-3-3sigma in serum of sporadic breast cancer patients. *Onkologie* **30**, 14–19.

51. Sharma, G., Mirza, S., Prasad, C.P., Srivastava, A., Gupta, S.D., and Ralhan, R. (2007) Promoter hypermethylation of p16INK4A, p14ARF, CyclinD2 and Slit2 in serum and tumor DNA from breast cancer patients. *Life Sci.* **80**, 1873–1881.

52. Taback, B., Giuliano, A.E., Lai, R., Hansen, N., Singer, F.R., Pantel, K., and Hoon, D.S. (2006) Epigenetic analysis of body fluids and tumor tissues: application of a comprehensive molecular assessment for early-stage breast cancer patients. *Ann. N. Y. Acad. Sci.* **1075**, 211–221.

53. Müller, H.M., Widschwendter, A., Fiegl, H., Ivarsson, L., Goebel, G., Perkmann, E., Marth, C., and Widschwendter, M. (2003) DNA methylation in serum of breast cancer patients: an independent prognostic marker. *Cancer Res.* **63**, 7641–7645.

54. Papadopoulou, E., Davilas, E., Sotiriou, V., Georgakopoulos, E., Georgakopoulou, S., Koliopanos, A., Aggelakis, F., Dardoufas, K., Agnanti, N.J., Karydas, I., and Nasioulas, G. (2006) Cell-free DNA and RNA in plasma as a new molecular marker for prostate and breast cancer. *Ann. N. Y. Acad. Sci.* **1075**, 235–243.

55. Zamagni, C., Martoni, A., Cacciari, N., Bellanova, B., Vecchi, F., and Pannuti, F. (1992) CA-549 serum levels in breast cancer monitoring. *Int. J. Biol. Markers* **7**, 217–221.

56. Rakha, E.A., Boyce, R.W., Abd El-Rehim, D., Kurien, T., Green, A.R., Paish, E.C., Robertson, J.F., and Ellis, I.O. (2005) Expression of mucins (MUC1, MUC2, MUC3, MUC4, MUC5AC and MUC6) and their prognostic significance in human breast cancer. *Mod. Pathol.* **18**, 1295–1304.

57. Giovanella, L., Ceriani, L., Giardina, G., Bardelli, D., Tanzi, F., and Garancini, S. (2002) Serum cytokeratin fragment 21.1 (CYFRA 21.1) as tumour marker for breast cancer: comparison with carbohydrate antigen 15.3 (CA 15.3) and carcinoembryonic antigen (CEA). *Clin. Chem. Lab. Med.* **40**, 298–303.

58. Eskelinen, M., Hippeläinen, M., Kettunen, J., Salmela, E., Penttilä, I., and Alhava, E. (1994) Clinical value of serum tumour markers TPA, TPS, TAG 12, CA 15-3 and MCA in breast

cancer diagnosis; results from a prospective study. *Anticancer Res.* **14**, 699–703.

59. Slamon, D.J., Leyland-Jones, B., Shak, S., Fuchs, H., Paton, V., Bajamonde, A., Fleming, T., Eierman, W., Wolter, J., Pegram, M., Baselga, J., and Norton, L. (2001) Use of chemotherapy plus a monoclonal antibody against HER2 for metastatic breast cancer that overexpresses HER2. *N. Engl. J. Med.* **344**, 783–792.

60. Kong, S.Y., Kang, J.H., Kwon, Y., Kang, H.S., Chung, K.W., Kang, S.H., Lee, D.H., Ro, J., and Lee, E.S. (2006) Serum HER-2 concentration in patients with primary breast cancer. *J. Clin. Pathol.* **59**, 373–376.

61. Quaranta, M., Daniele, A., Coviello, M., Savonarola, A., Abbate, I., Venneri, M.T., Paradiso, A., Stea, B., Zito, A., Labriola, A., and Schittulli, F. (2006) c-erbB-2 protein level in tissue and sera of breast cancer patients: a possibly useful clinical correlation. *Tumori* **92**, 311–317.

62. Imoto, S., Wada, N., Hasebe, T., Ochiai, A., and Kitoh, T. (2007) Serum c-erbB-2 protein is a useful marker for monitoring tumor recurrence of the breast. *Int. J. Cancer* **120**, 357–361.

63. Esteva, F.J., Cheli, C.D., Fritsche, H., Fornier, M., Slamon, D., Thiel, R.P., Luftner, D., and Ghani, F. (2005) Clinical utility of serum HER2/neu in monitoring and prediction of progression-free survival in metastatic breast cancer patients treated with trastuzumab-based therapies. *Breast Cancer Res.* **7**, R436–443.

64. Souder, C., Leitzel, K., Ali, S.M., Demers, L., Evans, D.B., Chaudri-Ross, H.A., Hackl, W., Hamer, P., Carney, W., and Lipton, A. (2006) Serum epidermal growth factor receptor/HER-2 predicts poor survival in patients with metastatic breast cancer. *Cancer* **107**, 2337–2345.

65. Bernstein, J.L., Godbold, J.H., Raptis, G., Watson, M.A., Levinson, B., Aaronson, S.A., and Fleming, T.P. (2005) Identification of mammaglobin as a novel serum marker for breast cancer. *Clin. Cancer Res.* **11**, 6528–6535.

66. Borgoño, C.A., Grass, L., Soosaipillai, A., Yousef, G.M., Petraki, C.D., Howarth, D.H., Fracchioli, S., Katsaros, D., and Diamandis, E.P. (2003) Human kallikrein 14: a new potential biomarker for ovarian and breast cancer. *Cancer Res.* **63**, 9032–9041.

67. Rodrigues, L.R., Teixeira, J.A., Schmitt, F.L., Paulsson, M., and Lindmark-Mänsson, H. The role of osteopontin in tumor progression and metastasis in breast cancer.

(2007) *Cancer Epidemiol. Biomarkers Prev.* **16**, 1087–1097.

68. Balogh, G.A., Mailo, D.A., Corte, M.M., Roncoroni, P., Nardi, H., Vincent, E., Martinez, D., Cafasso, M.E., Frizza, A., Ponce, G., Vincent, E., Barutta, E., Lizarraga, P., Lizarraga, G., Monti, C., Paolillo, E., Vincent, R., Quatroquio, R., Grimi, C., Maturi, H., Aimale, M., Spinsanti, C., Montero, H., Santiago, J., Shulman, L., Rivadulla, M., Machiavelli, M., Salum, G., Cuevas, M.A., Picolini, J., Gentili, A., Gentili, R., and Mordoh, J. (2006) Mutant p53 protein in serum could be used as a molecular marker in human breast cancer. *Int. J. Oncol.* **28**, 995–1002.

69. Bianco, C., Strizzi, L., Mancino, M., Rehman, A., Hamada, S., Watanabe, K., De Luca, A., Jones, B., Balogh, G., Russo, J., Mailo, D., Palaia, R., D'Aiuto, G., Botti, G., Perrone, F., Salomon, D.S., and Normanno, N. (2006) Identification of cripto-1 as a novel serologic marker for breast and colon cancer. *Clin. Cancer Res.* **12**, 5158–5164.

70. Tworoger, S.S., Eliassen, A.H., Sluss, P., and Hankinson, S.E. (2007) A prospective study of plasma prolactin concentrations and risk of premenopausal and postmenopausal breast cancer. *J. Clin. Oncol.* **25**, 1482–1488.

71. Baglietto, L., English, D.R., Hopper, J.L., Morris, H.A., Tilley, W.D., and Giles, G.G. (2007) Circulating insulin-like growth factor-I and binding protein-3 and the risk of breast cancer. *Cancer Epidemiol. Biomarkers Prev.* **16**, 763–768.

72. Nguyen, M. (1997) Angiogenic factors as tumor markers. *Invest. New Drug* **15**, 29–37.

73. Granato, A.M., Nanni, O., Falcini, F., Folli, S., Mosconi, G., De Paola, F., Medri, L., Amadori, D., and Volpi, A. (2004) Basic fibroblast growth factor and vascular endothelial growth factor serum levels in breast cancer patients and healthy women: useful as diagnostic tools? *Breast Cancer Res.* **6**, R38–45.

74. Bozcuk, H., Uslu, G., Samur, M., Yildiz, M., Ozben, T., Ozdoğan, M., Artaç, M., Altunbaş, H., Akan, I., and Savaş, B. (2004) Tumour necrosis factor-alpha, interleukin-6, and fasting serum insulin correlate with clinical outcome in metastatic breast cancer patients treated with chemotherapy. *Cytokine* **27**, 58–65.

75. Eichbaum, M.H., de Rossi, T.M., Kaul, S., Bruckner, T., Schneeweiss, A., and Sohn, C. (2007) Serum levels of hepatocyte growth factor/scatter factor in patients with liver

metastases from breast cancer. *Tumour Biol.* **28**, 36–44.

76. Dehqanzada, Z.A., Storrer, C.E., Hueman, M.T., Foley, R.J., Harris, K.A., Jama, Y.H., Shriver, C.D., Ponniah, S., and Peoples, G.E. (2007) Assessing serum cytokine profiles in breast cancer patients receiving a HER2/neu vaccine using Luminex technology. *Oncol. Rep.* **17**, 687–694.

77. Caine, G.J., Stonelake, P.S., Lip, G.Y., and Blann, A.D. (2007) Changes in plasma vascular endothelial growth factor, angiopoietins, and their receptors following surgery for breast cancer. *Cancer Lett.* **248**, 131–136.

78. Granato, A.M., Frassineti, G.L., Giovannini, N., Ballardini, M., Nanni, O., Maltoni, R., Amadori, D., and Volpi, A. (2006) Do serum angiogenic growth factors provide additional information to that of conventional markers in monitoring the course of metastatic breast cancer? *Tumour Biol.* **27**, 302–308.

79. Lipton, A., Ali, S.M., Leitzel, K., Demers, L., Evans, D.B., Hamer, P., Brown-Shimer, S., Pierce, K., and Carney, W. (2007) Elevated plasma tissue inhibitor of metalloproteinase-1 level predicts decreased response and survival in metastatic breast cancer. *Cancer* **109**, 1933–1939.

80. Kuvaja, P., Talvensaari-Mattila, A., Pääkkö, P., and Turpeenniemi-Hujanen, T. (2006) Low serum level of pro-matrix metalloproteinase 2 correlates with aggressive behavior in breast carcinoma. *Hum. Pathol.* **37**, 1316–1323.

81. Sheen-Chen, S.M., Eng, H.L., Huang, C.C., and Chen, W.J. (2004) Serum levels of soluble E-selectin in women with breast cancer. *Br. J. Surg.* **91**, 1578–1581.

82. Disis, M.L., Pupa, S.M., Gralow, J.R., Dittadi, R., Menard, S., and Cheever, M.A. (1997) High-titer HER-2/neu protein-specific antibody can be detected in patients with early-stage breast cancer. *J. Clin. Oncol.* 15, 3363–3367.

83. von Mensdorff-Pouilly, S., Gourevitch, M.M., Kenemans, P., Verstraeten, A.A., Litvinov, S.V., van Kamp, G.J., Meijer, S., Vermorken, J., and Hilgers, J. (1996) Humoral immune response to polymorphic epithelial mucin (MUC-1) in patients with benign and malignant breast tumours. *Eur. J. Cancer* **32A**, 1325–1331.

84. Bachelot, T., Ratel, D., Menetrier-Caux, C., Wion, D., Blay, J.Y., and Berger, F. (2006) Autoantibodies to endostatin in patients with breast cancer: correlation to endostatin levels and clinical outcome. *Br. J. Cancer* **94**, 1066–1070.

85. Müller, M., Meyer, M., Schilling, T., Ulsperger, E., Lehnert, T., Zentgraf, H., Stremmel, W., Volkmann, M., and Galle, P.R. (2006) Testing for anti-p53 antibodies increases the diagnostic sensitivity of conventional tumor markers. *Int. J. Oncol.* **29**, 973–980.

86. Fernández-Madrid, F., Tang, N., Alansari, H., Granda, J.L., Tait, L., Amirikia, K.C., Moroianu, M., Wang, X., and Karvonen, R.L. (2004) Autoantibodies to annexin XI-A and other autoantigens in the diagnosis of breast cancer. Cancer Res. **64**, 5089–5096.

87. Harman, S.M., Gucciardo, F., Heward, C.B., Granstrom, P., Barclay-White, B., Rogers, L.W., and Ibarra, J.A. (2005) Discrimination of breast cancer by anti-malignin antibody serum test in women undergoing biopsy. *Cancer Epidemiol. Biomarkers Prev.* **14**, 2310–2315.

88. Minenkova, O., Pucci, A., Pavoni, E., De Tomassi, A., Fortugno, P., Gargano, N., Cianfriglia, M., Barca, S., De Placido, S., Martignetti, A., Felici, F., Cortese, R., and Monaci, P. (2003) Identification of tumor-associated antigens by screening phage-displayed human cDNA libraries with sera from tumor patients. *Int. J. Cancer* **106**, 534–544.

89. Paik, S., Shak, S., Tang, G., Kim, C., Baker, J., Cronin, M., Baehner, F.L., Walker, M.G., Watson, D., Park, T., Hiller, W., Fisher, E., Wickerham, D.L., Bryant. J., and Wolmark, N. (2004) A multigene assay to predict recurrence of Tamoxifen-treated, node-negative breast cancer. *N. Engl. J. Med.* **351**, 2817–2826.

90. Buyse, M., Loi, S., van't Veer, L., Viale, G., Delorenzi, M., Glas, A.M., d'Assignies, M.S., Bergh, J., Lidereau, R., Ellis, P., Harris, A., Bogaerts, J., Therasse, P., Floore, A., Amakrane, M., Piette, F., Rutgers, E., Sotiriou, C., Cardoso, F., Piccart, M.J., and TRANSBIG Consortium. (2006) Validation and clinical utility of a 70-gene prognostic signature for women with node-negative breast cancer. *J. Natl. Cancer Inst.* **98**, 1183–1192.

91. Fan, C., Oh, D.S., Wessels, L., Weigelt, B., Nuyten, D.S., Nobel, A.B., van't Veer, L.J., and Perou, C.M. (2006) Concordance among gene-expression–based predictors for breast cancer. *N. Engl. J. Med.* **355**, 560–569.

92. Rui, Z., Jian-Guo, J., Yuan-Peng, T., Hai, P., and Bing-Gen, R. (2003) Use of serological proteomic methods to find biomarkers

associated with breast cancer. *Proteomics* **3**, 433–439.

93. Li, J., Zhang, Z., Rosenzweig, J., Wang, Y.Y., and Chan, D.W. (2002) Proteomics and bioinformatics approaches for identification of serum biomarkers to detect breast cancer. *Clin. Chem.* **48**, 1296–1304.

94. Mathelin, C., Cromer, A., Wendling, C., Tomasetto, C., and Rio, M.C. (2006) Serum biomarkers for detection of breast cancers: A prospective study. *Breast Cancer Res. Treat.* **96**, 83–90.

95. Li, J., Orlandi, R., White, C.N., Rosenzweig, J., Zhao, J., Seregni, E., Morelli, D., Yu, Y., Meng, X.Y., Zhang, Z., Davidson, N.E., Fung, E.T., and Chan, D.W. (2005) Independent validation of candidate breast cancer serum biomarkers identified by mass spectrometry. *Clin. Chem.* **51**, 2229–2235.

96. Shi, Q., Harris, L.N., Lu, X., Li, X., Hwang, J., Gentleman, R., Iglehart, J.D., and Miron, A. (2006) Declining plasma fibrinogen alpha fragment identifies HER2-positive breast cancer patients and reverts to normal levels after surgery. *J. Proteome Res.* **5**, 2947–2955.

97. Lin, S.M. and Kibbe, W.A. (2005) Irrational exuberance in clinical proteomics. *Clin. Cancer Res.* **11**, 7963–7964.

98. Davis, M.A. and Hanash, S. (2006) High-throughput genomic technology in research and clinical management of breast cancer. Plasma-based proteomics in early detection and therapy. *Breast Cancer Res.* **8**, 217.

99. Kirmiz, C., Li, B., An, H.J., Clowers, B.H., Chew, H.K., Lam, K.S., Ferrige, A., Alecio, R., Borowsky, A.D., Sulaimon, S., Lebrilla, C.B., and Miyamoto, S. (2007) A serum glycomics approach to breast cancer biomarkers. *Mol. Cell Proteomics* **6**, 43–55.

100. Petrakis, N.L. (1993) Nipple aspirate fluid in epidemiologic studies of breast disease. *Epidemiol. Rev.* **15**, 188–195.

101. Brooks, M.N. (2003) Will the analysis of nipple fluid and breast cells be useful in the clinical care of the breast patient? *Women's Oncol. Rev.* **3**, 179–186.

102. Liu, Y., Wang, J.L., Chang, H., Barsky, S.H., and Nguyen, M. (2000) Breast cancer diagnosis with nipple fluid bFGF. *Lancet* **356**, 567.

103. Sartippour, M.R., Zhang, L., Lu, M., Wang, H., and Brooks, M.N. (2005) Nipple fluid basic fibroblast growth factor in breast patients. *Cancer Epidemiol. Biomarkers Prev.* **4**, 2995–2998.

104. Hsiung, R., Zhu, W., Klein, G., Qin, W., Rosenberg, A., Park, P., Rosato, E., and Sauter, E. (2002) High basic fibroblast growth factor levels in nipple aspirate fluid are correlated with breast cancer. *Cancer J.* **8**, 308–310.

105. Black, M.H., Magklara, A., Obiezu, C., Levesque, M.A., Sutherland, D.J.A., Tindall, D.J., Young, C.Y.F., Sauter, E.R., and Diamandis, E.P. (2000) Expression of a prostate-associated protein, human glandular kallikrein (hK2), in breast tumours and in normal breast secretions. *Br. J. Cancer* **82**, 361–367.

106. Sauter, E.R., Welch, T., Magklara, A., Klein, G., and Diamandis, E.P. (2002) Ethnic variation in kallikrein expression in nipple aspirate fluid. *Int. J. Cancer* **100**, 678–682.

107. Kuerer, H.M., Thompson, P.A., Krishnamurthy, S., Fritsche, H.A., Marcy, S.M., Babiera, G.V., Singletary, S.E., Cristofanilli, M., Sneige, N., and Hunt, K.K. (2003) High and differential expression of HER-2/neu extracellular domain in bilateral ductal fluids from women with unilateral invasive breast cancer. *Clin. Cancer Res.* **9**, 601–605.

108. Sauter, E.R., Chervoneva, I., Diamandis, A., Khosravi, J.M., Litwin, S., and Diamandis, E.P. (2002) Prostate specific antigen and insulin like growth factor binding protein-3 in nipple aspirate fluid are associated with breast cancer. *Cancer Detect. Prevent.* **26**, 149–157.

109. Qin, W., Zhu, W., Wagner-Mann, C., Folk, W., and Sauter, E.R. (2003) Association of uPA, PAT-1, and uPAR in nipple aspirate fluid (NAF) with breast cancer. *Cancer J.* **9**, 293–301.

110. Alexander, H., Stegner, A.L., Wagner-Mann, C., Du Bois, G.C., Alexander, S., and Sauter, E.R. (2004) Proteomic analysis to identify breast cancer biomarkers in nipple aspirate fluid. *Clin. Cancer Res.* **10**, 7500–7510.

111. Li, J., Zhao, J., Yu, X., Lange, J., Kuerer, H., Krishnamurthy, S., Schilling, E., Khan, S.A., Sukumar, S., and Chan, D.W. (2005) Identification of biomarkers for breast cancer in nipple aspiration and ductal lavage fluid. *vClin. Cancer Res.* **11**, 8312–8320.

112. Mannello, F., Tonti, G.A., Pagliarani, S., Benedetti, S., Canestrari, F., Zhu, W., Qin, W., and Sauter, E.R. (2007) The 8-epimer of prostaglandin F(2alpha), a marker of lipid peroxidation and oxidative stress, is decreased in the nipple aspirate fluid of women with breast cancer. *Int. J. Cancer* **120**, 1971–1976.

113. Paweletz, C.P., Trock, B., Pennanen, M., Tsangaris, T., Magnant, C., Liotta, L.A., and Petricoin, E.F. 3rd. (2001) Proteomic

patterns of nipple aspirate fluids obtained by SELDI-TOF: potential for new biomarkers to aid in the diagnosis of breast cancer. *Dis. Markers* **17**, 301–307.

114. Sauter, E.R., Zhu, W., Fan, X.J., Wassell, R.P., Chervoneva, I., and Du Bois, G.C. (2002) Proteomic analysis of nipple aspirate fluid to detect biologic markers of breast cancer. *Br. J. Cancer* **86**, 1440–1443.

115. Pawlik, T.M., Hawke, D.H., Liu, Y., Krishnamurthy, S., Fritsche, H., Hunt, K.K., and Kuerer, H.M. (2006) Proteomic analysis of nipple aspirate fluid from women with early-stage breast cancer using isotope-coded affinity tags and tandem mass spectrometry reveals differential expression of vitamin D binding protein. *BMC Cancer* **6**, 68.

116. He, J., Gornbein, J., Shen, D., Lu, M., Rovai, L.E., Shau, H., Katz, J., Whitelegge, J.P., Faull, K.F., and Chang, H.R. (2007) Detection of breast cancer biomarkers in nipple aspirate fluid by SELDI-TOF and their identification by combined liquid chromatography-tandem mass spectrometry. *Int. J. Oncol.* **30**, 145–154.

117. Sauter, E.R., Wagner-Mann, C., Ehya, H., and Klein-Szanto, A. (2007) Biologic markers of breast cancer in nipple aspirate fluid and nipple discharge are associated with clinical findings. *Cancer Detect. Prev.* **31**, 50–58.

118. Dooley, W.C., Ljung, B.M., Veronesi, U., Cazzaniga, M., Elledge, R.M., O'shaughnessy, J.A., Kuerer, H.M., Hung, D.T., Khan, S.A., Phillips, R.F., Ganz, P.A., Euhus, D.M., Esserman, L.J., Haffty, B.G., King, B.L., Kelley, M.C., Anderson, M.M., Schmit, P.J., Clark, R.R., Kass, F.C., Anderson, B.O., Troyan, S.L., Arias, R.D., Quiring, J.N., Love, S.M., Page, D.L., and King, E.B. (2001) Ductal lavage for detection of cellular atypia in women at high risk for breast cancer. *J. Natl. Cancer Inst.* **93**, 1624–1632.

119. Khan, S.A., Wiley, E.L., Rodriguez, N., Baird, C., Ramakrishnan, R., Nayar, R., Bryk, M., Bethke, K.B., Staradub, V.L., Wolfman, J., Rademaker, A., Ljung, B.M., and Morrow, M. (2004) Ductal lavage finding in women with known breast cancer undergoing mastectomy. *J. Natl. Cancer Inst.* **96**, 1510–1517.

120. Ozanne, E.M. and Esserman, L.J. (2004) Evaluation of breast cancer risk assessment techniques: a cost effectiveness analysis. *Cancer Epidemiol. Biomarker Prev.* **13**, 2043–2052.

121. Wrensch, M.R., Petrakis, N.L., King, E.B., Lee, M.M., and Miike, R. (1993) Breast cancer risk associated with abnormal cytology in nipple aspirates of breast fluid and

prior history of breast biopsy. *Am. J. Epidemiol.* **37**, 829–833.

122. Wrensch, M.R., Petrakis, N.L., Miike, R., King, E.B., Chew, K., Neuhaus, J., Lee, M.M., and Rhys, M. (2001) Breast cancer risk in women with abnormal cytology in nipple aspirates of breast fluid. *J. Natl. Cancer Inst.* **93**, 1791–1798.

123. Fabian, C.J., Kimler, B.F., Zalles, C.M., Klemp, J.R., Kamel, S., Zeiger, S., and Mayo, M.S. (2000) Short-term breast cancer prediction by random periareolar fine-needle aspiration cytology and the gail risk model. *J. Natl. Cancer Inst.* **92**, 1217–1227.

124. Motomura, K., Koyama, H., Noguchi, S., Inaji, H., and Azuma, C. (1995) Detection of c-erbB-2 gene amplification in nipple discharge by means of polymerase chain reaction. *Breast Cancer Res. Treat.* **33**, 89–92.

125. King, B.L., Tsai, S.C., Gryga, M.E., D'Aquila, T.G., Seelig, S.A., Morrison, L.E., Jacobson, K.K.B., Legator, M.S., Ward, D.C., Rimm, D.L., and Phillips, R.F. (2003) Detection of chromosomal instability in paried breast surgery and ductal lavage specimens by interphase fluorescence in situ hybridization. *Clin. Cancer Res.* **9**, 1509–1516.

126. Zhu, W., Qin, W., Ehya, H., Lininger, J., and Sauter, E. (2003) Microsatellite changes in nipple aspirate fluid and breast tissue from women with breast carcinoma or its precursors. *Clin. Cancer Res.* **9**, 3029–3033.

127. Rao, J.Y., Apple, S.K., Jin, T.S., Lin, S., Nieberg, R.K., and Hirtschowitz, S.L. (2000) Comparative polymerase chain reaction analysis of c-myc amplification on archival breast fine needle aspiration materials. *Cancer Epidemiol. Biomarkers Prev.* **9**, 175–179.

128. Heselmeyer-Haddad, K., Chaudhri, N., Stoltzfus, P., Cheng, J.C., Wilber, K., Morrison, L., Auer, G., and Ried, T. (2002) Detection of chromosomal aneuploidies and gene copy number changes in fine needle aspirates is a specific, sensitive, and objective genetic test for the diagnosis of breast cancer. *Cancer Res.* **62**, 2365–2369.

129. Wu, J.T., Zhang, P., and Bentz, J.S. (2000) Quantification of HER2 oncoprotein in fine-needle aspirates of the breast. *Ann. Clin. Lab Sci.* **30**, 49–56.

130. Ball, H.M., Hupp, T.R., Ziyaie, D., Purdie, C.A., Kernohan, N.M., and Thompson, A.M. (2001) Differential p53 protein expression in breast cancer fine needle aspirates: the potential for in vivo monitoring. *Br. J. Cancer* **85**, 1102–1105.

Chapter 14

Epidemiology of Brain Tumors

Hiroko Ohgaki

Abstract

Gliomas account for more than 70% of all brain tumors, and of these, glioblastoma is the most frequent and malignant histologic type (World Health Organization [WHO] grade IV). There is a tendency toward a higher incidence of gliomas in highly developed, industrialized countries. Some reports indicate that Caucasians have a higher incidence than African or Asian populations. With the exception of pilocytic astrocytomas (WHO grade I), the prognosis of glioma patients is still poor. Fewer than 3% of glioblastoma patients are still alive at 5 years after diagnosis, older age being the most significant and consistent prognostic factor of poorer outcome. Gliomas are components of several inherited tumor syndromes, but the prevalence of these syndromes is very low. Many environmental and lifestyle factors including several occupations, environmental carcinogens, and diet have been reported to be associated with an elevated glioma risk, but the only factor unequivocally associated with an increased risk is therapeutic X-irradiation. In particular, children treated with X-irradiation for acute lymphoblastic leukemia show a significantly elevated risk of developing gliomas and primitive neuroectodermal tumors, often within 10 years after therapy. Significant correlation between G:C→A:T transitions in the *TP53* gene and promoter methylation of the *O6*-methylguanine-DNA methyltransferase (MGMT) gene in gliomas have been reported in several studies, suggesting the possible involvement of O^6-methylguanine DNA adducts, which may be produced by exogenous or endogenous alkylating agents in the development of gliomas.

Key words: Glioma, incidence, survival, occupation, *N*-nitroso compounds, cellular phone, hereditary syndrome, *TP53* mutations.

1. Incidence

The age-adjusted incidence rates of brain tumors tend to be highest in developed, industrial countries (*1, 2*). In Western Europe, North America, and Australia, there are about 6–11 new cases of primary intracranial tumors (including meningiomas) per

M. Verma (ed.), *Methods of Molecular Biology, Cancer Epidemiology, vol. 472*
© 2009 Humana Press, a part of Springer Science + Business Media, Totowa, NJ
Book doi: 10.1007/978-1-60327-492-0

100,000 population per year in men and 4–11 new cases in women (*1, 2*). Population-based incidence rates for each histologic type of glioma in the USA and Europe (Switzerland) are shown in **Table 14.1** (*3–5*).

The lower incidence in developing countries may be partly due to under-ascertainment (*6*), but ethnic differences in susceptibility to development of brain tumors cannot be excluded. Caucasians are more frequently affected than people of African or Asian descent (*7–10*). An ethnic analysis of 8,947 cases of primary central nervous system (CNS) tumors registered during 1971 to 1985 at the Armed Forces Institute of Pathology (AFIP), Washington, DC showed that gliomas were twice as frequent in whites as in blacks (*9*). Central Brain Tumor Registry of the United States (CBTRUS) data indicate that the incidence rates of glioblastomas, other gliomas, and germ-cell tumors are approximately twice as high in whites as in blacks, whereas the incidence of meningiomas, lymphomas, pituitary tumors, and craniopharyngiomas do not differ significantly (*10*). A population-based study on primary intracranial tumors in Kumamoto prefecture suggests that, in Japan, gliomas are about half as frequent as in the USA (*8*).

There has been some controversy regarding a possible increase of approximately 1–2% per year in the incidence of brain tumors (*11, 12*) during the 1980s and 1990s, particularly in the elderly (*13–15*) but also in children (*16*). This increase may be due to the introduction of high-resolution neuroimaging, which has greatly improved the clinical diagnosis of neurological diseases (*17–19*). However, some studies show a true tendency toward increased rates, independent of higher levels of ascertainment due to diagnostic improvements (*20*). A population-based study in the USA showed increases in lymphomas and ependymomas, but not in glioblastomas, astrocytomas, or oligodendrogliomas (*21*). A study in Nordic countries showed that the increase in incidence was confined to the late 1970s and early 1980s, which coincided with introduction of improved diagnostic methods, and this increase was largely confined to the oldest age group (*22*). After 1983 and during a period of increasing use of mobile phones, the incidence has remained relatively stable (*22*). The study on the trends in incidence rates of childhood cancer in Sweden showed significant changes for low-grade glioma/astrocytoma (+2.10%; 95% confidence interval [CI], 1.41–2.80) and benign brain tumors (+3.77%; 95% CI, 2.47–5.10) over the period 1960 to 1998 (*23*). Population-based incidence data from the Netherlands Cancer Registry showed a stable incidence of both childhood and adult gliomas (*24*). In adult gliomas, a significantly increasing incidence of high-grade astrocytoma was balanced by simultaneous decreases in low-grade astrocytoma, astrocytoma with unknown malignancy grade, and glioma of uncertain histology. Thus, these time trends may be at least in part explained by

Table 14.1
Population-based data of incidence rates and survival of patients with gliomas

Tumor	WHO grade	Region	Incidence rates*	Mean age	Median (months)	Survival 1 year	Survival 2 years	Survival 5 years	References
Pilocytic astrocytoma	I	USA	0.23	17		95%	93%	89%	http://www.cbtrus.org
		Zurich	0.39	20		100%	100%	100%	Burkhard et al. [5]
Low-grade diffuse astrocytoma	II	USA	0.13	47		73%	60%	45%	http://www.cbtrus.org
		Zurich	0.26	41	67	92%	88%	58%	Okamoto et al. [4]
Anaplastic astrocytoma	III	USA	0.49	50		60%	43%	28%	http://www.cbtrus.org
		Zurich	0.25	44	20	65%	43%	11%	Unpublished data
Glioblastoma	IV	USA	2.96	62		28%	8%	3%	http://www.cbtrus.org
		Zurich	3.39	61	4.9	18%	3%	1%	Ohgaki et al. [3]
Oligodendroglioma	II	USA	0.34	42		88%	80%	66%	http://www.cbtrus.org
		Zurich	0.27	40	139	98%	96%	78%	Okamoto et al. [4]
Anaplastic oligodendroglioma	III	USA	0.10	46		75%	57%	38%	http://www.cbtrus.org
		Zurich	0.11	49	16	50%	45%	30%	Unpublished data
Oligoastrocytoma	II	Zurich	0.10	40	79	95%	90%	70%	Okamoto et al. [4]
Anaplastic oligoastrocytoma	III	Zurich	0.08	46	18	63%	44%	13%	Unpublished data
Ependymoma / anaplastic ependymoma	II / III	USA	0.23	35		86%	79%	66%	http://www.cbtrus.org

* Incidence rates (per 100,000 person per year) in 1992–1997 in the United States adjusted to the 2000 US population (data for USA are from CBTRUS data [10]. Incidence rates in Zurich, Switzerland in 1980–1994 adjusted to the 2000 US population

improvements in detection and diagnostic precision. Similar find-ings have been reported by Hoffman et al. (*25*), who analyzed data from six collaborating cancer registries of the CBRTUS in 1985–1999.

2. Mortality and Survival

In North America, Western Europe, and Australia, the mortality rates from nervous system tumors (all histological types includ-ing meningiomas) are approximately 4–7 per 100,000 persons per year in men and 3–5 per 100,000 in women (*1, 2*). Mortality rates are similar to incidence rates in most geographical areas. Regional changes in the ratio between incidence and mortality usually reflect differences in the success of disease management (*2, 26*).

Survival of glioma patients is still poor, with the exception of pilocytic astrocytoma (*3, 5*) (**Fig. 14.1; Table 14.1**). The cumulative 5-, 10-, 15-, and 20- year survival rates among all individuals initially diagnosed with a supratentorial low-grade glioma reported to the Surveillance, Epidemiology, and End Results (SEER) program of the National Cancer Institute in 1973–2001 were 59.9%, 42.6%, 41.9%, and 26.0%, respectively (*27*). The 5-year survival rate of glioblastoma patients is < 3% (*3*). Older age at diagnosis is the most significant and consistent

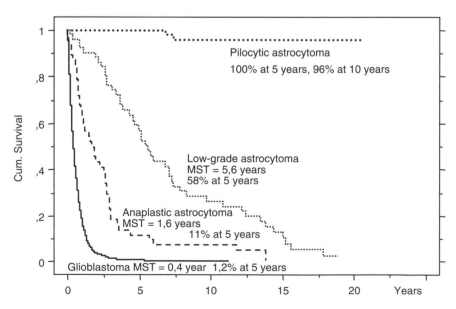

Fig. 14.1. Survival of patients with astrocytic brain tumors. *Cum*, cumulative; *MST*, mean survival time.

prognostic factor for poorer survival, and that is true for all age groups with glioblastomas (3). A study of >30,000 patients from a cancer registry in England and Wales showed that high socio-economic status is associated with longer survival among adult glioma patients (28). According to the data from the same cancer registry, survival improved by 16% in adult gliomas between 1971–1975 and 1986–1990 (29). Retrospective statistical analysis for glioma patients who underwent surgery at an institution in Germany showed a clear reduction of the perioperative morbidity and mortality rates in patients who underwent surgery in 1986–1995 than those in 1965–1974 (30). However, for the postoperative duration of survival, no significant difference was demonstrated for gliomas, indicating that the introduction of modern diagnostic modalities and surgical procedures has not improved the outcome in glioma patients (30). Survival of children with glioma diagnosed in Europe varied among countries, but there is a positive trend in survival probability for cases diagnosed after 1982 compared with those diagnosed before 1981 (31).

3. Occupation

3.1. Chemical Exposure

Epidemiological studies have revealed increased brain tumor risks associated with certain occupations. The somewhat increased incidence of gliomas in anatomists (32), pathologists (33, 34), and embalmers (35) has suggested a role of formaldehyde, but in an industrial setting, exposure to this weak carcinogen was not associated with increased brain tumor risk (32). Other occupations reportedly associated with elevated glioma risk include physicians (36–38); firefighters (36, 38), and farmers (37, 39, 40). Some studies point to an increased glioma risk factors such as the use of plastics (39, 41), rubber products (39, 41), and arsenic, mercury, and petroleum products (42). A large case–control study in the USA showed a significant excess brain tumor risk with high levels of lead exposure (43). Workers who showed blood lead concentrations ≥ 1.4 µmol/L had a twofold increase in risk of nervous system tumors compared with those with concentrations of 0.7 µmol/L (44). In contrast, other studies failed to show increased risk of gliomas in workers exposed to lead (45, 46). Occupational exposure to vinyl chloride causes angiosarcoma of the liver, but it may also carry a weakly enhanced risk of developing glioblastomas among workers with an average exposure period of 21 years (47). Polycyclic aromatic hydrocarbons and non-arsenical insecticides were suggested as possible occupational carcinogens associated with an excess risk of brain tumors (48).

3.2. Parental Occupation

Some studies suggest, but do not prove, a causal relationship between parental occupation and CNS tumor incidence in their offspring. In a population-based case–control study conducted in the USA, parents who worked in the chemical industry were at increased risk of having children with astroglial tumors (49). An international population-based case–control study conducted in seven countries showed an increased risk associated with agricultural work for all childhood brain tumors combined and for glial tumors (50). Paternal occupation as a driver or mechanic and maternal work in an environment related to motor vehicles were also associated with increased risk for all childhood brain tumors and astroglial tumors (50). More case mothers compared with control mothers were employed in the textile industry (50). Large international population-based case–control studies showed that paternal preconceptional occupational exposure to polycyclic aromatic hydrocarbons was associated with increased risks of all childhood brain tumors and astroglial tumors (51).

3.3. Socioeconomic Status

Occupational sectors with a higher socioeconomic status have been found to be associated with increased incidence of gliomas and meningiomas in women (42). Some studies have shown a slightly elevated risk of gliomas in "white collar" workers, including social science professionals (52), financial workers, managers, and people with higher socioeconomic status (41). Inskip et al. (53) reported positive associations with level of education for low-grade glioma and acoustic neuroma, but not for high-grade glioma or meningioma. These observations, although inconclusive, corroborate descriptive epidemiological studies showing a general trend toward higher brain tumor incidence rates in industrialized countries with a higher socioeconomic status.

4. Diet

N-Nitroso compounds may be detected in nitrite-preserved food or formed in the stomach after uptake of their chemical precursors, nitrate/nitrite and secondary amines (54). Formation of nitroso compounds from precursors are inhibited by vitamins C and E (54). Since some *N*-nitroso compounds are potent neurocarcinogens in experimental animals (55), many epidemiological studies have been carried out to assess the possible role of diets containing *N*-nitroso compounds and their precursors. High intake of cured meat, cooked ham, processed pork, and fried bacon, which contain high levels of nitrite, was associated with elevated glioma risk in adults (56–58). A meta-analysis of nine published studies yielded an increased relative risk of glioma development among adults frequently ingesting cured meat (*59*). An inverse association was noted for frequent intake of fruits, fresh vegetables, and vitamin C (*56*, *58*). However, other studies showed only limited support for the role of *N*-nitroso compounds (*59–61*). In a population-based case–control study of adult gliomas in Nebraska, there was a protective effect of dark yellow vegetables and beans, while no association was seen for dietary sources of preformed nitrosamines or high-nitrate vegetables (*61*). Overall, the available data were considered insufficient to establish a dose–response relationship.

In several studies, higher consumption of cured meats and processed meats by mothers during pregnancy was associated with elevated risk of astrocytic gliomas in their children (*62–64*). Increased risk (twofold to threefold) was observed in offspring of mothers who consumed 3 mg nitrite per day from cured meats throughout pregnancy (*65*). An inverse association of development of brain tumors including gliomas in children was observed with the intake of fruit and fresh vegetables and of vitamin C by mothers during pregnancy (*63*, *66*). A meta-analysis of cured meat consumption during pregnancy, pooling data from six reports containing data on maternal intake of cured meat of all types (*67*), yielded a relative risk of 1.68 (95% CI, 1.30–2.17).

Another dietary factor with a suggestive but not proven positive association for gliomas is high protein intake (*68*). Nutrients reported to be inversely associated with glioma risk include total fat and cholesterol (*68*), high dietary calcium intake for women (*69*), high sodium intake (*68*), and high dietary antioxidant and high intake of certain phytoestrogens (*70*).

5. Smoking

In adults, no causal link has been detected between cigarette smoking and the development of gliomas (*58*, *71*). A population-based case–control study carried out in seven countries as part of the Surveillance of Environmental Aspects Related to Cancer in Humans (SEARCH) program showed a weak association of paternal smoking with the risk of childhood astroglial tumors compared with nonsmoking, non-occupationally-exposed fathers (*51*). However, another study showed no significant association between parental tobacco smoking and the incidence of childhood brain tumors (*72*). The International Agency for Research on Cancer (IARC) Monographs evaluation did not list the nervous system as a target organ for tobacco-induced carcinogenesis in humans (*73*).

6. Therapeutic X-Irradiation

Therapeutic X-irradiation constitutes the only environmental factor unequivocally associated with an increased risk of brain tumors. Several studies have shown increased brain tumor risks (gliomas, primitive neuroectodermal tumors [PNETs]) in children who received prophylactic CNS irradiation for acute lymphoblastic leukemia (ALL) (74–80). Brain tumors may develop as early as 7–9 years after irradiation (77, 80). A high risk was most evident in children younger than 5 or 6 years at the time of the ALL diagnosis (76, 79). A large retrospective cohort study of 9,720 children treated for ALL in 1972–1988 showed that, of 43 second neoplasms diagnosed, 24 were CNS neoplasms in children who had previously undergone irradiation, which represented a 7-fold excess of all cancers and a 22-fold excess of CNS neoplasms (gliomas and PNETs) (76).

A cohort of 4,400 children treated for various cancers in France and the UK was followed up to assess risks of subsequent brain tumors in relation to radiotherapy and chemotherapy (78). Elevated risks of subsequent brain tumors were found for CNS tumors and neurofibromatosis (78). Neglia et al. (81) assessed subsequent primary neoplasms of the CNS occurring within a cohort of >14,000 5-year survivors of childhood cancer, demonstrating that radiation exposure was associated with increased risk of subsequent glioma and meningioma. For glioma, the excess relative risk was highest among children exposed at younger than 5 years of age. The higher risk of subsequent glioma in children irradiated at a very young age may reflect greater susceptibility of the developing brain to radiation (81). Even low-dose therapeutic radiation for the treatment of tinea capitis may result in subsequent development of brain tumors (82, 83).

7. Electromagnetic Fields

A weak association of brain tumors with occupational exposure to magnetic fields has been observed in some studies (84, 85); others failed to reveal a significantly elevated risk in electrical utility workers (86, 87). A population-based study in the San Francisco Bay area (USA) revealed no association between adult gliomas and residential power-frequency electromagnetic field exposures (88). The available evidence is insufficient to causally link electromagnetic fields with an increase in the incidence of childhood brain tumors (89–91).

8. Mobile Phones

Cellular phones operate at radio frequencies, a form of electro magnetic energy located in the spectrum between FM radio waves and the waves used in microwave ovens, radar, and satellite stations. The recent rapid worldwide increase in mobile phone use has generated considerable media attention with respect to a possible link between cellular phones and brain tumors, but no consistent association has so far been found (*92–98*). The only positive finding published to date came from a case–control study in Sweden on 649 adult patients with malignant brain tumors diagnosed from January 1997 to June 2000 (*99*). For ipsilateral (same side) radiofrequency exposure, use of analog mobile phones was associated with an odds ratio (OR) of 1.85 (95% CI, 1.16–2.96) for all malignant brain tumors. For astrocytoma, this risk was 1.95 (95% CI, 1.12–3.39).

9. Medical History

9.1. Head Injury

There have been many case reports on the occurrence of gliomas after a head injury at the same site (*100*). Epidemiological studies have found a weak but inconsistent or nonsignificant association with adult and perinatal traumatic head injury (*101, 102*) or combined perinatal and adult head trauma (*103*).

9.2. Allergy

Several studies have shown a significant inverse association between gliomas and allergic diseases or allergic conditions such as asthma and eczema (*104–107*), with a significant dose–response relationship for increasing numbers of allergens (*106*). A hospital-based case–control study in the USA showed a significant inverse association between gliomas and history of any allergy or autoimmune disease, whereas no association was evident for meningiomas and acoustic neuromas (*105*). In a population-based case–control study in the UK, reduced risk was observed in subjects reporting a history of asthma, hay fever, eczema, and other allergies (*108*). The decreased risk of glioma in patients reporting a history of allergic conditions suggests an influence of immunological factors on the development of gliomas. It has been reported that total immunoglobulin E levels were lower in adults with glioma than control subjects (*109*), and this may be at least in part due to interleukin (IL)-13 polymorphisms (*110*).

9.3. Acute Infections

Epidemiological studies on common acute infections in adults and subsequent cancer development found these infections to be associated with reduced risks for glioma (*111*). Risk reduction increased with the frequency of infections, with febrile infections affording the greatest protection (*111*). Subjects who reported a history of infectious diseases such as colds and flu, showed a 30% reduction in risk of brain tumors (*104*). In a study of the San Francisco Bay area (USA), glioma patients were less likely than control subjects to report a history of chickenpox, and they had also lower level of immunoglobulin G to varicella zoster virus (*112*).

10. SV40

It is well known that simian virus (SV)-40 was iatrogenically introduced on a large scale into human populations between 1955 and 1962 through SV40-contaminated polio vaccines (*113*). SV40 sequences have been identified in a variety of human neoplasms, suggesting the possibility of an etiological role. In brain tumors, SV40 sequences have been detected at an overall frequency of approximately 35% (*113–116*), while surrounding non-tumorous brain tissue rarely contained SV40 (*114, 115*). SV40 sequences were seen in 25–26% of brain tumors of Swiss patients, while they were not detectable in brain tumors of similar histological types from Finland, a country where SV40-contaminated polio vaccine was not used (*117*). These suggest that SV40 in human brain tumors did indeed originate from contaminated polio vaccine, and that SV40 is sufficiently able to spread in human populations so that it is still commonly present 40 years after cessation of the use of the contaminated vaccine. A meta-analysis of 13 published studies showed that brain tumor samples were almost four times more likely to have evidence of SV40 infection than were those from control samples (*118*).

However, there appears to be no selective increase in the incidence of brain tumors in populations that received SV40-contaminated vaccine, incidence rates of brain tumors being similar in countries that did or did not use SV40-contaminated vaccine (*117*).

11. Hereditary Tumor Syndromes

11.1 Li-Fraumeni Sydrome

Several familial cancer syndromes are associated with gliomas (*119*). Li-Fraumeni syndrome is an autosomal dominant disorder and is characterized by multiple primary neoplasms in children and young adults, with a predominance of soft-tissue sarcomas, osteosarcomas, and breast cancer, and an increased incidence of brain tumors, leukemia, and adrenocortical adenoma. Approximately 70% of Li-Fraumeni cases carry a *TP53* germline mutation. Approximately 13% of neoplasms in families with germline *TP53* mutations are brain tumors, and astrocytic gliomas are predominant (*120*).

11.2. Neurofibromatosis Type 1

Neurofibromatosis Type 1 (NF1) is an autosomal dominant disorder characterized by multiple neurofibromas, malignant peripheral nerve sheath tumors, optic nerve gliomas and other astrocytomas, multiple café-au-lait spots, axillary and inguinal freckling, and iris hamartomas. The prevalence of this disease is 1 per 3,000 newborns (*121*). The majority of gliomas in NF1 patients are pilocytic astrocytomas of the optic nerve (*122*). Other gliomas observed at an increased frequency in NF1 patients include diffuse astrocytomas and glioblastomas.

11.3. Neurofibromatosis Type 2

Neurofibromatosis Type 2 (NF2) is an autosomal dominant disorder characterized by neoplastic and dysplastic lesions of Schwann cells, meningeal cells, and glial cells. The prevalence of this disease is approximately 1 per 40,000 newborns (*123*). Approximately 80% of gliomas that develop in NF2 patients are spinal intramedullary or cauda equina tumors, particularly ependymomas (*124*), with an additional 10% of gliomas occurring in the medulla (*125*).

11.4. Turcot Syndrome

Turcot syndrome is an autosomal dominant disorder characterized by adenomatous colorectal polyps or colon carcinomas and by malignant neuroepithelial tumors. Turcot syndrome type 1 patients carry germline mutations in DNA mismatch repair genes such as *hPMS2*, *hMSH2*, or *hMLH1*, presenting with glioblastoma and hereditary nonpolyposis colorectal carcinoma, whereas Turcot syndrome type 2 patients carry a germline mutation of the *APC* gene, suffer from familial adenomatous polyposis (FAP), and typically develop medulloblastomas (*126*).

The occurrence of gliomas in individuals with hereditary syndromes supports the hypothesis of a genetic predisposition to brain tumors. However, syndromes resulting from mutations in high-penetrance genes are rare (*119*).

12. Familial Clustering

Family members of glioma patients may be more susceptible to glioma development than the general population. Malmer et al. (*127*) carried out a population-based study of the occurrence of familial astrocytoma among first-degree relatives of patients with astrocytoma diagnosed in 1985–1993 in Sweden. A significantly increased risk was shown for astrocytomas but not for other histological types of brain tumor (*127*). Another study from the same group suggested that familial clustering occurs in approximately 5% of glioma cases and that 1% have a possible autosomal dominant inheritance (*128*). Hemminki et al. (*129*) observed that 2.1% of a series of brain tumor patients had parents with nervous system tumors. In a study with a large series of brain tumor patients, including 5,088 relatives of 639 probands diagnosed with a glioma in 1992–1995, segregation analysis demonstrated that a multigenic Mendelian model was favored (*130*). In contrast, a population-based retrospective study in Iceland showed no significant increase in glioma among relatives of glioma patients (*131*).

13. Genetic Polymorphisms

Polymorphisms in genes encoding enzymes involved in the metabolism of chemical carcinogens or DNA repair may be associated with higher susceptibility to glioma development. In a case–control study, logistic regression analysis showed GSTT1-null and CYP2D6 poor metabolizer status are risk factors for both astrocytomas and meningiomas (*132*). A population-based case–control study of adult gliomas in the San Francisco Bay area (USA) showed that increased risk of oligodendrogliomas was associated with the GSTT1-null genotype (*133*). There was a significant increase in the frequency of the functional GSTM1 allele in high-grade pediatric astrocytomas, and a significant increase in the frequency of the rare GSTP1 variant 114 Val/Val (*134*). Similarly, the GSTP1 105 Val/Val genotype was associated with increased glioma incidence (*135*). In contrast, there was no significant association between null genotypes of GSTM1, GSTT1, and CYP1A1 and risk of gliomas (*136*). Adult glioma patients were significantly more likely than control subjects to be homozygous for the silent AA variant at codon 156 of the *ERCC2* gene, which encodes a protein essential for nucleotide excision repair (*137*).

14. TP53 Mutations as Etiological Molecular Fingerprint

Among *TP53* mutations identified in astrocytic brain tumors, G:C→A:T transitions are the most frequent, and they are predominantly located at CpG sites (*3, 120*). A similar pattern is seen in colon cancer, sarcomas, lymphomas, and germline *TP53* mutations (*119*). This is particularly true for low-grade astrocytomas and the secondary glioblastomas derived from them (*138*).

The best-characterized mechanism of G:C→A:T transitions at CpG sites is deamination of 5-methylcytosine at CpG sites, resulting in substitution of 5-methylcytosine by thymine. This occurs spontaneously or is factor-mediated, e.g., through the action of oxygen radicals or of nitric oxide produced by nitric oxide synthase under conditions of chronic inflammation (*139*). Since all CpG sites in exons 5–8 of the *TP53* gene are methylated in healthy human tissues (*140*), factors that affect the rate of deamination may influence the acquisition of G:C→A:T mutations. However, other mechanisms may also play roles. One possible mechanism of acquisition of G:C→A:T mutations is due to alkylating agents, since promoter methylation of the O^6-methylguanine-DNA methyltransferase (MGMT) gene is significantly associated with the presence of G:C→A:T mutations in gliomas (*138, 141–143*). MGMT specifically removes promutagenic alkyl groups from the O^6 position of guanine in DNA (*144*). Lack of MGMT in the histologically normal perifocal brain is frequent and age-dependent in brain tumor patients, while lack of MGMT in the normal brain is infrequent in patients without tumors (*145*). DNA methylation may be caused by *N*-nitroso compounds in food or tobacco (see above) (*54*). O^6-Methylguanine may be also produced through non-enzymatic methylation by *S*-adenosylmethionine (SAM) (*146*). Kang et al. (*147*) reported that O^6-methylguanine is present in leucocytes (0.7–4.6 adducts/10^8 guanine) and in the liver (1.1–6.7 adducts/10^7 guanine) of healthy volunteers. However, the level of O^6-methylguanine in human brain remains to be assessed.

References

1. Parkin, D.M., Whelan, S.L., Feraly, J., Teppo, L., Thomas, D.B. (2002) Cancer Incidence in Five Continents. Vol VIII, IARC Press, Lyon, France.

2. Feraly, J., Bray, F., Pisani, P., Parkin, D.M. (2000) Globocan 2000: Cancer Incidence, Mortality and Prevalence Worldwide. IARC Press, Lyon, France.

3. Ohgaki, H., Dessen, P., Jourde, B., Horstmann, S., Nishikawa, T., Di Patre, P. L., Burkhard, C., Schuler, D., Probst-Hensch, N. M., Maiorka, P. C., Baeza, N., Pisani, P., Yonekawa, Y., Yasargil, M. G., Lutolf, U. M., and Kleihues, P. (2004) Genetic pathways to glioblastoma: a population-based study. Cancer Res. 64, 6892–6899.

4. Okamoto, Y., Di Patre, P. L., Burkhard, C., Horstmann, S., Jourde, B., Fahey, M., Schuler, D., Probst-Hensch, N. M., Yasargil, M. G., Yonekawa, Y., Lutolf, U., Kleihues, P., and Ohgaki, H. (2004) Population-based study on incidence, survival rates, and genetic alterations of low-grade astrocytomas and oligodendrogliomas. Acta Neuropathol. 108, 49–56.

5. Burkhard, C., Di Patre, P. L., Schüler, D., Yasargil, M. G., Lütolf, U., Kleihues, P., and Ohgaki, H. (2003) A population-based study on the incidence and survival of patients with pilocytic astrocytoma. J Neurosurg. 98, 1170–1174.

6. Stiller, C. A. and Nectoux, J. (1994) International incidence of childhood brain and

spinal tumours. Int. J. Epidemiol. 23, 458–464.

7. McLendon, R. E., Robinson, J. S., Jr., Chambers, D. B., Grufferman, S., and Burger, P. C. (1985) The glioblastoma multiforme in Georgia, 1977–1981. Cancer. 56, 894–897.

8. Kuratsu, J., Takeshima, H., and Ushio, Y. (2001) Trends in the incidence of primary intracranial tumors in Kumamoto, Japan. Int J Clin Oncol. 6, 183–191.

9. Fan, K. J. and Pezeshkpour, G. H. (1992) Ethnic distribution of primary central nervous system tumors in Washington, DC, 1971 to 1985. J. Natl. Med. Assoc. 84, 858–863.

10. Central Brain Tumor Registry of the United States (CBTRUS; http://www.cbtrus.org).

11. Muir, C. S., Storm, H. H., and Polednak, A. (1994) Brain and other nervous system tumors. Cancer Surv. 19/20, 369–392.

12. Preston-Martin, S., Lewis, S., Winkelmann, R., Borman, B., Auld, J., and Pearce, N. (1993) Descriptive epidemiology of primary cancer of the brain, cranial nerves, and cranial meninges in New Zealand, 1948–88. Cancer Causes Control. 4, 529–538.

13. Boyle, P., Maisonneuve, P., Saracci, R., and Muir, C. S. (1990) Is the increased incidence of primary malignant brain tumors in the elderly real? J. Natl. Cancer Inst. 82, 1594–1596.

14. Greig, N. H., Ries, L. G., Yancik, R., and Rapoport, S. I. (1990) Increasing annual incidence of primary malignant brain tumors in the elderly. J. Natl. Cancer Inst. 82, 1621–1624.

15. Shugg, D., Allen, B. J., Blizzard, L., Dwyer, T., and Roder, D. (1994) Brain cancer incidence, mortality and case survival: observations from two Australian cancer registries. Int. J. Cancer. 59, 765–770.

16. Swensen, A. R. and Bushhouse, S. A. (1998) Childhood cancer incidence and trends in Minnesota, 1988–1994. Minn. Med. 81, 27–32.

17. Legler, J. M., Ries, L. A., Smith, M. A., Warren, J. L., Heineman, E. F., Kaplan, R. S., and Linet, M. S. (1999) Brain and other central nervous system cancers: recent trends in incidence and mortality. J. Natl. Cancer Inst. 91, 1382–1390.

18. Modan, B., Wagener, D. K., Feldman, J. J., Rosenberg, H. M., and Feinleib, M. (1992) Increased mortality from brain tumors: a combine outcome of diagnostic technology and change of attitude toward the elderly? Am. J. Epidemiol. 135, 1349–1357.

19. Christensen, H. C., Kosteljanetz, M., and Johansen, C. (2003) Incidences of gliomas and meningiomas in Denmark, 1943 to 1997. Neurosurgery. 52, 1327–1333.

20. Werner, M. H., Phuphanich, S., and Lyman, G. H. (1995) Increasing incidence of primary brain tumors in the elderly in Florida. Cancer Control. 2, 309–314.

21. Jukich, P. J., McCarthy, B. J., Surawicz, T. S., Freels, S., and Davis, F. G. (2001) Trends in incidence of primary brain tumors in the United States, 1985–1994. Neuro-oncol. 3, 141–151.

22. Lonn, S., Klaeboe, L., Hall, P., Mathiesen, T., Auvinen, A., Christensen, H. C., Johansen, C., Salminen, T., Tynes, T., and Feychting, M. (2004) Incidence trends of adult primary intracerebral tumors in four Nordic countries. Int. J. Cancer. 108, 450–455.

23. Dreifaldt, A. C., Carlberg, M., and Hardell, L. (2004) Increasing incidence rates of childhood malignant diseases in Sweden during the period 1960–1998. Eur. J. Cancer. 40, 1351–1360.

24. Houben, M. P., Aben, K. K., Teepen, J. L., Schouten-Van Meeteren, A. Y., Tijssen, C. C., Van Duijn, C. M., and Coebergh, J. W. (2006) Stable incidence of childhood and adult glioma in The Netherlands, 1989–2003. Acta Oncol. 45, 272–279.

25. Hoffman, S., Propp, J. M., and McCarthy, B. J. (2006) Temporal trends in incidence of primary brain tumors in the United States, 1985–1999. Neuro-oncol. 8, 27–37.

26. Ferlay, J., Bray, F., Sankila, R., Parkin, D.M. (1999) EUCAN 1999: Cancer Incidence, Mortality and Prevalence in the European Union. IARC Press, Lyon, France.

27. Claus, E. B. and Black, P. M. (2006) Survival rates and patterns of care for patients diagnosed with supratentorial low-grade gliomas: data from the SEER program, 1973–2001. Cancer. 106, 1358–1363.

28. Tseng, J. H., Merchant, E., and Tseng, M. Y. (2006) Effects of socioeconomic and geographic variations on survival for adult glioma in England and Wales. Surg. Neurol. 66, 258–263.

29. Tseng, M. Y. and Tseng, J. H. (2005) Survival analysis for adult glioma in England and Wales. J. Formos Med. Assoc. 104, 341–348.

30. Oertel, J., von Buttlar, E., Schroeder, H. W., and Gaab, M. R. (2005) Prognosis of

gliomas in the 1970s and today. Neurosurg. Focus. 18, e12

31. Magnani, C., Aareleid, T., Viscomi, S., Pastore, G., and Berrino, F. (2001) Variation in survival of children with central nervous system (CNS) malignancies diagnosed in Europe between 1978 and 1992: the EUROCARE study. Eur. J. Cancer. 37, 711–721.

32. Stroup, N. E., Blair, A., and Erikson, G. E. (1986) Brain cancer and other causes of death in anatomists. J. Natl. Cancer Inst. 77, 1217–1224.

33. Harrington, J. M. and Oakes, D. (1984) Mortality study of British pathologists 1974–1980. Brit. J. Ind. Med. 41, 188–191.

34. Hall, A., Harrington, J. M., and Aw, T. C. (1991) Mortality study of British pathologists. Am. J. Ind. Med. 20, 83–89.

35. Walrath, J. and Fraumeni, J. J. (1984) Cancer and other causes of death among embalmers. Cancer Res. 44, 4638–4641.

36. Krishnan, G., Felini, M., Carozza, S. E., Miike, R., Chew, T., and Wrensch, M. (2003) Occupation and adult gliomas in the San Francisco Bay Area. J. Occup. Environ. Med. 45, 639–647.

37. De Roos, A. J., Stewart, P. A., Linet, M. S., Heineman, E. F., Dosemeci, M., Wilcosky, T., Shapiro, W. R., Selker, R. G., Fine, H. A., Black, P. M., and Inskip, P. D. (2003) Occupation and the risk of adult glioma in the United States. Cancer Causes Control. 14, 139–150.

38. Carozza, S. E., Wrensch, M., Miike, R., Newman, B., Olshan, A. F., Savitz, D. A., Yost, M., and Lee, M. (2000) Occupation and adult gliomas. Am. J. Epidemiol. 152, 838–846.

39. Zheng, T., Cantor, K. P., Zhang, Y., Keim, S., and Lynch, C. F. (2001) Occupational risk factors for brain cancer: a population-based case-control study in Iowa. J. Occup. Environ. Med. 43, 317–324.

40. Khuder, S. A., Mutgi, A. B., and Schaub, E. A. (1998) Meta-analyses of brain cancer and farming. Am. J. Ind. Med. 34, 252–260.

41. Preston-Martin, S., Mack, W., and Henderson, B. E. (1989) Risk factors for gliomas and meningiomas in males in Los Angeles County. Cancer Res. 49, 6137–6143.

42. Navas-Acien, A., Pollan, M., Gustavsson, P., and Plato, N. (2002) Occupation, exposure to chemicals and risk of gliomas and meningiomas in Sweden. Am. J. Ind. Med. 42, 214–227.

43. Cocco, P., Dosemeci, M., and Heineman, E. F. (1998) Brain cancer and occupational exposure to lead. J. Occup. Environ. Med. 40, 937–942.

44. Anttila, A., Heikkila, P., Nykyri, E., Kauppinen, T., Pukkala, E., Hernberg, S., and Hemminki, K. (1996) Risk of nervous system cancer among workers exposed to lead. J. Occup. Environ. Med. 38, 131–136.

45. Wong, O., and Harris, F. (2000) Cancer mortality study of employees at lead battery plants and lead smelters, 1947–1995. Am. J. Ind. Med. 38, 255–270.

46. Rajaraman, P., Stewart, P. A., Samet, J. M., Schwartz, B. S., Linet, M. S., Zahm, S. H., Rothman, N., Yeager, M., Fine, H. A., Black, P. M., Loeffler, J., Shapiro, W. R., Selker, R. G., and Inskip, P. D. (2006) Lead, genetic susceptibility, and risk of adult brain tumors. Cancer Epidemiol Biomarkers Prev. 15, 2514–2520.

47. Moss, A. R. (1985) Occupational exposure and brain tumors. J. Toxicol. Environ. Health. 16, 703–711.

48. Siemiatycki, J., Richardson, L., Straif, K., Latreille, B., Lakhani, R., Campbell, S., Rousseau, M. C., and Boffetta, P. (2004) Listing occupational carcinogens. Environ Health Perspect. 112, 1447–1459.

49. McKean-Cowdin, R., Preston-Martin, S., Pogoda, J. M., Holly, E. A., Mueller, B. A., and Davis, R. L. (1998) Parental occupation and childhood brain tumors: astroglial and primitive neuroectodermal tumors. J. Occup. Environ. Med. 40, 332–340.

50. Cordier, S., Mandereau, L., Preston-Martin, S., Little, J., Lubin, F., Mueller, B., Holly, E., Filippini, G., Peris-Bonet, R., McCredie, M., Choi, N. W., and Arsla, A. (2001) Parental occupations and childhood brain tumors: results of an international case-control study. Cancer Causes Control. 12, 865–874.

51. Cordier, S., Monfort, C., Filippini, G., Preston-Martin, S., Lubin, F., Mueller, B. A., Holly, E. A., Peris-Bonet, R., McCredie, M., Choi, W., Little, J., and Arslan, A. (2004) Parental exposure to polycyclic aromatic hydrocarbons and the risk of childhood brain tumors: The SEARCH International Childhood Brain Tumor Study. Am. J. Epidemiol. 159, 1109–1116.

52. Brownson, R. C., Reif, J. S., Chang, J. C., and Davis, J. R. (1990) An analysis of occupational risks for brain cancer. Am. J. Public Health. 80, 169–172.

53. Inskip, P. D., Tarone, R. E., Hatch, E. E., Wilcosky, T. C., Fine, H. A., Black, P. M., Loeffler, J. S., Shapiro, W. R., Selker, R. G., and Linet, M. S. (2003) Sociodemographic

indicators and risk of brain tumours. Int. J. Epidemiol. 32, 225–233.

54. Lijinsky, W. (1992) Chemistry and Biology of N-Nitroso Compounds. Cambridge University Press, New York.

55. Kleihues, P., Wiestler, O. D., Ohgaki, H., and Aguzzi, A. (1998) Animal models of tumors of the nervous system, in The Gliomas (Berger, M. S., and Wilson, C. eds.) W.B. Saunders, Philadelphia, pp. 124–133.

56. Lee, M., Wrensch, M., and Miike, R. (1997) Dietary and tobacco risk factors for adult onset glioma in the San Francisco Bay Area (California, USA). Cancer Causes Control. 8, 13–24.

57. Boeing, H., Schlehofer, B., Blettner, M., and Wahrendorf, J. (1993) Dietary carcinogens and the risk for glioma and meningioma in Germany. Int. J. Cancer. 53, 561–565.

58. Blowers, L., Preston-Martin, S., and Mack, W. J. (1997) Dietary and other lifestyle factors of women with brain gliomas in Los Angeles County (California, USA). Cancer Causes Control. 8, 5–12.

59. Huncharek, M., Kupelnick, B., and Wheeler, L. (2003) Dietary cured meat and the risk of adult glioma: a meta-analysis of nine observational studies. J. Environ. Pathol. Toxicol. Oncol. 22, 129–137.

60. Giles, G. G., McNeil, J. J., Donnan, G., Webley, C., Staples, M. P., Ireland, P. D., Hurley, S. F., and Salzberg, M. (1994) Dietary factors and the risk of glioma in adults: results of a case-control study in Melbourne, Australia. Int. J. Cancer. 59, 357–362.

61. Chen, H., Ward, M. H., Tucker, K. L., Graubard, B. I., McComb, R. D., Potischman, N. A., Weisenburger, D. D., and Heineman, E. F. (2002) Diet and risk of adult glioma in eastern Nebraska, United States. Cancer Causes Control. 13, 647–655.

62. Bunin, G. R., Kuijten, R. R., Boesel, C. P., Buckley, J. D., and Meadows, A. T. (1994) Maternal diet and risk of astrocytic glioma in children: a report from the Childrens Cancer Group (United States and Canada). Cancer Causes Control. 5, 177–187.

63. Preston-Martin, S., Pogoda, J. M., Mueller, B. A., Holly, E. A., Lijinsky, W., and Davis, R. L. (1996) Maternal consumption of cured meats and vitamins in relation to pediatric brain tumors. Cancer Epidemiol Biomarkers Prev. 5, 599–605.

64. Kuijten, R. R., Bunin, G. R., Nass, C. C., and Meadows, A. T. (1990) Gestational and familial risk factors for childhood astrocytoma:

results of a case-control study. Cancer Res. 50, 2608–2612.

65. Pogoda, J. M. and Preston-Martin, S. (2001) Maternal cured meat consumption during pregnancy and risk of paediatric brain tumour in offspring: potentially harmful levels of intake. Public Health Nutr. 4, 183–189.

66. Preston-Martin, S., Pogoda, J. M., Mueller, B. A., Lubin, F., Holly, E. A., Filippini, G., Cordier, S., Peris-Bonet, R., Choi, W., Little, J., and Arslan, A. (1998) Prenatal vitamin supplementation and risk of childhood brain tumors. Int. J. Cancer Suppl. 11, 17–22.

67. Huncharek, M. and Kupelnick, B. (2004) A meta-analysis of maternal cured meat consumption during pregnancy and the risk of childhood brain tumors. Neuroepidemiology. 23, 78–84.

68. Kaplan, S., Novikov, I., and Modan, B. (1997) Nutritional factors in the etiology of brain tumors: potential role of nitrosamines, fat, and cholesterol. Am. J. Epidemiol. 146, 832–841.

69. Tedeschi-Blok, N., Schwartzbaum, J., Lee, M., Miike, R., and Wrensch, M. (2001) Dietary calcium consumption and astrocytic glioma: the San Francisco Bay Area Adult Glioma Study, 1991–1995. Nutr. Cancer. 39, 196–203.

70. Tedeschi-Blok, N., Lee, M., Sison, J. D., Miike, R., and Wrensch, M. (2006) Inverse association of antioxidant and phytoestrogen nutrient intake with adult glioma in the San Francisco Bay Area: a case-control study. BMC Cancer. 6, 148.

71. Zheng, T., Cantor, K. P., Zhang, Y., Chiu, B. C., and Lynch, C. F. (2001) Risk of brain glioma not associated with cigarette smoking or use of other tobacco products in Iowa. Cancer Epidemiol Biomarkers Prev. 10, 413–414.

72. Norman, M. A., Holly, E. A., Ahn, D. K., Preston-Martin, S., Mueller, B. A., and Bracci, P. M. (1996) Prenatal exposure to tobacco smoke and childhood brain tumors: results from the United States West Coast childhood brain tumor study. Cancer Epidemiol Biomarkers Prev. 5, 127–133.

73. IARC Working Group on the Evaluation of Carcinogenic Risks to Humans. (2004) Tobacco smoke and involuntary smoking. IARC, Lyon, France.

74. Relling, M. V., Rubnitz, J. E., Rivera, G. K., Boyett, J. M., Hancock, M. L., Felix, C. A., Kun, L. E., Walter, A. W., Evans, W. E., and Pui, C. H. (1999) High incidence of

secondary brain tumours after radiotherapy and antimetabolites. Lancet. 354, 34–39.

75. Rosso, P., Terracini, B., Fears, T. R., Jankovic, M., Fossati, B. F., Arrighini, A., Carli, M., Cordero, d. M., Garre, M. L., and Guazzelli, C. (1994) Second malignant tumors after elective end of therapy for a first cancer in childhood: a multicenter study in Italy. Int. J. Cancer. 59, 451–456.

76. Neglia, J. P., Meadows, A. T., Robison, L. L., Kim, T. H., Newton, W. A., Ruymann, F. B., Sather, H. N., and Hammond, G. D. (1991) Second neoplasms after acute lymphoblastic leukemia in childhood. N. Engl. J. Med. 325, 1330–1336.

77. Nygaard, R., Garwicz, S., Haldorsen, T., Hertz, H., Jonmundsson, G. K., Lanning, M., and Moe, P. J. (1991) Second malignant neoplasms in patients treated for childhood leukemia. A population-based cohort study from the Nordic countries. The Nordic Society of Pediatric Oncology and Hematology (NOPHO). Acta Paediatr Scand. 80, 1220–1228.

78. Little, M. P., De Vathaire, F., Shamsaldin, A., Oberlin, O., Campbell, S., Grimaud, E., Chavaudra, J., Haylock, R. G., and Muirhead, C. R. (1998) Risks of brain tumour following treatment for cancer in childhood: modification by genetic factors, radiotherapy and chemotherapy. Int. J. Cancer. 78, 269–275.

79. Walter, A. W., Hancock, M. L., Pui, C. H., Hudson, M. M., Ochs, J. S., Rivera, G. K., Pratt, C. B., Boyett, J. M., and Kun, L. E. (1998) Secondary brain tumors in children treated for acute lymphoblastic leukemia at St Jude Children's Research Hospital. J. Clin. Oncol. 16, 3761–3767.

80. Brustle, O., Ohgaki, H., Schmitt, H. P., Walter, G. F., Ostertag, H., and Kleihues, P. (1992) Primitive neuroectodermal tumors after prophylactic central nervous system irradiation in children. Association with an activated K-ras gene. Cancer. 69, 2385–2392.

81. Neglia, J. P., Robison, L. L., Stovall, M., Liu, Y., Packer, R. J., Hammond, S., Yasui, Y., Kasper, C. E., Mertens, A. C., Donaldson, S. S., Meadows, A. T., and Inskip, P. D. (2006) New primary neoplasms of the central nervous system in survivors of childhood cancer: a report from the Childhood Cancer Survivor Study. J. Natl. Cancer Inst. 98, 1528–1537.

82. Soffer, D., Gomori, J. M., Pomeranz, S., and Siegal, T. (1990) Gliomas following low-dose irradiation to the head report of three cases. J. Neurooncol. 8, 67–72.

83. Ron, E., Modan, B., Boice, J. D., Jr., Alfandary, E., Stovall, M., Chetrit, A., and Katz, L. (1988) Tumors of the brain and nervous system after radiotherapy in childhood. N. Engl. J. Med. 319, 1033–1039.

84. Savitz, D. A. and Loomis, D. P. (1995) Magnetic field exposure in relation to leukemia and brain cancer mortality among electric utility workers. Am. J. Epidemiol. 141, 123–134.

85. Villeneuve, P. J., Agnew, D. A., Johnson, K. C., and Mao, Y. (2002) Brain cancer and occupational exposure to magnetic fields among men: results from a Canadian population-based case-control study. Int. J. Epidemiol. 31, 210–217.

86. Armstrong, B., Thierault, G., Guenel, P., Deadman, J., Goldberg, M., and Heroux, P. (1994) Association between exposure to pulsed electromagnetic fields and cancer in electric utility workers in Quebec, Canada, and France. Am. J. Epidemiol. 140, 805–820.

87. Thierault, G., Goldberg, M., Miller, A. B., Armstrong, B., Guenel, P., Deadman, J., Imbernon, E., To, T., Chevalier, A., Cyr, D., et al. (1994) Cancer risks associated with occupational exposure to magnetic fields among electric utility workers in Ontario and Quebec, Canada and France: 1970–1989. Am. J. Epidemiol. 139, 550–572.

88. Wrensch, M., Yost, M., Miike, R., Lee, G., and Touchstone, J. (1999) Adult glioma in relation to residential power frequency electromagnetic field exposures in the San Francisco Bay area. Epidemiology. 10, 523–527.

89. Kheifets, L. I., Sussman, S. S., and Preston-Martin, S. (1999) Childhood brain tumors and residential electromagnetic fields (EMF). Rev. Environ. Contam. Toxicol. 159, 111–129.

90. Gurney, J. G., Mueller, B. A., Davis, S., Schwartz, S. M., Stevens, R. G., and Kopecky, K. J. (1996) Childhood brain tumor occurrence in relation to residential power line configurations, electric heating sources, and electric appliance use. Am. J. Epidemiol. 143, 120–128.

91. Preston-Martin, S., Navidi, W., Thomas, D., Lee, P. J., Bowman, J., and Pogoda, J. (1996) Los Angeles study of residential magnetic fields and childhood brain tumors. Am. J. Epidemiol. 143, 105–119.

92. Johansen, C., Boice, J., Jr., McLaughlin, J., and Olsen, J. (2001) Cellular telephones and cancer--a nationwide cohort study in Denmark. J. Natl. Cancer Inst. 93, 203–207.

93. Muscat, J. E., Malkin, M. G., Thompson, S., Shore, R. E., Stellman, S. D., McRee, D., Neugut, A. I., and Wynder, E. L. (2000) Handheld cellular telephone use and risk of brain cancer. JAMA. 284, 3001–3007.

94. Inskip, P. D., Tarone, R. E., Hatch, E. E., Wilcosky, T. C., Shapiro, W. R., Selker, R. G., Fine, H. A., Black, P. M., Loeffler, J. S., and Linet, M. S. (2001) Cellular-telephone use and brain tumors. N. Engl. J. Med. 344, 79–86.

95. Schuz, J., Bohler, E., Berg, G., Schlehofer, B., Hettinger, I., Schlaefer, K., Wahrendorf, J., Kunna-Grass, K., and Blettner, M. (2006) Cellular phones, cordless phones, and the risks of glioma and meningioma (Interphone Study Group, Germany). Am. J. Epidemiol. 163, 512–520.

96. Hepworth, S. J., Schoemaker, M. J., Muir, K. R., Swerdlow, A. J., van Tongeren, M. J., and McKinney, P. A. (2006) Mobile phone use and risk of glioma in adults: case-control study. BMJ. 332, 883–887.

97. Lahkola, A., Auvinen, A., Raitanen, J., Schoemaker, M. J., Christensen, H. C., Feychting, M., Johansen, C., Klaeboe, L., Lonn, S., Swerdlow, A. J., Tynes, T., and Salminen, T. (2007) Mobile phone use and risk of glioma in 5 North European countries. Int. J. Cancer. 120, 1769–1775.

98. Lonn, S., Ahlbom, A., Hall, P., and Feychting, M. (2005) Long-term mobile phone use and brain tumor risk. Am. J. Epidemiol. 161, 526–535.

99. Hardell, L., Mild, K. H., and Carlberg, M. (2002) Case-control study on the use of cellular and cordless phones and the risk for malignant brain tumours. Int. J. Radiat. Biol. 78, 931–936.

100. Lantos, P. L., Louis, D. N., Rosenblum, M. K., and Kleihues, P. (2002) Tumours of the Nervous System, in Greenfield's Neuropathology (Graham, D. I., and Lantos, P. L. eds.) Arnold, London, pp. 767–1052.

101. Hochberg, F., Toniolo, P., and Cole, P. (1984) Head trauma and seizures as risk factors of glioblastoma. Neurology. 34, 1511–1514.

102. Schlehofer, B., Blettner, M., Becker, N., Martinsohn, C., and Wahrendorf, J. (1992) Medical risk factors and the development of brain tumors. Cancer. 69, 2541–2547.

103. Gurney, J. G., Preston-Martin, S., McDaniel, A. M., Mueller, B. A., and Holly, E. A. (1996) Head injury as a risk factor for brain tumors in children: results from a multicenter case-control study. Epidemiology. 7, 485–489.

104. Schlehofer, B., Blettner, M., Preston-Martin, S., Niehoff, D., Wahrendorf, J., Arslan, A., Ahlbom, A., Choi, W. N., Giles, G. G., Howe, G. R., Little, J., Menegoz, F., and Ryan, P. (1999) Role of medical history in brain tumour development. Results from the international adult brain tumour study. Int. J. Cancer. 82, 155–160.

105. Brenner, A. V., Linet, M. S., Fine, H. A., Shapiro, W. R., Selker, R. G., Black, P. M., and Inskip, P. D. (2002) History of allergies and autoimmune diseases and risk of brain tumors in adults. Int. J. Cancer. 99, 252–259.

106. Wiemels, J. L., Wiencke, J. K., Sison, J. D., Miike, R., McMillan, A., and Wrensch, M. (2002) History of allergies among adults with glioma and controls. Int. J. Cancer. 98, 609–615.

107. Schwartzbaum, J., Jonsson, F., Ahlbom, A., Preston-Martin, S., Lonn, S., Soderberg, K. C., and Feychting, M. (2003) Cohort studies of association between self-reported allergic conditions, immune-related diagnoses and glioma and meningioma risk. Int. J. Cancer. 106, 423–428.

108. Schoemaker, M. J., Swerdlow, A. J., Hepworth, S. J., McKinney, P. A., van Tongeren, M., and Muir, K. R. (2006) History of allergies and risk of glioma in adults. Int. J. Cancer. 119, 2165–2172.

109. Wiemels, J. L., Wiencke, J. K., Patoka, J., Moghadassi, M., Chew, T., McMillan, A., Miike, R., Barger, G., and Wrensch, M. (2004) Reduced immunoglobulin E and allergy among adults with glioma compared with controls. Cancer Res. 64, 8468–8473.

110. Wiemels, J. L., Wiencke, J. K., Kelsey, K. T., Moghadassi, M., Rice, T., Urayama, K. Y., Miike, R., and Wrensch, M. (2007) Allergy-related polymorphisms influence glioma status and serum IgE levels. Cancer Epidemiol Biomarkers Prev. 16, 1229–1235.

111. Hoption Cann, S. A., van Netten, J. P., and van Netten, C. (2006) Acute infections as a means of cancer prevention: opposing effects to chronic infections? Cancer Detect Prev. 30, 83–93.

112. Wrensch, M., Weinberg, A., Wiencke, J., Miike, R., Sison, J., Wiemels, J., Barger, G., DeLorenze, G., Aldape, K., and Kelsey, K. (2005) History of chickenpox and shingles and prevalence of antibodies to varicella-zoster virus and three other herpesviruses among adults with glioma and controls. Am. J. Epidemiol. 161, 929–938.

113. Carbone, M., Rizzo, P., and Pass, H. I. (1997) Simian virus 40, poliovaccines and

human tumors: a review of recent developments. Oncogene. 15, 1877–1888.

114. Huang, H., Reis, R., Yonekawa, Y., Lopes, J. M., Kleihues, P., and Ohgaki, H. (1999) Identification in human brain tumors of DNA sequences specific for SV40 large T antigen. Brain Pathol. 9, 33–44.

115. Martini, F., Iaccheri, L., Lazzarin, L., Carinci, P., Corallini, A., Gerosa, M., Iuzzolino, P., Barbanti-Brodano, G., and Tognon, M. (1996) SV40 early region and large T antigen in human brain tumors, peripheral blood cells, and sperm fluids from healthy individuals. Cancer Res. 56, 4820–4825.

116. Vilchez, R. A., and Butel, J. S. (2004) Emergent human pathogen simian virus 40 and its role in cancer. Clin. Microbiol. Rev. 17, 495–508.

117. Ohgaki, H., Huang, H., Haltia, M., Vainio, H., and Kleihues, P. (2000) More about: Cell and molecular biology of Simian Virus 40: Implications for human infections and disease. J. Natl. Cancer Inst. 92, 495–496.

118. Vilchez, R. A., Kozinetz, C. A., Arrington, A. S., Madden, C. R., and Butel, J. S. (2003) Simian virus 40 in human cancers. Am. J. Med. 114, 675–684.

119. Louis, D.N., Ohgaki, H., Wiestler O.D., Cavenee, W.K. (eds.) (2007) WHO Classification of Tumours of the Central Nervous System. IARC, Lyon, France.

120. Ohgaki, H., Olivier, M., and Hainaut, P. (2007) Li-Fraumeni syndrome and TP53 germline mutations, in WHO Classification of Tumours of the Central Nervous System. In: Louis, D. N., Ohgaki, H., Wiestler, O. D., and Cavenee, W. K. (eds.) IARC, Lyon, France, pp. 222–225.

121. von Deimling, A. and Perry, A. (2007) Neurofibromatosis type 1, in WHO Classification of Tumours of the Central Nervous System. In: Louis, D. N., Ohgaki, H., Wiestler, O. D., and Cavenee, W. K. (eds.) IARC, Lyon, France, pp. 206–209.

122. Lewis, R. A., Gerson, L. P., Axelson, K. A., Riccardi, V. M., and Whitford, R. P. (1984) von Recklinghausen neurofibromatosis. II. Incidence of optic gliomata. Ophthalmology. 91, 929–935.

123. Stemmer-Rachamimov, A. O., Wiestler, O. D., and Louis, D. N. (2007) Neurofibromatosis type 2, in WHO Classification of Tumours of the Central Nervous System. In: Louis, D. N., Ohgaki, H., Wiestler, O. D., and Cavenee, W. K. (eds.) IARC, Lyon, France, pp. 210–214.

124. Lamszus, K., Lachenmayer, L., Heinemann, U., Kluwe, L., Finckh, U., Hoppner, W., Stavrou, D., Fillbrandt, R., and Westphal, M. (2001) Molecular genetic alterations on chromosomes 11 and 22 in ependymomas. Int. J. Cancer. 91, 803–808.

125. Rodriguez, H. A., and Berthrong, M. (1966) Multiple primary intracranial tumors in von Recklinghausen's neurofibromatosis. Arch. Neurol. 14, 467–475.

126. Cavenee, W. K., Burger, P. C., Leung, S. Y., and Van Meir, E. G. (2007) Turcot syndrome, in WHO Classification of Tumours of the Central Nervous System. In: Louis, D. N., Ohgaki, H., Wiestler, O. D., and Cavenee, W. K. (eds.) IARC, Lyon, France, pp. 229–231.

127. Malmer, B., Gronberg, H., Bergenheim, A. T., Lenner, P., and Henriksson, R. (1999) Familial aggregation of astrocytoma in northern Sweden: an epidemiological cohort study. Int. J. Cancer. 81, 366–370.

128. Malmer, B., Iselius, L., Holmberg, E., Collins, A., Henriksson, R., and Gronberg, H. (2001) Genetic epidemiology of glioma. Br. J. Cancer. 84, 429–434.

129. Hemminki, K., Kyyronen, P., and Vaittinen, P. (1999) Parental age as a risk factor of childhood leukemia and brain cancer in offspring. Epidemiology. 10, 271–275.

130. de Andrade, M., Barnholtz, J. S., Amos, C. I., Adatto, P., Spencer, C., and Bondy, M. L. (2001) Segregation analysis of cancer in families of glioma patients. Genet. Epidemiol. 20, 258–270.

131. O'Neill, B. P., Blondal, H., Yang, P., Olafsdottir, G. H., Sigvaldason, H., Jenkins, R. B., Kimmel, D. W., Scheithauer, B. W., Rocca, W. A., Bjornsson, J., and Tulinius, H. (2002) Risk of cancer among relatives of patients with glioma. Cancer Epidemiol Biomarkers Prev. 11, 921–924.

132. Elexpuru-Camiruaga, J., Buxton, N., Kandula, V., Dias, P. S., Campbell, D., McIntosh, J., Broome, J., Jones, P., Inskip, A., Alldersea, J. (1995) Susceptibility to astrocytoma and meningioma: influence of allelism at glutathione S-transferase (GSTT1 and GSTM1) and cytochrome P-450 (CYP2D6) loci. Cancer Res. 55, 4237–4239.

133. Kelsey, K. T., Wrensch, M., Zuo, Z. F., Miike, R., and Wiencke, J. K. (1997) A population-based case-control study of the CYP2D6 and GSTT1 polymorphisms and malignant brain tumors. Pharmacogenetics. 7, 463–468.

134. Ezer, R., Alonso, M., Pereira, E., Kim, M., Allen, J. C., Miller, D. C., and Newcomb,

E. W. (2002) Identification of glutathione S-transferase (GST) polymorphisms in brain tumors and association with susceptibility to pediatric astrocytomas. J. Neurooncol. 59, 123–134.

135. De Roos, A. J., Rothman, N., Inskip, P. D., Linet, M. S., Shapiro, W. R., Selker, R. G., Fine, H. A., Black, P. M., Pittman, G. S., and Bell, D. A. (2003) Genetic polymorphisms in GSTM1, -P1, -T1, and CYP2E1 and the risk of adult brain tumors. Cancer Epidemiol Biomarkers Prev. 12, 14–22.

136. Trizna, Z., de Andrade, M., Kyritsis, A. P., Briggs, K., Levin, V. A., Bruner, J. M., Wei, Q., and Bondy, M. L. (1998) Genetic polymorphisms in glutathione S-transferase mu and theta, N-acetyltransferase, and CYP1A1 and risk of gliomas. Cancer Epidemiol Biomarkers Prev. 7, 553–555.

137. Caggana, M., Kilgallen, J., Conroy, J. M., Wiencke, J. K., Kelsey, K. T., Miike, R., Chen, P., and Wrensch, M. R. (2001) Associations between ERCC2 polymorphisms and gliomas. Cancer Epidemiol Biomarkers Prev. 10, 355–360.

138. Nakamura, M., Watanabe, T., Yonekawa, Y., Kleihues, P., and Ohgaki, H. (2001) Promoter hypermethylation of the DNA repair gene MGMT in astrocytomas is frequently associated with G:C–A:T mutations of the TP53 tumor suppressor gene. Carcinogenesis. 22, 1715–1719.

139. Ohshima, H. and Bartsch, H. (1994) Chronic infections and inflammatory processes as cancer risk factors: possible role of nitric oxide in carcinogenesis. Mutat. Res. 305, 253–264.

140. Tornaletti, S. and Pfeifer, G. P. (1995) Complete and tissue-independent methylation of CpG sites in the p53 gene: implications for mutations in human cancers. Oncogene. 10, 1493–1499.

141. Bello, M. J., Alonso, M. E., Aminoso, C., Anselmo, N. P., Arjona, D., Gonzalez-Gomez, P., Lopez-Marin, I., de Campos, J. M., Gutierrez, M., Isla, A., Kusak, M. E., Lassaletta, L., Sarasa, J. L., Vaquero, J., Casartelli, C., and Rey, J. A. (2004) Hypermethylation of the DNA repair gene MGMT: association with TP53 G:C to A:T transitions in a series of 469 nervous system tumors. Mutat. Res. 554, 23–32.

142. Watanabe, T., Katayama, Y., Komine, C., Yoshino, A., Ogino, A., Ohta, T., and Fukushima, T. (2005) O6-methylguanine-DNA methyltransferase methylation and TP53 mutation in malignant astrocytomas and their relationships with clinical course. Int. J. Cancer. 113, 581–587.

143. Yin, D., Xie, D., Hofmann, W. K., Zhang, W., Asotra, K., Wong, R., Black, K. L., and Koeffler, H. P. (2003) DNA repair gene O6-methylguanine-DNA methyltransferase: promoter hypermethylation associated with decreased expression and G:C to A:T mutations of p53 in brain tumors. Mol. Carcinog. 36, 23–31.

144. Pegg, A. E. (2000) Repair of O^6-alkylguanine by alkyltransferases. Mutat. Res. 462, 83–100.

145. Silber, J. R., Blank, A., Bobola, M. S., Mueller, B. A., Kolstoe, D. D., Ojemann, G. A., and Berger, M. S. (1996) Lack of the DNA repair protein O^6-methylguanine-DNA methyltransferase in histologically normal brain adjacent to primary human brain tumors. Proc. Natl. Acad. Sci. USA. 93, 6941–6946.

146. De Bont, R. and van Larebeke, N. (2004) Endogenous DNA damage in humans: a review of quantitative data. Mutagenesis. 19, 169–185.

147. Kang, H., Konishi, C., Kuroki, T., and Huh, N. (1995) Detection of O6-methylguanine, O4-methylthymine and O4-ethylthymine in human liver and peripheral blood leukocyte DNA. Carcinogenesis. 16, 1277–1280.

Chapter 15

Mammographic Density: A Heritable Risk Factor for Breast Cancer

Norman F. Boyd, Lisa J. Martin, Johanna M. Rommens, Andrew D. Paterson, Salomon Minkin, Martin J. Yaffe, Jennifer Stone, and John L. Hopper

Abstract

The appearance of the breast on mammography varies among women, reflecting variations in tissue composition. Stroma and epithelium attenuate x-rays more than fat and appear light on a mammogram, which we refer to here as "mammographic density," while fat appears dark. We show evidence that mammographic density is a strong risk factor for breast cancer, and that risk of breast cancer is four to five times greater in women with density in more than 75% of the breast, compared with those with little or no density. Density in more than 50% of the breast may account for a large proportion of breast cancers.

Density is influenced by age, parity, body mass index, and menopause but these factors account for only 20–30% of the variation in density in the population. Twin studies have shown that percent mammographic density, at a given age, is highly heritable, and that inherited factors explain 63% of the variance. Mammographic density has the characteristics of a quantitative trait, and may be influenced by genes that are easier to identify than those associated with breast cancer itself. The genes that influence mammographic density may also be associated with risk of breast cancer, and their identification is also likely to provide insights into the biology of the breast, and to identify potential targets for preventive strategies.

Key words: Breast cancer, heritable factors, mammography density.

1. Introduction

Breast cancer is the most common cancer in women, and a leading cause of cancer death in most Western countries (1). Despite extensive research, the causes of most cases of breast cancer remain unknown, although there is strong evidence that risk of the disease is influenced by both genetic and environmental factors. The tendency

M. Verma (ed.), *Methods of Molecular Biology, Cancer Epidemiology, vol. 472*
© 2009 Humana Press, a part of Springer Science + Business Media, Totowa, NJ
Book doi: 10.1007/978-1-60327-492-0

of breast cancers to cluster in some families, the twofold to three-fold increase in risk of disease associated with having an affected first-degree relative, and the higher risk within monozygotic twin pairs suggest that genes are associated with susceptibility to the disease *(2)*. The known genetic factors associated with susceptibility, including mutations in *BRCA1* and *BRCA2*, account for at most 25% of familial risk, and less than 5% of breast cancer risk overall *(3–6)*. The causes of most cases of the disease remain unexplained and are likely to be heterogeneous.

Mammographic density is one of the strongest known risk factors for the disease. Mammographic density refers to variations in the radiological appearance of the breast among women, which reflect variations in breast tissue composition, and is illustrated in **Fig. 15.1**. Women who have >75% of their breast area as dense tissue (**Fig. 15.1F**) have a risk of breast cancer four to six times greater than women of the same age with no density (**Fig. 15.1A**) *(7, 8)*.

Mammographic density differs from other risk factors for the disease in a number of ways. In addition to a family history of breast cancer, several menstrual, reproductive, and anthropometric variables are known to influence risk of breast cancer, and also influence density (*see* below), but the differences in risk associated with these risk factors are small compared with density, and the

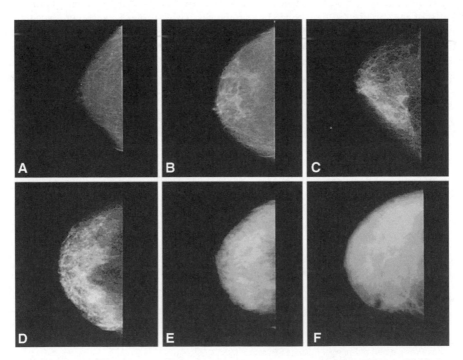

Fig. 15.1. Examples of categories of percent mammographic density estimated by radiologists. (**A**) 0%; (**B**) <10%; (**C**) <25%; (**D**) <50%; (**E**) <75%; and (**F**) ≥75%.

risk associated with density is independent of them. Mammographic density has wide variation across the population, even for women of the same age, and is associated with a substantial gradient of risk across the population, and may therefore account for a substantial fraction of the disease (*see* below).

In this chapter, we describe briefly the evidence that mammographic density is a risk factor for breast cancer, the histological basis for mammographic density, and the factors that are associated with variations in mammographic density, including the evidence that genetic factors have a major influence in explaining the large population variance of mammographic density.

2. Mammographic Density and Breast Cancer Risk

In 1976, Wolfe described a method of classifying variations in the appearance of the mammogram comprised of four categories that were associated with different risks of breast cancer (*9, 10*). The categories were designated N, for a breast comprised mainly of fat, DY for a breast mostly dense, and P1 and P2 for linear densities of different extent, indicating "ductal prominence." Other methods of classifying breast tissue as seen on mammography have been introduced, including a Breast Imaging Reporting and Data System (BIRADS) classification (*11*) and a classification proposed by Tabar (*12*). Various approaches have been taken to generate a quantitative measure of the degree to which the mammogram is dense, including estimation of percent density by radiologists and measurement of the area of the breast and density by planimetry or by a computer-assisted method applied to digitized images.

McCormack and dos Santos Silva have reviewed the data on the association of mammographic density with risk of breast cancer in a meta-analysis of aggregate data for >14,000 cases and 226,000 noncases from 42 studies (*13*). Associations were most consistent in studies conducted in the general population (rather than in symptomatic women), were stronger for percentage density than for Wolfe categories or the BIRADS classification, and were stronger in studies of incident than of prevalent cancer. No differences in the breast cancer risk associated with mammographic density were observed by age or menopausal status at mammography or by ethnicity. Mammographic density has been shown to influence risk of breast cancer in Caucasians, African Americans, Asian Americans, and Asians (*14*).

Although extensive mammographic density is associated with an increased risk of breast cancer, it also makes the detection of cancer by mammography more difficult. The influence of density on risk according to method of cancer detection has been studied in three nested case–control studies with 1,112 age-matched case–control pairs from screened populations (The Canadian National Breast Screening Programme, and the population-based screening programs of Ontario and British Columbia). The association of measured percent density in the baseline mammogram with risk of breast cancer was examined according to method of cancer detection, time since the initiation of screening, and age *(15)*.

As shown in **Table 15.1**, compared with women with density (estimated by radiologists) in less than 10% of the mammogram, women of the same age with more than 75% density had, after adjustment for other risk factors, an increased risk of breast cancer (odds ratio (OR) = 4.7; 95% confidence interval [CI]: 3.0–7.4), whether detected by screening (OR = 3.5; 95% CI: 2.0–6.2), or detected within 12 months of a negative screening examination (OR = 17.8; 95% CI: 4.8–65.9). Increased risks of breast cancer, for both screen-detected and nonscreen-detected breast cancer, persisted for at least 8 years after entry, and were greater in younger than in older women. The continuous computer-assisted measure showed a higher level of percent density in the baseline mammogram of women who later developed breast cancer, whether screen or nonscreen detected, up to 8 years after entry (*see* **Fig. 15.2**).

For women younger than the median age of 56 years, 26% of all breast cancers and 50% of cancers detected within 12 months of a negative screen were attributable to density in 50% or more of the mammogram. These data thus show that more extensive mammographic density is strongly associated with greater risk of breast cancer detected by screening, and with a marked increase in risk of detection between screens. As in other studies *(14, 16, 17)*, risk of breast cancer was associated positively with the area of dense tissue, but the gradient in risk was smaller than for percent density (data not shown).

The optimal approach to detecting breast cancer in women with dense breast tissue remains to be determined, but there is evidence that digital mammography improves cancer detection in women with extensive mammographic density *(18)*.

3. Breast Tissue and Mammographic Density

Studies of breast sections prepared from mastectomy specimens or biopsies and thus selected for the presence of suspected breast disease, have shown that epithelial and stromal proliferation were associated with mammographic density. Their findings are described in detail in reference *(19)*. Breast tissue obtained at

Table 15.1
Mammographic density and risk of breast cancer according to method of detection: unmatched analysis, radiologists' classification of density

		Categories of percent density (%)					
		No. of pairs[a]	<10	10 to <25	25 to <50	50 to <75	≥75	P value[b]
All	Case	1,112	230	272	336	178	96	
	Control	1,112	362	270	290	144	46	
	OR[c] (95% CI)		1	1.75 (1.4, 2.2)	2.06 (1.6, 2.6)	2.43 (1.8, 3.3)	4.74 (3.0, 7.4)	<0.0001
Screen detected	Case	717	173	171	219	102	52	
	Control	717	242	162	196	88	29	
	OR[c] (95% CI)		1	1.65 (1.2, 2.2)	1.77 (1.3, 2.4)	1.98 (1.3, 2.9)	3.52 (2.0, 6.2)	<0.0001
Non-screen detected <12 months[d]	Case	124	12	22	33	32	25	
	Control	124	35	29	29	23	8	
	OR[c] (95% CI)		1	2.11 (0.9, 5.2)	3.61 (1.5, 8.7)	5.65 (2.1, 15.3)	17.81 (4.8, 65.9)	<0.0001
Non-screen detected ≥12 months[e]	Case	262	43	79	80	42	18	
	Control	262	82	79	62	30	9	
	OR[c] (95% CI)		1	2.00 (1.2, 3.4)	2.64 (1.5, 4.6)	3.13 (1.6, 6.2)	5.68 (2.1, 15.5)	<0.0001

[a] Nine pairs were excluded from the screen or non-screen group analysis because of missing information on detection (n = 1), or the last mammogram date (n = 8). [b] P value for the Cochran-Armitage trend test. [c] Adjusted for age, BMI, age at menarche, parity, number of live births, age at first birth, menopausal status, age at menopause, hormone replacement therapy (ever/never), breast cancer in first-degree relatives (0, 1, 2+), study (NBSS, OBSP, SMPBC) and observation time (<2 years, 2–4 years, >4 years). [d] Cancers detected within 12 months of the last screening date. [e] Cancers detected 12 months or more after the last screening date

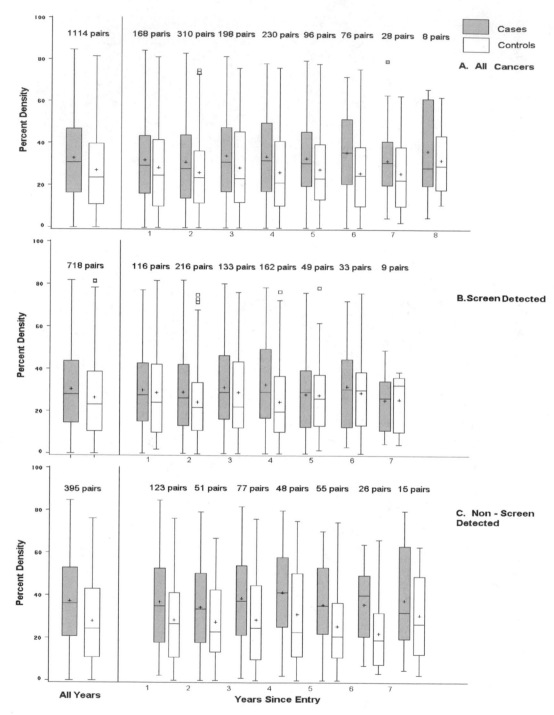

Fig. 15.2. Distribution of percent density, by computer-assisted measure, in the baseline mammogram of cases and controls, according to year of diagnosis of breast cancer and method of detection. Distributions are shown as boxplots, in which the box shows the interquartile range of the data, and the lines extend 1.75 times the length of the box (previously published in New Engl J (15)).

forensic autopsy by Dr. Sue Bartow and colleagues *(20)*, and hence unselected for breast disease, was studied by Li et al. *(21)*. Randomly selected tissue blocks were taken from breast tissue slices obtained by subcutaneous mastectomy, and quantitative microscopy was used to determine the proportions of the biopsy occupied by cells (estimated by nuclear area), glandular structures, and collagen. Percent mammographic density was estimated in the original study by a radiologist in the (Faxitron) x-ray image of the tissue slice from which the biopsy was taken.

Figure 15.3 shows the association between percent density, age and the breast tissue measurements made from histological sections, expressed as a percentage of the total area of the section, and percent mammographic density. Greater percent mammographic density was associated with a significantly greater total nuclear area, a greater nuclear area of both epithelial and non-epithelial cells, a greater proportion of the area of collagen, and a greater area of glandular structures. The area of collagen explained 29% of the variance in percent density, and the other tissue measurements accounted for between 4 and 7% of the variance in percent density. Also, age, body weight, parity and number of births, and menopausal status, all factors that are associated with variations in mammographic density in these and other data (discussed below), were associated with variations in one or more of these tissue features.

These findings suggest that stimuli to breast tissue growth may be in part responsible for the tissue features associated with mammographic density. Growth factors and stromal matrix proteins in breast tissue have been examined in formalin-fixed paraffin blocks of breast tissue (N = 92) surrounding benign lesions, half from breasts with little or no density, and half from breasts with extensive density *(22)*, with the groups matched for age at the time of biopsy. Sections were stained for cell nuclei, total collagen, the stromal matrix regulatory protein, tissue inhibitor of metalloproteinase (TIMP)-3, and the growth factors transforming growth factor (TGF)-α and insulin-like growth factor (IGF)-I, and the area of immunoreactive staining measured using quantitative microscopy. As in the study of Li et al., breast tissue from subjects with extensive densities had a greater nuclear area ($p = 0.007$), as well as larger stained areas of total collagen ($p = 0.003$). In addition, stained areas on immunohistochemistry for TIMP-3 ($p = 0.08$) and IGF-I ($p = 0.02$) were greater in subjects with extensive density. These differences were greater in women aged younger than 50 years.

IGF-I is a known mitogen for breast epithelium that is produced in the breast stroma (as well as by the liver), that is thought to have an important role in mammary carcinogenesis *(12)*. The amount of stromal matrix is determined by the opposing actions of metalloproteinases and their inhibitors, TIMPs. The associations of density with the area of staining for IGF-I and TIMP-3

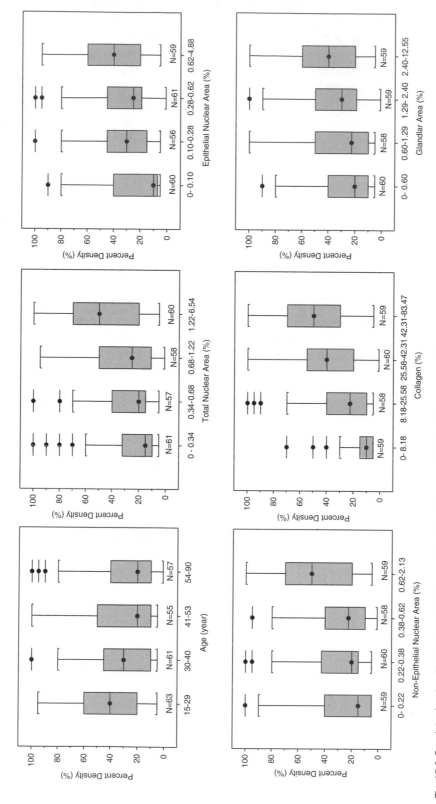

Fig. 15.3. Boxplots showing the associations of percent density with age and histological measures. The median is shown by a *horizontal line*, the interquartile range by the *columns*, 1.5 times the interquartile range by the *whiskers*, and outliers are shown separately. *P* values from linear regression, using continuous variables adjusted for age, were: age ($p = 0.04$); total nuclear area ($p < 0.001$); epithelial nuclear area ($p < 0.001$); non-epithelial nuclear area ($p < 0.001$); collagen ($p < 0.001$), and glandular area ($p < 0.001$) (previously published Cancer Epi Bio Prev – (21)).

may reflect respectively the influence of these factors on cell proliferation and inhibition of matrix degradation.

4. Sources of Variation in Mammographic Density

Detailed descriptions of the associations of risk factors with mammographic density can be found elsewhere *(19, 23, 24)*. The average level of percent mammographic density declines with increasing age, reflecting the age-related differences in breast tissue composition referred to in the previous section. Both absolute and percent mammographic density is less extensive in women who are parous, and in those with a larger number of live births. Postmenopausal women have consistently been found to have less extensive mammographic density than premenopausal women, and a longitudinal study of the effects of the menopause on mammographic density showed that percent density was reduced on average by about 8% over the menopause *(25)*. A family history of breast cancer is associated with more extensive mammographic density, after adjustment for age and other potential influences *(26)*.

In addition to the decline with increasing age, and the effects of parity and menopause referred to above, percent mammographic density has consistently been found to be inversely associated with body weight *(23, 24, 27)*. The association of percent mammographic density is consistent with other data that show leanness to be associated with an increased risk of premenopausal breast cancer, but not with the evidence that obesity is a risk factor for breast cancer after the menopause *(28)*, suggesting that the effect of obesity on risk is not mediated through density.

The effects of body size and percent mammographic density on breast cancer risk have been examined in the nested case–control studies in screening programs referred to above *(29)* by examining the effect of each factor on risk of breast cancer, before and after adjustment for the other *(30)*. In all subjects, before adjustment for mammographic density, breast cancer risk in the highest quintile of body mass index (BMI), compared with the lowest, was 1.04 (95% CI: 0.8–1.4). BMI was associated positively with breast cancer risk in postmenopausal women, and negatively in premenopausal women. After adjustment for density, the risk associated with BMI in all subjects increased to 1.60 (95% CI: 1.27–2013;2.2), and was positive in both menopausal groups. Adjustment for BMI increased breast cancer risk in women with 75% or greater density compared with 0% increased from 4.25 (95% CI: 1.6–11.1) to 5.86 (95% CI: 2.2–15.6). These effects of adjustment on risk are seen because BMI and percent mammographic density are strongly and negatively correlated.

These results show that BMI and percent mammographic density are independent risk factors for breast cancer, and suggest that they are likely to operate through different pathways.

The strong negative correlation between BMI and percent mammographic density will lead to underestimation of the effects on risk of either pathway if confounding is not controlled.

Height has been shown to be positively associated with percent mammographic density (31), and with an increased risk of breast cancer (32).

Blood levels of estradiol and testosterone, either total or free, have not consistently been shown to be associated with percent mammographic density (33–37), suggesting that these hormones may influence risk through pathways that are unrelated to density. Percent mammographic density has been found to be positively associated with serum IGF-I levels in premenopausal women (38–40) in three of five studies (41, 42), and one study found an association in postmenopausal women (43). Results with IGF-binding protein (IGFBP)-3 and the ratio of IGF-I to IGFBP-3 have been inconsistent. Prolactin levels have been found to be positively associated with the area of dense tissue in premenopausal women in one study (39), with percent mammographic density in postmenopausal women in two studies (37, 39), and, in a further study, statistical significance was lost after adjustment for other variables (34). Both IGF-I and prolactin levels are influenced by age, parity, and number of births in a manner similar to the way these factors are associated with mammographic density (44, 45).

5. Heritability

The factors described above that influence percent mammographic density account for only 20–30% of the variation observed in the population (24). Early suggestions that genetic factors might explain a proportion of variation (i.e., the heritability) of percent mammographic density came from relatively small studies of mother–daughter sets (46) and twins (47).

To determine the proportions of the variances in mammographic density measures that could be explained by genetic factors, we carried out two independent twin studies (48). Within a twin pair, monozygous twins share all of their genes, while dizygous twins share on average half of their genes. Differences in a trait between monozygous twins are thus due to environmental factors (and measurement error), and differences between dizygous twins may be due either to genetic or environmental factors (and measurement error). The classic twin model makes the critical assumption that the degree of environmental influence on a trait of interest, both within and between twin pairs, is the same for monozygous and dizygous pairs. Given these assumptions, a difference in the correlation for a trait between monozygous and dizygous twin pairs is consistent with the existence of one or more genetic factors that influence variation in the trait.

Twin pairs aged 40–70 years and living in Australia or North America were recruited, and information was collected using the same questionnaires on the factors known to be associated with variations in mammographic density. Mammograms from each member of each twin pair were digitized and measured using the computer-assisted method shown above, by one observer, blinded to zygosity and twin pairing. The results of these twin studies are shown in **Tables 15.2** and **15.3**.

After adjustment for age, age at menarche, parity, number of live births, menopausal status, and BMI, the variances in percent density, shown in **Table 15.2**, were almost identical in both

Table 15.2
Estimates of residual variance, correlations between monozygotic pairs of twins and dizygotic pairs of twins, and heritability of the percentage of dense tissue, adjusted for age and other covariates (previously published in New Engl J (our ref 48))

Variable	Australia	North America	Combined studies
Residual variance (σ^2)	306.40 ± 13.97	306.00 ± 18.61	310.00 ± 11.33
Correlation coefficient for monozygotic pairs	0.61 ± 0.03	0.67 ± 0.03	0.63 ± 0.02
Correlation coefficient for dizygotic pairs	0.25 ± 0.06	0.27 ± 0.08	0.27 ± 0.05
Heritability	0.60 ± 0.03	0.67 ± 0.04	0.63 ± 0.02

Plus-minus values are estimate ± standard error. The mean percentage of dense tissue was adjusted for age, BMI, age at menarche, cessation or continuation of menstruation, parity, and in parous women, number of live births and age at first birth. The symbol σ^2 denotes the residual variance, in units of the square of the percentage of dense tissue

Table 15.3
Estimates (standard error) of the cross-trait correlation between dense and nondense area in the same individual and the cross-trait cross-twin correlation between dense area in one twin and nondense area in the other twin

Bivariate model: log dense and log nondense	Correlation in same individual	Cross-correlation between individuals	
		Monozygous pairs	Dizygous pairs
Mean adjusted for age	–0.35 (0.023)	–0.26 (0.026)	–0.14 (0.034)
Mean adjusted for age and covariates	–0.31 (0.023)	–0.20 (0.027)	–0.08 (0.036)

samples. The correlations between twin pairs in percent mammographic density in Australia and North America, shown in Table 2, were, respectively, 0.61 (s.e.= 0.03) and 0.67 (0.03) for monozygotic twin pairs, and 0.25 (0.06) and 0.27 (0.08) for dizygotic twin pairs, and 0.25 (standard error = 0.06) and 0.27 (standard error = 0.08) for dizygotic twin pairs. These data thus provide an almost exact replication of evidence that is consistent with a strong genetic influence on the population variance of "age and covariate adjusted percent mammographic density," which is the risk factor for breast cancer.

The classic twin model also assumes that variance for a given population can be partitioned into three components representing unmeasured effects, namely additive genetic effects, the effects of environmental factors that are shared by or common to twin pairs, and individual specific environmental effects that include measurement error.

Analysis of the components of variance showed that the best-fitting model included only components for the additive genetic factors, and person-specific environmental factors. The proportion of the residual variation accounted for by additive genetic factors (heritability) was estimated to be 60% (95% CI: 54–66%) from Australian twins, 67% (95% CI: 59–75%) from North American twins, and 63% (95% CI: 59–67%) when the studies were combined (48).

The dense and nondense areas of the mammogram each showed evidence of heritability that was similar in magnitude to that found above for percent mammographic density (49). After adjusting for measured determinants, the estimates of heritability as shown in **Table 15.3** were 65% (95% CI: 60–70%) for the dense area and 66% (95% CI: 61–71%) for the nondense area. **Table 15.3** also shows the correlations of measured dense and nondense areas within the same individual, and between individuals in each twin pair. The correlations (and standard errors) between the two adjusted traits were –0.35 (0.023) in the same individual, –0.26 (0.026) across monozygotic pairs, and –0.14 (0.034) across dizygotic pairs. About two thirds of the negative correlation between age- and covariate-adjusted dense and nondense areas is explained by the same genetic factors influencing both traits, but in opposite directions. Genetic factors thus appear to play a large role in explaining variation not only in percent mammographic density as a whole, but also in its components, the areas of dense and nondense tissue.

Many of the factors associated with differences in mammographic density, including age at menarche and menopause, and BMI, are known to be at least in part heritable, but the estimates of heritability given for mammographic density were generated after adjusting for the effects of these factors. Heritability, however, refers to explaining the variation within a population, and both twin studies were carried out in populations that are predominately European in origin and living in "Western" environments, so our findings do not exclude the possibility of a greater influence of environmental factors at levels of exposure that lie outside the range usually seen in Western societies.

It is unknown whether, as with other quantitative traits, multiple genes determine mammographic density variation at a given age or, as recent work suggests, that the inheritance of variants in one or more major genes may be responsible (a major gene is defined here to mean a gene for which there are mutations associated with a large effect on an individual's trait, even though it may be rare for an individual to have a mutation). A segregation analysis of nuclear family data by Pankow et al. suggested a single mode of inheritance of effect associated with one or more major genes, but could not distinguish between dominant, recessive, or co-dominant models *(50)*.

The search for genes associated with mammographic density is in its infancy, and few have been found to date and replications are rare. The preliminary results from one genome-wide sibling-pair linkage study showed evidence for linkage at a region on chromosome 6 *(51)*. In the association studies of candidate genes carried out to date, variants in genes concerned with estrogen metabolism *(52–55)*, the estrogen *(56)* and androgen receptors *(57)*, IGFBP-3 *(58)*, IGF *(59)*, growth hormone *(60)*, and *IISD3B1 (54, 61)* have been found to show at least some evidence for being associated with mammographic density. To date, few of these findings have been replicated *(54, 61)*, and some that have been replicated *(52, 53)* have also been contradicted *(54, 55, 61)*. Several large-scale genome-wide linkage and association studies of candidate genes are in progress and can be expected to report their findings within the next few years.

6. Summary and Conclusions

There is now extensive evidence that percent mammographic density is a risk factor for breast cancer, independent of other risk factors, and associated with large relative and attributable risks for the disease. Percent mammographic density reflects variations in the tissue composition of the breast, and is positively associated with collagen and epithelial and non-epithelial cells and negatively associated with fat. Mammographic density has wide variation across the population, even for women of the same age, and is associated with a substantial gradient of risk. Extensive mammographic density is relatively common, and estimates of the associated attributable risk suggest that about a third of breast cancer is attributable to (in an epidemiological sense) to density in more than 50% of the breast compared to little or no density in women aged less than 56 (15). Current estimates of risk are however based on two-dimensional measurement of the mammogram, rather than tissue volumes, and they may underestimate the true underlying risk gradient.

All risk factors for breast cancer must ultimately exert their influence by an effect on the breast and these findings suggest that, for at least some risk factors, this influence includes an effect on the number of cells and the quantity of collagen in the breast that is reflected in differences in percent mammographic density.

The hypothesis that we have developed from the observations described above is discussed elsewhere (63) and illustrated in **Fig. 15.4**. We postulate that many of the genetic and environmental factors that influence risk of breast cancer affect the proliferative activity and quantity of stromal and epithelial tissue in the breast, and that these effects are reflected in differences in mammographic density among women of the same age. The evidence cited above shows that the environmental influences include menstrual and reproductive factors, as well as anthropometric variables, but these factors explain only 20–30% of the variance in percent density. The two twin studies show that most of the remaining variance after adjusting for these factors is explained by as yet unidentified genetic factors.

We propose that these inherited and environmental factors influence breast tissue composition, at least in part, through effects on the levels of exposure to hormones and growth factors that are mitogens in the breast, and include IGF-I and prolactin, resulting in greater proliferative activity and greater quantities of stromal and epithelial tissue. Greater quantities of

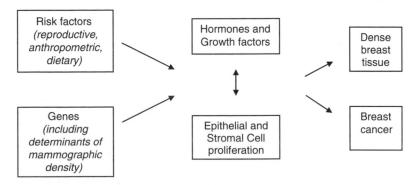

Fig. 15.4. Summary of biological hypotheses. It is postulated that the combined effects of cell proliferation (mitogenesis), and genetic damage to proliferating cells by mutagens (mutagenesis), may underlie the increased risk of breast cancer associated with extensive mammographic density (63).

cells, together with greater proliferative activity, are associated with an increase in susceptibility to mutagens, and an increased risk of breast cancer.

As noted above, the quantity of stromal and epithelial tissue is reflected by the dense area of the mammogram. While it has been shown that the dense area is also related to risk of breast cancer, percent density appears to be the stronger risk factor *(8, 14)*. The nondense area in the mammogram, which reflects fat, may also provide information about risk, and most risk factors for breast cancer that influence mammographic density have opposite effects on the dense and nondense areas of the mammogram *(62)*. Genetic factors appear to play a large role in explaining variation in the mammographic areas of both dense and nondense tissue, and about two thirds of the negative correlation between dense and nondense area is explained by the same genetic factors influencing both traits, but in opposite directions.

Whether percent mammographic density is the optimal method of combining the information about risk that is contained in the measured dense and nondense components of the mammographic image remains to be determined.

As described, mammographic density is highly heritable, and thus meets criteria for an intermediate phenotype. Mammographic density is a continuous trait, with a wide unimodal and approximately normal distribution and is thus likely to be influenced by multiple genes. The genetic variants that influence the tissue composition of the breast are therefore likely individually to have modest effects on risk of breast cancer, but their combined effects could be substantial. Perhaps more importantly, finding the genes involved in mammographic density measures may lead to new insights into the biological and etiological pathways that underpin this biomarker and help to explain why it is such a strong risk factor for breast cancer.

References

1. Muir C, Waterhouse T, Mack J, Powell S, Whelan S. Cancer Incidence in Five Continents. Volume VI ed. IARC Scientific Publication, 1992.

2. Pharoah PD, Antoniou AC, Bobrow M, Zimmern RL, Easton D, Ponder AJ. Polygenic susceptibility of breast cancer and implications for prevention. Nat Genet 2002; 31(1):33–36.

3. Malone KE, Daling JR, Thompson JD, O'Brien CA, Francisco LV, Ostrander EA. BRCA1 mutations and breast cancer in the general population. JAMA 1998; 279(12):922–929.

4. Newman B, Mu H, Butler LM, Millikan R, Moorman PG, King M-C. Frequency of breast cancer attributable to BRCA1 in a population-based series of American women. JAMA 1998; 279(12): 915–921.

5. Peto J, Collin N, Barfoot R, et al. Prevalence of BRCA1 and BRCA2 gene mutations in patients with early-onset breast cancer. J Natl Cancer Inst 2001; 91(11):943–949.

6. Dite GS, Jenkins MA, Southey MC, et al. Familial risks, early-onset breast cancer, and BRCA1 and BRCA2 germline mutations. J Natl Cancer Inst 2003; 95(6):448–457.

7. Boyd NF, Byng JW, Jong RA, et al. Quantitative classification of mammographic densities and breast cancer risk: Results from the Canadian National Breast Screening Study. J Natl Cancer Inst 1995; 87(9):670–675.

8. Byrne C, Schairer C, Wolfe J, et al. Mammographic features and breast cancer risk: Effects with time, age, and menopause status. J Natl Cancer Inst 1995; 87(21):1622–1629.

9. Wolfe JN. Risk for breast cancer development determined by mammographic parenchymal pattern. Cancer 1976; 37(5):2486–2492.

10. Wolfe JN. Breast patterns as an index of risk for developing breast cancer. Am J Roentgenol 1976; 126(6):1130–1139.

11. Kerlikowske K, Grady D, Barclay J, et al. Variability and accuracy in mammographic interpretation using the American college of radiology breast imaging reporting and data system. J Natl Cancer Inst 1998; 90(23):1801–1809.

12. Gram IT, Funkhouser E, Tabar L. The Tabar classification of mammographic parenchymal patterns. Eur J Radiol 1997; 24(2):131–136.

13. McCormack VA, dos Santos Silva I. Breast density and parenchymal patterns as markers of breast cancer risk: A meta-analysis. Cancer Epidemiol Biomarkers Prev 2006; 15(6):1159–1169.

14. Ursin G, Wu AH, Bernstein L, et al. Mammographic density and breast cancer in three ethnic groups. Cancer Epidemiol Biomarkers Prev 2003; 12(4):332–338.

15. Boyd NF, Guo H, Martin LJ, et al. Mammographic density and the risk and detection of breast cancer. N Engl J Med 2007; 356(3):227–236.

16. Byrne C, Schairer C, Wolfe J, et al. Mammographic features and breast cancer risk: Effects with time, age, and menopause status. J Natl Cancer Inst 1995; 87(21):1622–1629.

17. Torres-Mejia G, De Stavola B, Allen D, et al. Mammographic features and subsequent risk of breast cancer: A comparison of qualitative and quantitative evaluations in the Guernsey prospective studies. Cancer Epidemiol Biomarkers Prev 2005; 14(5):1052–1059.

18. Pisano ED, Gatsonis C, Hendrick E, et al. Diagnostic performance of digital versus film mammography for breast-cancer screening. N Engl J Med 2005; 353(17):1773–1783.

19. Boyd NF, Lockwood GA, Byng J, Tritchler DL, Yaffe M. Mammographic densities and breast cancer risk. Cancer Epidemiol Biomarkers Prev 1998; 7(12):1133–1144.

20. Bartow SA, Mettler FA Jr, Black WC III. Correlations between radiographic patterns and morphology of the female breast. Rad Patterns Morph 1997; 13:263–275.

21. Li T, Sun L, Miller N, et al. The association of measured breast tissue characteristics with mammographic density and other risk factors for breast cancer. Cancer Epidemiol Biomarkers Prev 2005; 14(2):343–349.

22. Guo YP, Martin LJ, Hanna W, et al. Growth factors and stromal matrix proteins associated with mammographic densities. Cancer Epidemiol Biomarkers Prev 2001; 10(3):243–248.

23. Grove JS, Goodman MJ, Gilbert F, Mi MP. Factors associated with mammographic pattern. Br J Radiol 1985; 58(685):21–25.

24. Vachon CM, Kuni CC, Anderson K. Association of mammographically defined percent breast density with epidemiologic risk factors for breast cancer (United States). Cancer Causes Control 2000; 11(7):653–662.

25. Boyd N, Martin L, Stone J, Little L, Minkin S, Yaffe M. A longitudinal study of the effects of menopause on mammographic features. Cancer Epidemiol Biomarkers Prev 2002; 11(10 Pt 1):1048–1053.

26. Ziv E, Shepherd J, Smith-Bindman R, Kerlikowske K. Mammographic breast density and family history of breast cancer. J Natl Cancer Inst 2005; 95(7):556–558.

27. Bartow SA, Pathak DR, Mettler FA, Key CR, Pike MC. Breast mammographic pattern: A concatenation of confounding and breast cancer risk factors. Am J Epidemiol 1995; 142(8):813–819.

28. Trentham-Dietz A, Newcomb PA, Storer BE, et al. Body size and risk of breast cancer. Am J Epidemiol 1997; 145(11):1011–1019.

29. Boyd NF, Guo H, Martin LJ, et al. Mammographic density and the risk and detection of breast cancer. N Engl J Med 2007; 356(3):227–236.

30. Boyd NF, Martin LJ, Sun L, et al. Body size, mammographic density and breast cancer risk. Cancer Epidemiol Biomarkers Prev 2006; 15(11):2086–2092.

31. Brisson J, Morrison AS, Kopans DB. Height and weight, mammographic features of breast tissue, and breast cancer risk. Am J Epidemiol 1984; 119(3):371–381.

32. Hunter DJ, Willett WC. Diet, body size, and breast cancer. Epidemiol Rev 1993; 15(1):110–132.

33. Noh JJ, Maskarinec G, Pagano I, Cheung LW, Stanczyk FZ. Mammographic densities

and circulating hormones: A cross-sectional study in premenopausal women. Breast 2006; 15(1):20–28.

34. Tamimi RM, Hankinson SE, Colditz GA, Byrne C. Endogenous sex hormone levels and mammographic density among postmenopausal women. Cancer Epidemiol Biomarkers Prev 2005; 14(11 (Pt 1)):2641–2647.

35. Aiello EJ, Tworoger SS, Yasui Y, et al. Associations among circulating sex hormones, insulin-like growth factor, lipids, and mammographic density in postmenopausal women. Cancer Epidemiol Biomarkers Prev 2005; 14(6):1411–1417.

36. Warren R, Skinner J, Sala E, et al. Associations among mammographic density, circulating sex hormones, and polymorphisms in sex hormone metabolism genes in postmenopausal women. Cancer Epidemiol Biomarkers Prev 2006; 15(8):1502–1508.

37. Greendale GA, Palla SL, Ursin G, et al. The association of endogenous sex steroids and sex steroid binding proteins with mammographic density: results from the Postmenopausal Estrogen/Progestin Interventions Mammographic Density Study. Am J Epidemiol 2005; 162(9):826–834.

38. Byrne C, Colditz GA, Pollak M, Willet WC, Speizer FE, Hankinson SE. Plasma insulin-like growth factor-I, insulin-like growth factor binding protein-3 and mammographic density. Cancer Res 2000; 60(14):3744–3748.

39. Boyd NF, Stone J, Martin LJ, et al. The association of breast mitogens with mammographic densities. Br J Cancer 2002; 87(8):876–882.

40. Diorio C, Pollak M, Byrne C, et al. Insulin-like growth factor-I, IGF-binding protein-3, and mammographic breast density. Cancer Epidemiol Biomarkers Prev 2005; 14(5):1065–1073.

41. Maskarinec G, Williams AE, Kaaks R. A cross-sectional investigation of breast density and insulin-like growth factor I. Int J Cancer 2003; 107(6):991–996.

42. dos Santos Silva I, Johnson N, De Stavola B, et al. The insulin-like growth factor system and mammographic features in premenopausal and postmenopausal women. Cancer Epidemiol Biomarkers Prev 2006; 15(3):449–455.

43. Bremnes Y, Ursin G, Bjurstam N, Rinaldi S, Kaaks R, Gram IT. Insulin-like growth factor and mammographic density in postmenopausal Norwegian women. Cancer Epidemiol Biomarkers Prev 2007; 16(1):57–62.

44. Holmes MD, Pollak MN, Hankinson SE. Lifestyle correlates of plasma insulin-like growth factor I and insulin-like growth factor binding protein 3 concentrations. Cancer Epidemiol Biomarkers Prev 2002; 11(9):862–867.

45. Eliassen AH, Tworoger SS, Hankinson SE. Reproductive factors and family history of breast cancer in relation to plasma prolactin levels in premenopausal and postmenopausal women. Int J Cancer 2007; 120(7):1536–1541.

46. Wolfe JN, Albert S, Belle S, Salane M. Familial influences on breast parenchymal patterns. Cancer 1980; 46(11):2433–2437.

47. Kaprio J, Alanko A, Kivisaari L. Mammographic patterns in twin pairs discordant for breast cancer. Br J Radiol 1987; 60(713):459–462.

48. Boyd NF, Dite GS, Stone J, et al. Heritability of mammographic density, a risk factor for breast cancer. N Engl J Med 2002; 347(12):886–894.

49. Stone J, Dite GS, Gunasekara A, et al. The heritability of mammographically dense and nondense breast tissue. Cancer Epidemiol Biomarkers Prev 2006; 15(4):612–617.

50. Pankow JS, Vachon CM, Kuni CC, et al. Genetic analysis of mammographic breast density in adult women: evidence of a gene effect. J Natl Cancer Inst 1997; 89(8):549–556.

51. Vachon CM, King RA, Atwood LD, Kuni CC, Sellers TA. Preliminary sibpair linkage analysis of percent mammographic density. J Natl Cancer Inst 1999; 91(20):1778–1779.

52. Hong C-C, Thompson HJ, Jiang C, et al. Val158Met Polymorphism in catechol-O-methyltransferase (COMT) gene associated with risk factors for breast cancer. Cancer Epidemiol Biomarkers Prev 2003; 12(9):838–847.

53. Maskarinec G, Luire G, Williams AE, Marchand L. An investigation of mammographic density and gene variants in healthy women. Int J Cancer 2004; 112(4):683–688.

54. Haiman CA, Bernstein L, Berg D, Ingles SA, Salane M, Ursin G. Genetic determinants of mammographic density. Breast Cancer Res 2002; 4(3):R5.

55. Haiman CA, Hankinson SE, De Vivo I, et al. Polymorphisms in steroid hormone pathway genes and mammographic density. Breast Cancer Research and Treatment 2003; 77(1):27–36.

56. Van Duijnhoven FJ, Bezemer ID, Peeters PH, et al. Polymorphisms in the estrogen receptor alpha gene and mammographic

density. Cancer Epidemiol Biomarkers Prev 2005; 14(11 Pt 1):2655–2660.

57. Lillie EO, Bernstein L, Ingles SA, et al. Polymorphism in the androgen receptor and mammographic density in women taking and not taking estrogen and progestin therapy. Cancer Res 2004; 64(4):1237–1241.

58. Lai JH, Vesprini D, Zhang W, Yaffe MJ, Pollak M, Narod SA. A polymorphic locus in the promoter region of the IGFBP3 gene is related to mammographic breast density. Cancer Epidemiol Biomarkers Prev 2004; 13(4):573–582.

59. Tamimi RM, Cox DG, Kraft P, et al. Common genetic variation in IGF1, IGFBP-1, and IGFBP-3 in relation to mammographic density: a cross-sectional study. Breast Cancer Res 2007; 9(1):R18.

60. Mulhall C, Hegele R, Cao H, Tritchler D, Yaffe M, Boyd NF. Mammographic density and the pituitary growth hormone and growth hormone releasing hormone receptor genes. Cancer Epidemiol Biomarkers Prev 2005; 14(11 Pt 1):2648–2654.

61. Stone J., Gurrin LC, Byrnes GB, et al. Mammographic density and candidate gene variants: a twins and sisters study. Cancer Epidemiol Biomarkers Prev 2007; 16(7):1479–1484.

62. Heng D, Gao F, Jong R, et al. Risk factors for breast cancer associated with mammographic features in Singaporean Chinese women. Cancer Epidemiol Biomarkers Prev 2004; 13(11 Pt 1):1751–1758.

63. Martin LJ, Boyd N. Potential mechanisms of breast cancer risk associated with mammographic density: hypotheses based on epidemiological evidence. Breast Cancer Res 2008; 10:1–14.

Chapter 16

Acquired Risk Factors for Colorectal Cancer

Otto S. Lin

Abstract

The risk of developing colorectal cancer (CRC) is influenced by several acquired risk factors, including environmental exposures and comorbid medical conditions that are partially genetic in nature. These risk factors are based on data almost exclusively derived from observational studies. Because of the possibility of bias due to confounding, these acquired risk factors should not be automatically assumed to be causative, and in fact some may not be truly independent risk factors. Acquired risk factors include the following categories: 1) dietary factors, 2) lifestyle factors, 3) side-effects of medical interventions, and 4) comorbid medical conditions.

Dietary factors that potentially increase the risk of CRC include low fruit, vegetable, or fiber intake, high red meat or saturated fat consumption, and exposure to caffeine or alcohol. Of these factors, the significance of low fruit, vegetable, and fiber intake has been called into question because of contradictory results from large observational studies and negative results from randomized trials. The association of high red meat or saturated fat consumption with increased CRC risk is supported by the preponderance of observational data. Lifestyle factors include lack of exercise and smoking. These risk factors are supported by observational data of moderate quality.

Medical interventions that may increase the risk of CRC include pelvic irradiation, cholecystectomy, and ureterocolic anastomosis after major surgery of the urinary and intestinal tracts. Aside from cholecystectomy, these risk factors are supported by observational data from small studies only, therefore their validity is not well established.

Finally, comorbid medical conditions that are associated with increased risk of CRC include Barrett's esophagus, human immunodeficiency virus infection, acromegaly, and inflammatory bowel disease. The association between inflammatory bowel disease and CRC is well established and it forms the basis for widely adopted colonoscopic surveillance recommendations from national medical organizations. The other factors are supported by limited observational data only and are still controversial.

Key words: Colorectal cancer, adenoma, risk factors, fiber, inflammatory bowel disease, surveillance.

M. Verma (ed.), *Methods of Molecular Biology, Cancer Epidemiology, vol. 472*
© 2009 Humana Press, a part of Springer Science+Business Media, Totowa, NJ
Book doi: 10.1007/978-1-60327-492-0

1. Introduction

The risk of developing colorectal cancer (CRC) is influenced by both environmental and genetic factors. This chapter reviews acquired risk factors, including environmental exposures and comorbid medical conditions that are associated with CRC. Genetic factors such as family history or genetic cancer syndromes (e.g., familial adenomatous polyposis) will not be discussed; however, we will cover some medical conditions associated with an increased the risk for CRC that may be partially genetic in nature (e.g., diabetes and inflammatory bowel disease [IBD]). Acquired risk factors are divided into the following categories: 1) dietary factors, 2) lifestyle factors, 3) side-effects of medical interventions, and 4) comorbid medical conditions.

2. Dietary Factors

2.1. Fruit, Vegetable, and Fiber Intake

Several epidemiologic studies have shown an association between a diet low in fruits and vegetables and increased risk of CRC (1, 2). It is hypothesized that the fiber, antioxidant vitamin, folic acid, micronutrient, or phytochemical (flavone) content in vegetables and fruits may exert a protective effect. The relative risk of CRC is approximately 0.5 when we compare groups with the highest vegetable and fruit intake to those with the lowest (2). Furthermore, some observational studies have noted an inverse relationship between dietary fiber consumption and risk of colorectal adenomas and/or CRC (3–6).

On the other hand, some studies have not shown this association. In an analysis that combined data from the Nurses Health Study (88,764 female subjects) and the Health Professionals Follow-up Study (47,325 male subjects), there was no significant association between the intake of fruits or vegetables and the incidence of CRC (7). Another study looking at data only from the Nurses Health Study also found no relationship between fiber intake and the risk of CRC or colorectal adenoma (8). Moreover, two large randomized controlled studies in the USA concluded that fiber supplementation had no significant protective effect against the development of metachronous adenomas in patients who had undergone colonoscopic polypectomy (9, 10). More recently, the Women's Health Initiative Trial also found no protective effect of a low fat, high fiber and high fruit and vegetable content diet against CRC development (11). Formal meta-analyses have corroborated these findings. For example, a Cochrane systematic review of five studies concluded that increased dietary fiber did not appear to reduce the incidence or recurrence of colorectal adenoma over a 4-year period *(12)*. Similarly, a meta-analysis of 13 prospective cohort studies found that dietary fiber intake was not an independent risk factor for CRC *(13)*. The reasons for the discrepancies among the available studies are unclear. At present, the degree of protection from the consumption of vegetables, fruits, or dietary fiber remains unsettled.

2.2. Red Meat and Saturated Fat Intake

Some studies have suggested that a diet high in red meat, animal fat, or cholesterol content may be associated with CRC development, especially in the left colon *(14–19)*. In one study, subjects in the highest quartile of cholesterol consumption had a significantly higher risk of CRC compared with subjects in the lowest quartile (relative risk of 3.26), even after adjusting for other variables such as fruit and vegetable intake *(15)*. Most studies have not shown a similarly increased risk for poultry meat. However, it should be noted that there are also some studies that have failed to find a significant relationship between red meat intake and CRC *(20)*. Although the data are not completely consistent, the bulk of the available evidence supports the view that red meat consumption is associated with an increased risk of CRC, as shown by a systematic review *(21)*.

2.3. Alcohol

An association between heavy alcohol consumption and increased risk of CRC has been reported in several observational studies *(22, 23)* as well as meta-analyses *(24)*. As with most epidemiologic associations, there were contradicting data as well *(25, 26)*. A pooled analysis of eight cohort studies estimated that the CRC risk was increased slightly (relative risk of 1.41) in those whose alcohol consumption exceeded 45 g/day *(27)*. The risk was increased to a lesser degree in those with alcohol consumption between 30 to 45 g/day. This phenomenon may be the result of decreased folate absorption and intake in alcoholic patients *(28, 29)*.

2.4. Caffeine

The relationship between caffeine consumption and CRC is unresolved. Although a link between low rates of coffee consumption and an elevated risk of CRC was reported in a meta-analysis of 12 case–control studies *(30)*, data from the Nurses Health Study and the Health Professionals Follow-up Study did not support this *(7)*.

3. Lifestyle Factors

3.1. Physical Activity

Observational data suggest that inadequate regular physical activity is associated with increased risk of CRC, an effect that may interact with high energy intake, obesity, and the metabolic syndrome *(31–33)*.

In one study, sedentary workers had a significantly increased risk of CRC compared with those engaged in light or heavy physical activity *(34)*. The mechanism for the apparent protective effect of physical activity is not known.

3.2. Cigarette Smoking   Smoking has been associated with increased CRC incidence and mortality in some studies *(35–37)*.

4. Previous Medical Interventions

4.1. Pelvic Irradiation   Previous exposure to pelvic radiation may be associated with a higher risk of CRC after a 5- to 10-year lag period *(38)*. A history of radiation therapy for prostate cancer correlated with an increased risk of rectal cancer in a large retrospective study *(39)*. The magnitude of risk was similar to that observed in patients with a family history of colorectal neoplasia, suggesting that tighter surveillance may be appropriate. However, whether such increased screening would improve CRC outcomes and prognosis is unclear.

4.2. Cholecystectomy   A relationship between cholecystectomy and right-sided colon cancer has been described in some reports. Patients who had undergone cholecystectomy demonstrated a slightly increased risk of right-sided colon cancer (with a standardized incidence ratio of 1.16) but not left-sided cancer *(40)*. However, discordant data have also been published *(41, 42)*. Although publication bias needs to be kept in mind, the results of meta-analyses have in general supported this association with proximal colon cancers *(43, 44)*.

4.3. Ureterocolic Anastomosis   A few studies have reported an apparently increased risk of colorectal neoplasia near ureterocolic anastomoses after major surgery of the urinary or intestinal tract *(45, 46)*. The presumed mechanism is exposure of colonic mucosa to carcinogenic substances from the urinary system.

5. Concurrent Medical Conditions

5.1. Barrett's Esophagus   An association between CRC and Barrett's esophagus has been proposed *(47–49)*, but conflicting data are also available *(50–55)*. Pooling of data in formal meta-analysis has supported the increased risk of CRC in patients with Barrett's esophagus *(56)*.

This apparent association may be due to bias and confounding because patients with Barrett's esophagus and CRC share many risk factors.

5.2. Human Immunodeficiency Virus Infection

Some studies have shown an increase in the incidence of colorectal neoplasia in patients infected with the human immunodeficiency virus *(57)*. This is thought to be a result of increased susceptibility to carcinogenesis due to chronic immunosuppression.

5.3. Diabetes Mellitus

Diabetes mellitus may be associated with an elevated risk of CRC *(33, 58–60)*. A meta-analysis of 15 studies found a significantly increased risk of CRC in diabetic patients compared with nondiabetic control subjects (relative risk of 1.30) *(61)*. One possible explanation linking diabetes to CRC is hyperinsulinemia because insulin and insulin-like growth factor are important growth factors for colonic mucosal cells and stimulate colonic neoplastic cells *(62)*. A relationship between serum levels of C-peptide, an indicator of insulin production, and CRC risk was reported from the Physicians' Health Study *(63)*. Chronic insulin therapy may also increase the risk of CRC in diabetic individuals. A case–control study estimated that the age- and sex-adjusted risk of CRC associated with more than 1 year of insulin use was 2.1 *(64)*.

5.4. Acromegaly

There is some evidence that colorectal adenomas occur with increased frequency in acromegalic patients *(65, 66)*. A prospective controlled study found that adenomatous polyps occurred in 22% of male acromegalic patients compared with 8% of control subjects *(65)*. Patients with acromegaly were more likely to have multiple and proximal adenomas. Reduced expression of the peroxisome proliferator-activated receptor gene has been implicated in such patients.

5.5. Inflammatory Bowel Disease

Patients with chronic IBD involving the colon are at significantly increased risk for CRC *(67, 68)*, and special colonoscopic surveillance measures are recommended for such individuals *(69–71)*.

In ulcerative colitis (UC), the risk of CRC depends on the duration and extent of disease. The risk is highest in those with extensive colitis or "pancolitis," with a standardized incidence ratio of 2.4 according to a population-based study in the USA *(72)*. Compared with age-matched controls, the risk begins to increase 8–10 years following the onset of UC symptoms *(73)*. Overall, the approximate cumulative incidence of CRC is 5–10% after 20 years, 12–20% after 30 years, and 30% after 35 years of UC *(67, 73)*. However, in a Danish study, the risk of CRC in patients with long-standing UC was not different from that of the general population, a finding that may be a reflection of the more aggressive surgical approach in Europe toward patients poorly responsive to medical treatment *(74)*. It is believed that the risk of CRC increases after 15–20 years (approximately 10 years later than in pancolitis) in patients with left-sided colitis distal to the splenic flexure *(75)*. However, some studies on patients with left-sided colitis have described rates of CRC similar to those seen in patients with pancolitis *(76)*. Most authorities agree that patients with limited ulcerative proctitis are not at increased risk for CRC, and therefore do not require special surveillance *(77)*.

Several factors may influence the risk of CRC in IBD patients. For example, the risk is increased in those with early onset of disease (prior to age 15 years). One study reported that "backwash ileitis" was an independent risk factor for CRC *(78)*, but subsequent studies have not confirmed this association *(79, 80)*. The severity of inflammation may also be an important marker of CRC risk, as suggested by case–control studies *(79)*. A meta-analysis concluded that there is an increased risk of CRC in patients with UC complicated by primary sclerosing cholangitis (PSC), when compared with UC patients without PSC *(81)*. In patients with PSC and UC, the colon cancer was more likely to occur in the proximal colon, suggesting a possible carcinogenic role of bile acids.

Earlier reports found no increased risk of CRC in patients with Crohn's disease (CD), but these did not adjust for disease duration and extent. More recent studies have reported that the risk of CRC in long-standing CD involving the colon is probably comparable to that of UC *(68, 82–84)*. In a population-based study from Sweden, the relative risk of CRC was 5.6 in CD patients with disease restricted to the colon *(68)*. Increased risk of CRC in CD patients has been reported in other studies *(85, 86)*. CRC in CD develops over a similar time frame as in UC *(87, 88)*. The median duration of disease prior to the diagnosis of CRC was comparable for CD and UC (15 and 18 years, respectively); however, the median age at diagnosis of CRC was somewhat older in CD (55 years) than in UC (43 years).

The mean age of onset for IBD-associated CRC is lower than that for sporadic CRC (45 versus 60 years). Unlike CRC associated with CD, which is evenly distributed between the right and left colon, CRC associated with UC is more common in the rectum and sigmoid colon *(87)*. Synchronous tumors are much more common in patients with IBD than in those with sporadic CRC. Furthermore, poorly differentiated, anaplastic, and mucinous carcinomas are more common in IBD-associated CRC. Despite this, there are conflicting data as to whether patients with IBD-associated CRC have a worse prognosis compared with patients with sporadic CRC *(89, 90)*. Interestingly, some studies suggest that the prognosis for IBD-associated CRC is similar to (or better than) that for sporadic CRC when matched for stage *(91, 92)*.

Although no large randomized controlled trials have proven that intensive colonoscopic surveillance reduces mortality, surveillance is widely practiced and recommended by guidelines from various societies *(69–71)*. For UC, it is generally recommended that colonoscopic surveillance should begin after 8 years in patients with pancolitis, and after 15 years in patients with colitis involving the left colon. Colonoscopy should be repeated every 1 to 2 years. Two to four random colonic biopsy specimens every 10 cm should be taken with additional samples of suspicious areas. Patients with PSC (including those who have undergone orthotopic liver transplant) may need more frequent colonoscopy. For CD involving substantial areas of the colon, the UC surveillance strategy discussed above also applies, according to most guidelines.

It is generally accepted that CRC in IBD is preceded by dysplastic changes. Thus, dysplasia may be a marker for coexisting and subsequent malignancy. This hypothesis serves as the rationale for colonoscopic surveillance. There is agreement that the finding of high-grade dysplasia warrants prompt colectomy because of the high risk of synchronous CRC. The approach to low-grade dysplasia seen in random colonic biopsies is more controversial, although some institutions currently also recommend colectomy for patients with definite low-grade dysplasia confirmed by at least two expert pathologists *(93)*. This is justified by the high rate of progression from low-grade to high-grade dysplasia or CRC, estimated to be 53% at 5 years *(94)*. However, other studies have not shown such a high rate of progression *(95–97)*. IBD patients who have dysplasia associated with a lesion or mass (DALM) are also at high risk for CRC and may benefit from prophylactic colectomy *(98, 99)*. Whereas non-adenoma-like DALMs are an indication for colectomy, sporadic adenomas may be removed endoscopically with close follow-up. As mentioned above, there have been no randomized trials showing a direct mortality benefit from surveillance. However, there is evidence from retrospective studies that cancers tend to be detected at earlier stages during surveillance and that IBD patients diagnosed with CRC after they developed symptoms had worse prognosis than those detected during surveillance *(100, 101)*. Also, a case–control study found that the incidence of CRC was reduced by surveillance colonoscopy *(102)*.

6. Conclusions

In summary, numerous acquired risk factors for CRC have been reported in the medical literature. These risk factors are based on data almost exclusively derived from prospective, retrospective, or cross-sectional observational studies, large case series or retrospective case–control studies. Because of the possibility of bias and confounding in such studies, these risk factors should not be automatically assumed to be causative, and in fact some may not be truly independent risk factors. This review serves to highlight the need for additional high-quality studies, preferably prospective, interventional, and randomized (if feasible), in order to further investigate the importance of each of these risk factors.

References

1. Terry P, Giovannucci E, Michels KB, Bergkvist L, Hansen H, Holmberg L, et al. (2001) Fruit, vegetables, dietary fiber, and risk of colorectal cancer. J Natl Cancer Inst 93, 525–533.

2. Slattery ML, Boucher KM, Caan BJ, Potter JD, and Ma KN. Eating patterns and risk of colon cancer. (1998) Am J Epidemiol 148, 4–16.

3. Negri E, Franceschi S, Parpinel M, and La Vecchia C. (1998) Fiber intake and risk of colorectal cancer. Cancer Epidemiol Biomarkers Prev 7, 667–671.

4. Peters U, Sinha R, Chatterjee N, Subar AF, Ziegler RG, Kulldorff M, et al. (2003) Dietary fibre and colorectal adenoma in a colorectal cancer early detection programme. Lancet 361, 1491–1495.

5. Bingham SA, Day NE, Luben R, Ferrari P, Slimani N, Norat T, et al. (2203) Dietary fibre in food and protection against colorectal cancer in the European Prospective Investigation into Cancer and Nutrition (EPIC): an observational study. Lancet 361, 1496–1501.

6. Larsson SC, Giovannucci E, Bergkvist L, and Wolk A. (2005) Whole grain consumption and risk of colorectal cancer: a population-based cohort of 60,000 women. Br J Cancer 92, 1803–1807.

7. Michels KB, Edward G, Joshipura KJ, Rosner BA, Stampfer MJ, Fuchs CS, et al. (2000) Prospective study of fruit and vegetable consumption and incidence of colon and rectal cancers. J Natl Cancer Inst 92, 1740–1752.

8. Fuchs CS, Giovannucci EL, Colditz GA, Hunter DJ, Stampfer MJ, Rosner B, et al. (1999) Dietary fiber and the risk of colorectal cancer and adenoma in women. N Engl J Med 340, 169–176.

9. Schatzkin A, Lanza E, Corle D, Lance P, Iber F, Caan B, et al. (2000) Lack of effect of a low-fat, high-fiber diet on the recurrence of colorectal adenomas. Polyp Prevention Trial Study Group. N Engl J Med 342, 1149–1155.

10. Alberts DS, Martinez ME, Roe DJ, Guillen-Rodriguez JM, Marshall JR, van Leeuwen JB, et al. (2000) Lack of effect of a high-fiber cereal supplement on the recurrence of colorectal adenomas. Phoenix Colon Cancer Prevention Physicians' Network. N Engl J Med 342, 1156–1162.

11. Beresford SA, Johnson KC, Ritenbaugh C, Lasser NL, Snetselaar LG, Black HR, et al. (2006) Low-fat dietary pattern and risk of colorectal cancer: the Women's Health Initiative Randomized Controlled Dietary Modification Trial. JAMA 295, 643–654.

12. Asano T and McLeod RS. (2002) Dietary fibre for the prevention of colorectal adenomas and carcinomas. Cochrane Database Syst Rev 2, CD003430.

13. Park Y, Hunter DJ, Spiegelman D, Bergkvist L, Berrino F, van den Brandt PA, et al. (2005) Dietary fiber intake and risk of colorectal cancer: a pooled analysis of pros-pective cohort studies. JAMA 294, 2849–2857.

14. Chao A, Thun MJ, Connell CJ, McCullough ML, Jacobs EJ, Flanders WD, et al. (2005) Meat consumption and risk of colorectal cancer. JAMA 293, 172–182.

15. Jarvinen R, Knekt P, Hakulinen T, Rissanen H, and Heliovaara M. (2001) Dietary fat, cholesterol and colorectal cancer in a prospective study. Br J Cancer 85, 357–361.

16. Butler LM, Sinha R, Millikan RC, Martin CF, Newman B, Gammon MD, et al. (2003) Heterocyclic amines, meat intake, and association with colon cancer in a population-based study. Am J Epidemiol 157, 434–445.

17. Larsson SC, Rafter J, Holmberg L, Bergkvist L, and Wolk A. (2005) Red meat consumption and risk of cancers of the proximal colon, distal colon and rectum: the Swedish Mammography Cohort. Int J Cancer 113, 829–834.

18. Norat T, Bingham S, Ferrari P, Slimani N, Jenab M, Mazuir M, et al. (2005) Meat, fish, and colorectal cancer risk: the European Prospective Investigation into cancer and nutrition. J Natl Cancer Inst 97, 906–916.

19. Willett WC, Stampfer MJ, Colditz GA, Rosner BA, and Speizer FE. (1990) Relation of meat, fat, and fiber intake to the risk of colon cancer in a prospective study among women. N Engl J Med 323, 1664–1672.

20. Sanjoaquin MA, Appleby PN, Thorogood M, Mann JI, and Key TJ. (2004) Nutrition, lifestyle and colorectal cancer incidence: a prospective investigation of 10998 vegetarians and non-vegetarians in the United Kingdom. Br J Cancer 90, 118–121.

21. Sandhu MS, White IR, and McPherson K. (2001) Systematic review of the prospective cohort studies on meat consumption and colorectal cancer risk: a meta-analytical approach. Cancer Epidemiol Biomarkers Prev 10, 439–446.

22. Pedersen A, Johansen C, and Gronbaek M. (2003) Relations between amount and type of alcohol and colon and rectal cancer in a Danish population based cohort study. Gut 52, 861–867.

23. Shimizu N, Nagata C, Shimizu H, Kametani M, Takeyama N, Ohnuma T, et al. (2003) Height, weight, and alcohol consumption in relation to the risk of colorectal cancer in Japan: a prospective study. Br J Cancer 88, 1038–1043.

24. Longnecker MP, Orza MJ, Adams ME, Vioque J, and Chalmers TC. (1990) A meta-analysis of alcoholic beverage consumption in relation to risk of colorectal cancer. Cancer Causes Control 1, 59–68.

25. Gapstur SM, Potter JD, and Folsom AR. (1994) Alcohol consumption and colon and rectal cancer in postmenopausal women. Int J Epidemiol 23, 50–57.

26. Ye W, Romelsjo A, Augustsson K, Adami HO, and Nyren O. (2003) No excess risk of colorectal cancer among alcoholics followed for up to 25 years. Br J Cancer 88, 1044–1046.

27. Cho E, Smith-Warner SA, Ritz J, van den Brandt PA, Colditz GA, Folsom AR, et al. (2004) Alcohol intake and colorectal cancer: a pooled analysis of 8 cohort studies. Ann Intern Med 140, 603–613.

28. Harnack L, Jacobs DR Jr, Nicodemus K, Lazovich D, Anderson K, and Folsom AR. (2002) Relationship of folate, vitamin B-6, vitamin B-12, and methionine intake to incidence of colorectal cancers. Nutr Cancer 43, 152–158.

29. Giovannucci E, Rimm EB, Ascherio A, Stampfer MJ, Colditz GA, and Willett WC. (1995) Alcohol, low-methionine–low-folate diets, and risk of colon cancer in men. J Natl Cancer Inst 87, 265–273.

30. Giovannucci E. (1998) Meta-analysis of coffee consumption and risk of colorectal cancer. Am J Epidemiol 147, 1043–1052.

31. Colditz GA, Cannuscio CC, and Frazier AL. (1997) Physical activity and reduced risk of colon cancer: implications for prevention. Cancer Causes Control 8, 649–667.

32. Mao Y, Pan S, Wen SW, and Johnson KC. (2003) Physical inactivity, energy intake, obesity and the risk of rectal cancer in Canada. Int J Cancer 105, 831–837.

33. Nilsen TI and Vatten LJ. (2001) Prospective study of colorectal cancer risk and physical activity, diabetes, blood glucose and BMI: exploring the hyperinsulinaemia hypothesis. Br J Cancer 84, 417–422.

34. Colbert LH, Hartman TJ, Malila N, Limburg PJ, Pietinen P, Virtamo J, et al. (2001) Physical activity in relation to cancer of the colon and rectum in a cohort of male smokers. Cancer Epidemiol Biomarkers Prev 10, 265–268.

35. Sturmer T, Glynn RJ, Lee IM, Christen WG, and Hennekens CH. (2000) Lifetime cigarette smoking and colorectal cancer incidence in the Physicians' Health Study I. J Natl Cancer Inst 92, 1178–1181.

36. Chao A, Thun MJ, Jacobs EJ, Henley SJ, Rodriguez C, and Calle EE. (2000) Cigarette smoking and colorectal cancer mortality in the cancer prevention study II. J Natl Cancer Inst 92, 1888–1896.

37. Colangelo LA, Gapstur SM, Gann PH, and Dyer AR. (2004) Cigarette smoking and colorectal carcinoma mortality in a cohort with long-term follow-up. Cancer 100, 288–293.

38. Sandler RS and Sandler DP. (1983) Radiation-induced cancers of the colon and rectum: assessing the risk. Gastroenterology 84, 51–57.

39. Baxter NN, Tepper JE, Durham SB, Rothenberger DA, and Virnig BA. (2005) Increased risk of rectal cancer after prostate radiation: a population-based study. Gastroenterology 128, 819–824.

40. Lagergren J, Ye W, and Ekbom A. (2001) Intestinal cancer after cholecystectomy: is bile involved in carcinogenesis? Gastroenterology 121, 542–547.

41. Todoroki I, Friedman GD, Slattery ML, Potter JD, and Samowitz W. (1999) Cholecystectomy and the risk of colon cancer. Am J Gastroenterol 94, 41–46.

42. Mercer PM, Reid FD, Harrison M, and Bates T. (1995) The relationship between cholecystectomy, unoperated gallstone disease, and colorectal cancer. A necropsy study. Scand J Gastroenterol 30, 1017–1020.

43. Giovannucci E, Colditz GA, and Stampfer MJ. (1993) A meta-analysis of cholecystec-

tomy and risk of colorectal cancer. Gastro-enterology 105, 130–141.

44. Reid FD, Mercer PM, harrison M, and Bates T. (1996) Cholecystectomy as a risk factor for colorectal cancer: a meta-analysis. Scand J Gastroenterol 31, 160–169.

45. Stewart M, Macrae FA, and Williams CB. (1982) Neoplasia and ureterosigmoidostomy: a colonoscopy survey. Br J Surg 69, 414–416.

46. Azimuddin K, Khubchandani IT, Stasik JJ, Rosen L, and Riether RD. (1999) Neoplasia after ureterosigmoidostomy. Dis Colon Rectum 42, 1632–1638.

47. Siersema PD, Yu S, Sahbaie P, Steyerberg EW, Simpson PW, Kuipers EJ, et al. (2006) Colorectal neoplasia in veterans is associated with Barrett's esophagus but not with proton-pump inhibitor or aspirin/NSAID use. Gastrointest Endosc 63, 581–586.

48. Sontag SJ, Schnell TG, Chejfec G, O'Connell S, Stanley MM, Best W, et al. (1985) Barrett's oesophagus and colonic tumours. Lancet 1, 946–949.

49. Vaughan TL, Kiemeney LA, and McKnight B. (1995) Colorectal cancer in patients with esophageal adenocarcinoma. Cancer Epidemiol Biomarkers Prev 4, 93–97.

50. Tripp MR, Sampliner RE, Kogan FJ, and Morgan TR. (1986) Colorectal neoplasms and Barrett's esophagus. Am J Gastroenterol 81, 1063–1064.

51. Post AB, Achkar E, and Carey WD. (1993) Prevalence of colonic neoplasia in patients with Barrett's esophagus. Am J Gastroenterol 88, 877–880.

52. Cauvin JM, Goldfain D, Le Rhun M, Robaszkiewicz M, Cadiot G, Carpentier S, et al. (1995) Multicentre prospective controlled study of Barrett's oesophagus and colorectal adenomas. Groupe d'Etude de l'Oesophage de Barrett. Lancet 346, 1391–1394.

53. Laitakari R, Laippala P, and Isolauri J. (1995) Barrett's oesophagus is not a risk factor for colonic neoplasia: a case-control study. Ann Med 27, 499–502.

54. Poorman JC, Lieberman DA, Ippoliti AF, Weber LJ, and Weinstein WM. (1997) The prevalence of colonic neoplasia in patients with Barrett's esophagus: prospective assessment in patients 50–80 years old. Am J Gastroenterol 92, 592–596.

55. Lagergren J and Nyren O. (1999) No association between colon cancer and adenocarcinoma of the oesophagus in a population based cohort study in Sweden. Gut 44, 819–821.

56. Howden CW and Hornung CA. (1995) A systematic review of the association between Barrett's esophagus and colon neoplasms. Am J Gastroenterol 90, 1814–1819.

57. Bini EJ, Park J, and Francois F. (2006) Use of flexible sigmoidoscopy to screen for colorectal cancer in HIV-infected patients 50 years of age and older. Arch Intern Med 166, 1626–1631.

58. La Vecchia C, Negri E, Decarli A, and Franceschi S. (1997) Diabetes mellitus and colorectal cancer risk. Cancer Epidemiol Biomarkers Prev 6, 1007–1010.

59. Hu FB, Manson JE, Liu S, Hunter D, Colditz GA, Michels KB, et al. (1999) Prospective study of adult onset diabetes mellitus (type 2) and risk of colorectal cancer in women. J Natl Cancer Inst 91, 542–547.

60. Yang YX, Hennessy S, and Lewis JD. (2005) Type 2 diabetes mellitus and the risk of colorectal cancer. Clin Gastroenterol Hepatol 3, 587–594.

61. Larsson SC, Orsini N, and Wolk A. (2005) Diabetes mellitus and risk of colorectal cancer: a meta-analysis. J Natl Cancer Inst 97, 1679–1687.

62. Ma J, Pollak MN, Giovannucci E, Chan JM, Tao Y, Hennekens CH, et al. (1999) Prospective study of colorectal cancer risk in men and plasma levels of insulin-like growth factor (IGF)-I and IGF-binding protein-3. J Natl Cancer Inst 91, 620–625.

63. Ma J, Giovannucci E, Pollak M, Leavitt A, Tao Y, Gaziano JM, et al. (2004) A prospective study of plasma C-peptide and colorectal cancer risk in men. J Natl Cancer Inst 96, 546–553.

64. Yang YX, Hennessy S, and Lewis JD. (2004) Insulin therapy and colorectal cancer risk among type 2 diabetes mellitus patients. Gastroenterology 127, 1044–1050.

65. Delhougne B, Deneux C, Abs R, Chanson P, Fierens H, Laurent-Puig P, et al. (1995) The prevalence of colonic polyps in acromegaly: a colonoscopic and pathological study in 103 patients. J Clin Endocrinol Metab 80, 3223–3226.

66. Fukuda I, Hizuka N, Murakami Y, Itoh E, Yasumoto K, Sata A, et al. (2001) Clinical features and therapeutic outcomes of 65 patients with acromegaly at Tokyo Women's Medical University. Intern Med 40, 987–992.

67. Ekbom A, Helmick C, Zack M, and Adami HO. (1990) Ulcerative colitis and colorectal cancer. A population-based study. N Engl J Med 323, 1228–1233.

68. Ekbom A, Helmick C, Zack M, and Adami HO. (1990) Increased risk of large-bowel cancer in Crohn's disease with colonic involvement. Lancet 336, 357–359.

69. Hommes DW and van Deventer SJ. (2004) Endoscopy in inflammatory bowel diseases. Gastroenterology 126, 1561–1573.

70. Eaden JA and Mayberry JF. (2002) Guidelines for screening and surveillance of asymptomatic colorectal cancer in patients with inflammatory bowel disease. Gut 51 Suppl 5:V10–12.

71. Kornbluth A and Sachar DB. (2004) Ulcerative colitis practice guidelines in adults (update): American College of Gastroenterology, Practice Parameters Committee. Am J Gastroenterol 99, 1371–1385.

72. Jess T, Loftus EV Jr, Velayos FS, Harmsen WS, Zinsmeister AR, Smyrk TC, et al. (2006) Risk of intestinal cancer in inflammatory bowel disease: a population-based study from Olmsted county, Minnesota. Gastroenterology 130, 1039–1046.

73. Gyde SN, Prior P, Allan RN, Stevens A, Jewell DP, Truelove SC, et al. (1988) Colorectal cancer in ulcerative colitis: a cohort study of primary referrals from three centres. Gut 29, 206–217.

74. Winther KV, Jess T, Langholz E, Munkholm P, and Binder V. (2004) Long-term risk of cancer in ulcerative colitis: a population-based cohort study from Copenhagen County. Clin Gastroenterol Hepatol 2, 1088–1095.

75. Greenstein AJ, Sachar DB, Smith H, Pucillo A, Papatestas AE, Kreel I, et al. (1979) Cancer in universal and left-sided ulcerative colitis: factors determining risk. Gastroenterology 77, 290–294.

76. Nugent FW, Haggitt RC, and Gilpin PA. (1991) Cancer surveillance in ulcerative colitis. Gastroenterology 100, 1241–1248.

77. Levin B. (1992) Inflammatory bowel disease and colon cancer. Cancer 70, 1313–1316.

78. Heuschen UA, Hinz U, Allemeyer EH, Stern J, Lucas M, Autschbach F, et al. (2001) Backwash ileitis is strongly associated with colorectal carcinoma in ulcerative colitis. Gastroenterology 120, 841–847.

79. Rutter M, Saunders B, Wilkinson K, Rumbles S, Schofield G, Kamm M, et al. (2004) Severity of inflammation is a risk factor for colorectal neoplasia in ulcerative colitis. Gastroenterology 126, 451–459.

80. Haskell H, Andrews CW Jr, Reddy SI, Dendrinos K, Farraye FA, Stucchi AF, et al. (2005) Pathologic features and clinical significance of "backwash" ileitis in ulcerative colitis. Am J Surg Pathol 29, 1472–1481.

81. Soetikno RM, Lin OS, Heidenreich PA, Young HS, and Blackstone MO. (2002) Increased risk of colorectal neoplasia in patients with primary sclerosing cholangitis and ulcerative colitis: a meta-analysis. Gastrointest Endosc 56, 48–54.

82. Rubio CA and Befrits R. (1997) Colorectal adenocarcinoma in Crohn's disease: a retrospective histologic study. Dis Colon Rectum 40, 1072–1078.

83. Friedman S, Rubin PH, Bodian C, Goldstein E, Harpaz N, and Present DH. (2001) Screening and surveillance colonoscopy in chronic Crohn's colitis. Gastroenterology 120, 820–826.

84. Maykel JA, Hagerman G, Mellgren AF, Li SY, Alavi K, Baxter NN, et al. (2006) Crohn's colitis: the incidence of dysplasia and adenocarcinoma in surgical patients. Dis Colon Rectum 49, 950–957.

85. Gyde SN, Prior P, Macartney JC, Thompson H, Waterhouse JA, and Allan RN. (1980) Malignancy in Crohn's disease. Gut 21, 1024–1029.

86. Greenstein AJ, Sachar DB, Smith H, Janowitz HD, and Aufses AH, Jr. (1981) A comparison of cancer risk in Crohn's disease and ulcerative colitis. Cancer 48, 2742–2745.

87. Choi PM and Zelig MP. (1994) Similarity of colorectal cancer in Crohn's disease and ulcerative colitis: implications for carcinogenesis and prevention. Gut 35, 950–954.

88. Gillen CD, Walmsley RS, Prior P, Andrews HA, and Allan RN. (1994) Ulcerative colitis and Crohn's disease: a comparison of the colorectal cancer risk in extensive colitis. Gut 35, 1590–1592.

89. Jensen AB, Larsen M, Gislum M, Skriver MV, Jepsen P, Norgaard B, et al. Survival after colorectal cancer in patients with ulcerative colitis: a nationwide population-based Danish study. Am J Gastroenterol 2006;101(6):1283–1287.

90. Larsen M, Mose H, Gislum M, Skriver MV, Jepsen P, Norgard B, et al. (2007) Survival after colorectal cancer in patients with Crohn's disease: A nationwide population-based Danish follow-up study. Am J Gastroenterol 102, 163–167.

91. Sugita A, Greenstein AJ, Ribeiro MB, Sachar DB, Bodian C, Panday AK, et al. (1993) Survival with colorectal cancer in ulcerative colitis. A study of 102 cases. Ann Surg 218, 189–195.

92. Heimann TM, Oh SC, Martinelli G, Szporn A, Luppescu N, Lembo CA, et al. (1992) Colorectal carcinoma associated with ulcerative colitis: a study of prognostic indicators. Am J Surg 164, 13–17.

93. Gorfine SR, Bauer JJ, Harris MT, and Kreel I. (2000) Dysplasia complicating chronic ulcerative colitis: is immediate colectomy warranted? Dis Colon Rectum 43, 1575–1581.

94. Ullman T, Croog V, Harpaz N, Sachar D, and Itzkowitz S. (2003) Progression of flat low-grade dysplasia to advanced neoplasia in patients with ulcerative colitis. Gastroenterology 125, 1311–1319.

95. Lim CH, Dixon MF, Vail A, Forman D, Lynch DA, and Axon AT. (2003) Ten year follow up of ulcerative colitis patients with and without low grade dysplasia. Gut 52, 1127–1132.

96. Jess T, Loftus EV Jr, Velayos FS, Harmsen WS, Zinsmeister AR, Smyrk TC, et al. (2006) Incidence and prognosis of colorectal dysplasia in inflammatory bowel disease: a population-based study from Olmsted County, Minnesota. Inflamm Bowel Dis 12, 669–676.

97. Befrits R, Ljung T, Jaramillo E, and Rubio C. (2002) Low-grade dysplasia in extensive, long-standing inflammatory bowel disease: a follow-up study. Dis Colon Rectum 45, 615–620.

98. Blackstone MO, Riddell RH, Rogers BH, and Levin B. (1981) Dysplasia-associated lesion or mass (DALM) detected by colonoscopy in long-standing ulcerative colitis: an indication for colectomy. Gastroenterology 80, 366–374.

99. Connell WR, Lennard-Jones JE, Williams CB, Talbot IC, Price AB, and Wilkinson KH. (1994) Factors affecting the outcome of endoscopic surveillance for cancer in ulcerative colitis. Gastroenterology 107, 934–944.

100. Choi PM, Nugent FW, Schoetz DJ Jr, Silverman ML, and Haggitt RC. (1993) Colonoscopic surveillance reduces mortality from colorectal cancer in ulcerative colitis. Gastroenterology 105, 418–424.

101. Karlen P, Kornfeld D, Brostrom O, Lofberg R, Persson PG, and Ekbom A. (1998) Is colonoscopic surveillance reducing colorectal cancer mortality in ulcerative colitis? A population based case control study. Gut 42, 711–714.

102. Velayos FS, Loftus EV Jr, Jess T, Harmsen WS, Bida J, Zinsmeister AR, et al. (2006) Predictive and protective factors associated with colorectal cancer in ulcerative colitis: A case-control study. Gastroenterology 130, 1941–1949.

Chapter 17

Aberrant Crypt Foci in Colon Cancer Epidemiology

Sharad Khare, Kamran Chaudhary, Marc Bissonnette, and Robert Carroll

Abstract

Colonic carcinogenesis is characterized by progressive accumulations of genetic and epigenetic derangements. These molecular events are accompanied by histological changes that progress from mild cryptal architectural abnormalities in small adenomas to eventual invasive cancers. The transition steps from normal colonic epithelium to small adenomas are little understood. In experimental models of colonic carcinogenesis aberrant crypt foci (ACF), collections of abnormal appearing colonic crypts, are the earliest detectable abnormality and precede adenomas. Whether in fact ACF are precursors of colon cancer, however, remains controversial. Recent advances in magnification chromoendoscopy now allow these lesions to be identified in vivo and their natural history ascertained.

While increasing lines of evidence suggest that dysplastic ACF harbor a malignant potential, there are few prospective studies to confirm causal relationships and supporting epidemiological studies are scarce. It would be very useful, for example, to clarify the relationship of ACF incidence to established risks for colon cancer, including age, smoking, sedentary lifestyle, and Western diets. In experimental animal models, carcinogens dose-dependently increase ACF, whereas most chemopreventive agents reduce ACF incidence or growth. In humans, however, few agents have been validated to be chemopreventive of colon cancer. It remains unproven, therefore, whether human ACF could be used as reliable surrogate markers of efficacy of chemopreventive agents. If these lesions could be used as reliable biomarkers of colon cancer risk and their reductions as predictors of effective chemopreventive agents, metrics to quantify ACF could greatly facilitate the study of colonic carcinogenesis and chemoprevention.

Key words: Aberrant crypt foci, colon cancer.

1. Introduction

Colorectal cancers (CRC) are the second leading cause of cancer-related deaths in men and women in the United States *(1)*. Both genetic and environmental factors are thought to play roles in tumor development *(2)*. Host modifiable factors such as Western style diet, sedentary lifestyle, and smoking are believed to

M. Verma (ed.), *Methods of Molecular Biology, Cancer Epidemiology, vol. 472*
© 2009 Humana Press, a part of Springer Science + Business Media, Totowa, NJ
Book doi: 10.1007/978-1-60327-492-0

contribute more than 50% to the risk of these malignancies (3, 4). Unfortunately, studies to test specific agents or interventions that might prevent CRC are complicated by the relative infrequency of cancer in the general population and the long premalignant phase prior to the occurrence of detectable tumors. The incidence of CRC among men and women combined is approximately 50 per 100,000, or only 0.05% (5). Thus, while CRC is the most common gastrointestinal malignancy in developed countries, even these malignancies occur relatively infrequently. CRC carries an excessively high morbidity and mortality given the fact that endoscopic screening can reduce colon cancer incidence by as much as 90% (6). The effectiveness of endoscopic screening, however, is dependent on the removal of adenomas (7). The genetic and histological characteristics of these premalignant lesions have been well characterized. Retrospective and prospective studies support the use of adenomas as surrogate intermediates of colon cancer for epidemiological and cancer chemoprevention studies (8). There are, however, limitations on the use of adenomas as surrogate biomarkers for colon cancer. The most obvious limitation is the relative infrequency of transformation from small adenomas to cancers because few adenomas progress to cancer. To count the recurrence of all adenomas could lead to false inferences in prevention trials and epidemiological studies. For example, the intervention might not block adenoma recurrence, but prevent growth of established adenomas or their progression to cancer. While inhibiting colon cancer occurrence is the gold standard for prevention therapy, the infrequency of this occurrence and the long premalignant time interval would require an enormous number of individuals and periods of follow-up lasting many years. Factors such as the large cohort size required, noncompliance and drop out over time, and high costs make studies employing cancer as an end point impractical. Even polyp recurrence requires a long period of follow-up, with a minimum of 3–5 years. The focus on adenoma removal also limits cancer prevention to an endoscopic approach. From a public health prospective, the cost effectiveness of such an endoscopic approach for average risk individuals remains controversial. A second reason why adenomas are not ideal as biomarkers stems from the fact that some cancers arise from flat and depressed lesions that would be missed in studies using recurrent polyps as endpoints (9–11). For all of these reasons there is much interest in identifying and validating other surrogate biomarkers in colonic carcinogenesis for epidemiologic studies and cancer prevention trials (12). The development of a safe and cost-effective agent to inhibit tumorigenesis could also allow a non-endoscopic approach to prevent this malignancy.

To overcome the problems of using adenomas or cancers as endpoints, earlier more prevalent and potentially more reversible lesions than polyps have been sought as biomarkers. Ideally, such biomarkers could be reverted or their progression blocked by appropriate host modifiable factors such as diet changes, increased exercise, tobacco cessation, or use of an effective and well-tolerated chemopreventive agent. In this regard, increased understanding of the pathogenesis of earlier stages of malignant transformation might suggest better targets for chemoprevention. These insights could lead to improved methods to identify individuals at increased risk for adenoma development and/or simpler and safer methods to prevent colon cancer.

Aberrant crypt foci (ACF) have been identified as biomarkers of colonic carcinogenesis and putative precursors of colon cancers (13). Numerous studies have been carried out using animal models or human pathologic specimens to investigate the role of ACF in colonic carcinogenesis. These lesions are frequently present in individuals with sporadic colon cancer and also in familial adenomatous polyposis (FAP) syndrome, an autosomal dominant form of hereditary colon cancer (14). Individuals with FAP have a germ line mutation in the *apc* gene, which is also the most common mutation in sporadic human colon cancer. Further, ACF are the earliest microscopic lesions to appear in the colonic mucosa of mice treated with chemical carcinogens, such as azoxymethane (AOM) (15, 16). The AOM rodent model is one of the most widely used preclinical models to screen agents for chemopreventive efficacy. More than 180 dietary interventions and pharmacologic agents have been shown to reduce ACF in models of chemical colonic carcinogenesis (17). Importantly, many agents that block ACF growth also prevent tumor development in the AOM model. ACF have been studied in human colons that were surgically resected (18) or examined in situ with image magnification chromoendoscopy (19–21). Individuals with a history of advanced adenomas or colon cancer, or older individuals, have been shown to have a higher incidence of ACF. Preliminary evidence suggests ACF are rapidly reversible with pharmacologic agents such as sulindac or aspirin. This has led to the proposal that these lesions could be utilized as surrogate intermediate biomarkers to predict colon cancer risk (22–24) and to assess the efficacy of chemopreventive agents.

2. ACF Morphology/ Histology

ACF were identified in human colonic mucosa 4 years after initial reports of these lesions in carcinogen-treated animals (25). In resected colonic surgical specimens fixed flat in formalin, human ACF were found to have similar morphological characteristics to those in experimental animals: 1) component ACF crypts were larger than normal crypts, 2) pericryptal spaces were expanded, 3) crypts stained darker than adjacent crypts, and 4) crypt orifices differed in configuration from circular openings of normal crypts *(22, 25–29)* (**Fig. 17.1**). ACF varied in size from a single crypt to multiple abnormal crypts, sometimes with more than 150–200 crypts per focus. ACF are usually elevated, but can be depressed

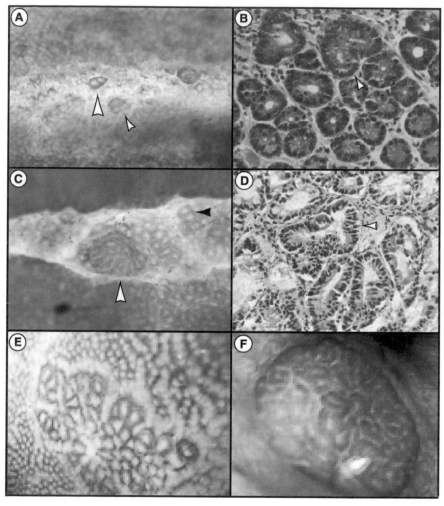

Fig. 17.1. (A) Whole mount preparations of the distal colon of an AOM-treated mouse. The methylene blue stain identifies nondysplastic ACF (*white arrows*) with small rounded crypts (×40) (B) Hematoxylin and eosin staining shows that the rounded ACF are composed of enlarged crypts with loss of mucin (*white arrow*) but otherwise possess normal cellular features (×400). (C) The dysplastic ACF (white arrow) compared with nondysplastic ACF (*black arrow*) are larger and the crypts are elongated (×40). (D) Hematoxylin and eosin stains display the marked nuclear atypia, loss of cell polarity, and the increase in mitoses consistent with high-grade dysplasia (*white arrow*) (×400). (E) Human rectum stained by methylene blue. A nondysplastic ACF with enlarged rounded and oval shaped crypts is at the center of the field. The relative size difference from the normal background crypts and increased pericryptal staining are identifying features (×35). (F) Human rectum with dysplastic ACF composed of indented crypts. The elevated surface in contrast to the surrounding healthy mucosa is more apparent in the larger ACF lesions (×35).

relative to adjacent mucosa. It is important to emphasize that ACF must be identified in situ in the colon, and not from histological sections. The criteria that define ACF require identification of specific surface features that cannot be reliably appreciated in histological sections.

Recently, investigators have described dysplastic crypts that differed from conventional ACF in the colons of carcinogen-treated rodents. These included β-catenin-accumulated ACF *(30, 31)*, flat-appearing ACF *(32)*, or mucin-depleted ACF *(33)*. These newly described lesions appear to exhibit stronger associations with the development of tumors than conventional ACF. Some of these lesions appear to be variants of conventional ACF, while others are reported to have normal surface features when stained in situ, but are dysplastic in histological sections. Conventional ACF are heterotypical in histology, with features ranging from hyperplastic to dysplastic. Nondysplastic crypts are 1.5–2.5 times larger than surrounding crypts, often with rounded lumens and mucin depletion. On scanning electron microscopy, ACF possess larger luminal openings and flatter mucosal surfaces. The latter occurs because of loss of microvilli *(34)*. Colonic epithelial cells of dysplastic ACF show loss of basal nuclear polarity and increased proliferation *(27)*. Dysplastic ACF often possess slit-like, irregular, or closed lumens. Dysplastic crypt cells within ACF may be focally localized, with adjacent cells in the same focus showing only hyperproliferativechanges. Some ACF exhibit a serrated luminal pattern and may constitute a distinct group from hyperplastic or dysplastic ACF *(28, 35)*. Recent studies suggest there may be staining differences between dysplastic and nondysplastic ACF *(36)*. Dysplastic ACF might provide ideal premalignant structures to elucidate causally important steps early in colonic carcinogenesis. Differential staining could also allow more rapid and accurate detection of precursor lesions for chemoprevention studies.

3. Molecular Abnormalities in ACF

Numerous genetic and epigenetic changes have been identified in ACF that are also present in colon cancers, including frequent K-*ras* mutations *(37)* and rare *apc* mutations *(38)* or microsatellite instability (MSI) *(39)*. While many of the molecular abnormalities in ACF overlap in humans and experimental animals, there are also differences reported *(40–43)*. Two major pathways to colon cancer have been distinguished by differences in molecular abnormalities in the *apc* gene and DNA mismatch repair genes.

Nearly 70% of sporadic colon cancers possess truncating nonsense mutations in one *apc* allele, with deletion of the second allele by loss of heterozygosity (LOH). The finding of LOH in ACF with normal expressions of APC and β-catenin proteins suggests that LOH can occur very early in colon neoplasia and perhaps even before APC mutations *(44)*. Half of the remaining sporadic tumors express activating mutations in β-catenin, a downstream effector of Wnt/APC signaling. Another smaller subset of sporadic colon cancers (10–20%) possesses defects in DNA mismatch repair genes and exhibits MSI. A comparable fraction of ACF exhibit MSI, suggesting that at least some MSI tumors might arise from ACF *(45–47)*.

Inactivating mutations in the *apc* gene, or alternatively activating mutations in β-catenin, are believed to be critical "gate keeper" events in colonic adenoma formation *(48, 49)*. APC and β-catenin are part of the Wnt pathway that controls cell fate determination in embryogenesis and postnatal colonic proliferation. Together, these mutations distinguish neoplastic lesions with malignant potential *(50)* from hyperplastic polyps with little or no malignant potential *(51)*. Somatic APC mutations were infrequent in sporadic ACF and identified only in dysplastic lesions *(38)*. Jen et al. found an *apc* mutation in only 1 (5%) of 20 ACF and this ACF was dysplastic *(52)*. In the largest study of sporadic ACF in colon cancer reported to date, APC mutations as assessed by in vitro protein transcription translation assays were absent in 21 nondysplastic ACF and 15 dysplastic ACF isolated from healthy individuals or individuals with sporadic adenomas or cancers. In contrast, adenomas from these same subjects had a high prevalence (6 [75%] of 8) of APC mutations. Truncating APC mutations were found in 7 of 7 ACF and 11 of 11 adenomas examined from FAP individuals. Thus, *apc* mutations in ACF are common in individuals with FAP, but rare in sporadic ACF *(14)*.

In contrast to infrequent *apc* mutations in sporadic ACF, the reported frequency of K-ras mutations has ranged from 13–95% *(41)*. These wide differences might reflect differences in populations studied, or use of K-ras mutation assays of varying sensitivity *(14, 53, 54)*. Several studies suggest K-ras mutations are more frequent in small hyperproliferative lesions compared with large dysplastic lesions *(14, 35)*. In a recent study, we reported that approximately 20% of large human ACF had K-ras mutations and a comparable fraction of ACF had activated wild-type Ras, the protein encoded by *ras (55)*. Regulated (nonmutant) Ras can be activated by upstream signals including growth factors. We demonstrated that epidermal growth factor receptor (EGFR) signaling was upregulated in a subset of large hyperproliferative human ACF. We speculated that this increased EGFR signaling activated wild-type Ras *(55)*. In more recent studies, we demonstrated that EGFR signals were increased in the AOM model and activated wild-type Ras *(56)*.

4. ACF Formation and Links to Colon Cancer

ACF prevalence has been compared in surgical colonic resections for malignant and benign disease. ACF densities were highest in individuals with FAP, followed by individuals with CRC. The lowest ACF densities were found in colons resected for benign diseases such as diverticulosis *(22)*. In vivo studies using magnification chromoendoscopy have confirmed more frequent ACF in individuals with a history of colonic adenomas or cancer *(13, 19, 57)*. ACF densities were also higher in colons from individuals with cancer of the rectum and sigmoid colon, compared with colons resected for right-sided cancers *(28, 58, 59)*. ACF numbers were also greater in individuals from regions with high colon cancer incidence, compared with those from regions with low colon cancer incidence *(18)*.

Human ACF are monoclonal in origin *(60)*. Human ACF also aberrantly expressed carcinoembryonic antigen (CEA), a molecular marker of colon cancer *(61)*. CEA was strongly expressed in 39 (93%) of 42 ACF from 15 patients with sporadic or hereditary colon cancer. The expression in adjacent normal mucosa was absent or faint. CEA expression related to ACF size but not with dysplasia *(62)*. Evidence of variable expression of other oncoproteins has also been demonstrated in ACF by immunohistochemistry *(12)*.

As noted earlier, the incidence of APC mutations in ACF differs in individuals with FAP compared with those with sporadic colon cancer. In FAP individuals, germ line mutations occurred in one allele *(63)* with a mutation or deletion of the 2nd allele in more than half of ACF *(14)*. In contrast, in individuals with sporadic colonic carcinomas, APC or β-catenin mutations were rare in ACF *(14)*, but frequent in adenomas and cancers *(50)*. Nuclear accumulation of β-catenin occurs not only with APC or β-catenin mutations, but also with wild-type β-catenin, reflecting signal-induced changes. In this regard, recent studies suggest that silencing of secreted frizzled-related protein (SFRP), an inhibitor of Wnt signaling, could be an early event in human ACF *(64)*. It should be noted that loss-of-function mutations in *apc* might not be functionally equivalent to gain-of-function mutations in β-catenin. In this regard, β-catenin mutations occurred in 12% of small adenomas, but in only 5% of large adenomas and 1% of cancers *(65)*. This suggests that APC, but not β-catenin mutations provide a selective growth advantage for large adenomas *(50, 65)*.

Furthermore, there is evidence that Wnt signals, but not activating β-catenin mutations, can increase Cox-2 expression *(66, 67)*. Wild-type APC has also been shown to suppress Cox-2 *(68)*. These findings emphasize the non-equivalence between inactivating *apc* mutations and activating β-catenin mutations.

The largest study to date compared K-ras frequency in ACF from individuals with FAP to those with sporadic ACF. In FAP individuals, K-ras mutations in codon 12 or 13 occurred with low frequency (1 [13%] of 8), whereas K-ras mutations were common in sporadic ACF (106 [80%] of 133) *(14)*. In small adenomas (<1 cm), the authors also reported a higher rate of K-ras mutations compared with previous reports, which ranged from 9 to 22%. Thus, small ACF and adenomas appear to have higher rates of K-ras mutations compared with larger lesions. Perhaps signals that activate wild-type Ras provide a selective growth advantage for lesions more likely to become tumors. An alternative explanation suggests that most hyperplastic polyps that commonly possess K-ras mutations (~60%) are derived from hyperplastic ACF *(69, 70)*. This could account for the common association of ACF and hyperplastic polyps in rectal mucosa.

Even prior to molecular characterizations, adenomas were suggested to be precursors of colon cancers by their parallel distributions and the presence of carcinoma in situ in some adenomas *(71, 72)*. In contrast, ACF and colon cancers do not follow parallel distributions, but, rather, ACF are predominantly found in the left colon *(13, 73, 74)* and only very rarely contain foci of carcinoma in situ *(75)*. Thus, if ACF were precursors of colon cancer, it would appear more likely that left colon cancers rather than right colon cancers arise from ACF. In this regard, different etiologies and molecular pathways have been postulated for right- and left-sided colon cancers *(76)*.

5. ACF as Surrogate Intermediates in Colon Cancer Epidemiology

Can ACF serve as surrogate biomarkers of colonic carcinogenesis for purposes of risk stratification or testing chemopreventive efficacy of new agents? Abundant lines of evidence in animal studies and growing evidence in humans suggests that even if ACF are not precursors of colon cancers, these lesions might serve as reliable biomarkers of a cancer-prone colon and could be exploited to assess the chemopreventive efficacy of interventions. More ACF were reported in patients with a family history of CRC or with a personal history of advanced adenomas compared with individuals without these risk factors. Investigators have also reported that ACF numbers, size, and/or histological progression were significantly increased in individuals with CRC or adenomas (77). These lesions increase in overall number with age (13, 78), analogous to colon cancer risk (79). Regional differences in ACF frequency also paralleled differences in colon cancer incidence. Taken together, these data are consistent with ACF as biomarkers and perhaps precursors of colon cancer.

Current guidelines recommend initiating screening at a younger age for persons with a strong family history (genetic predisposition) of colon cancer. In animal studies, genetic (strain-dependent) differences in sensitivity to develop ACF have confirmed that these lesions are under genetic control (80). Studies comparing ACF from susceptible and resistant strains have also demonstrated potentially important differences in gene expression patterns (81). Differences in ACF incidence might, therefore, serve as predictive biomarkers of relative cancer risk when comparing populations of different genetic backgrounds. The effects of dietary fat, alcohol consumption, and smoking habits on ACF prevalence would also be interesting since these host modifiable factors are associated with increased risk of CRC. Could reduction of these risk factors be shown to lead to regression of ACF? Such potentially quantifiable changes in ACF numbers could have major implications with respect to public health care initiatives to decrease colon cancer incidence. In this regard, sulindac (13) and aspirin (82) have been reported to cause regression of ACF within a few months. These findings suggest that ACF could be used to rapidly screen the effectiveness of interventions (e.g., smoking cessation or dietary changes) (83) or to assess the chemopreventive efficacy of promising new agents.

ACF identification should not be viewed as a colonic Pap smear, as their presence does not guarantee a coexisting colon cancer. Rather, the presence of large and dysplastic ACF could identify colonic mucosa that is at risk to develop colon cancer, analogous to "field cancerization" described in the aerodigestive system of smokers (84). Such preneoplastic changes within the bronchial epithelium of smokers have been used to identify high-risk individuals for interventions being studied to prevent lung cancer (85). Similarly, the presence of large and dysplastic ACF could help risk-stratify the population. For example, to rationalize limited health care resources, one could target individuals harboring dysplastic ACF for increased endoscopic surveillance. Furthermore, cohorts of such individuals could serve as "reagent grade" test populations to assess the efficacy of potential chemopreventive agents.

Targeting individuals at increased risk for this malignancy is an important goal for effective colon cancer chemoprevention. But how do we identify an effective agent? Several hundred compounds with potential chemopreventive efficacy have been tested in preclinical studies (86). Similar to recent studies with aspirin

(ASA), to adequately test any one of these agents in an adenoma prevention trial that is powered to detect a 50% reduction in polyps would probably require 3–5 years, involve multiple institutions, and necessitate enrollment of 600–1,200 subjects *(87, 88)*. In contrast, we estimate that a chromoendoscopy study to assess reductions in ACF in response to a single agent using a double-blinded, placebo-controlled design could likely be completed in 1–2 years at a single institution and require only 150–250 subjects. Such a study could provide sufficient power to detect a 50% reduction in these lesions. This type of limited ACF study could also provide a cost-effective method to initially screen promising agents or interventions that could then be examined in larger and more definitive adenoma prevention trials. ACF studies in humans using image magnification chromoendoscopy could thus exploit the insights from 20 years of animal research in colon cancer to incorporate this biomarker into the clinical arena in a timely and cost-effective manner.

References

1. Jemal, A., Murray, T., Samuels, A., Ghafoor, A., Ward, E., and Thun, M. J. (2003) Cancer statistics 2003. *CA Cancer J Clin.* **53**, 5–26.

2. Fernandez, E., Gallus, S., La Vecchia, C., Talamini, R., Negri, E., and Franceschi, S. (2004) Family history and environmental risk factors for colon cancer. *Cancer Epidemiol Biomarkers Prev.* **13**, 658–661.

3. Lieberman, D. A., Prindiville, S., Weiss, D. G., and Willett, W. (2003) Risk factors for advanced colonic neoplasia and hyperplastic polyps in asymptomatic individuals. *JAMA* **290**, 2959–2967.

4. Emmons, K. M., McBride, C. M., Puleo, E., Pollak, K. I., Clipp, E., Kuntz, K., Marcus, B. H., Napolitano, M., Onken, J., Farraye, F., and Fletcher, R. (2005) Project PREVENT: a randomized trial to reduce multiple behavioral risk factors for colon cancer. *Cancer Epidemiol Biomarkers Prev.* **14**, 1453–1459.

5. Schatzkin, A. (2000) Intermediate markers as surrogate endpoints in cancer research. *Hematol Oncol Clin North Am.* **14**, 887–905.

6. Winawer, S. J., Zauber, A. G., Ho, M. N., O'Brien, M. J., Gottlieb, L. S., Sternberg, S. S., Waye, J. D., Schapiro, M., Bond, J. H., Panish, J. F., and et al. (1993) Prevention of colorectal cancer by colonoscopic polypectomy. The National Polyp Study Workgroup. *N Engl J Med.* **329**, 1977–1981.

7. Kinzler, K. W. and Vogelstein, B. (1996) Lessons from hereditary colorectal cancer. *Cell* **87**, 159–170.

8. Winawer, S. J. (2005) Screening of colorectal cancer. *Surg Oncol Clin N Am.* **14**, 699–722.

9. Hurlstone, D. P., Fujii, T., and Lobo, A. J. (2002) Early detection of colorectal cancer using high-magnification chromoscopic colonoscopy. *Br J Surg.* **89**, 272–282.

10. Hurlstone, D. P., Karajeh, M., Sanders, D. S., Drew, S. K., and Cross, S. S. (2005) Rectal aberrant crypt foci identified using high-magnification-chromoscopic colonoscopy: biomarkers for flat and depressed neoplasia. *Am J Gastroenterol.* **100**, 1283–1289.

11. Ross, A. S. and Waxman, I. (2006) Flat and depressed neoplasms of the colon in Western populations. *Am J Gastroenterol.* **101**, 172–180.

12. Srivastava, S., Verma, M., and Henson, D. E. (2001) Biomarkers for early detection of colon cancer. *Clin Cancer Res.* **7**, 1118–1126.

13. Takayama, T., Katsuki, S., Takahashi, Y., Ohi, M., Nojiri, S., Sakamaki, S., Kato, J., Kogawa, K., Miyake, H., and Niitsu, Y. (1998) Aberrant crypt foci of the colon as precursors of adenoma and cancer. *N Engl J Med.* **339**, 1277–1284.

14. Takayama, T., Ohi, M., Hayashi, T., Miyanishi, K., Nobuoka, A., Nakajima, T., Satoh, T., Takimoto, R., Kato, J., Sakamaki, S., and

Niitsu, Y. (2001) Analysis of K-ras, APC, and beta-catenin in aberrant crypt foci in sporadic adenoma, cancer, and familial adenomatous polyposis. *Gastroenterology* **121**, 599–611.

15. Bird, R. P. (1987) Observation and quantification of aberrant crypts in the murine colon treated with a colon carcinogen: preliminary findings. *Cancer Lett.* **37**, 147–151.

16. McLellan, E. A. and Bird, R. P. (1988) Aberrant crypts: potential preneoplastic lesions in the murine colon. *Cancer Research* **48**, 6187–6192.

17. Corpet, D. E. and Tache, S. (2002) Most effective colon cancer chemopreventive agents in rats: a systematic review of aberrant crypt foci and tumor data, ranked by potency. *Nutr Cancer* **43**, 1–21.

18. Roncucci, L., Modica, S., Pedroni, M., Tamassia, M. G., Ghidoni, M., Losi, L., Fante, R., Di Gregorio, C., Manenti, A., Gafa, L., and Ponz de Leon, M. (1998) Aberrant crypt foci in patients with colorectal cancer. *Br J Cancer* **77**, 2343–2348.

19. Yokota, T., Sugano, K., Kondo, H., Saito, D., Sugihara, K., Fukayama, N., Ohkura, H., Ochiai, A., and Yoshida, S. (1997) Detection of aberrant crypt foci by magnifying colonoscopy. *Gastrointest Endosc.* **46**, 61–65.

20. Hurlstone, D. P. and Cross, S. S. (2005) Role of aberrant crypt foci detected using high-magnification-chromoscopic colonoscopy in human colorectal carcinogenesis. *J Gastroenterol Hepatol.* **20**, 173–181.

21. Seike, K., Koda, K., Oda, K., Kosugi, C., Shimizu, K., Nishimura, M., Shioiri, M., Takano, S., Ishikura, H., and Miyazaki, M. (2006) Assessment of rectal aberrant crypt foci by standard chromoscopy and its predictive value for colonic advanced neoplasms. *Am J Gastroenterol.* **101**, 1362–1369.

22. Roncucci, L., Stamp, D., Medline, A., Cullen, J. B., and Bruce, W. R. (1991) Identification and quantification of aberrant crypt foci and microadenomas in the human colon. *Hum Pathol.* **22**, 287–294.

23. Rao, A. V., Janezic, S. A., Friday, D., and Kendall, C. W. (1992) Dietary cholesterol enhances the induction and development of colonic preneoplastic lesions in C57BL/6J and BALB/cJ mice treated with azoxymethane. *Cancer Lett.* **63**, 249–257.

24. Kendall, C. W., Koo, M., Sokoloff, E., and Rao, A. V. (1992) Effect of dietary oxidized cholesterol on azoxymethane-induced colonic preneoplasia in mice. *Cancer Lett.* **66**, 241–248.

25. Pretlow, T. P., Barrow, B. J., Ashton, W. S., O'Riordan, M. A., Pretlow, T. G., Jurcisek, J. A., and Stellato, T. A. (1991) Aberrant crypts: putative preneoplastic foci in human colonic mucosa. *Cancer Res.* **51**, 1564–1567.

26. Roncucci, L., Pedroni, M., Fante, R., Di Gregorio, C., and Ponz de Leon, M. (1993) Cell kinetic evaluation of human colonic aberrant crypts. (Colorectal Cancer Study Group of the University of Modena and the Health Care District 16, Modena, Italy). *Cancer Res.* **53**, 3726–3729.

27. Di Gregorio, C., Losi, L., Fante, R., Modica, S., Ghidoni, M., Pedroni, M., Tamassia, M. G., Gafa, L., Ponz de Leon, M., and Roncucci, L. (1997) Histology of aberrant crypt foci in the human colon. *Histopathology* **30**, 328–334.

28. Shpitz, B., Bomstein, Y., Mekori, Y., Cohen, R., Kaufman, Z., Neufeld, D., Galkin, M., and Bernheim, J. (1998) Aberrant crypt foci in human colons: distribution and histomorphologic characteristics. *Hum Pathol.* **29**, 469–475.

29. Bouzourene, H., Chaubert, P., Seelentag, W., Bosman, F. T., and Saraga, E. (1999) Aberrant crypt foci in patients with neoplastic and nonneoplastic colonic disease. *Hum Pathol.* **30**, 66–71

30. Yamada, Y., Yoshimi, N., Hirose, Y., Kawabata, K., Matsunaga, K., Shimizu, M., Hara, A., and Mori, H. (2000) Frequent beta-catenin gene mutations and accumulations of the protein in the putative preneoplastic lesions lacking macroscopic aberrant crypt foci appearance, in rat colon carcinogenesis. *Cancer Res.* **60**, 3323–3327.

31. Yamada, Y., Yoshimi, N., Hirose, Y., Matsunaga, K., Katayama, M., Sakata, K., Shimizu, M., Kuno, T., and Mori, H. (2001) Sequential analysis of morphological and biological properties of beta-catenin-accumulated crypts, provable premalignant lesions independent of aberrant crypt foci in rat colon carcinogenesis. *Cancer Res.* **61**, 1874–1878.

32. Paulsen, J. E., Loberg, E. M., Olstorn, H. B., Knutsen, H., Steffensen, I. L., and Alexander, J. (2005) Flat dysplastic aberrant crypt foci are related to tumorigenesis in the colon of azoxymethane-treated rat. *Cancer Res.* **65**, 121–129.

33. Caderni, G., Femia, A. P., Giannini, A., Favuzza, A., Luceri, C., Salvadori, M., and Dolara, P. (2003) Identification of mucin-depleted foci in the unsectioned colon of azoxymethane-treated rats: correlation with carcinogenesis. *Cancer Res.* **63**, 2388–2392.

34. Vaccina, F., Scorcioni, F., Pedroni, M., Tamassia, M. G., De Leon, M. P., De Pol, A., Marzona, L., and Roncucci, L. (1998) Scanning electron microscopy of aberrant crypt foci in human colorectal mucosa. *Anticancer Res.* **18**, 3451–3456.

35. Otori, K., Sugiyama, K., Hasebe, T., Fukushima, S., and Esumi, H. (1995) Emergence of adenomatous aberrant crypt foci (ACF) from hyperplastic ACF with concomitant increase in cell proliferation. *Cancer Research* **55**, 4743–4746.

36. Ochiai, M., Watanabe, M., Nakanishi, M., Taguchi, A., Sugimura, T., and Nakagama, H. (2005) Differential staining of dysplastic aberrant crypt foci in the colon facilitates prediction of carcinogenic potentials of chemicals in rats. *Cancer Lett.* **220**, 67–74.

37. Losi, L., Roncucci, L., di Gregorio, C., de Leon, M. P., and Benhattar, J. (1996) K-ras and p53 mutations in human colorectal aberrant crypt foci. *J Pathol.* **178**, 259–263.

38. Otori, K., Konishi, M., Sugiyama, K., Hasebe, T., Shimoda, T., Kikuchi-Yanoshita, R., Mukai, K., Fukushima, S., Miyaki, M., and Esumi, H. (1998) Infrequent somatic mutation of the adenomatous polyposis coli gene in aberrant crypt foci of human colon tissue. *Cancer* **83**, 896–900.

39. Greenspan, E. J., Cyr, J. L., Pleau, D. C., Levine, J., Rajan, T. V., Rosenberg, D. W., and Heinen, C. D. (2007) Microsatellite instability in aberrant crypt foci from patients without concurrent colon cancer. *Carcinogenesis* **28**, 769–776.

40. Cheng, L. and Lai, M. D. (2003) Aberrant crypt foci as microscopic precursors of colorectal cancer. *World J Gastroenterol.* **9**, 2642–2649.

41. Pretlow, T. P. and Pretlow, T. G. (2005) Mutant KRAS in aberrant crypt foci (ACF): initiation of colorectal cancer? *Biochim Biophys Acta* **1756**, 83–96.

42. Alrawi, S. J., Schiff, M., Carroll, R. E., Dayton, M., Gibbs, J. F., Kulavlat, M., Tan, D., Berman, K., Stoler, D. L., and Anderson, G. R. (2006) Aberrant crypt foci. *Anticancer Res.* **26**, 107–119.

43. Gupta, A. K., Pretlow, T. P., and Schoen, R. E. (2007) Aberrant crypt foci: what we know and what we need to know. *Clin Gastroenterol Hepatol.* **5**, 526–533.

44. Luo, L., Shen, G. Q., Stiffler, K. A., Wang, Q. K., Pretlow, T. G., and Pretlow, T. P. (2006) Loss of heterozygosity in human aberrant crypt foci (ACF), a putative precursor of colon cancer. *Carcinogenesis* **27**, 1153–1159.

45. Augenlicht, L. H., Richards, C., Corner, G., and Pretlow, T. P. (1996) Evidence for genomic instability in human colonic aberrant crypt foci. *Oncogene* **12**, 1767–1772

46. Heinen, C. D., Shivapurkar, N., Tang, Z., Groden, J., and Alabaster, O. (1996) Microsatellite instability in aberrant crypt foci from human colons. *Cancer Res.* **56**, 5339–5341.

47. Gryfe, R., Kim, H., Hsieh, E. T., Aronson, M. D., Holowaty, E. J., Bull, S. B., Redston, M., and Gallinger, S. (2000) Tumor microsatellite instability and clinical outcome in young patients with colorectal cancer. *N Engl J Med.* **342**, 69–77.

48. Polakis, P. (1999) The oncogenic activation of beta-catenin. *Curr Opin Genet Dev.* **9**, 15–21.

49. Giles, R. H., van Es, J. H., and Clevers, H. (2003) Caught up in a Wnt storm: Wnt signaling in cancer. *Biochim Biophys Acta* **1653**, 1–24.

50. Powell, S. M., Zilz, N., Beazer-Barclay, Y., Bryan, T. M., Hamilton, S. R., Thibodeau, S. N., Vogelstein, B., and Kinzler, K. W. (1992) APC mutations occur early during colorectal tumorigenesis. *Nature* **359**, 235–237.

51. Iwamoto, M., Ahnen, D. J., Franklin, W. A., and Maltzman, T. H. (2000) Expression of beta-catenin and full-length APC protein in normal and neoplastic colonic tissues. *Carcinogenesis* **21**, 1935–1940.

52. Jen, J., Powell, S. M., Papadopoulos, N., Smith, K. J., Hamilton, S. R., Vogelstein, B., and Kinzler, K. W. (1994) Molecular determinants of dysplasia in colorectal lesions. *Cancer Res.* **54**, 5523–5526.

53. Smith, A. J., Stern, H. S., Penner, M., Hay, K., Mitri, A., Bapat, B. V., and Gallinger, S. (1994) Somatic APC and K-ras codon 12 mutations in aberrant crypt foci from human colons. *Cancer Res.* **54**, 5527–5530.

54. Shivapurkar, N., Tang, Z., Ferreira, A., Nasim, S., Garett, C., and Alabaster, O. (1994) Sequential analysis of K-*ras* mutations in aberrant crypt foci and colonic tumors induced by azoxymethane in Fischer-344 rats on high-risk diet. *Carcinogenesis* **15**, 775–778.

55. Cohen, G., Mustafi, R., Chumsangsri, A., Little, N., Nathanson, J., Cerda, S., Jagadeeswaran, S., Dougherty, U., Joseph, L., Hart, J., Yerian, L., Tretiakova, M., Yuan, W., Obara, P., Khare, S., Sinicrope, F. A.,

Fichera, A., Boss, G. R., Carroll, R., and Bissonnette, M. (2006) Epidermal growth factor receptor signaling is up-regulated in human colonic aberrant crypt foci. *Cancer Res.* **66**, 5656–5664.

56. Fichera, A., Little, N., Jagadeeswaran, S., Dougherty, U., Sehdev, A., Mustafi, R., Cerda, S., Yuan, W., Khare, S., Tretiakova, M., Gong, C., Tallerico, M., Cohen, G., Joseph, L., Hart, J., Turner, J. R., and Bissonnette, M. (2007) Epidermal growth factor receptor signaling is required for microadenoma formation in the mouse azoxymethane model of colonic carcinogenesis. *Cancer Res.* **67**, 827–835.

57. Adler, D. G., Gostout, C. J., Sorbi, D., Burgart, L. J., Wang, L., and Harmsen, W. S. (2002) Endoscopic identification and quantification of aberrant crypt foci in the human colon. *Gastrointest Endosc.* **56**, 657–662.

58. Yamashita, N., Minamoto, T., Ochiai, A., Onda, M., and Esumi, H. (1995) Frequent and characteristic K-ras activation in aberrant crypt foci of colon. Is there preference among K-ras mutants for malignant progression? *Cancer* **75**, 1527–1533.

59. Siu, I. M., Pretlow, T. G., Amini, S. B., and Pretlow, T. P. (1997) Identification of dysplasia in human colonic aberrant crypt foci. *Am J Pathol.* **150**, 1805–1813.

60. Siu, I. M., Robinson, D. R., Schwartz, S., Kung, H. J., Pretlow, T. G., Petersen, R. B., and Pretlow, T. P. (1999) The identification of monoclonality in human aberrant crypt foci. *Cancer Res.* **59**, 63–66.

61. Gold, P., Shuster, J., and Freedman, S. O. (1978) Carcinoembryonic antigen (CEA) in clinical medicine: historical perspectives, pitfalls and projections. *Cancer* **42**, 1399–1405.

62. Pretlow, T. P., Roukhadze, E. V., O'Riordan, M. A., Chan, J. C., Amini, S. B., and Stellato, T. A. (1994) Carcinoembryonic antigen in human colonic aberrant crypt foci. *Gastroenterology* **107**, 1719–1725.

63. Miyoshi, Y., Ando, H., Nagase, H., Nishisho, I., Horii, A., Miki, Y., Mori, T., Utsunomiya, J., Baba, S., Petersen, G., and et al. (1992) Germ-line mutations of the APC gene in 53 familial adenomatous polyposis patients. *Proc Natl Acad Sci U S A* **89**, 4452–4456.

64. Qi, J., Zhu, Y. Q., Luo, J., and Tao, W. H. (2006) Hypermethylation and expression regulation of secreted frizzled-related protein genes in colorectal tumor. *World J Gastroenterol.* **12**, 7113–7117.

65. Samowitz, W. S., Powers, M. D., Spirio, L. N., Nollet, F., van Roy, F., and Slattery, M. L. (1999) b-catenin mutations are more frequent in small colorectal adenomas than in larger adenomas and invasive carcinomas. *Cancer Res.* **59**, 1442–1444.

66. Howe, L. R., Subbaramaiah, K., Chung, W. J., Dannenberg, A. J., and Brown, A. M. (1999) Transcriptional activation of cyclooxygenase-2 in Wnt-1-transformed mouse mammary epithelial cells. *Cancer Res.* **59**, 1572–1577.

67. Bissonnette, M., Khare, S., von Lintig, F. C., Wali, R. K., Nguyen, L., Zhang, Y., Hart, J., Skarosi, S., Varki, N., Boss, G. R., and Brasitus, T. A. (2000) Mutational and nonmutational activation of p21ras in rat colonic azoxymethane-induced tumors: effects on mitogen-activated protein kinase, cyclooxygenase-2, and cyclin D1. *Cancer Res.* **60**, 4602–4609.

68. Eisinger, A. L., Nadauld, L. D., Shelton, D. N., Peterson, P. W., Phelps, R. A., Chidester, S., Stafforini, D. M., Prescott, S. M., and Jones, D. A. (2006) The adenomatous polyposis coli tumor suppressor gene regulates expression of cyclooxygenase-2 by a mechanism that involves retinoic acid. *J Biol Chem.* **281**, 20474–20482.

69. Bjerknes, M., Cheng, H., Hay, K., and Gallinger, S. (1997) APC mutation and the crypt cycle in murine and human intestine. *Am J Pathol.* **150**, 833–839.

70. Otori, K., Oda, Y., Sugiyama, K., Hasebe, T., Mukai, K., Fujii, T., Tajiri, H., Yoshida, S., Fukushima, S., and Esumi, H. (1997) High frequency of K-ras mutations in human colorectal hyperplastic polyps. *Gut* **40**, 660–663.

71. Hill, M. J., Morson, B. C., and Bussey, H. J. (1978) Aetiology of adenoma—carcinoma sequence in large bowel. *Lancet* **1**, 245–247.

72. Day, D. W. and Morson, B. C. (1978) The adenoma-carcinoma sequence. *Major Probl Pathol.* **10**, 58–71.

73. Granqvist, S. (1981) Distribution of polyps in the large bowel in relation to age. A colonoscopic study. *Scand J Gastroenterol.* 16, 1025–1031.

74. Devesa, S. S. and Chow, W. H. (1993) Variation in colorectal cancer incidence in the United States by subsite of origin. *Cancer* **71**, 3819–3826.

75. Konstantakos, A. K., Siu, I. M., Pretlow, T. G., Stellato, T. A., and Pretlow, T. P. (1996) Human aberrant crypt foci with carcinoma in situ from a patient with sporadic colon cancer. *Gastroenterology* **111**, 772–777.

76. Boland, C. R., Sinicrope, F. A., Brenner, D. E., and Carethers, J. M. (2000) Colorectal cancer prevention and treatment. *Gastroenterology* **118**, 115–128.

77. Stevens, R. G., Swede, H., Heinen, C. D., Jablonski, M., Grupka, M., Ross, B., Parente, M., Tirnauer, J. S., Giardina, C., Rajan, T. V., Rosenberg, D. W., and Levine, J. (2007) Aberrant crypt foci in patients with a positive family history of sporadic colorectal cancer. *Cancer Lett.* **248**, 262–268.

78. Rudolph, R. E., Dominitz, J. A., Lampe, J. W., Levy, L., Qu, P., Li, S. S., Lampe, P. D., Bronner, M. P., and Potter, J. D. (2005) Risk factors for colorectal cancer in relation to number and size of aberrant crypt foci in humans. *Cancer Epidemiol Biomarkers Prev.* **14**, 605–608.

79. Armitage, P. and Doll, R. (1954) The age distribution of cancer and a multi-stage theory of carcinogenesis. *Br J Cancer* **8**, 1–12.

80. Papanikolaou, A., Wang, Q. S., Papanikolaou, D., Whiteley, H. E., and Rosenberg, D. W. (2000) Sequential and morphological analyses of aberrant crypt foci formation in mice of differing susceptibility to azoxymethane-induced colon carcinogenesis. *Carcinogenesis* **21**, 1567–1572.

81. Nambiar, P. R., Nakanishi, M., Gupta, R., Cheung, E., Firouzi, A., Ma, X. J., Flynn, C., Dong, M., Guda, K., Levine, J., Raja, R., Achenie, L., and Rosenberg, D. W. (2004) Genetic signatures of high- and low-risk aberrant crypt foci in a mouse model of sporadic colon cancer. *Cancer Res.* **64**, 6394–6401.

82. Shpitz, B., Klein, E., Buklan, G., Neufeld, D., Nissan, A., Freund, H. R., Grankin, M., and Bernheim, J. (2003) Suppressive effect of aspirin on aberrant crypt foci in patients with colorectal cancer. *Gut* **52**, 1598–1601.

83. Moxon, D., Raza, M., Kenney, R., Ewing, R., Arozullah, A., Mason, J. B., and Carroll, R. E. (2005) Relationship of aging and tobacco use with the development of aberrant crypt foci in a predominantly African-American population. *Clin Gastroenterol Hepatol.* **3**, 271–278.

84. Slaughter, D. P., Southwick, H. W., and Smejkal, W. (1953) Field cancerization in oral stratified squamous epithelium; clinical implications of multicentric origin. *Cancer* **6**, 963–968.

85. Benner, S. E., Hong, W. K., Lippman, S. M., Lee, J. S., and Hittelman, W. M. (1992) Intermediate biomarkers in upper aerodigestive tract and lung chemoprevention trials. *J Cell Biochem Suppl.* **16G**, 33–38.

86. Wattenberg, L. W. (1985) Chemoprevention of cancer. *Cancer Res.* **45**, 1–8.

87. Sandler, R. S., Halabi, S., Baron, J. A., Budinger, S., Paskett, E., Keresztes, R., Petrelli, N., Pipas, J. M., Karp, D. D., Loprinzi, C. L., Steinbach, G., and Schilsky, R. (2003) A randomized trial of aspirin to prevent colorectal adenomas in patients with previous colorectal cancer. *N Engl J Med.* **348**, 883–890.

88. Baron, J. A., Cole, B. F., Sandler, R. S., Haile, R. W., Ahnen, D., Bresalier, R., McKeown-Eyssen, G., Summers, R. W., Rothstein, R., Burke, C. A., Snover, D. C., Church, T. R., Allen, J. I., Beach, M., Beck, G. J., Bond, J. H., Byers, T., Greenberg, E. R., Mandel, J. S., Marcon, N., Mott, L. A., Pearson, L., Saibil, F., and van Stolk, R. U. (2003) A randomized trial of aspirin to prevent colorectal adenomas. *N Engl J Med.* **348**, 891–899.

Chapter 18

Determinants of Incidence of Primary Fallopian Tube Carcinoma (PFTC)

Annika Riska and Arto Leminen

Abstract

Primary fallopian tube carcinoma (PFTC) is a rare malignancy, but its incidence has been rising during the last decades and varies between 2.9/1,000,000 and 5.7/1,000,000. The epidemiology of PFTC has been sparsely studied. In Finland, the incidence rate has been rising during the last decades. The rise has been highest in the cities, in higher social classes, and in certain specific occupations. Parity gives protection against this disease, as does a previous sterilization procedure. Earlier thoughts of a previous salpingitis as a possible promoter of PFTC seem not to hold. Previous infections such as *Chlamydia trachomatis* infections or human papillomavirus infections cannot be regarded as risk factors. In this chapter, we clarify the possible epidemiological factors behind this disease.

Key words: Primary fallopian tube carcinoma, sociodemographic determinants, parity, *Chlamydia trachomatis*, human papillomavirus, sterilization.

1. Introduction

Primary fallopian tube carcinoma (PFTC) is a rare malignancy accounting for 0.3–1.6% of female genital tract malignancies in Western countries (*1–3*). It was first described by Renaud in 1847. According to Ricci, a case recorded by Renaud is in an unpublished manuscript in the library of the Royal College of Surgeons (*4*). Later it was reported by Rokitansky in 1861, but it was Orthmann who described PFTC as its own entity in 1886 (*5*). PFTC resembles ovarian carcinoma. The fallopian tube and ovary both develop from the Müllerian duct in organogenesis, the two diseases have a similar pattern of spread, they are diagnosed and treated similarly, and the prognosis is also quite alike.

M. Verma (ed.), *Methods of Molecular Biology, Cancer Epidemiology, vol. 472*
© 2009 Humana Press, a part of Springer Science + Business Media, Totowa, NJ
Book doi: 10.1007/978-1-60327-492-0

Histologically, more than 90% of the cases are serous adenocarcinomas and the histological appearance resembles that of ovarian serous carcinomas. Occasional cases of endometrioid, clear cell, transitional cell, and glassy cell carcinomas have been reported *(6)*. So far, fewer than 2,500 cases have been reported in different studies worldwide, most of the reports being case reports. Although the etiological factors of PFTC have been largely unknown, they have been considered to be similar to those of ovarian carcinoma. During the last years, we have studied the possible protective and risk factors for PFTC. We have tried to find out why the incidence has been rising during the last decades.

2. The Incidence of PFTC and its Sociodemographic Determinants

Incidence refers to the number of new cases developing during some specific time interval. An average annual incidence rate of 3.6 of PFTC cases per million women per year was reported by Rosenblatt et al. *(7)*. Incidence rates were examined for epithelial malignant fallopian tube neoplasms diagnosed between 1973 and 1984 and reported to nine population-based cancer registries in the United States. Age-specific incidence followed a pattern similar to that observed for ovarian and endometrial neoplasms, rising rapidly during the reproductive years and flattening out thereafter. The incidence rate varied by race, with Caucasian women (including Hispanics) having a 14% higher rate than African Americans. During the period 1995–1999, the Surveillance, Epidemiology, and End Results (SEER) program reported an age-adjusted incidence rate of 3.3/1,000,000 among Caucasian women *(8)*. In Denmark, the incidence rate around 1980 was 2.9/1,000,000 *(9)*.

We studied the incidence rates of PFTC in Finland between the years 1953 and 1997 using the Finnish Cancer Registry. More than 99% of all cancer cases have been reported to the Finnish Cancer Registry since 1953 *(10)*. The Registry obtains information from hospitals and other institutions with inpatient beds, general practitioners, pathology and cytology laboratories, and from death certificates with cancer diagnoses. In the 1990s, about 95% of the cases were based on the death certificate data only *(11)*. The age-adjusted incidence of PFTC in Finland increased from 1.2/1,000,000 in 1953–1957 to 5.4/1,000,000 in 1993–1997, indicating a 4.5-fold increase, corresponding to a 7-fold increase in the absolute number of new cases **(Table 18.1)** *(3)*. Some part of the rise of incidence may be explained by the earlier difficulties in separating the advanced cases of PFTC and ovarian carcinoma histologically from each other. The main increase was in the oldest

Table 18.1

Annual number of new cases and female population at risk, and incidence rates per 1,000,000 for primary fallopian tube carcinoma in Finland by period of diagnosis

Period	n	Population	Rate[a]
1953–1957	15	11,011,700	1.2
1958–1962	31	11,508,000	2.3
1963–1967	47	11,888,100	3.3
1968–1972	40	11,933,500	2.5
1973–1977	39	12,174,800	2.4
1978–1982	46	12,378,000	2.7
1983–1987	69	12,655,100	3.6
1988–1992	90	12,869,900	4.3
1993–1997	108	13,119,000	5.4

[a] Adjusted for age to the world standard population From ref. [3]

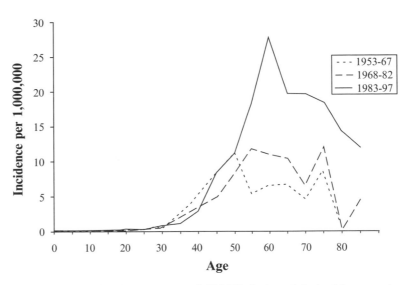

Fig. 18.1 Age-specific incidence rates per/1,000,000 of primary fallopian tube cancer in Finland expressed in 15-year periods from 1953 to 1997 [3].

age groups. During 1953–1967, the peak incidence occurred in groups aged 50–54 years, whereas during 1983–1997, the incidence was highest in the group between 60 and 64 years of age. The age patterns in Finland and Denmark resemble each other, with peak incidence occurring between the ages of 60 and 64 years (**Fig. 18.1**), whereas in the USA, the peak incidence has been highest between the ages of 70 and 74 years. In our materials from case–control hospital-based studies in Finland, the mean age of the patients has been 61 years (range, 40–82 years) *(12, 13)* and in our multicenter study of second primary cancers after first PFTC, including data from 13 cancer registries in Europe, Australia, Canada, and Singapore, at the time of diagnosis of PFTC, 18.9% of patients were 21–49 years, 28.8% were 50–59 years, and 52.3% were 60–92 years of age *(14)*.

In a study from the United Kingdom, incidence in patients with PFTC was studied in the catchment area of the Royal United Hospital (RUH) in Bath between 1999 and 2004. They found an incidence rate of 5.7/1,000,000/year, which resembles our findings. Their data suggested a relative increase in the number of patients with PFTC over the study period. The incidence of ovarian cancer increased during this period also, but the latter change was much smaller *(15)*. These findings support our findings of a true increase in incidence of PFTC, and not an increase caused by better diagnostic methods.

Social class. Finland organized an official census of the Finnish population on the last day of 1970 *(16)*. All residents in Finland were expected to complete a comprehensive questionnaire including information on occupation, which was coded into more than 400 occupational categories. The response rate was 98% *(17)*. Also four social classes were defined on the basis of education, occupation, industrial status, and industry groupings *(16, 18)*. Financially dependent persons (e.g., housewives and students) were classified by the occupation of their supporter. The four social classes were defined as follows:

Class I.   Managers and other higher administrative or clerical employees, farmers owning more than 50 hectares of land.

Class II. Lower administrative or clerical employees, small-scale entrepreneurs, farmers owning 15 to 49.9 hectares of land.

Class III. Skilled and specialized workers, farmers owning 5 to 14.9 hectares of land.

Class IV. Laborers, farm and forestry workers, institution inmates, farmers owning <5 hectares of land, and retired persons whose former occupation was unknown.

The cancer records of the Finnish Cancer Registry from 1971 to 1995 for persons born in 1906–1945 were linked with the census data *(3)*. The expected numbers of cases were calculated by multiplying the stratum-specific number of person-years by the respective calendar period and birth cohort-specific incidence rate of all Finnish women. The standardized incidence ratio (SIR) values were the ratio of the observed to the expected number of cases. The methods for calculating the SIRs in relation to occupation and social class have been described in detail by Pukkala *(19)*. The confidence intervals (CI) were defined with the assumption that the observed number of cases followed a Poisson distribution.

In the study, 268 cases of PFTC were detected in 1971–1995 in women born 1906–1945, for whom information on social class were available from the Population Census. The incidence rate of PFTC was greatest in the higher social classes (**Table 18.2**): the ratio of combined SIR of classes I and II compared with that of class IV was 1.8 (95% CI, 1.2–2.6). In Finland, in upper social classes, the incidence of breast and endometrial cancer cases has also been higher than in lower social classes, but for endometrial cancer, the positive social class association disappeared in the early 1980s. For cancers of the vulva and ovary, no clear differences by social class have been observed *(20)*.

Place of residence. During the follow-up period between the years 1953 and 1997 in Finland, the incidence of PFTC was highest in the main cities, but the relative rise was higher in rural areas than in the cities, perhaps reflecting the adoption of an urban lifestyle factor in rural areas. Part of the variation between these areas could be explained by changes in parity. The lower incidence rates in rural areas could reflect the influence of environmental and lifestyle factors in the etiology of PFTC. It could also reflect the differences in availability of health care services between rural and urban areas.

Occupation. We also studied the incidence of PFTC in different occupational branches. The incidence of PFTC was high in various occupations in health care, technical, physical and social

Table 18.2
Number of women born between 1906 and 1945 in the cohort in 1970; and observed and expected numbers and standardized incidence ratios (SIRs) of primary fallopian tube carcinomas observed during 1971–1995 among women, by social class

Social class	Observed	Expected	SIR (95% CI)	Women in cohort (N)
I	25	20	1.27 (0.81–1.87)	88,737
II	95	74	1.28 (1.04–1.57)	405,654
III	114	128	0.89 (0.74–1.06)	595,805
IV	34	46	0.73 (0.51–1.02)	177,474
Total	268	268	1.00 (reference)	1,267,670

Modified from ref. [3]

Table 18.3
Observed number of cases and standardized incidence ratios (SIRs) with 95% confidence intervals (CIs) for PFTC in the main occupational categories from 1971 through 1995, women born from 1906 through 1945

Occupation	Observed	SIR (95% CI)
"Academic" work[a]	37	1.63 (1.15–2.25)
Administrative and clerical work	35	1.60 (1.12–2.23)
All economically active persons	180	1.11 (0.96–1.28)
Transport and communications	6	1.09 (0.40–2.37)
Whole population	268	1.00 (0.88–1.12)
Services	32	1.00 (0.69–1.42)
Sales professions	16	0.98 (0.56–1.59)
Industrial and construction work	27	0.95 (0.63–1.38)
Economically inactive[b]	88	0.83 (0.66–1.02)
Farming, forestry, and fishing	27	0.79 (0.52–1.14)

[a] Technical, physical science, social science, humanistic, and artistic work. [b] >50% housewives From ref. [3].

science, humanistic and artistic work, as well as administrative and clerical work (Table 18.3). In specific occupations, increased risks of PFTC were observed among private secretaries (SIR 4.4; 95% CI, 1.4–10), nurses (SIR 4.0; 95% CI, 2.1–7.0), hairdressers and barbers (SIR 3.9; 95% CI, 1.3–9.2), and bookkeepers and accountants (SIR 3.6; 95% CI, 1.6–7.1).

The differences in incidence among women in different occupations are difficult to explain, but part of the variation may be explained by real occupational exposures even though we do not have any linkage studies on the occupational carcinogenic agents and PFTC yet. We do know that among ovarian cancer patients there have been detected indications of elevated risks for aromatic hydrocarbon solvents, leather dust, man-made vitreous fibers, and high levels of asbestos, diesel, and gasoline (21). The lower incidence rates among workers in the fields of farming, forestry, and fishing might be explained by environmental and lifestyle factors.

3. Protective and Risk Factors of PFTC

In case—controls studies, associations with low parity and infertility among PFTC patients have been reported. The nulliparity rate among PFTC patients has varied between 17 and 45% (2, 6, 15, 22) and the infertility rate has been up to 31% (2, 6, 23).

In our previous study, the relationship among parity, a previous sterilization procedure, and a previous hysterectomy and the risk of PFTC was evaluated (14). We selected all women reported to have had PFTC in 1975–2004 (n = 573) from the Finnish Cancer Registry. Ten age-matched controls per case (n = 5,473) were randomly selected from the Finnish Central Population Registry (CPR) for each PFTC patient. The control subject had to be alive at the time when diagnosis of the PFTC was completed. The dates of birth of children of PFTC patients and control subjects were collected from the CPR.

The CPR has covered information on all residents of Finland since 1967, and on their relatives since 1973 (24). It administers the Finnish system of unique identifiers (IDs). It was started in 1964, and by 1967 all Finnish citizens and permanent residents had received their own ID. These IDs are used in practically all Finnish registries, and we used them as linkage keys to combine information from various registries in this study. The sterilization, hysterectomy, and salpingectomy data were obtained from the Hospital Discharge Registry (HILMO). The linkage has been described in detail in our article by Riska et al. (14).

The strongest known protective factor as regards PFTC is parity. The protection gets stronger with increasing number of deliveries: odds ratio (OR) for one to two deliveries, 0.63 (95% CI, 0.44–0.91); and for at least three deliveries 0.32 (95% CI, 0.19–0.52) (25). In univariate analysis, an older age (≥35 years) at first birth is also protective. A previous sterilization gives a mild protection, but a previous hysterectomy does not. In our study, a previous cancer was a significant risk factor for PFTC (OR, 1.69; 95% CI, 1.08–2.67), especially a previous breast cancer (OR, 1.69; 95% CI, 1.08–2.67).

These present findings of the protective effect of parity on PFTC correlate with the results of studies on ovarian cancer (26–30). Each full-term pregnancy diminishes the risk of ovarian cancer by 15 to 20% (26, 27). Earlier studies have revealed varying results concerning the age at first birth on the risk of ovarian cancer. Some studies have revealed an increased risk of ovarian cancer at an older age at first birth (31), some a decreased risk (32–34), and some revealed no association at all (27, 35).

The protective effect of parity on PFTC may reflect the hormonal background for the disease as the high circulating levels of progesterone during pregnancy induce apoptosis of transformed epithelial cells *(36)*. In upper social classes, the number of deliveries has been lower than in lower social classes. This is in line with our results of the higher incidence of PFTC in upper social classes.

The mild protection effect of a previous sterilization procedure on PFTC is in line with the protection effect on ovarian cancer *(37–39)*. The protective effect has been theorized to be based on blocking of ascending carcinogenic factors from uterus to ovaries *(40, 41)*.

Our serological case–control studies of previous infections of *Chlamydia trachomatis* or human papillomavirus (HPV) on the risk PFTC *(12, 13)* do not confirm the earlier thoughts of a previous salpingitis to be a promoter for PFTC *(42)*, and so ascending factors other than infectious ones should be sought for risk factors for PFTC.

In 11 to 15% of PFTC patients there has been another malignancy before the diagnosis of PFTC *(2, 15, 25, 43)*, especially breast and colon cancer. This association between breast and PFTC might reflect the similar hormone responsiveness of these two cancers.

4. Conclusions and Future Prospects

PFTC is a rare but highly aggressive malignancy with 5-year survival rates varying between 22 and 57%. Only 4% of the PFTC are diagnosed preoperatively. The incidence of PFTC has been rising, especially in upper social classes and among women living in large cities. In certain occupations, there is a risk for this disease, but studies on the specific carcinogenic agents have not yet been performed. Parity is a clear protective factor for PFTC. Factors other than infectious ones should be sought for this disease. As it seems that this carcinoma is hormonally reactive, studies of the effect of hormone-replacement therapy as a possible risk factor should be performed.

References

1. Nordin, A. J. (1994) Primary Carcinoma of the Fallopian Tube: A 20-Year Literature Review. *Obstet. Gynecol. Surv.* **49**, 349–361.

2. Baekelandt, M., Jorunn Nesbakken, A., Kristensen, G. B., Trope, C. G., and Abeler, V. M. (2000) Carcinoma of the Fallopian Tube. *Cancer.* **89**, 2076–2084.

3. Riska, A., Leminen, A., and Pukkala, E. (2003) Sociodemographic Determinants of Incidence of Primary Fallopian Tube Carcinoma, Finland 1953–97. *Int. J. Cancer.* **104**, 643–645.

4. Ricci, J. V. (1945) *One Hundred Years of Gynecology.* Blakiston, Philadelphia.

5. Orthmann, E. G. (1888) Primareskarzinom in Einertuberkulosen. *Zeitschrift für Geburtshülfe und Gynäkologie.* **15**, 211–237.

6. Alvarado-Cabrero, I., Young, R. H., Vamvakas, E. C., and Scully, R. E. (1999) Carcinoma of the Fallopian Tube: A Clinicopathological

Study of 105 Cases with Observations on Staging and Prognostic Factors. *Gynecol. Oncol.* 72, 367–379.

7. Rosenblatt, K. A., Weiss, N. S., and Schwartz, S. M. (1989) Incidence of Malignant Fallopian Tube Tumors. *Gynecol. Oncol.* 35, 236–239.

8. National Cancer Institute. (2001) *SEER Program. 12 Geographic Areas for 1995–1999*. National Cancer Institute, Cancer Statistics Branch, Bethesda, MD.

9. Pfeiffer, P., Mogensen, H., Amtrup, F., and Honore, E. (1989) Primary Carcinoma of the Fallopian Tube. A Retrospective Study of Patients Reported to the Danish Cancer Registry in a Five-Year Period. *Acta Oncol.* 28, 7–11.

10. Teppo, L., Pukkala, E., and Lehtonen, M. (1994) Data Quality and Quality Control of a Population-Based Cancer Registry. Experience in Finland. *Acta Oncol.* 33, 365–369.

11. Finnish Cancer Registry. Institute for statistical and epidemiological cancer research. (2000) Cancer Incidence in Finland 1996 and 1997. Cancer statistics of the national research and development centre for welfare and health, Helsinki: Cancer Society of Finland.

12. Riska, A., Finne, P., Alfthan, H., Anttila, T., Jalkanen, J., Sorvari, T., Stenman, U. H., Paavonen, J., and Leminen, A. (2006) Past Chlamydial Infection is Not Associated with Primary Fallopian Tube Carcinoma. *Eur. J. Cancer.* 42, 1835–1838.

13. Riska, A., Finne, P., Koskela, P., Alfthan, H., Jalkanen, J., Lehtinen, M., Sorvari, T., Stenman, U. H., Paavonen, J., and Leminen, A. (2007) Human Papillomavirus Infection and Primary Fallopian Tube Carcinoma: A Seroepidemiological Study. *BJOG.* 114, 425–429.

14. Riska, A., Pukkala, E., Scelo, G., Mellemkjaer, L., Hemminki, K., Weiderpass, E., McBride, M. L., Pompe-Kirn, V., Tracey, E., Brewster, D. H., Kliewer, E. V., Tonita, J. M., Kee-Seng, C., Jonasson, J. G., Martos, C., Boffetta, P., and Brennan, P. (2007) Second Primary Malignancies in Females with Primary Fallopian Tube Cancer. *Int. J. Cancer.* 120, 2047–2051.

15. Clayton, N. L., Jaaback, K. S., and Hirschowitz, L. (2005) Primary Fallopian Tube Carcinoma—the Experience of a UK Cancer Centre and a Review of the Literature. *J. Obstet. Gynaecol.* 25, 694–702.

16. Central Statistical Office of Finland. (1974) *Population Census 1970: Occupation and Social Position*. Central Statistical Office of Finland, Helsinki.

17. Sauli, H. (1979) Occupational Mortality in 1971–75. *Studies.* 54. Central Statistical Office of Finland, Helsinki.

18. Rauhala, U. (1966) *Social Structures of the Finnish Society*. Ministry of Social Affairs and Health, Helsinki.

19. Pukkala, E. (1995) *Cancer Risk by Social Class and Occupation: A Survey of 109 000 Cancer Cases among Finns of Working Age. Contributions to Epidemiology and Biostatistics*. Karger, Basel.

20. Pukkala, E. and Weiderpass, E. (1999) Time Trends in Socio-Economic Differences in Incidence Rates of Cancers of the Breast and Female Genital Organs (Finland, 1971–1995). *Int. J. Cancer.* 81, 56–61.

21. Vasama-Neuvonen, K., Pukkala, E., Paakkulainen, H., Mutanen, P., Weiderpass, E., Boffetta, P., Shen, N., Kauppinen, T., Vainio, H., and Partanen, T. (1999) Ovarian Cancer and Occupational Exposures in Finland. *Am. J. Ind. Med.* 36, 83–89.

22. Hellstrom, A. C., Silfversward, C., Nilsson, B., and Pettersson, F. (1994) Carcinoma of the Fallopian Tube. A Clinical and Histopathologic Review. The Radiumhemmet Series. *Int. J. Gynecol. Cancer.* 4, 395–400.

23. Peters, W. A., 3rd, Andersen, W. A., Hopkins, M. P., Kumar, N. B., and Morley, G. W. (1988) Prognostic Features of Carcinoma of the Fallopian Tube. *Obstet. Gynecol.* 71, 757–762.

24. Gissler, M. and Haukka, J. (2004) Finnish Health and Social Welfare Registers in Epidemiological Research. 14, 1–8.

25. Riska, A., Sund, R., Pukkala, E., Gissler, M., and Leminen, A. (2007) Parity, Tubal Sterilization, Hysterectomy and Risk of Primary Fallopian Tube Carcinoma in Finland, 1975–2004. *Int. J. Cancer.* 120, 1351–1354.

26. Adami, H. O., Hsieh, C. C., Lambe, M., Trichopoulos, D., Leon, D., Persson, I., Ekbom, A., and Janson, P. O. (1994) Parity, Age at First Childbirth, and Risk of Ovarian Cancer. *Lancet.* 344, 1250–1254.

27. Risch, H. A., Marrett, L. D., and Howe, G. R. (1994) Parity, Contraception, Infertility, and the Risk of Epithelial Ovarian Cancer. *Am. J. Epidemiol.* 140, 585–597.

28. Albrektsen, G., Heuch, I., and Kvale, G. (1996) Further Evidence of a Dual Effect of a Completed Pregnancy on Breast Cancer Risk. *Cancer Causes Control.* 7, 487–488.

29. Riman, T., Persson, I., and Nilsson, S. (1998) Hormonal Aspects of Epithelial Ovarian Cancer: Review of Epidemiological Evidence. *Clin. Endocrinol. (Oxf).* 49, 695–707.

30. Hinkula, M., Pukkala, E., Kyyronen, P., and Kauppila, A. (2006) Incidence of Ovarian Cancer of Grand Multiparous Women—A Population-Based Study in Finland. *Gynecol. Oncol.* **103**, 207–211.

31. Booth, M., Beral, V., and Smith, P. (1989) Risk Factors for Ovarian Cancer: A Case-Control Study. *Br. J. Cancer.* **60**, 592–598.

32. Purdie, D., Green, A., Bain, C., Siskind, V., Ward, B., Hacker, N., Quinn, M., Wright, G., Russell, P., and Susil, B. (1995) Reproductive and Other Factors and Risk of Epithelial Ovarian Cancer: An Australian Case-Control Study. Survey of Women's Health Study Group. *Int. J. Cancer.* **62**, 678–684.

33. Cooper, G. S., Schildkraut, J. M., Whittemore, A. S., and Marchbanks, P. A. (1999) Pregnancy Recency and Risk of Ovarian Cancer. *Cancer Causes Control.* **10**, 397–402.

34. Titus-Ernstoff, L., Perez, K., Cramer, D. W., Harlow, B. L., Baron, J. A., and Greenberg, E. R. (2001) Menstrual and Reproductive Factors in Relation to Ovarian Cancer Risk. *Br. J. Cancer.* **84**, 714–721.

35. Hankinson, S. E., Colditz, G. A., Hunter, D. J., Willett, W. C., Stampfer, M. J., Rosner, B., Hennekens, C. H., and Speizer, F. E. (1995) A Prospective Study of Reproductive Factors and Risk of Epithelial Ovarian Cancer. *Cancer.* **76**, 284–290.

36. Rodriguez, G. C., Walmer, D. K., Cline, M., Krigman, H., Lessey, B. A., Whitaker, R. S., Dodge, R., and Hughes, C. L. (1998) Effect of Progestin on the Ovarian Epithelium of Macaques: Cancer Prevention through Apoptosis? *J. Soc. Gynecol. Investig.* **5**, 271–276.

37. Green, A., Purdie, D., Bain, C., Siskind, V., Russell, P., Quinn, M., and Ward, B. (1997) Tubal Sterilisation, Hysterectomy and Decreased Risk of Ovarian Cancer. Survey of Women's Health Study Group. *Int. J. Cancer.* **71**, 948–951.

38. Miracle-McMahill, H. L., Calle, E. E., Kosinski, A. S., Rodriguez, C., Wingo, P. A., Thun, M. J., and Heath, C. W., Jr. (1997) Tubal Ligation and Fatal Ovarian Cancer in a Large Prospective Cohort Study. *Am. J. Epidemiol.* **145**, 349–357.

39. Kjaer, S. K., Mellemkjaer, L., Brinton, L. A., Johansen, C., Gridley, G., and Olsen, J. H. (2004) Tubal Sterilization and Risk of Ovarian, Endometrial and Cervical Cancer. A Danish Population-Based Follow-Up Study of More than 65,000 Sterilized Women. *Int. J. Epidemiol.* **33**, 596–602.

40. Cramer, D. W. and Welch, W. R. (1983) Determinants of Ovarian Cancer Risk. II. Inferences regarding Pathogenesis. *J. Natl. Cancer Inst.* **71**, 717–721.

41. Cornelison, T. L., Natarajan, N., Piver, M. S., and Mettlin, C. J. (1997) Tubal Ligation and the Risk of Ovarian Carcinoma. *Cancer Detect. Prev.* **21**, 1–6.

42. Gungor, T., Keskin, H. L., Zergeroglu, S., Keskin, E. A., Yalcin, H., Aydogdu, T., and Kucukozkan, T. (2003) Tuberculous Salpingitis in Two of Five Primary Fallopian Tube Carcinomas. *J. Obstet. Gynaecol.* **23**, 193–195.

43. Riska, A., Alfthan, H., Finne, P., Jalkanen, J., Sorvari, T., Stenman, U. H., and Leminen, A. (2006) Preoperative Serum hCGbeta as a Prognostic Marker in Primary Fallopian Tube Carcinoma. *Tumour Biol.* **27**, 43–49.

Chapter 19

The Changing Epidemiology of Lung Cancer

Chee-Keong Toh

Abstract

The 20th century witnessed the scourge of lung cancer as the disease rapidly rose the ranks to become the commonest cause of cancer mortality in the world. Epidemiological evidence conclusively associated cigarette smoking with the causation of lung cancer in the 1950s. Since then and the few decades after, lung cancer of the squamous cell or small cell histological subtypes was mainly diagnosed among male smokers in developed countries. As we move into the 21st century, the incidence of lung cancer is unlikely to abate but the burden will shift from the developed to the less-developed countries. Other epidemiological changes of lung cancer include the narrowing of the gap between men and women affected by the disease, predominance of the adenocarcinoma histological subtypes as well as more never-smokers afflicted with the disease. Unless we eliminate tobacco smoking completely, lung cancer will continue its wrath into the 21st century.

Key words: Lung cancer, epidemiology, women, never-smokers, developing countries, adenocarcinoma.

1. Introduction

Lung cancer started out as a rare disease and became the commonest cause of cancer mortality in the world toward the end of the 20th century (1). Epidemiological studies in the 1950s (2, 3) linked the causal association between cigarette smoke with lung cancer and this was followed by conclusive reports from the Advisory Committee to the Surgeon General of the Public Health Service, USA (4) as well as the Royal College of Physicians, London, UK (5) in the 1960s. As lung cancer incidence parallels that of past smoking trends, with a rough estimate of a 20-year lag period, we are beginning to see a decline in the rates of lung cancer among the developed countries, which reflects the

M. Verma (ed.), *Methods of Molecular Biology, Cancer Epidemiology, vol. 472*
© 2009 Humana Press, a part of Springer Science + Business Media, Totowa, NJ
Book doi: 10.1007/978-1-60327-492-0

encouraging decline in smoking prevalence in the 1980s. Other than this decrease in lung cancer incidence, we are observing a change in the ratio of the sexes inflicted with the disease. In the initial report of the Advisory Committee to the US Surgeon General *(4)*, the conclusion was limited to men as there was not enough evidence to implicate the lung cancer-causing effect of smoke on women. Since then, lung cancer has not only been proven to cause lung cancer in women *(6)*, but has also risen to become the commonest cause of cancer death among women. In 2002, almost half of the lung cancer cases were found in the developing countries, a significant change from 1980 when most cases occurred in the developed countries *(1)*. The histological subtype of lung cancer has also shifted from a predominance of squamous cell carcinoma (SCC) and small cell lung cancer (SCLC) to that of adenocarcinoma toward the latter half of the 20th century *(7)*, which is a likely consequence of the changing composition of cigarette smoke. Without doubt, lung cancer occurs mainly in smokers, but recently it appears that a not insignificant proportion of never-smokers are afflicted with this disease *(8)*. This is especially seen in studies involving women from Asian countries along the Pacific Rim. Thus, the established epidemiology of lung cancer in the 1950s being that of a disease of male smokers with SCC in developed countries is slowly, but surely, showing signs of change toward that of a cancer that includes women, never-smokers, adenocarcinoma, and the developing countries at the beginning of the 21th century.

2. Women and Lung Cancer

The initial illusion in the 1950s that women may be immune to smoking-related diseases was due solely to the fact that women's cigarette use lagged behind that of men *(8)*. Men took up smoking at the early decades of the 20th century. In 1923, it was already reported that 51.8% of males aged 18 years and older smoked cigarettes. Lung cancer incidence and mortality in men started to rise in the 1930s and by the time of the landmark epidemiological studies in 1950s, the men examined in these studies were already longtime cigarette smokers. On the other hand, widespread cigarette use among women started about 25 years later. About 18% of women were regular cigarette smokers in 1935 as compared with 33.3% in 1965. Thus, there were not many women included in the analysis of the 1950–1960s reports and those women smokers included were only in their 20s and 30s. By 1980, the first US Surgeon General report on women and smoking *(8)* had enough evidence to conclude that women smokers face the same risks as men smokers for lung cancer. The lung cancer epidemic in women began in the 1970s and surpassed breast cancer to become the commonest cause of cancer death among women in the 1980s.

As tobacco smoking remains the main etiologic agent for lung cancer, it is of increasing concern that the smoking prevalence among women is not showing signs of significant decline over the past years, unlike that of men **(Fig. 19.1)**. In 1965, 51.1% of US men and 33.3% of US women were regular smokers. By 1998, smoking prevalence among men had dropped by half to 26.4%, while that for women had declined by a third to 22% *(9)*. The smoking prevalence among adolescent girls is also worrying. Based on the 1991–2001 Youth Risk Behavior Survey, USA, the percentage of high school girls who reported current smoking was 27.3% in 1991 and at 27.7% in 2001. There was no change for the 10 years between 1991 and 2001, and there was no difference between the boys and girls *(10)*. In the 2002 US survey of high school students, 55.3% of girls reported having ever used cigarettes *(11)*. Globally, in the Global Youth Tobacco Survey, it was found that although boys are more likely than girls to be current tobacco smokers, the difference between them is smaller than that between men and women *(12)*.

Initiating cigarettes is a prelude to continuing the habit and this portends a big problem in the future as more girls light up in their adolescence. Factors influencing smoking among girls include parental and peer smoking habits, educational level, and socioeconomic status. They are more likely than boys to perceive that

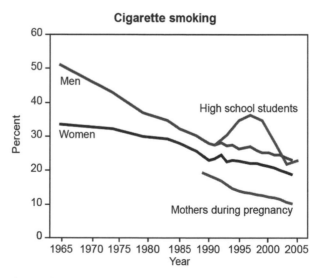

Sources: Centers for Disease Control and Prevention, National Center for Health Statistics, *Health, United States, 2006*, Figure 10. Data from the National Health Interview Survey, Youth Risk Behavior Survey, National Vital Statistics System.

Fig. 19.1. Cigarette smoking among men, women, high school students, and mothers during pregnancy: United States, 1965–2005.

smoking can have beneficial effects on the control of weight and negative moods *(9)*. The tobacco industry has turned these factors to their advantage to entice women into smoking using slim, attractive models to enforce the theme of social desirability and independence with cigarettes. Furthermore, studies have found that women may be less successful than men in their attempts to stop smoking. Using data from the National Health Interview Surveys (NHIS) USA 1965–1994, prevalence of cessation of smoking was consistently higher for men than for women *(13)*. The ability to quit smoking is dependent on psychological and behavioral factors such as personality, motivation, and social pressures. Sorensen et al. *(14)* found that men were more interested in quitting compared with women and women were less likely than men to perceive the health benefits of quitting. Men and women are different physiologically, psychologically, and behaviorally, and a good understanding of the reasons for women initiating smoking as well as quitting smoking is very important to reverse the increasing trend of women getting lung cancer.

The smoking patterns of the yesteryears are showing up now as the incidence of lung cancer starts to narrow between men and women. Compounding this problem is that recent research has suggested that women smokers may be more susceptible than their male counterparts in developing lung cancer. It has been noted that the increase in lung cancer incidence among women in the 1970s is more rapid than the corresponding increase among men in the 1930s *(8)*. Subsequently, many studies have attempted to answer the question of increased susceptibility among women, but results have been inconclusive. In the 1980s, McDuffie et al. *(15)* reported that "women developed primary lung cancer at an earlier age while smoking for fewer years than men. " Similar to that, other groups also reported a higher risk of lung cancer among women based on case–control studies *(16–19)*. Reports from the baseline computed tomography (CT) lung cancer screening of men and women smokers also suggested a higher risk among women *(20)*. Notwithstanding the positive studies, there are studies that refute this stand. A report from Copenhagen *(21)* based on three prospective population-based studies of 30,874 subjects did not find any difference in rate ratio (RR) of developing lung cancer between men and women (RR, 0.8; 95% confidence interval [CI], 0.3–2.1), while a large recent analysis of prospective data from former and current-smokers *(22)* reported that the hazard ratio in women ever-smokers for lung cancer compared with men was 1.11 (95% CI, 0.95–1.31). Further studies have attempted to find reasons for the increased susceptibility of women to tobacco smoke. Some studies suggested that the hormonal environment has a role to play *(23–25)*, while others have looked at the way the different sexes metabolize carcinogens *(26, 27)*. Recently, epidermal growth factor receptor (EGFR)-activating mutations in the tyrosine kinase (TK) domains were found to be more common among lung tumors of never-smokers, adenocarcinoma, patients of East Asian ethnicity, and women, suggesting that women may be at a higher risk for this particular type of non-small cell lung cancer (NSCLC) *(28, 29)*.

At this point in time, there is no conclusive evidence that women are at an increased susceptibility to lung cancer *(9)*. Our focus should be to curb the initiation of smoking among adolescent girls and to promote and advise smoking cessation among women. It is likely that the lung cancer incidence rate will normalize between the sexes as women continue to smoke just as much as men. The possible increased susceptibility of women to cigarette smoke, if present, will only contribute slightly if at all, to the increase in lung cancer cases among them.

3. Never-smokers and Lung Cancer

Although smoking is definitely a cause of lung cancer, there is evidence that a not insignificant proportion of lung cancer patients are never-smokers, especially among Asian women *(8)*. Clinical observations suggest that there may be an increasing number of never-smokers afflicted with the disease, but there are no definitive data because literature on this topic is sparse. Recently, interest has been fueled by the differential response of never-smokers to EGFR TK inhibitors as well as the more frequent finding of activating EGFR mutations in the lung tumors of never-smokers.

In 1979, Enstrom suggested that factors other than smoking may have an effect on lung cancer mortality *(30)*. He reported that the lung cancer mortality rate among never-smokers had risen between 1914 and 1968 with a relative increase of 15-fold and 7-fold for white men and women aged 35–84 years, respectively. In a large Swedish study based on a nationwide health care program among construction workers, Boffetta et al. *(31)* found that the rates of lung cancer among never-smokers increased from 1.5/100,000 to 5.4/100,000 during the periods 1976–1980 to 1991–1995. In a more recent study based on two American Cancer Society Cancer Prevention Study (CPS) cohorts during 1959–1972 (CPS-I) and 1982–2000 (CPS II), the lung cancer death rate was higher in CPS-II than CPS-I among women never-smokers and the increase among white women was statistically significant only in those ages 70–84 years *(32)*. But there was no difference between the two time periods among men never-smokers. In an Italian study, the authors studied differences in indirect estimates of lung cancer death rates over two time periods, 1956–1958 and 1987–1989, and found an increase in the rates not attributable to active smoking, which suggested that factors other than smoking may play an important role in causing lung cancer *(33)*. However, some studies based on hospital records did not see any change in the percentage of nonsmokers afflicted with lung cancer. In the late 1980s, a study in a single institution in the USA found that 11% of their patients with NSCLC were nonsmokers *(34)*. Subsequently, in another retrospective analysis of data from three South California counties from 1999 to 2003, the authors found that 9.7% of the NSCLC patients were never-smokers *(35)*. These studies on never-smokers need to be interpreted and compared with caution because they are confounded by the way the smoking history is taken as well as differences in classification of never-smokers. This is illustrated in the study by Peto et al. *(36)* who compared two case–control studies performed in two time periods, 1948–1952 and 1988–1993, separately. In the 1950s study, 0.5% of lung cases and 4.5% of controls among men were nonsmokers while in the 1990s, 0.5% of lung cases and 19% of controls among men were nonsmokers. As for the women, 37% of cases and 54.6% of controls in 1950s were nonsmokers, while 7.6% of cases and 50.3% of controls in the 1990s were nonsmokers. Although the results could suggest that the proportion of never-smokers with lung cancer does not reflect that of the population, it may also mean that the documentation of smoking status is highly varied and can differ between various studies. This stems from the fact that smoking history is subject to recall biases and self-reported reliability and a small misclassification of smokers among nonsmokers would substantially affect the lung cancer rates.

Recently, Wakelee et al. *(37)* performed an analysis using data from six large cohort populations in the USA to estimate the lung cancer incidence among never-smokers. This is one of a few studies that estimated incidence rates instead of mortality rates among never-smokers with lung cancer. The authors found that the truncated age-adjusted incidence rates of lung cancer among never-smokers aged 40–79 years ranged from 14.4 to 20.8 per 100,000 person-years in women and 4.8 to 13.7 per 100,000 person years in men. This gives us an idea of the magnitude of the problem, as the numbers are comparable to the incidence rates of myeloma in men and cervical cancer in women. As this is the first study on incidence rate in the USA, there are no previous studies to compare with to determine if the incidence is indeed rising.

While we are unable to conclusively determine if lung cancer among never-smokers is increasing, there is evidence to suggest that lung cancer in never-smokers may be a biologically different disease from smokers *(38)*. Many epidemiological studies have found that the characteristics of lung cancer among never-smokers are significantly different from that of smokers *(8, 39, 40)*. Consistent findings include a higher proportion of women, adenocarcinoma, as well as an earlier age at diagnosis among the never-smokers. Some studies have also reported better survival among never-smokers *(8, 41, 42)*. Further support came from differences in genetic profile of the tumors, including EGFR-activating mutations and differential response to treatment with oral EGFR TK inhibitors between smokers and never-smokers *(29, 43–45)*. There are also studies to suggest increased familial risk among relatives of never-smokers with lung cancer *(46–48)*. However, due to a similar shared environment, whether the aggregation of cancer within a family is the result of tobacco smoking exposure in the same household or truly a higher predisposition of the individuals may be difficult to determine. Other nonsmoking factors such as the role of human papilloma virus (HPV) *(49)*, cooking oil fumes *(50)*, and diet *(51)* have been proposed but none has been confirmed.

Whether there will be an epidemic of lung cancer among nonsmokers is difficult to predict, as we do not yet know if any factors other than smoking are involved. For now, it is important that we keep a close watch on the trend by collecting more data to form a base for future comparison.

4. Histopathology of Lung Cancer

In the early part of the century, SCC was the predominant histological subtype of lung cancer and SCLC was the next most frequent. It was first noticed in the 1960s and 1970s in the USA that the incidence of the more peripheral adenocarcinoma was rising *(52, 53)*. These were mainly hospital-based studies but subsequent population based studies also confirmed the trend *(54)*. Now, adenocarcinoma has usurped the throne to be the most common histological subtype of lung cancer **(Fig. 19.2)** *(55)*. This shift is similarly seen in Asia *(56)* and Europe *(57)*. The change was attributed to several reasons such as detection bias, advances in diagnostic techniques, as well as changes in histological classification and pathological techniques. In the earlier years, the diagnosis of lung cancer was usually made in smokers with pulmonary symptoms and these patients tend to have centrally located SCC. McFarlane et al. *(58)* found that 28% of lung cancers were not diagnosed antemortem and, among them, the proportion of women and nonsmokers were higher. As adenocarcinoma usually occurs in the periphery and are more common among women and never-smokers, the incidence may have been previously underestimated because they go undiagnosed and undetected *(59)*. With the ability to diagnose peripheral lesions using CT scanning and advances in diagnostic techniques such

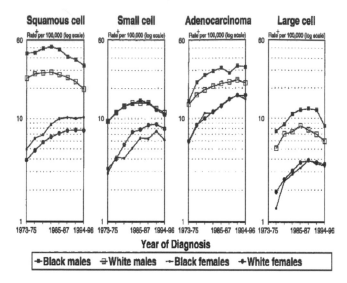

Fig. 19.2. Cancer of the lung and bronchus: Surveillance, Epidemiology, and End Results (SEER) incidence rates by histologic types, sex, race, and ethnicity, all ages, 1973–1996. Adapted from Wingo et al. *(73)*.

as flexible bronchoscopy and transthoracic needle aspiration, the histological diagnosis of adenocarcinoma may have picked up in the 1980s. In addition, the increase in the use of mucin staining since the 1980s may have resulted in the increased diagnosis of adenocarcinoma. Kung et al. *(60)* found that more than half of the large cell carcinoma was retyped into adenocarcinoma when the 1981 World Health Organization (WHO) classification was used instead of the 1967 WHO classification. Arguments against the above reasons are that these changes in diagnostic advances and techniques happened mainly in the 1980s but the shift has been noted in the 1960s and 1970s. The more likely explanation for the change is the change in composition and design of cigarettes. Thun et al. *(61)* analyzed data from the Connecticut Tumor Registry and two American Cancer Society studies and found that the increase in adenocarcinoma followed a clear birth cohort pattern that parallels gender and generational changes in smoking, which suggests that the changes are more consistent with changes in smoking behavior and cigarette design.

After the landmark studies *(2, 3)* that concluded a dose–response relationship between the number of cigarettes smoked and lung cancer as well as animal studies that found tar to be tumorigenic on mouse skin *(62)*, tobacco companies began to find ways to reduce the yield of tar and nicotine in cigarettes. Significant changes can be seen from the sales-weighted average smoke yield of tar and nicotine of US cigarettes **(Fig. 19.3)**. From 1953 to 1996, the tar and nicotine yields decreased from 38 and 2.7 mg to 12 and 0.85 mg, respectively. Filter cigarettes sales also

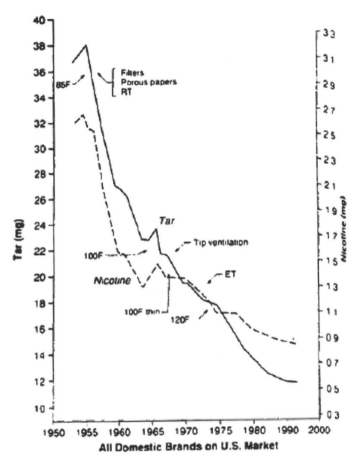

Fig. 19.3. Sales-weighted average tar and nicotine deliveries, 1953–1993, USA. Adapted from Hoffmann et al. *(74)*. *RT*, reconstituted tobacco; *F*, filter; *ET*, expanded tobacco.

increased from 1950 to 1997. All these changes in the design of the cigarettes have resulted in changes in smoke composition as well as the smoking patterns of smokers. The smoke composition has shifted toward an increase in tobacco-specific nitrosamines and a decrease in the polycyclic aromatic hydrocarbons *(63)*. Nitrosamines have been shown in animal studies to induce adenoca *(64)*. In addition, smoking low-nicotine cigarettes causes smokers to inhale more intensely and deeply to satisfy their craving *(65)*, and this results in possibly more deposition of the carcinogens in the periphery of the lungs.

There is likely a shift toward a true increase in the proportion of adenoca of the lung that is due to the changing cigarette. Some of the increase may have been contributed to somewhat by detection bias due to advances in diagnostic abilities and technologies. The proportion of adenoca will continue to increase as more people smoke filtered, low-tar or low-nicotine cigarettes. Although there are studies that suggest that smoking low-tar and filter-tip cigarettes is associated with less lung cancer risks *(66)*, there are also studies that refute this *(67)*. In a large study, Harris et al. *(67)* found that the increase in lung cancer risk is similar in people who smoke medium tar, low-tar, or very low-tar cigarettes. More importantly, all current smokers have a much higher risk of lung cancer than people who never smoked or stopped smoking regardless of the amount of tar in the brand. It must be realized that there can be no "safe cigarette" no matter how the tobacco industry pushes for the idea of a less harmful cigarette.

5. Developing Countries and Lung Cancer

Lung cancer was second in incidence after stomach cancer in the worldwide estimates of cancer incidence in 1985. By 1990, lung cancer became the most common cancer in the world, with 1.04 million new cases, about 42% of which occurred in the developing countries *(68)*. Due to the high fatality of the disease, lung cancer is the leading cause of cancer death and contributes to over 900,000 cancer deaths in the world *(69)*. This is likely to be an underestimate of the true rates as many cases can go undiagnosed and unreported in developing countries with unsatisfactory health care system. As the incidence of lung cancer in developed countries such as the USA begins to decline, the incidence in developing countries is rising. This is due to falling smoking rates in the high-income countries where public campaigns and regulation help to control the smoking rates. Unfortunately, in many developing countries, poor literacy and poor health care systems have impeded public campaigns against smoking, and smoking rates in many developing countries remain high. This is particularly disturbing in China, which is the world's most populous country and unfortunately also has one of the highest smoking rates in the world.

The smoking prevalence among men in China is 63% in the 1996 national prevalence survey, which reaffirms the high smoking rate seen in the 1984 survey *(70)*. With a population of 1.2 billion, one third of current smokers in the world would be residing in China *(71)*. It is estimated that the mortality from smoking-related diseases will hit 1 million in the first decade of 21st century and will be expected to double in 20 years time if smoking rates are not reduced *(72)*. While the cigarette consumption in the USA is declining, the sales volume in China has grown since 1981. In 1994, 1.7 trillion cigarettes were produced in China and about 900 million were imported. It is worrying that although the smoking rate among women in China is low at 3.8 %, more than half (53.5%) reported that they were exposed to environ-

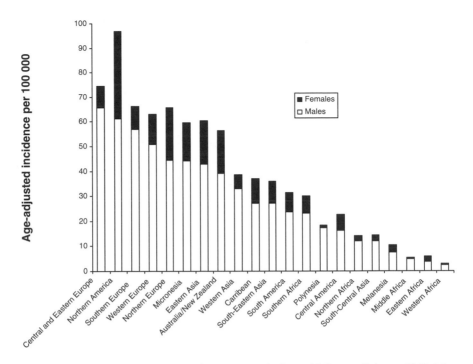

Fig. 19.4. Age-adjusted incidence rates for lung cancer in the world. Source: Globocan 2002 database (www-dep.iarc.fr/globocan/database.htm).

mental tobacco smoke at least 15 minutes per day on more than 1 day per week *(70)*.

From the experience in developed countries, lung cancer incidence will follow the trend of smoking 20 years later. As the smoking prevalence does not abate in the developing countries, lung cancer incidence in these countries will continue to rise toward the first half of the 21st century. At the moment, lung cancer is commonest in developed countries in North America and Europe, intermediate in Australia/New Zealand and Eastern Asia, and least common in Africa and South America **(Fig. 19.4)**. However, the epidemiology is changing and, by the middle of the 21st century, more than half of lung cancer cases will come from the developing countries. Hopefully, as the international community, including 145 countries, ratify the WHO Framework Convention on Tobacco Control (FCTC), the war against the tobacco industry can be won.

6. Conclusion

Despite the encouraging decline in smoking prevalence since the 1980s, it has leveled off toward the end of the 1990s. This would mean that the lung cancer decline would plateau off sometime in 2020 given the lag-time period but unfortunately this decline will only be seen in the developed countries. With the increasing numbers of smokers in the developing countries toward the later half of the 20th century, we will be unlikely to see a decline in the incidence of lung cancer worldwide, but will witness a shift in the burden of lung cancer toward the developing countries. In the foreseeable future, we will also see that the disease will inflict both men and women in equal proportions and a higher proportion of never-smokers with adenocarcinoma of the lung. Lung cancer will continue its scourge into the 21st century. While research is now focused on gene–environmental associations to understand those at risk of this disease, particularly the women and nonsmokers, as well as curtailing mortality with improved screening, earlier detection and new treatment modalities, we are still far from winning the battle against lung cancer as the clear "vector" of the disease is still rampant. Hopefully, with the international commitment toward the WHO FCTC, we will push ahead toward adopting clean-air policies in many countries. The tobacco industry will also adapt to these social changes and target more vulnerable groups like children and women. The world needs to cooperate to stem out the "vector" of the disease. It may be a mammoth task but it will be one of the greatest gifts we can give to our future generation as we prevent millions of unnecessary premature deaths.

References

1. Parkin DM, Bray F, Ferlay J, Pisanin P. (2005) Global cancer statistics, 2002. CA Cancer J Clin. **55**, 74–108.

2. Doll R, Hill AB. (1950) Smoking and carcinoma of the lung; preliminary report. Br Med J. **2**, 739–748.

3. Wynder EL, Graham EA. (1950) Tobacco smoking as a possible etiologic factor in bronchiogenic carcinoma; a study of 684 proved cases. JAMA. **143**, 329–336.

4. US Department of Health Education, and Welfare (DHEW). (1964) Smoking and health: a report of the Advisory Committee to the Surgeon General of the Public Health Service. DHEW-Public Health Service Publication No. 1103. Washington, DC: US Government Printing Office.

5. Royal College of Physicians of London. (1962) Smoking and health: summary of a report of the Royal College of Physicians of London on smoking in relation to cancer of the lung and other disease. Publication No. S2-70. Pitman Medical Publishing, LTD, London, UK.

6. US Department of Health and Human Services (US-DHHS). (1980) The health consequences of smoking for women: a report of the Surgeon General. US-DHHS, Public Health Service, Office of the Assistant Secretary for Health, Office of Smoking and Health.

7. Devasa SS, Shaw GL, Blot WJ. (1991) Changing patterns of lung cancer incidence by histological type. Cancer Epidemiol Biomarkers Prev **1**, 29–34.

8. Toh CK, Gao F, Lim WT, Leong SS, Fong KW, Yap SP, Hsu AA, Eng P, Koong HN, Thiruganam A, Tan EH. (2006) Never-smokers with lung cancer: epidemiologic evidence of a distinct disease entity. J Clin Oncol. **24**, 2245–2251.

9. US Department of Health and Human Services (US-DHHS). (2001) Women and smoking: a report of the Surgeon General. US-DHHS, Public Health Service, Office of the Surgeon General.

10. Center for Disease Control and Prevention. (2002) Trends in cigarette smoking among high school students–United States, 1991–2001. Morb Mortal Wkly Rep. *51*, 409–412.

11. Center for Disease Control and Prevention. (2003) Tobacco use among middle and high school students–United States, 2002. Morb Mortal Wkly Rep. **52**, 1096–1098.

12. Warren CW, Jones NR, Eriksen MP, Asma S, for the Global Tobacco Surveillance System (GTSS) Collaborative Group. (2006) Patterns of global tobacco use in young people and implications for future chronic disease burden in adults. Lancet. **367**, 749–753.

13. Husten CG, Shelton DM, Chrismon JH, Lin YC, Mower P, Powell FA. (1997) Cigarette smoking and smoking cessation among older adults: United States, 1965–94. Tob Control. **6**, 175–180.

14. Sorensen G, Pechacek TF. (1987) Attitudes toward smoking cessation among men and women. J Behav Med. **10**, 129–137.

15. McDuffie HH, Klaassen DJ, Dosman JA. (1987) Female-male differences in patients with primary lung cancer. Cancer. **59**, 1825–1830.

16. Brownson RC, Chang JC, Davis JR. (1992) Gender and histologic type variations in smoking-related risk of lung cancer. Epidemiology. **3**, 61–64.

17. Risch HA, Howe GR, Jain M, Burch JD, Holowaty EJ, Miller AB. (1993) Are female smokers at higher risk for lung cancer than male smokers? A case-control analysis by histologic type. Am J Epidemiol. 138, 281–293.

18. Harris RE, Zang EA, Anderson JI, Wynder EL. (1993) Race and sex differences in lung cancer risk associated with cigarette smoking. Int J Epidemiol. **22**, 592–599.

19. Zang EA, Wynder EL. (1996) Differences in lung cancer risk between men and women: examination of the evidence. J Natl Cancer Inst. **88**, 183–192.

20. International Early Lung Cancer Action Program Investigators. (2006) Women's susceptibility to tobacco carcinogens and survival after diagnosis of lung cancer. JAMA. **296**, 180–184.

21. Prescott E, Osler M, Hein HO, Borch-Johnsen K, Lange P, Schnohr P, Vestbo J. (1998) Gender and smoking-related risk of lung cancer. The Copenhagen Center for Prospective Population Studies. Epidemiology. **9**, 79–83.

22. Bain C, Feskanich D, Speizer FE, Thun M, Hertzmark E, Rosner BA, Colditz GA. (2004) Lung cancer rates in men and women with comparable histories of smoking. J Natl Cancer Inst. **96**, 826–834.

23. Taioli E, Wynder EL. (1994) Re: Endocrine factors and adenocarcinoma of the lung in women. J Natl Cancer Inst. **86**, 869–870.

24. Gao YT, Blot WJ, Zheng W, Ershow AG, Hsu CW, Levin LI, Zhang R, Fraumeni JF Jr. (1987) Lung cancer among Chinese women. Int J Cancer. **40**, 604–609.

25. Seow A, Poh WT, Teh M, Eng P, Wang YT, Tan WC, Chia KS, Yu MC, Lee HP. (2002) Diet, reproductive factors and lung cancer risk among Chinese women in Singapore: evidence for a protective effect of soy in nonsmokers. Int J Cancer. **97**, 365–371.

26. Mollerup S, Berge G, Baera R, Skaug V, Hewer A, Phillips DH, Stangeland L, Haugen A. (2004) Sex differences in risk of lung cancer: expression of genes in the PAH bioactivation pathway in relation to smoking and bulky DNA adducts. Int J Cancer. **119**, 741–744.

27. Dresler CM, Fratelli C, Babb J, Everley L, Evans AA, Clapper ML. (2000) Gender differences in genetic susceptibility for lung cancer. Lung Cancer. **30**, 153–160.

28. Shigematsu H, Lin L, Takahashi T, Nomura M, Suzuki M, Wistuba II, Fong KM, Lee H, Toyooka S, Shimizu N, Fujisawa T, Feng Z, Roth JA, Herz J, Minna JD, Gazdar AF. (2005) Clinical and biological features associated with epidermal growth factor receptor gene mutations in lung cancers. J Natl Cancer Inst. **97**, 339–346.

29. Tokumo M, Toyooka S, Kiura K, Shigematsu H, Tomii K, Aoe M, Ichimura K, Tsuda T, Yano M, Tsukuda K, Tabata M, Ueoka H, Tanimoto M, Date H, Gazdar AF, Shimizu N. (2005) The relationship between epidermal growth factor receptor mutations and clinicopathologic features in non-small-cell lung cancers. Clin Cancer Res. **11**, 1167–1173.

30. Enstrom JE. (1979) Rising lung cancer mortality among nonsmokers. J Natl Cancer Inst. **62**, 755–760.

31. Boffetta P, Jarvholm B, Brennan P, Nyren O. (2001) Incidence of lung cancer in a large cohort of non-smoking men from Sweden. Int J Cancer. **94**, 591–593.

32. Thun MJ, Henly SJ, Burns D, Jemal A, Shanks TG, Calle EE. (2006) Lung cancer death rates in lifelong nonsmokers. J Natl Cancer Inst. **98**:691–699.

33. Forastiere F, Perucci CA, Arca M, Axelson O. (1993) Indirect estimates of lung cancer death rates in Italy not attributable to active smoking. Epidemiology. **4**, 502–510.

34. Sridhar KS, Raub WA Jr. (1992) Present and past smoking history and other predisposing factors in 100 lung cancer patients. Chest. **101**, 19–25.

35. Zell JA, Ou SH, Ziogas A, Anton-Culver H. (2005) Epidemiology of bronchioloalveolar carcinoma: improvement in survival after release of the 1999 WHO classification of lung tumors. J Clin Oncol. **23**, 8396–8405.

36. Peto R, Darby S, Deo H, Silcocks P, Whitley E, Doll R. (2000) Smoking, smoking cessation, and lung cancer in the UK since 1950: combination of national statistics with two case-control studies. BMJ. **321**, 323–329.

37. Wakelee HA, Chang ET, Gomez SL, Keegan TH, Feskanich D, Clarke CA, Holmberg L, Yong LC, Kolonel LN, Gould MK, West DW. (2007) Lung cancer incidence in never smokers. J Clin Oncol. **25**, 472–478.

38. Toh CK, Lim WT. (2007) Lung cancer in never smokers. J Clin Path. **60**, 337–340.

39. Koo LC, Ho JH. (1990) Worldwide epidemiological patterns of lung cancer in nonsmokers. Int J Epidemiol. **19** (Suppl 1), S14–23.

40. Chen CJ, Wu HY, Chuang YC, Chang AS, Luh KT, Chao HH, Chen KY, Chen SG, Lai GM, Huang HH. (1990) Epidemiologic characteristics and multiple risk factors of lung cancer in Taiwan. Anticancer Res. **10**, 971–976.

41. Nordquist LT, Simon GR, Cantor A, Alberts WM, Bepler G. (2004) Improved survival in never-smokers vs current smokers with primary adenocarcinoma of the lung. Chest. **126**, 347–351.

42. Tsao AS, Liu D, Lee JJ, Spitz M, Hong WK. (2006) Smoking affects treatment outcome in patient with advanced nonsmall cell lung cancer. Cancer. **106**, 2428–2436.

43. Suzuki H, Takahashi T, Kuroishi T, Suyama M, Ariyoshi Y, Takahashi T, Ueda R. (1992) p53 mutations in non-small cell lung cancer in Japan: association between mutations and smoking. Cancer Res. **52**, 734–736.

44. Powell CA, Spira A, Derti A, DeLisi C, Liu G, Borczuk A, Busch S, Sahasrabudhe S, Chen Y, Sugarbaker D, Bueno R, Richards WG, Brody JS. (2003) Gene expression in lung adenocarcinomas of smokers and nonsmokers. Am J Respir Cell Mol Biol. **29**, 157–162.

45. Toyooka S, Tokumo M, Shigematsu H, Matsuo K, Asano H, Tomii K, Ichihara S, Suzuki M, Aoe M, Date H, Gazdar AF, Shimizu N. (2006) Mutational and epigenetic evidence for independent pathways for lung adenocarcinoma arising in smokers and never smokers. Cancer Res. **66**, 1371–1375.

46. Bromen K, Pohlabeln H, Jahn I, Ahrens W, Jockel KH. (2000) Aggregation of lung cancer in families: results from a population-based case-control study in Germany. Am J Epidemiol. **152**, 497–505.

47. Schwartz AG, Rothrock M, Yang P. (1999) Increased cancer risk among relatives of nonsmoking lung cancer cases. Genet Epidemiol. **17**, 1–15.

48. Gorlova OY, Zhang Y, Schabath MB, Lei L, Zhang Q, Amos CI, Spitz MR. (2006) Never smoker and lung cancer risk: a case-control study of epidemiological factors. Int J Cancer. **118**, 1798–1804.

49. Cheng YW, Chiou HL, Sheu GT, Hsieh LL, Chen JT, Chen CY, Su JM, Lee H. (2001) The association of human papillomavirus 16/18 infection with lung cancer among nonsmoking Taiwanese women. Cancer Res. **61**, 2799–2803.

50. Ko YC, Cheng LS, Lee CH, Huang JJ, Huang MS, Kao EL, Wang HZ, Lin HJ. (2000) Chinese food cooking and lung cancer in women nonsmokers. Am J Epidemiol. **151**, 140–147.

51. Brennan P, Butler J, Agudo A, Benhamou S, Darby S, Fortes C, Jockel KH, Kreuzer M, Nyberg F, Pohlabeln H, Saracci R, Wichman HE, Boffetta P. (2000) Joint effect of diet and environmental tobacco smoke on risk of lung cancer among nonsmokers. J Natl Cancer Inst. **92**, 426–427.

52. Vincent RG, Pickren JW, Lane WW, Bross I, Takita H, Houten L, Gutierrez AC, Rzepka T. (1977) The changing histopathology of lung cancer: a review of 1682 cases. Cancer. **39**, 1647–1655.

53. Valaitis J, Warren S, Gamble D. (1981) Increasing incidence of adenocarcinoma of the lung. Cancer. **47**, 1042–1046.

54. Dodds L, Davis S, Polissar L. (1986) A population-based study of lung cancer incidence trends by histologic type, 1974–81. J Natl Cancer Inst. **76**, 21–29.

55. Travis WD, Travis LB, Devesa SS. (1995). Lung Cancer. Cancer. **75**(1 Supp), 191–202.

56. Ikeda T, Kurita Y, Inutsuka S, Tanaka K, Nakanishi Y, Shigematsu N, Nobutomo K. (1991) The changing pattern of lung cancer by histological type–a review of 1151 cases from a university hospital in Japan, 1970–1989. Lung Cancer. **7**, 157–164.

57. Janssen-Heijnen ML, Nab HW, van Reek J, van der Heijden LH, Schipper R, Coebergh JW. (1995) Striking changes in smoking behaviour and lung cancer incidence by histological type in south-east Netherlands, 1960–1991. Eur J Cancer. **31A**, 949–952.

58. McFarlane MJ, Feinstein AR, Wells CK. (1986) Clinical features of lung cancer discovered as a postmortem "surprise. " Chest. **90**, 520–523.

59. Wells CK, Feinstein AR. (1988) Detection bias in the diagnostic pursuit of lung cancer. Am J Epidemiol. **128**, 1016–1026.

60. Kung IT, So KF, Lam TH. (1984) Lung cancer in Hong Kong Chinese: mortality and histological types, 1973–1982. Br J Cancer. **50**, 381–388.

61. Thun MJ, Lally CA, Flannery JT, Calle EE, Dana Flanders W, Health CW Jr. (1997) Cigarette smoking and changes in the histopathology of lung cancer. J Natl Cancer Inst. **89**, 1580–1586.

62. Wynder El, Graham EA, Croninger AB. (1953) Experimental production of carcinoma with cigarette tar. Cancer Res. **13**, 855–864.

63. Fischer S, Spiegelhalder B, Preussmann R. (1989) Influence of smoking parameters on the delivery of tobacco-specific nitrosamines in cigarette smoke–a contribution to relative risk evaluation. Carcinogenesis. **10**, 1059–1066.

64. Hecht SS. (1997) Tobacco smoke carcinogens and lung cancer. J Natl Cancer Inst. **89**, 1580–1586.

65. Djordjevic MV, Hoffmann D, Hoffmann I. (1997) Nicotine regulates smoking patterns. Prev Med. **26**, 435–440.

66. Kabat KC. (2003) Fifty years' experience of reduced-tar cigarettes: what do we know about their health effects? Inhal Toxicol. **15**, 1059–1102.

67. Harris JE, Thun MJ, Mondul AM, Calle EE. (2004) Cigarette tar yields in relation to mortality from lung cancer in the cancer prevention study II prospective cohort, 1982–8. BMJ. **328**, 72.

68. Parkin DM, Pisani P, Ferlay J. (1999) Estimates of the worldwide incidence of 25 major cancers in 1990. Int J Cancer. **80**, 827–841.

69. Pisani P, Parkin DM, Bray F, Ferlay J. (1999) Estimates of the worldwide mortality from 25 cancers in 1990. Int J Cancer. **83**, 18–29.

70. Yang G, Fan L, Tan J, Qi G, Zhang Y, Samet JM, Taylor CE, Becker K, Xu J. (1999) Smoking in China: findings of the 1996 National Prevalence Survey. JAMA. **282**, 1247–1253.

71. Wright AA, Katz IT. (2007) Tobacco tightrope–balancing disease prevention and economic development in China. N Engl J Med. **356**, 1493–1496.

72. Liu BQ, Peto R, Chen ZM, Boreham J, Wu YP, Li JY, Colin Campbell T, Chen JS. (1998) Emerging tobacco hazards in China: 1. Retrospective proportional mortality study of one million deaths. BMJ. **317**, 1411–1422.

73. Wingo PA, Ries LAG, Giovino GA, Miller DS, Rosenberg HM, Shopland DR, Thun MJ, Edwards BK. (1999) Annual report to the nation on the status of cancer, 1973–1996, with a special section on lung cancer and tobacco smoking. J Natl Cancer Inst. **91**, 675–690.

74. Hoffmann D, Hoffmann I, El-Bayoumy K. The less harmful cigarette: a controversial issue. A tribute to Ernst L. Wynder. (2001) Chem Res Toxicol. **14**, 767–790.

Chapter 20

Epidemiology of Ovarian Cancer

Jennifer Permuth-Wey and Thomas A. Sellers

Abstract

Ovarian cancer represents the sixth most commonly diagnosed cancer among women in the world, and causes more deaths per year than any other cancer of the female reproductive system. Despite the high incidence and mortality rates, the etiology of this disease is poorly understood. Established risk factors for ovarian cancer include age and having a family history of the disease, while protective factors include increasing parity, oral contraceptive use, and oophorectomy. Lactation, incomplete pregnancies, and surgeries such as hysterectomy and tubal ligation may confer a weak protective effect against ovarian cancer. Infertility may contribute to ovarian cancer risk among nulliparous women. Other possible risk factors for ovarian cancer include postmenopausal hormone-replacement therapy and lifestyle factors such as cigarette smoking and alcohol consumption. Many of the causes of ovarian cancer are yet to be identified. Additional research is needed to better understand the etiology of this deadly disease.

Key words: Ovarian cancer, epidemiology, risk factors, histology, reproductive history.

1. Introduction

Ovarian cancer is the sixth most commonly diagnosed cancer among women in the world, accounting for nearly 4% of all female cancers *(1)*. Ovarian cancer also represents the second leading gynecologic cancer, following cancer of the uterine corpus, and causes more deaths per year than any other cancer of the female reproductive system *(1, 2)*. An estimated 1 in 70 women in the United States will develop ovarian cancer in their lifetime *(3)*. On a worldwide basis, an estimated 204,000 new cases are diagnosed and 125,000 women die of ovarian cancer annually *(1, 2)*. In 2007, approximately 22,430 new cases of ovarian cancer will be diagnosed and 15,280 ovarian cancer-related

M. Verma (ed.), *Methods of Molecular Biology, Cancer Epidemiology, vol. 472*
© 2009 Humana Press, a part of Springer Science+Business Media, Totowa, NJ
Book doi: 10.1007/978-1-60327-492-0

deaths are expected in the United States *(3, 4)*. Mortality is high because women typically present with late-stage disease when the overall 5-year relative survival rate is 45% *(4)*. Thus, the public health burden is significant. Despite the high incidence and mortality rates, the etiology of this lethal disease is not completely understood. Research to identify the causes of ovarian cancer is sorely needed, as such knowledge could inform strategies for risk assessment, prevention, surveillance, early detection, and treatment. The purpose of this chapter is to review some of the established and suspected epidemiologic risk factors for ovarian cancer. We divide this chapter into four sections: the pathologic classification of ovarian cancer, descriptive epidemiology, risk factors and protective factors for ovarian cancer, and summary and conclusions.

2. Pathological Classification of Ovarian Cancer

Nearly all benign and malignant ovarian tumors originate from one of three cell types: epithelial cells, stromal cells, and germ cells. In developed countries, more than 90% of malignant ovarian tumors are epithelial in origin, 5–6% of tumors constitute sex cord-stromal tumors, and 2–3% are germ cell tumors *(2)*. The pathology and classification of ovarian tumors are described in detail by Chen et al. *(5)*. Epidemiologic studies have suggested etiologic differences in these three cell types *(6)*. Most epidemiologic research, including the present review, focuses on epithelial ovarian cancers because they are the predominant subtype. Malignant epithelial ovarian cancers are known as carcinomas, and can be classified into four main categories: serous, mucinous, endometrioid, and clear cell *(7)*. Within each of these categories are tumors of uncertain malignant behavior (known as "borderline tumors" or "tumors of low malignant potential") that contain microscopic features of malignancy without frank invasion into surrounding stroma. Such borderline tumors are usually not included in the published statistics of most cancer-reporting systems *(6)*. However, the risk factors for epithelial ovarian cancer seem to apply similarly for borderline and invasive epithelial tumors, although the mean age at diagnosis is earlier among women with borderline tumors *(8, 9)*.

It is important to point out that epithelial ovarian cancers themselves may reflect a heterogeneous group of diseases. Many studies have investigated etiologic differences according to the histologic subtype of ovarian cancer *(8–14)*. We will comment on some of these study findings throughout this chapter.

3. Descriptive Epidemiology

Ovarian cancer incidence exhibits wide geographic variation, as shown in **Fig. 20.1** *(1)*. The highest age-adjusted incidence rates are observed in developed parts of the world, including North America and Western and Northern Europe, with rates in these areas exceeding 10 per 100,000, except for Japan (6.4 per 100,000). Rates are intermediate in South America (7.7 per 100,000), and lowest in Asia and Africa. Migration from countries with low rates to those with high rates results in greater risk *(15, 16)*, underscoring the importance of nongenetic factors. However, even within the United States, racial differences in risk are apparent that mimic the observed international variation. Rates are highest among whites (14.3 per 100,000), intermediate for Hispanics (11.5 per 100,000), and lowest among blacks (10.1 per 100,000) and Asians (9.7 per 100,000) *(4)*. In most parts of North America and Europe, the incidence of ovarian cancer was constant in the decades prior to the 1990s, and has gradually declined since that time *(4, 17–19)*. In the United States, there has also been a gradual decline in ovarian cancer-related mortality for all races combined *(19)*.

Several reasons have been proposed to explain both the geographic variation in incidence rates and the trends in incidence and mortality. Such reasons include differences in oral contraceptive (OC) use practices and pregnancy history along with variations in the frequency of prophylactic oophorectomy *(17, 20, 21)*. Additionally, changes that have impacted medical care such as improvements in diagnosis and treatment, better access to care for minorities and underserved populations, and improved levels of general health awareness may explain the trends *(22)*.

The incidence of ovarian cancer increases with age, with a median age at diagnosis of 63 years **(Fig. 20.2)** *(4)*. Over 80% of ovarian cancers occur after age 45 years.

4. Risk Factors and Preventive Factors

4.1. Family History

One of the most significant risk factors for ovarian cancer is a family history of the disease. It is estimated that approximately 7% of women with ovarian cancer have a positive family history of the disease *(23)*. First-degree relatives of ovarian cancer probands have a threefold to sevenfold increased risk, especially if multiple relatives are affected and at an early age at onset *(24–28)*.

It is clear that a subset of ovarian cancers occur as part of a hereditary cancer syndrome that is inherited in an autosomal

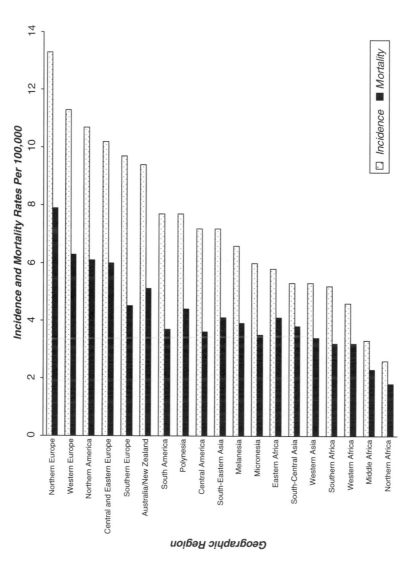

Fig. 20.1. Worldwide ovarian cancer incidence and mortality rates (rates are per 100,000 and are age adjusted according to the world standard population). From ref. *(1)*.

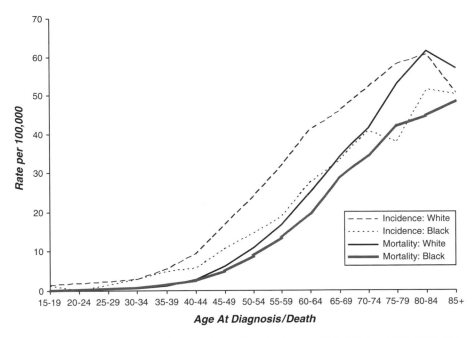

Fig. 20.2. Ovarian cancer: age-specific incidence and mortality rates by race, United States, 1975–2004. Rates are per 100,000 and are age adjusted to the 2000 US standard population. From ref. *(4)*.

dominant pattern. The majority of hereditary ovarian cancers can be attributed to mutations in the *BRCA1* and *BRCA2* genes *(29, 30)*. According to data from the Breast Cancer Linkage Consortium, the risk of ovarian cancer through age 70 years is up to 44% in *BRCA1* families *(31)* and approaches 27% in *BRCA2* families *(32)*. Mutation screening of population-based series of ovarian cancer cases has shown that 10–15% of ovarian cancers can be explained by mutations in the *BRCA1* and *BRCA2* genes *(33–41)*. In addition, ovarian cancer also occurs in families with hereditary non-polyposis colorectal cancer syndrome (HNPCC), also known as Lynch syndrome II *(42)*. The genetic defects underlying HNPCC (the mismatch repair genes *hMLH1*, *hMSH2*, *hPMS1*, *hPMS2*, and *hMSH6*) *(42, 43)* may account for roughly 2% of epithelial ovarian cancers *(44)* and confer up to a 12% lifetime risk of ovarian cancer *(45–47)*. Overall, mutations in highly penetrant genes account for 10–15% of epithelial ovarian cancers *(48, 49)*. It is generally held that most of the inherited component of ovarian cancer may be attributed to low penetrant variants that have yet to be identified.

4.2. Hormonal Risk Factors

Hormones such as estrogen and progesterone are believed to be involved in promoting ovarian carcinogenesis. An extensive review of the hormonal etiology of epithelial ovarian cancer *(50)* concluded that there are two, not necessarily mutually exclusive, hypotheses that reflect what is currently known about the disease. The "incessant ovulation" hypothesis proposes that the number of ovulatory cycles increases the rate of cellular division associated with the repair of the surface epithelium after each ovulation, thereby increasing the likelihood of spontaneous mutations that may promote carcinogenesis (51). The second hypothesis, often referred to as the "gonadotropin hypothesis," posits that gonadotropins such as luteinizing hormone and follicle-stimulating hormone overstimulate the ovarian epithelium, causing increased proliferation and subsequent malignant transformation (52). The epidemiology of ovarian cancer does not help clearly distinguish between these two hypotheses.

The following sections review the epidemiologic data on both endogenous correlates of reproductive hormone exposure and exogenous sources of hormones, specifically, OCs and hormone-replacement therapy (HRT). For a more detailed summary of the hormonal aspects of ovarian cancer, the reader is referred to a review by Riman et al. (53).

4.2.1. Menstrual Factors and Gynecologic Surgery

In support of the incessant ovulation hypothesis, early age at menarche and late age at menopause should increase the risk for ovarian cancer due to an increased number of ovulatory cycles. On the other hand, according to the gonadotropin hypothesis, a late age at menopause delays the surge of postmenopausal gonadotropin hormones, possibly reducing ovarian cancer risk.

Numerous epidemiologic studies have examined the relation between lifetime menstrual history and ovarian cancer risk. The majority of studies have identified slightly increased risks among women whose menarche occurred prior to age 12 years as compared with those having menarche after age 14 years, with odds ratios (OR) ranging from 1.1–1.5 (20, 54–63). For example, in a collaborative analysis of 12 United States case–control studies conducted between 1956 and 1986, data from 2,197 white ovarian cancer cases and 8,893 white controls was used to examine the relationship between reproductive and menstrual characteristics, exogenous estrogen use, and prior pelvic surgeries (59). No consistent trends in risk were identified with onset of menses before 12 years of age. The relationship between age of menarche and ovarian cancer risk was also studied in the Nurses' Health Study, a prospective cohort study of 121,700 female registered nurses aged 30–55 years in 1976 when the study began (62). Only a small, statistically insignificant protective effect from undergoing menarche younger than age 12 years was identified. One Chinese study identified a significant protection with late age at menarche (after age 18 years) (64), while another study showed a slight increased risk with late age at menarche (65). Several studies have identified no association between age at menarche and ovarian cancer risk (51, 55, 66–69).

With regard to the relationship between age at natural menopause and ovarian cancer risk, the data are inconsistent. Numerous case–control studies have identified an association between late age at menopause and the risk of ovarian cancer, with OR ranging from 1.4 to 4.6 in the highest category of age at menopause *(54–56, 60, 64, 65, 69)*. Other case–control studies *(59, 61, 67, 68, 70–72)* and several cohort studies *(62, 66)* found no such association. The collaborative analysis by Whittemore et al., for example, showed an OR of 1.1 (95% CI, 0.71–1.3) for menopause occurring after the age of 55 years *(59)*.

There are various explanations for the conflicting results regarding the relationship between ages at menarche and menopause and ovarian cancer risk *(21)*. Besides the role of chance, it has been proposed that these differences may be explained through real differences between populations. Additionally, it is possible that the definition of menarche and menopause can be subject to recall and misclassification bias. It has also been pointed out that various populations have different age distributions, and that some studies may have failed to adjust for age or other covariates in the analysis. In summary, it can be inferred from the available evidence that if early age at menarche and late age at menopause increase the risk of ovarian cancer, the magnitude is likely small.

Several gynecologic procedures appear to influence the risk for ovarian cancer. It is well established that among high-risk women, bilateral prophylactic oophorectomy reduces ovarian cancer risk by at least 90% *(73)*. Numerous studies have identified a reduced risk of ovarian cancer associated with either a hysterectomy or tubal ligation (without oophorectomy), with the protective effect for each of these procedures ranging from 30 to 40% *(54, 63, 74–78)*. Furthermore, these studies have demonstrated that the risk reduction from these procedures seems to last for at least 10–15 years, which goes against the hypothesis that screening bias (due to selective removal of subclinical ovarian tumors) can explain the protective effect against ovarian cancer *(72, 75, 79, 80)*. Although it is uncertain how these procedures reduce the risk of ovarian cancer, it has been proposed that removal of the uterus and/or blockage of the tubes may prevent potential carcinogens from ascending the genital tract *(20)*. Ascending infections of the ovary have also been proposed as the mechanism by which talcum powder *(81)* and pelvic inflammatory disease *(82)* may increase ovarian cancer risk. Additionally, it has been proposed that these procedures may decrease ovarian cancer risk by decreasing blood flow to the ovaries *(80)*.

4.2.2. Pregnancy

The association between pregnancy and ovarian cancer risk has been studied extensively. Pregnancy causes anovulation and suppresses secretion of pituitary gonadotropins. In agreement with both the incessant ovulation and the gonadotropin hypotheses, pregnancy is expected to reduce the risk of ovarian cancer. One of the most consistent findings is the protective effect of full-term pregnancies on ovarian cancer risk. Parous women are estimated to have a 30–60% lower risk for ovarian cancer compared with nulliparous women *(21, 51, 54, 60, 64–68, 71, 83–86)*. Furthermore, each additional full-term pregnancy is estimated to lower ovarian cancer risk by approximately 15% *(59, 66, 87)*. The influence of age at first birth on ovarian cancer risk is uncertain. While many case–control studies with hospital controls have shown positive associations with late age at first birth (≥30 years of age) *(54, 58, 59, 67, 69, 83, 88–91)*, a reduced risk with late age at first birth has been identified in some case-control studies with population controls *(57, 59, 92)*.

It is unclear whether incomplete pregnancies such as spontaneous or induced abortions impact ovarian cancer risk. It has been suggested that such studies may be biased due to inaccurate reporting of spontaneous or induced pregnancies, although it is unknown whether the accuracy differs between women with and without ovarian cancer *(53)*. Many investigations have identified that an increased number of incomplete pregnancies may have a weak protective effect on ovarian cancer risk *(51, 54, 58, 59, 65, 66, 93–95)*, while other investigations have showed a slightly increased risk with one or more incomplete pregnancies *(68, 86)*. In other studies, incomplete pregnancies had no impact on ovarian cancer risk *(57, 60, 61, 63, 67, 71, 83, 85)*. Induced abortions were found to be protective in several studies *(66, 94, 95)*, while other investigations did not find an increased risk with induced abortion *(57, 69, 93)*. With regard to spontaneous abortions and ovarian cancer risk, positive *(61, 83, 93)*, inverse *(63)*, and null associations *(64, 85, 94)* have been identified.

It is yet to be determined whether nulliparity and low parity per se, rather than difficulty becoming pregnant due to female infertility, are relevant to the development of ovarian cancer. Infertility is an outcome resulting from a heterogenous group of biologically distinct conditions ranging from genital tract infections and tubal disturbances to medical conditions such as endometriosis and polycystic ovarian syndrome *(96, 97)*. Infertility appears to be associated with increased ovarian cancer risk in most studies *(54, 59, 63, 67, 71, 83, 85, 86, 91, 96)*, but not all *(66, 98)*. Infertility seems to pose the greatest risk among women who remain nulliparous, while periods of temporary infertility among parous women are of little concern *(54, 59, 63, 67, 85)*. For example, in a large Canadian case–control study in which most nulliparous women were so by choice, infertility did not appear to impact ovarian cancer risk among parous women, while a slightly elevated risk was observed in a small group of infertile nulliparous women (OR = 2.5; 95% CI, 0.6–4.1) *(63)*.

Possible reasons for the inconsistent results may include the failure to examine the various types of infertility separately, as each relates to ovarian cancer risk. Furthermore, it has been demonstrated that some factors such as a personal history of endometriosis *(99–101)* or polycystic ovarian syndrome *(102)* may influence both infertility and ovarian cancer risk. There have been differences in the definition of infertility used across studies, including physician-diagnosed infertility, self-reported infertility, and periods of unprotected intercourse without becoming pregnant *(53)*. Another methodological concern relates to the potential effect of fertility drug exposure. Some studies suggest that women with a prior history of fertility drug use who remain nulliparous are at an elevated risk for ovarian tumors, particularly tumors of low malignant potential *(59, 103)*. On the other hand, numerous studies have not implicated fertility drugs in increasing ovarian cancer risk *(96–98, 104–106)*. Early detection bias may explain the discrepant findings, as early-stage cancers may be overdiagnosed in infertile women due to the close medical surveillance *(107)*.

4.2.3. Lactation

Lactation suppresses secretion of pituitary gonadotropins and leads to anovulation, particularly in the initial months after delivery *(6)*. If the incessant ovulation and gonadotropin hypotheses are true, lactation should reduce the risk of ovarian cancer. Although the majority of studies have identified a slight decrease in ovarian cancer risk with lactation, with OR approximating 0.6–0.7 *(59, 60, 63, 84–86, 108–110)*, some studies have not *(57, 61, 71)*. Despite the conflicting results, the overall impression is that lactation protects against epithelial ovarian cancer, especially in the first few months following delivery.

4.2.4. Oral Contraceptives

The protection of combined OCs against ovarian cancer risk is one of the most established and significant epidemiologic observations on a public health scale. This is not surprising, as OC use is anticipated to decrease ovarian cancer risk according to both the incessant ovulation and gonadotropin hypotheses. Early studies that relate to the protective effect of OCs on ovarian cancer risk include women who used high estrogen and progestin OC formulations that were introduced in the 1960s. From the mid-1970s, the hormone content in OCs decreased, and in the early 1980s, the sequential OC compounds (biphasic and triphasic) were introduced *(111)*.

The overall estimated protection is approximately 30–40% in ever OC users, and a steady inverse relation is observed with duration of use *(59, 63, 112–115)*. OC use is estimated to reduce a woman's ovarian cancer risk by at least 5% per year, with about a 50% reduction in risk for long-term use of 10 years or greater *(116)*. The favorable effect of OCs against ovarian cancer risk also seems to persist after OC use has ceased *(71, 84, 114, 117–120)*. Moreover, the risk reduction is not confined to any particular type of combined OC formulation *(121, 122)* or to any histological type of ovarian cancer, although the inverse relation is less consistent for mucinous cancers *(9, 11, 14, 123)*. Few epidemiologic studies have evaluated the link between progestin-only contraceptives and ovarian cancer, mostly due to the rarity of this exposure compared with combination OCs. Findings from these studies *(84, 114, 124)* suggest a protective effect of the progestin-only OCs, but further evaluation is needed.

The inverse relation between OC use and ovarian cancer has been observed whether or not other forms of contraception were also used, and across various strata of parity, ages at diagnosis, marital status, and other selected menstrual and reproductive risk factors *(122)*. It has also been observed that potential selection or indication biases, including selective exclusion of OC use by smokers and by women at risk of liver and thromboembolic diseases were also unlikely to alter the association between OC use and ovarian cancer risk *(122)*.

The protection afforded by OC use corresponds to the avoidance of approximately 3,000–5,000 ovarian cancer cases and 2,000–3,000 deaths per year in both Europe *(17)* and in North America *(125)*. The use of OCs therefore has implications for individual risk assessment and on a public health scale.

4.2.5. Hormone-Replacement Therapy

Despite the growing body of literature that has evaluated whether postmenopausal HRT alters ovarian cancer risk, this question remains unanswered. It has been postulated that HRT may reduce ovarian cancer risk by decreasing the secretion of gonadotropins. However, the reduced levels are still above those of premenopausal women *(126)*. On the other hand, it has also been postulated that postmenopausal HRT may increase ovarian cancer risk due to increased estrogen-induced proliferation of ovarian cells *(127)*.

Most studies on the topic have focused on unopposed estrogen therapy. In the collaborative reanalysis of 12 US case–control studies, no association was identified with duration of HRT use in either hospital-based (OR = 0.90 for a 5-year increment of use; $p = 0.37$) or population-based (OR = 1.10 for a 5-year increment of use; $p = 0.21$) studies *(59)*. Several case–control studies *(128, 129)* and meta-analyses *(130, 131)* also failed to identify a statistically significant trend with duration of use, although a few studies have identified a positive association or suggested a positive trend *(11, 132)*. Several prospective studies have demonstrated that longer durations of HRT use were associated with ovarian cancer risk or death *(133–136)*. For example, in the National Institute of Health AARP Diet and Health Study Cohort *(137)*, ovarian cancer risk was increased among unopposed estrogen users of ≥10 years, but not among users of <10 years.

Only recently have studies had sufficient statistical power to evaluate associations between combined estrogen and progestin use and ovarian cancer risk. A Swedish case–control study (n = 655 cases) found that while use of estrogen plus sequential progestin was associated with an increased risk for ovarian cancer, estrogen plus continuous progestin was not *(123)*. However, results from the Women's Health Initiative (WHI), a randomized clinical trial of estrogen plus continuous progestin, revealed an increase in ovarian cancer risk (relative risk [RR] = 1.58; 95% CI, 0.77–3.24), although the increase was not statistically significant due to a limited sample size of only 32 ovarian cancer cases *(138)*.

Data collected on HRT use as part of the Nurses' Health Study cohort were recently analyzed *(139)*. Compared with never-users of any type of HRT, both current and past HRT users of 5 or more years had a significantly elevated risk for ovarian cancer (RR = 1.41; 95% CI, 1.07–1.86) and (RR = 1.52; 95% CI, 1.01–2.27), respectively. Based on their statistical modeling, the authors concluded that the significant increase in risk appeared to be driven largely by duration rather than by status of use. Although use of unopposed estrogen was associated with a 25% increased risk of ovarian cancer (*P* for trend <0.0001; 95% CI for 5-year increment of use, 12–38% increase), use of estrogen plus progestin was not (RR for 5-year increment of use = 1.04; 95% CI, 0.82–1.32). In the United Kingdom Million Women Study *(140)*, 2,273 incident ovarian cancers were observed among 948,576 postmenopausal women who did not have a prior cancer history or a bilateral oophorectomy. For current users of HRT, incidence of ovarian cancer increased with increasing duration of use, but did not differ significantly by type of preparation used, its constituents, or mode of administration. Past users of HRT were not at an increased risk (RR = 0.98; 95% CI, 0.88–1.11).

Some studies that have evaluated HRT use in relation to ovarian cancer risk have pointed to an increased risk only for certain histologic subtypes of ovarian cancer. For example, data from the Nurses' Health Study cohort observed that the association with unopposed estrogen was slightly stronger for endometrioid tumors, which is consistent with other studies *(129, 141)*. A link between unopposed estrogen and the development of endometrioid ovarian tumors is biologically plausible because endometrioid tumors are histologically similar to endometrial tissue *(142)*, and unopposed estrogen use increases the risk of endometrial cancer *(127)*. However, in the United Kingdom Million Women Study *(140)*, although risks associated with HRT varied significantly according to tumor histology (*p* < 0.0001), the relative risk for current versus never users of HRT was greater for serous than for mucinous, endometrioid, or clear cell tumors (RR = 1.53 [95% CI, 1.31–1.79]; RR = 0.72 [95%

CI, 0.52–1.00]; RR = 1.05 [95% CI, 0.77–1.43]; or RR = 0.77 [95% CI, 0.48–1.23]), respectively.

It can be inferred from the available evidence that if an association exists between HRT use and ovarian cancer risk, the magnitude is probably moderate. Findings suggest that women should be counseled about the potential increase in ovarian cancer risk with long-term use of unopposed estrogen. Evidence is insufficient to say whether estrogen plus progestin or very short durations of unopposed estrogen therapy are associated with an increased risk. Since many women are exposed to HRT several years before the peak age-specific incidence of ovarian cancer, even a small change in risk may have a significant impact on the number of ovarian cancer cases.

4.3. Anthropometric Factors

The previous sections highlighting the importance of hormonal factors raise questions about other potential influences on circulating levels of estrogens. One area of great interest is on body mass index (BMI), a measure of body fat calculated as weight in kilograms divided by height in meters squared. The rationale for such studies includes the fact that for postmenopausal women the predominant source of circulating estrogens is aromatization of androgens in adipose tissue *(50, 143)*.

Studies of the relation between *current* BMI and ovarian cancer risk among postmenopausal women are inconclusive. Increases in risk with increasing BMI have been identified in several case–control studies *(144–146)*, but others have found no association *(147–149)* or even an inverse association *(150, 151)*. Alternatively, the majority of recent studies that have examined the relation between ovarian cancer incidence and reported BMI during *adolescence/young adulthood* have yielded less conflicting results. For example, while the Netherlands Cohort Study on Diet and Cancer *(152)* did not detect a significant association between BMI at age 20 years and ovarian cancer risk, other studies, including those involving participants from the Nurses' Health Study and the Iowa Women's Health Study, have detected a positive association *(144, 147–149)*. Two recently published studies, a US hospital-based case–control study *(153)* and a systematic review and meta-analysis *(154)*, also concluded that being obese or overweight in the premenopausal years (<50 years of age) is associated with an increased risk of ovarian cancer *(154)*, suggesting a possible influence of menopausal status on the endogenous hormonal environment.

It is becoming increasingly evident that although BMI is an appropriate measure of adiposity in young and middle-aged women, it may not be as adequate for postmenopausal women *(143)*. As women age, they may lose lean body mass while maintaining the same weight, decreasing the validity of BMI as a measure of central adiposity. It has been suggested that abdominal adiposity measured by waist-to-hip ratio may be a more appropriate measure of obesity *(155, 156)*.

4.4. Diet and Nutrition

The previous section on anthropometric factors and ovarian cancer raises questions about the role of dietary factors and energy intake (balance) in the etiology of ovarian cancer. Ecological studies serve as the basis for most of the suggested links between diet and ovarian cancer risk *(157)*. Based on these data, it was hypothesized that a high intake of fat, milk, and eggs may increase risk, and high intakes of fruits and vegetables may lower risk. Despite numerous analytical epidemiologic studies on various aspects of diet, the findings remain inconsistent.

An extensive review of the epidemiologic literature pertaining to the dietary determinants of ovarian cancer *(157)* concluded that vegetables but not fruits are likely to lower risk. A protective effect for whole grain food consumption and consumption of low-fat milk is also suggested by the results. However, the association between specific fats and oils, fish and meats, and certain milk products are inconsistent and await further investigation before firm conclusions can be made. Similarly, although several studies have examined coffee and tea consumption in relation to ovarian cancer risk, the findings are inconsistent *(65, 69, 158–162)*.

4.5. Exercise and Physical Activity

The potential health benefits of exercise are well established. Thus, it is not surprising that lack of exercise and sedentary behavior have been hypothesized to increase ovarian cancer risk. Although several previous studies have found a protective effect of physical activity *(163, 164)*, more recent studies have not. For example, in the Women's Lifestyle and Health Study *(165)*, a prospective European study of physical activity in different periods of life, physical activity at age 14 or 30 years did not afford any protection from ovarian cancer nor did consistently high levels of activity from younger ages. Results were similar for borderline and invasive tumors, and for different subgroups of women classified according to known risk factors for ovarian cancer. The association between physical activity, sedentary behavior, and ovarian cancer risk was also recently examined in the American Cancer Society Prevention Study II Nutrition Cohort *(166)*, a prospective cohort of cancer incidence and mortality, using information obtained at baseline in 1992. No overall association was observed between measures of past physical activity or with recreational physical activity at baseline and ovarian cancer risk for the highest category of physical activity compared with none (hazard ratio = 0.73; 95% CI, 0.40–1.34). However, among the women in the American Cancer Society Prevention Study II Nutrition Cohort *(166)*, a prolonged duration of sedentary behavior was associated with an increase risk for ovarian cancer (≥ 6 hours per day versus <3 hours per day; hazard ratio = 1.55; 95% CI, 1.08–2.22; p-trend = 0.01). Sedentary behaviors were also associated with an increase in ovarian cancer risk in a Chinese case–control study *(167)*.

Based on the available evidence, it can be inferred that high levels of sedentary behavior may increase ovarian cancer risk, but it is unclear whether light or moderate physical activity alters ovarian cancer risk. It has been suggested that future studies should be directed toward different types (occupational, recreational, household) and components (frequency, intensity, and duration) of activity and their relation to ovarian cancer risk *(165, 166)*. Additionally, the association between physical activity and sedentary behavior should be further evaluated at various periods in life. Even though questions remain unanswered regarding the relationship between exercise and physical activity and ovarian cancer risk, when considering the additional benefits of exercise on weight control, bone density, and heart disease, the promotion of regular activity to women should be encouraged.

4.6. Other Lifestyle Factors

4.6.1. Cigarette Smoking

Cigarette smoking is a modifiable cause of many types of cancer, but whether it impacts a woman's risk of ovarian cancer is unclear. The majority of early reports concluded that smoking was not associated with an increased risk of ovarian cancer *(85, 162, 168, 169)*. Recent studies that have examined the relation between smoking and ovarian cancer by histologic subtype report that smoking may actually increase the risk for the invasive mucinous tumors but not other subtypes *(10, 13, 170)*. A recently published systematic literature review and meta-analysis on the topic *(171)* concluded that there is a significant doubling of risk of mucinous ovarian cancer in current smokers compared with never-smokers (summary RR = 2.1; 95% CI, 1.7–2.7), but no increased risk of serous (summary RR = 1.0; 95% CI, 0.8–1.2) or endometrioid (summary RR = 0.8; 95% CI, 0.6–1.1) cancers, and a significant risk reduction for clear cell cancers (summary RR = 0.6; 95% CI, 0.3–0.9). The risk of mucinous cancer increased in a dose–response relationship, but returned to that of never-smokers within 20–30 years of stopping smoking. Histologically, mucinous ovarian tumors resemble mucinous gastrointestinal cancers, some of which (pancreatic cancer, gastric cancer) have been classified as smoking-related cancers *(171)*. These findings suggest that smoking may be one of the few modifiable risk factors offering primary prevention of mucinous ovarian cancer.

4.6.2. Alcohol Consumption

Consistent evidence that moderate alcohol consumption increases breast cancer risk, presumably by increasing levels of circulating hormones *(172)*, infers that alcohol consumption may also impact the development of other hormone-related cancers, such as ovarian cancer. Alcohol consumption, a common and modifiable exposure, has been investigated as a possible cause of ovarian cancer in numerous epidemiologic studies. However, findings from case–control and cohort studies have been conflicting, with published reports of null *(60, 85, 160, 162, 173, 174)*, positive *(65, 175, 176)*, and inverse associations *(177–179)*.

Several studies have explored whether some of the observed inconsistency reflect differences in risk by the type of alcohol consumed (wine, beer, or alcohol) *(176, 177)*, or histologic subtype of the tumor *(176, 177, 179)*. In a large population-based case–control study *(180)*, consumption of beer (not liquor or wine) during early adulthood (20–30 years of age) was associated with a moderately increased risk of invasive ovarian cancer, with the association limited to serous tumors (OR = 1.52; 95% CI, 1.01–2.30), though results for other histological subtypes were based on sparse data. This risk was associated with regular consumption (1 or more drinks per day), and there was no evidence of a dose-response relationship. Although there was no association between wine consumption and ovarian cancer risk in the large population-based study by Peterson et al. *(180)*, a recent publication involving the California Teachers Study cohort *(181)* revealed that regular consumption of wine in early adulthood (ages 18–22 years or 30–35 years or at baseline) was associated with a moderately increased ovarian cancer risk.

Data from the Netherlands Cohort Study on Diet and Cancer found no association between alcohol consumption in the form of wine, beer, or liquor and ovarian cancer risk *(182)*. A recently published pooled analysis of 10 cohort studies that included over 500,000 women and 2,001 incident ovarian cancer cases also found no association between total alcohol intake (pooled multivariate RR = 1.12; 95% CI, 0.86–1.44 comparing ≥30 to 0 g day of alcohol) or alcohol intake from wine, beer, or spirits and ovarian cancer risk *(183)*.

In summary, the literature tends to suggest that if alcohol intake does influence risk of ovarian cancer, the magnitude is small and possibly limited to particular histologic subtypes.

5. Summary and Conclusions

Ovarian cancer represents a fairly common malignancy among women. Due to the inability to detect this type of cancer at an early stage, ovarian cancer causes more deaths per year than any other gynecologic malignancy. Ovarian cancer therefore represents a significant public health problem. This chapter describes the magnitude of the problem and summarizes the results of epidemiologic studies in order to identify risk factors for the disease.

Although many of the risk factors in **Table 20.1** cannot be modified, reflecting the contribution of genetics and unavoidable

Table 20.1
Summary of risk factors for ovarian cancer by strength of evidence

Established risk factors	Possible risk factors	Suspected risk factors
Age	Early age at menarche	Hormone-replacement therapy
Family history	Late age at menopause	Dietary fat
Nulliparity	Infertility	Obesity
Oral contraceptive use (protective)	Lactation (protective)	Sedentary lifestyle
Oophorectomy (protective)	Tubal ligation (protective)	Cigarette smoking
	Hysterectomy (protective)	Alcohol consumption
	Low vegetable intake	

exposures, a number of others can be altered. Increasing parity and OC use lower risk of ovarian cancer. The same is probably true, but to a weaker degree, from lactation and incomplete pregnancies. Infertility contributes to ovarian cancer risk among nulliparous women, while temporary fertility problems in parous women does not. Risks associated with postmenopausal HRT use require further investigation, especially since several studies suggest use may increase risk.

It is important to emphasize that the established risk factors confer neither large increases in risk nor account for all the variability in the incidence of this disease. Thus, many of the causes of ovarian cancer are yet to be identified. Additional research is needed to better understand the etiology of this deadly disease. This knowledge is necessary to reduce the public health burden from ovarian cancer.

References

1. Ferlay J., Bray F., Pisani P. and Parkin D.M. (2004) GLOBOCAN 2002: Cancer Incidence, Mortality, and Prevalence Worldwide IARC CancerBase No. 5. version 2.0, IARC Press, Lyon, France. http://www-dep.iarc.fr/.

2. Sankaranarayanan, R., and Ferlay, J. (2006) Worldwide burden of gynaecological cancer: the size of the problem. *Best Pract Res Clin Obstet Gynaecol* 20, 207–225

3. American Cancer Society. Cancer Facts and Figures 2006. Atlanta: American Cancer Society, 2006.

4. Ries, L. A. G., Harkins, D., Krapcho, M., Mariotto, A., Miller, B. A., Feuer, E. S., Clegg, L., Horner, M. J., Howlader, N., Eisner, M. P., Richman, M., Edwards, B. K. (eds). SEER Cancer Statistics Review, 1975–2004, National Cancer Institute. Bethesa, MD, http://seer.cancer.gov/csr/1975_2004/, based on November 2006 SEER data submission, posted to the SEER website 2007.

5. Chen, V. W., Ruiz, B., Killeen, J. L., Cote, T. R., Wu, X. C., and Correa, C. N. (2003)

Pathology and classification of ovarian tumors. *Cancer* **97**, 2631–2642

6. Weiss, N. S., Cook, L. S., Farrow, D. C., Rosenblatt, K. A. (1996) Ovarian Cancer. In: Schottenfeld, D., Fraumeni, J. F. (eds.) Cancer Epidemiology and Prevention. Oxford University Press, New York pp. 1040–1057.

7. Averette, H.E., Nguyen, H. (1995) Gynecologic Cancer. In: Murphy GP, Lawrence L, Lenhard RE (eds) American Cancer Society Textbook of Clinical Oncology, Atlanta, pp 552–579.

8. Eltabbakh, G. H., Natarajan, N., Piver, M. S., and Mettlin, C. J. (1999) Epidemiologic differences between women with borderline ovarian tumors and women with epithelial ovarian cancer. *Gynecol Oncol* **74**, 103–107.

9. Tung, K. H., Goodman, M. T., Wu, A. H., McDuffie, K., Wilkens, L. R., Kolonel, L. N., Nomura, A. M., Terada, K. Y., Carney, M. E., and Sobin, L. H. (2003) Reproductive factors and epithelial ovarian cancer risk by histologic type: a multiethnic case-control study. *Am J Epidemiol* **158**, 629–638.

10. Marchbanks, P. A., Wilson, H., Bastos, E., Cramer, D. W., Schildkraut, J. M., and Peterson, H. B. (2000) Cigarette smoking and epithelial ovarian cancer by histologic type. *Obstet Gynecol* **95**, 255–260.

11. Risch, H. A., Marrett, L. D., Jain, M., and Howe, G. R. (1996) Differences in risk factors for epithelial ovarian cancer by histologic type. Results of a case-control study. *Am J Epidemiol* **144**, 363–372.

12. Chiaffarino, F., Parazzini, F., Bosetti, C., Franceschi, S., Talamini, R., Canzonieri, V., Montella, M., Ramazzotti, V., Franceschi, S., and La Vecchia, C. (2007) Risk factors for ovarian cancer histotypes. *Eur J Cancer* **43**, 1208–1213.

13. Kurian, A. W., Balise, R. R., McGuire, V., and Whittemore, A. S. (2005) Histologic types of epithelial ovarian cancer: have they different risk factors? *Gynecol Oncol* **96**, 520–530.

14. Parazzini, F., Chiaffarino, F., Negri, E., Surace, M., Benzi, G., Franceschi, S., Fedele, L., and La Vecchia, C. (2004) Risk factors for different histological types of ovarian cancer. *Int J Gynecol Cancer* **14**, 431–436.

15. Herrinton, L. J., Stanford, J. L., Schwartz, S. M., and Weiss, N. S. (1994) Ovarian cancer incidence among Asian migrants to the United States and their descendants. *J Natl Cancer Inst* **86**, 1336–1339.

16. Kliewer, E. V. and Smith, K. R. (1995) Ovarian cancer mortality among immigrants in Australia and Canada. *Cancer Epidemiol Biomarkers Prev* **4**, 453–458.

17. Bray, F., Loos, A. H., Tognazzo, S., and La Vecchia, C. (2005) Ovarian cancer in Europe: Cross-sectional trends in incidence and mortality in 28 countries, 1953–2000. *Int J Cancer* **113**, 977–990.

18. Coleman, M. P., Esteve, J., Damiecki, P., Arslan, A., and Renard, H. (1993) Trends in cancer incidence and mortality. *IARC Sci Publ*, 1–806.

19. Howe, H. L., Wu, X., Ries, L. A., Cokkinides, V., Ahmed, F., Jemal, A., Miller, B., Williams, M., Ward, E., Wingo, P. A., Ramirez, A., and Edwards, B. K. (2006) Annual report to the nation on the status of cancer, 1975–2003, featuring cancer among U.S. Hispanic/Latino populations. *Cancer* **107**, 1711–1742.

20. Parazzini, F., Franceschi, S., La Vecchia, C., and Fasoli, M. (1991) The epidemiology of ovarian cancer. *Gynecol Oncol* **43**, 9–23.

21. La Vecchia, C. (2001) Epidemiology of ovarian cancer: a summary review. *Eur J Cancer Prev* **10**, 125–129.

22. Barnholtz-Sloan, J. S., Schwartz, A. G., Qureshi, F., Jacques, S., Malone, J., and Munkarah, A. R. (2003) Ovarian cancer: changes in patterns at diagnosis and relative survival over the last three decades. *Am J Obstet Gynecol* **189**, 1120–1127.

23. Nguyen, H. N., Averette, H. E., and Janicek, M. (1994) Ovarian carcinoma. A review of the significance of familial risk factors and the role of prophylactic oophorectomy in cancer prevention. *Cancer* **74**, 545–555.

24. Parazzini, F., Negri, E., La Vecchia, C., Restelli, C., and Franceschi, S. (1992) Family history of reproductive cancers and ovarian cancer risk: an Italian case-control study. *Am J Epidemiol* **135**, 35–40.

25. Stratton, J. F., Pharoah, P., Smith, S. K., Easton, D., and Ponder, B. A. (1998) A systematic review and meta-analysis of family history and risk of ovarian cancer. *Br J Obstet Gynaecol* **105**, 493–499.

26. Sutcliffe, S., Pharoah, P. D., Easton, D. F., and Ponder, B. A. (2000) Ovarian and breast cancer risks to women in families with two or more cases of ovarian cancer. *Int J Cancer* **87**, 110–117.

27. Ziogas, A., Gildea, M., Cohen, P., Bringman, D., Taylor, T. H., Seminara, D., Barker, D., Casey, G., Haile, R., Liao, S. Y., Thomas, D., Noble, B., Kurosaki, T., and Anton-Culver, H. (2000) Cancer risk

estimates for family members of a population-based family registry for breast and ovarian cancer. *Cancer Epidemiol Biomarkers Prev* 9, 103–111.

28. Negri, E., Pelucchi, C., Franceschi, S., Montella, M., Conti, E., Dal Maso, L., Parazzini, F., Tavani, A., Carbone, A., and La Vecchia, C. (2003) Family history of cancer and risk of ovarian cancer. *Eur J Cancer* 39, 505–510.

29. Frank, T. S., Manley, S. A., Olopade, O. I., Cummings, S., Garber, J. E., Bernhardt, B., Antman, K., Russo, D., Wood, M. E., Mullineau, L., Isaacs, C., Peshkin, B., Buys, S., Venne, V., Rowley, P. T., Loader, S., Offit, K., Robson, M., Hampel, H., Brener, D., Winer, E. P., Clark, S., Weber, B., Strong, L. C., Thomas, A., et al. (1998) Sequence analysis of BRCA1 and BRCA2: correlation of mutations with family history and ovarian cancer risk. *J Clin Oncol* 16, 2417–2425.

30. Narod, S., Ford, D., Devilee, P., Barkardottir, R. B., Eyfjord, J., Lenoir, G., Serova, O., Easton, D., and Goldgar, D. (1995) Genetic heterogeneity of breast-ovarian cancer revisited. Breast Cancer Linkage Consortium. *Am J Hum Genet* 57, 957–958.

31. Ford, D., Easton, D. F., Bishop, D. T., Narod, S. A., and Goldgar, D. E. (1994) Risks of cancer in BRCA1-mutation carriers. Breast Cancer Linkage Consortium. *Lancet* 343, 692–695.

32. Antoniou, A., Pharoah, P. D., Narod, S., Risch, H. A., Eyfjord, J. E., Hopper, J. L., Loman, N., Olsson, H., Johannsson, O., Borg, A., Pasini, B., Radice, P., Manoukian, S., Eccles, D. M., Tang, N., Olah, E., Anton-Culver, H., Warner, E., Lubinski, J., Gronwald, J., Gorski, B., Tulinius, H., Thorlacius, S., Eerola, H., Nevanlinna, H., Syrjakoski, K., Kallioniemi, O. P., Thompson, D., Evans, C., Peto, J., Lalloo, F., Evans, D. G., and Easton, D. F. (2003) Average risks of breast and ovarian cancer associated with BRCA1 or BRCA2 mutations detected in case Series unselected for family history: a combined analysis of 22 studies. *Am J Hum Genet* 72, 1117–1130.

33. Malander, S., Ridderheim, M., Masback, A., Loman, N., Kristoffersson, U., Olsson, H., Nilbert, M., and Borg, A. (2004) One in 10 ovarian cancer patients carry germ line BRCA1 or BRCA2 mutations: results of a prospective study in Southern Sweden. *Eur J Cancer* 40, 422–428.

34. Menkiszak, J., Gronwald, J., Gorski, B., Jakubowska, A., Huzarski, T., Byrski, T., Foszczynska-Kloda, M., Haus, O., Janiszewska, H., Perkowska, M., Brozek, I., Grzybowska, E., Zientek, H., Gozdz, S., Kozak-Klonowska, B., Urbanski, K., Miturski, R., Kowalczyk, J., Pluzanska, A., Niepsuj, S., Koc, J., Szwiec, M., Drosik, K., Mackiewicz, A., Lamperska, K., Strozyk, E., Godlewski, D., Stawicka, M., Wasko, B., Bebenek, M., Rozmiarek, A., Rzepka-Gorska, I., Narod, S. A., and Lubinski, J. (2003) Hereditary ovarian cancer in Poland. *Int J Cancer* 106, 942–945.

35. Pal, T., Permuth-Wey, J., Betts, J. A., Krischer, J. P., Fiorica, J., Arango, H., LaPolla, J., Hoffman, M., Martino, M. A., Wakeley, K., Wilbanks, G., Nicosia, S., Cantor, A., and Sutphen, R. (2005) BRCA1 and BRCA2 mutations account for a large proportion of ovarian carcinoma cases. *Cancer* 104, 2807–2816.

36. Risch, H. A., McLaughlin, J. R., Cole, D. E., Rosen, B., Bradley, L., Kwan, E., Jack, E., Vesprini, D. J., Kuperstein, G., Abrahamson, J. L., Fan, I., Wong, B., and Narod, S. A. (2001) Prevalence and penetrance of germline BRCA1 and BRCA2 mutations in a population series of 649 women with ovarian cancer. *Am J Hum Genet* 68, 700–710.

37. Stratton, J. F., Gayther, S. A., Russell, P., Dearden, J., Gore, M., Blake, P., Easton, D., and Ponder, B. A. (1997) Contribution of BRCA1 mutations to ovarian cancer. *N Engl J Med* 336, 1125–1130.

38. Takahashi, H., Behbakht, K., McGovern, P. E., Chiu, H. C., Couch, F. J., Weber, B. L., Friedman, L. S., King, M. C., Furusato, M., LiVolsi, V. A., and et al. (1995) Mutation analysis of the BRCA1 gene in ovarian cancers. *Cancer Res* 55, 2998–3002.

39. Anton-Culver, H., Cohen, P. F., Gildea, M. E., and Ziogas, A. (2000) Characteristics of BRCA1 mutations in a population-based case series of breast and ovarian cancer. *Eur J Cancer* 36, 1200–1208.

40. Bjorge, T., Lie, A. K., Hovig, E., Gislefoss, R. E., Hansen, S., Jellum, E., Langseth, H., Nustad, K., Trope, C. G., and Dorum, A. (2004) BRCA1 mutations in ovarian cancer and borderline tumours in Norway: a nested case-control study. *Br J Cancer* 91, 1829–1834.

41. Van Der Looij, M., Szabo, C., Besznyak, I., Liszka, G., Csokay, B., Pulay, T., Toth, J., Devilee, P., King, M. C., and Olah, E. (2000) Prevalence of founder BRCA1 and BRCA2 mutations among breast and ovarian cancer patients in Hungary. *Int J Cancer* 86, 737–740.

42. Lynch, H. T. and Smyrk, T. (1996) Hereditary nonpolyposis colorectal cancer (Lynch syndrome). An updated review. *Cancer* **78**, 1149–1167.

43. Marra, G., and Boland, C. R. (1995) Hereditary nonpolyposis colorectal cancer: the syndrome, the genes, and historical perspectives. *J Natl Cancer Inst* **87**, 1114–1125.

44. Malander, S., Rambech, E., Kristoffersson, U., Halvarsson, B., Ridderheim, M., Borg, A., and Nilbert, M. (2006) The contribution of the hereditary nonpolyposis colorectal cancer syndrome to the development of ovarian cancer. *Gynecol Oncol* **101**, 238–243.

45. Aarnio, M., Mecklin, J. P., Aaltonen, L. A., Nystrom-Lahti, M., and Jarvinen, H. J. (1995) Life-time risk of different cancers in hereditary non-polyposis colorectal cancer (HNPCC) syndrome. *Int J Cancer* **64**, 430–433.

46. Aarnio, M., Sankila, R., Pukkala, E., Salovaara, R., Aaltonen, L. A., de la Chapelle, A., Peltomaki, P., Mecklin, J. P., and Jarvinen, H. J. (1999) Cancer risk in mutation carriers of DNA-mismatch-repair genes. *Int J Cancer* **81**, 214–218.

47. Prat, J., Ribe, A., and Gallardo, A. (2005) Hereditary ovarian cancer. *Hum Pathol* **36**, 861–870.

48. Boyd, J. and Rubin, S. C. (1997) Hereditary ovarian cancer: molecular genetics and clinical implications. *Gynecol Oncol* **64**, 196–206.

49. Lynch, H. T., Casey, M. J., Shaw, T. G., and Lynch, J. F. (1998) Hereditary factors in gynecologic cancer. *Oncologist* **3**, 319–338.

50. Risch, H. A. (1998) Hormonal etiology of epithelial ovarian cancer, with a hypothesis concerning the role of androgens and progesterone. *J Natl Cancer Inst* **90**, 1774–1786.

51. Casagrande, J. T., Louie, E. W., Pike, M. C., Roy, S., Ross, R. K., and Henderson, B. E. (1979) "Incessant ovulation" and ovarian cancer. *Lancet* **2**, 170–173.

52. Cramer, D. W. and Welch, W. R. (1983) Determinants of ovarian cancer risk. II. Inferences regarding pathogenesis. *J Natl Cancer Inst* **71**, 717–721.

53. Riman, T., Persson, I., and Nilsson, S. (1998) Hormonal aspects of epithelial ovarian cancer: review of epidemiological evidence. *Clin Endocrinol (Oxf)* **49**, 695–707.

54. Booth, M., Beral, V., and Smith, P. (1989) Risk factors for ovarian cancer: a case-control study. *Br J Cancer* **60**, 592–598.

55. Franceschi, S., La Vecchia, C., Booth, M., Tzonou, A., Negri, E., Parazzini, F., Trichopoulos, D., and Beral, V. (1991) Pooled analysis of 3 European case-control studies of ovarian cancer: II. Age at menarche and at menopause. *Int J Cancer* **49**, 57–60.

56. Parazzini, F., La Vecchia, C., Negri, E., and Gentile, A. (1989) Menstrual factors and the risk of epithelial ovarian cancer. *J Clin Epidemiol* **42**, 443–448.

57. Purdie, D., Green, A., Bain, C., Siskind, V., Ward, B., Hacker, N., Quinn, M., Wright, G., Russell, P., and Susil, B. (1995) Reproductive and other factors and risk of epithelial ovarian cancer: an Australian case-control study. Survey of Women' Health Study Group. *Int J Cancer* **62**, 678–684.

58. Tavani, A., Negri, E., Franceschi, S., Parazzini, F., and La Vecchia, C. (1993) Risk factors for epithelial ovarian cancer in women under age 45. *Eur J Cancer* **29A**, 1297–1301.

59. Whittemore, A. S., Harris, R., and Itnyre, J. (1992) Characteristics relating to ovarian cancer risk: collaborative analysis of 12 US case-control studies. II. Invasive epithelial ovarian cancers in white women. Collaborative Ovarian Cancer Group. *Am J Epidemiol* **136**, 1184–1203.

60. Wu, M. L., Whittemore, A. S., Paffenbarger, R. S., Jr., Sarles, D. L., Kampert, J. B., Grosser, S., Jung, D. L., Ballon, S., Hendrickson, M., and Mohle-Boetani, J. (1988) Personal and environmental characteristics related to epithelial ovarian cancer. I. Reproductive and menstrual events and oral contraceptive use. *Am J Epidemiol* **128**, 1216–1227.

61. Wynder, E. L., Dodo, H., and Barber, H. R. (1969) Epidemiology of cancer of the ovary. *Cancer* **23**, 352–370.

62. Hankinson, S. E., Colditz, G. A., Hunter, D. J., Willett, W. C., Stampfer, M. J., Rosner, B., Hennekens, C. H., and Speizer, F. E. (1995) A prospective study of reproductive factors and risk of epithelial ovarian cancer. *Cancer* **76**, 284–290.

63. Risch, H. A., Marrett, L. D., and Howe, G. R. (1994) Parity, contraception, infertility, and the risk of epithelial ovarian cancer. *Am J Epidemiol* **140**, 585–597.

64. Shu, X. O., Brinton, L. A., Gao, Y. T., and Yuan, J. M. (1989) Population-based case-control study of ovarian cancer in Shanghai. *Cancer Res* **49**, 3670–3674.

65. Tzonou, A., Day, N. E., Trichopoulos, D., Walker, A., Saliaraki, M., Papapostolou, M., and Polychronopoulou, A. (1984) The

epidemiology of ovarian cancer in Greece: a case-control study. *Eur J Cancer Clin Oncol* **20**, 1045–1052.

66. Kvale, G., Heuch, I., Nilssen, S., and Beral, V. (1988) Reproductive factors and risk of ovarian cancer: a prospective study. *Int J Cancer* **42**, 246–251.

67. McGowan, L., Norris, H. J., Hartge, P., Hoover, R., and Lesher, L. (1988) Risk factors in ovarian cancer. *Eur J Gynaecol Oncol* **9**, 195–199.

68. Newhouse, M. L., Pearson, R. M., Fullerton, J. M., Boesen, E. A., and Shannon, H. S. (1977) A case control study of carcinoma of the ovary. *Br J Prev Soc Med* **31**, 148–153.

69. Polychronopoulou, A., Tzonou, A., Hsieh, C. C., Kaprinis, G., Rebelakos, A., Toupadaki, N., and Trichopoulos, D. (1993) Reproductive variables, tobacco, ethanol, coffee and somatometry as risk factors for ovarian cancer. *Int J Cancer* **55**, 402–407.

70. Annegers, J. F., Strom, H., Decker, D. G., Dockerty, M. B., and O'Fallon, W. M. (1979) Ovarian cancer: incidence and case-control study. *Cancer* **43**, 723–729.

71. Cramer, D. W., Hutchison, G. B., Welch, W. R., Scully, R. E., and Ryan, K. J. (1983) Determinants of ovarian cancer risk. I. Reproductive experiences and family history. *J Natl Cancer Inst* **71**, 711–716.

72. Hartge, P., Hoover, R., McGowan, L., Lesher, L., and Norris, H. J. (1988) Menopause and ovarian cancer. *Am J Epidemiol* **127**, 990–998.

73. Domchek, S. M. and Rebbeck, T. R. (2007) Prophylactic oophorectomy in women at increased cancer risk. *Curr Opin Obstet Gynecol* **19**, 27–30.

74. Green, A., Purdie, D., Bain, C., Siskind, V., Russell, P., Quinn, M., and Ward, B. (1997) Tubal sterilisation, hysterectomy and decreased risk of ovarian cancer. Survey of Women' Health Study Group. *Int J Cancer* **71**, 948–951.

75. Hankinson, S. E., Hunter, D. J., Colditz, G. A., Willett, W. C., Stampfer, M. J., Rosner, B., Hennekens, C. H., and Speizer, F. E. (1993) Tubal ligation, hysterectomy, and risk of ovarian cancer. A prospective study. *JAMA* **270**, 2813–2818.

76. Kreiger, N., Sloan, M., Cotterchio, M., and Parsons, P. (1997) Surgical procedures associated with risk of ovarian cancer. *Int J Epidemiol* **26**, 710–715.

77. Miracle-McMahill, H. L., Calle, E. E., Kosinski, A. S., Rodriguez, C., Wingo, P. A., Thun, M. J., and Heath, C. W., Jr. (1997) Tubal ligation and fatal ovarian cancer in a large prospective cohort study. *Am J Epidemiol* **145**, 349–357.

78. Rosenblatt, K. A. and Thomas, D. B. (1996) Reduced risk of ovarian cancer in women with a tubal ligation or hysterectomy. The World Health Organization Collaborative Study of Neoplasia and Steroid Contraceptives. *Cancer Epidemiol Biomarkers Prev* **5**, 933–935.

79. Weiss, N. S. and Harlow, B. L. (1986) Why does hysterectomy without bilateral oophorectomy influence the subsequent incidence of ovarian cancer? *Am J Epidemiol* **124**, 856–858.

80. Chiaffarino, F., Parazzini, F., Decarli, A., Franceschi, S., Talamini, R., Montella, M., and La Vecchia, C. (2005) Hysterectomy with or without unilateral oophorectomy and risk of ovarian cancer. *Gynecol Oncol* **97**, 318–322.

81. Huncharek, M., Geschwind, J. F., and Kupelnick, B. (2003) Perineal application of cosmetic talc and risk of invasive epithelial ovarian cancer: a meta-analysis of 11,933 subjects from sixteen observational studies. *Anticancer Res* **23**, 1955–1960.

82. Risch, H. A. and Howe, G. R. (1995) Pelvic inflammatory disease and the risk of epithelial ovarian cancer. *Cancer Epidemiol Biomarkers Prev* **4**, 447–451.

83. Joly, D. J., Lilienfeld, A. M., Diamond, E. L., and Bross, I. D. (1974) An epidemiologic study of the relationship of reproductive experience to cancer of the ovary. *Am J Epidemiol* **99**, 190–209.

84. (1987) Centers for Disease Control Cancer and Steroid Hormone Study. The reduction in risk of ovarian cancer associated with oral-contraceptive use. *N Engl J Med* **316**, 650–655.

85. Hartge, P., Schiffman, M. H., Hoover, R., McGowan, L., Lesher, L., and Norris, H. J. (1989) A case-control study of epithelial ovarian cancer. *Am J Obstet Gynecol* **161**, 10–16.

86. Nasca, P. C., Greenwald, P., Chorost, S., Richart, R., and Caputo, T. (1984) An epidemiologic case-control study of ovarian cancer and reproductive factors. *Am J Epidemiol* **119**, 705–713.

87. Adami, H. O., Hsieh, C. C., Lambe, M., Trichopoulos, D., Leon, D., Persson, I., Ekbom, A., and Janson, P. O. (1994) Parity, age at first childbirth, and risk of ovarian cancer. *Lancet* **344**, 1250–1254.

88. La Vecchia, C., Decarli, A., Franceschi, S., Regallo, M., and Tognoni, G. (1984) Age

at first birth and the risk of epithelial ovarian cancer. *J Natl Cancer Inst* **73**, 663–666.

89. Negri, E., Franceschi, S., Tzonou, A., Booth, M., La Vecchia, C., Parazzini, F., Beral, V., Boyle, P., and Trichopoulos, D. (1991) Pooled analysis of 3 European case-control studies: I. Reproductive factors and risk of epithelial ovarian cancer. *Int J Cancer* **49**, 50–56.

90. Franceschi, S., La Vecchia, C., Helmrich, S. P., Mangioni, C., and Tognoni, G. (1982) Risk factors for epithelial ovarian cancer in Italy. *Am J Epidemiol* **115**, 714–719.

91. Hildreth, N. G., Kelsey, J. L., LiVolsi, V. A., Fischer, D. B., Holford, T. R., Mostow, E. D., Schwartz, P. E., and White, C. (1981) An epidemiologic study of epithelial carcinoma of the ovary. *Am J Epidemiol* **114**, 398–405.

92. John, E. M., Whittemore, A. S., Harris, R., and Itnyre, J. (1993) Characteristics relating to ovarian cancer risk: collaborative analysis of seven U.S. case-control studies. Epithelial ovarian cancer in black women. Collaborative Ovarian Cancer Group. *J Natl Cancer Inst* **85** 142–147.

93. Chen, M. T., Cook, L. S., Daling, J. R., and Weiss, N. S. (1996) Incomplete pregnancies and risk of ovarian cancer (Washington, United States). *Cancer Causes Control* **7**, 415–420.

94. Mori, M., Harabuchi, I., Miyake, H., Casagrande, J. T., Henderson, B. E., and Ross, R. K. (1988) Reproductive, genetic, and dietary risk factors for ovarian cancer. *Am J Epidemiol* **128**, 771–777.

95. Negri, E., Franceschi, S., La Vecchia, C., and Parazzini, F. (1992) Incomplete pregnancies and ovarian cancer risk. *Gynecol Oncol* **47**, 234–238.

96. Mosgaard, B. J., Lidegaard, O., Kjaer, S. K., Schou, G., and Andersen, A. N. (1997) Infertility, fertility drugs, and invasive ovarian cancer: a case-control study. *Fertil Steril* **67**, 1005–1012.

97. Modan, B., Ron, E., Lerner-Geva, L., Blumstein, T., Menczer, J., Rabinovici, J., Oelsner, G., Freedman, L., Mashiach, S., and Lunenfeld, B. (1998) Cancer incidence in a cohort of infertile women. *Am J Epidemiol* **147**, 1038–1042.

98. Franceschi, S., La Vecchia, C., Negri, E., Guarneri, S., Montella, M., Conti, E., and Parazzini, F. (1994) Fertility drugs and risk of epithelial ovarian cancer in Italy. *Hum Reprod* **9**, 1673–1675.

99. Brinton, L. A., Sakoda, L. C., Sherman, M. E., Frederiksen, K., Kjaer, S. K., Graubard, B. I., Olsen, J. H., and Mellemkjaer, L. (2005) Relationship of benign gynecologic diseases to subsequent risk of ovarian and uterine tumors. *Cancer Epidemiol Biomarkers Prev* **14**, 2929–2935.

100. Edmondson, R. J. and Monaghan, J. M. (2001) The epidemiology of ovarian cancer. *Int J Gynecol Cancer* **11**, 423–429.

101. Vigano, P., Somigliana, E., Parazzini, F., and Vercellini, P. (2007) Bias versus causality: interpreting recent evidence of association between endometriosis and ovarian cancer. *Fertil Steril* **88**, 588–593.

102. Schildkraut, J. M., Schwingl, P. J., Bastos, E., Evanoff, A., and Hughes, C. (1996) Epithelial ovarian cancer risk among women with polycystic ovary syndrome. *Obstet Gynecol* **88**, 554–559.

103. Rossing, M. A., Daling, J. R., Weiss, N. S., Moore, D. E., and Self, S. G. (1994) Ovarian tumors in a cohort of infertile women. *N Engl J Med* **331**, 771–776.

104. Ness, R. B., Cramer, D. W., Goodman, M. T., Kjaer, S. K., Mallin, K., Mosgaard, B. J., Purdie, D. M., Risch, H. A., Vergona, R., and Wu, A. H. (2002) Infertility, fertility drugs, and ovarian cancer: a pooled analysis of case-control studies. *Am J Epidemiol* **155**, 217–224.

105. Potashnik, G., Lerner-Geva, L., Genkin, L., Chetrit, A., Lunenfeld, E., and Porath, A. (1999) Fertility drugs and the risk of breast and ovarian cancers: results of a long-term follow-up study. *Fertil Steril* **71**, 853–859.

106. Venn, A., Watson, L., Lumley, J., Giles, G., King, C., and Healy, D. (1995) Breast and ovarian cancer incidence after infertility and in vitro fertilisation. *Lancet* **346**, 995–1000.

107. Ayhan, A., Salman, M. C., Celik, H., Dursun, P., Ozyuncu, O., and Gultekin, M. (2004) Association between fertility drugs and gynecologic cancers, breast cancer, and childhood cancers. *Acta Obstet Gynecol Scand* **83**, 1104–1111.

108. Gwinn, M. L., Lee, N. C., Rhodes, P. H., Layde, P. M., and Rubin, G. L. (1990) Pregnancy, breast feeding, and oral contraceptives and the risk of epithelial ovarian cancer. *J Clin Epidemiol* **43**, 559–568.

109. Rosenblatt, K. A. and Thomas, D. B. (1993) Lactation and the risk of epithelial ovarian cancer. The WHO Collaborative Study of Neoplasia and Steroid Contraceptives. *Int J Epidemiol* **22**, 192–197.

110. Schneider, A. P., 2nd (1987) Risk factor for ovarian cancer. *N Engl J Med* **317**, 508–509.

111. Gerstman, B. B., Gross, T. P., Kennedy, D. L., Bennett, R. C., Tomita, D. K., and Stadel, B. V. (1991) Trends in the content and use of oral contraceptives in the United States, 1964–88. *Am J Public Health* **81**, 90–96.

112. Franceschi, S., Parazzini, F., Negri, E., Booth, M., La Vecchia, C., Beral, V., Tzonou, A., and Trichopoulos, D. (1991) Pooled analysis of 3 European case-control studies of epithelial ovarian cancer: III. Oral contraceptive use. *Int J Cancer* **49**, 61–65.

113. La Vecchia, C. and Franceschi, S. (1999) Oral contraceptives and ovarian cancer. *Eur J Cancer Prev* **8**, 297–304.

114. Rosenberg, L., Palmer, J. R., Zauber, A. G., Warshauer, M. E., Lewis, J. L., Jr., Strom, B. L., Harlap, S., and Shapiro, S. (1994) A case-control study of oral contraceptive use and invasive epithelial ovarian cancer. *Am J Epidemiol* **139**, 654–661.

115. Vessey, M. and Painter, R. (2006) Oral contraceptive use and cancer. Findings in a large cohort study, 1968–2004. *Br J Cancer* **95**, 385–389.

116. La Vecchia, C. (2006) Estrogen-progestogen replacement therapy and ovarian cancer: an update. *Eur J Cancer Prev* **15**, 490–492.

117. (1989) Epithelial ovarian cancer and combined oral contraceptives. The WHO Collaborative Study of Neoplasia and Steroid Contraceptives. *Int J Epidemiol* **18**, 538–545.

118. Beral, V., Hannaford, P., and Kay, C. (1988) Oral contraceptive use and malignancies of the genital tract. Results from the Royal College of General Practitioners' Oral Contraception Study. *Lancet* **2**, 1331–1335.

119. La Vecchia, C., Altieri, A., Franceschi, S., and Tavani, A. (2001) Oral contraceptives and cancer: an update. *Drug Saf* **24**, 741–754.

120. Rosenblatt, K. A., Thomas, D. B., and Noonan, E. A. (1992) High-dose and low-dose combined oral contraceptives: protection against epithelial ovarian cancer and the length of the protective effect. The WHO Collaborative Study of Neoplasia and Steroid Contraceptives. *Eur J Cancer* **28A**, 1872–1876.

121. Ness, R. B., Grisso, J. A., Klapper, J., Schlesselman, J. J., Silberzweig, S., Vergona, R., Morgan, M., and Wheeler, J. E. (2000) Risk of ovarian cancer in relation to estrogen and progestin dose and use characteristics of oral contraceptives. SHARE Study Group. Steroid Hormones and Reproductions. *Am J Epidemiol* **152**, 233–241.

122. La Vecchia, C. (2006) Oral contraceptives and ovarian cancer: an update, 1998–2004. *Eur J Cancer Prev* **15**, 117–124.

123. Riman, T., Dickman, P. W., Nilsson, S., Correia, N., Nordlinder, H., Magnusson, C. M., and Persson, I. R. (2002) Risk factors for invasive epithelial ovarian cancer: results from a Swedish case-control study. *Am J Epidemiol* **156**, 363–373.

124. Liang, A. P., Levenson, A. G., Layde, P. M., Shelton, J. D., Hatcher, R. A., Potts, M., and Michelson, M. J. (1983) Risk of breast, uterine corpus, and ovarian cancer in women receiving medroxyprogesterone injections. *JAMA* **249**, 2909–2912.

125. Wingo, P. A., Cardinez, C. J., Landis, S. H., Greenlee, R. T., Ries, L. A., Anderson, R. N., and Thun, M. J. (2003) Long-term trends in cancer mortality in the United States, 1930–1998. *Cancer* **97**, 3133–3275.

126. Mathur, R. S., Landgrebe, S. C., Moody, L. O., Semmens, J. P., and Williamson, H. O. (1985) The effect of estrogen treatment on plasma concentrations of steroid hormones, gonadotropins, prolactin and sex hormone-binding globulin in post-menopausal women. *Maturitas* **7**, 129–133.

127. Fraser, I. S. (1998) *Estrogens and progestogens in clinical practice*, New York, London.

128. Riman, T., Dickman, P. W., Nilsson, S., Correia, N., Nordlinder, H., Magnusson, C. M., Weiderpass, E., and Persson, I. R. (2002) Hormone replacement therapy and the risk of invasive epithelial ovarian cancer in Swedish women. *J Natl Cancer Inst* **94**, 497–504.

129. Weiss, N. S., Lyon, J. L., Krishnamurthy, S., Dietert, S. E., Liff, J. M., and Daling, J. R. (1982) Noncontraceptive estrogen use and the occurrence of ovarian cancer. *J Natl Cancer Inst* **68**, 95–98.

130. Coughlin, S. S., Giustozzi, A., Smith, S. J., and Lee, N. C. (2000) A meta-analysis of estrogen replacement therapy and risk of epithelial ovarian cancer. *J Clin Epidemiol* **53**, 367–375.

131. Garg, P. P., Kerlikowske, K., Subak, L., and Grady, D. (1998) Hormone replacement therapy and the risk of epithelial ovarian carcinoma: a meta-analysis. *Obstet Gynecol* **92**, 472–479.

132. Kaufman, D. W., Kelly, J. P., Welch, W. R., Rosenberg, L., Stolley, P. D., Warshauer, M. E., Lewis, J., Woodruff, J., and Shapiro, S. (1989) Noncontraceptive estrogen use and epithelial ovarian cancer. *Am J Epidemiol* **130**, 1142–1151.

133. Folsom, A. R., Anderson, J. P., and Ross, J. A. (2004) Estrogen replacement therapy and ovarian cancer. *Epidemiology* **15**, 100–104.

134. Lacey, J. V., Jr., Brinton, L. A., Leitzmann, M. F., Mouw, T., Hollenbeck, A., Schatzkin, A., and Hartge, P. (2006) Menopausal hormone therapy and ovarian cancer risk in the National Institutes of Health–AARP Diet and Health Study Cohort. *J Natl Cancer Inst* **98**, 1397–1405.

135. Lacey, J. V., Jr., Mink, P. J., Lubin, J. H., Sherman, M. E., Troisi, R., Hartge, P., Schatzkin, A., and Schairer, C. (2002) Menopausal hormone replacement therapy and risk of ovarian cancer. *JAMA* **288**, 334–341.

136. Rodriguez, C., Patel, A. V., Calle, E. E., Jacob, E. J., and Thun, M. J. (2001) Estrogen replacement therapy and ovarian cancer mortality in a large prospective study of US women. *JAMA* **285**, 1460–1465.

137. Lacey, J. V., Jr., Leitzmann, M., Brinton, L. A., Lubin, J. H., Sherman, M. E., Schatzkin, A., and Schairer, C. (2006) Weight, height, and body mass index and risk for ovarian cancer in a cohort study. *Ann Epidemiol* **16**, 869–876.

138. Anderson, G. L., Judd, H. L., Kaunitz, A. M., Barad, D. H., Beresford, S. A., Pettinger, M., Liu, J., McNeeley, S. G., and Lopez, A. M. (2003) Effects of estrogen plus progestin on gynecologic cancers and associated diagnostic procedures: the Women' Health Initiative randomized trial. *JAMA* **290**, 1739–1748.

139. Danforth, K. N., Tworoger, S. S., Hecht, J. L., Rosner, B. A., Colditz, G. A., and Hankinson, S. E. (2007) A prospective study of postmenopausal hormone use and ovarian cancer risk. *Br J Cancer* **96**, 151–156.

140. Beral, V., Bull, D., Green, J., and Reeves, G. (2007) Ovarian cancer and hormone replacement therapy in the Million Women Study. *Lancet* **369**, 1703–1710.

141. Risch, H. A. (1996) Estrogen replacement therapy and risk of epithelial ovarian cancer. *Gynecol Oncol* **63**, 254–257.

142. Kumar, V. and Robbins, S. L. (2007) *Robbins basic pathology*, Saunders/Elsevier, Philadelphia, PA.

143. Rodriguez, C., Calle, E. E., Fakhrabadi-Shokoohi, D., Jacobs, E. J., and Thun, M. J. (2002) Body mass index, height, and the risk of ovarian cancer mortality in a prospective cohort of postmenopausal women. *Cancer Epidemiol Biomarkers Prev* **11**, 822–828.

144. Lubin, F., Chetrit, A., Freedman, L. S., Alfandary, E., Fishler, Y., Nitzan, H., Zultan, A., and Modan, B. (2003) Body mass index at age 18 years and during adult life and ovarian cancer risk. *Am J Epidemiol* **157**, 113–120.

145. Farrow, D. C., Weiss, N. S., Lyon, J. L., and Daling, J. R. (1989) Association of obesity and ovarian cancer in a case-control study. *Am J Epidemiol* **129**, 1300–1304.

146. Purdie, D. M., Bain, C. J., Webb, P. M., Whiteman, D. C., Pirozzo, S., and Green, A. C. (2001) Body size and ovarian cancer: case-control study and systematic review (Australia). *Cancer Causes Control* **12**, 855–863.

147. Anderson, J. P., Ross, J. A., and Folsom, A. R. (2004) Anthropometric variables, physical activity, and incidence of ovarian cancer: The Iowa Women' Health Study. *Cancer* **100**, 1515–1521.

148. Engeland, A., Tretli, S., and Bjorge, T. (2003) Height, body mass index, and ovarian cancer: a follow-up of 1.1 million Norwegian women. *J Natl Cancer Inst* **95**, 1244–1248.

149. Fairfield, K. M., Willett, W. C., Rosner, B. A., Manson, J. E., Speizer, F. E., and Hankinson, S. E. (2002) Obesity, weight gain, and ovarian cancer. *Obstet Gynecol* **100**, 288–296.

150. Hirose, K., Tajima, K., Hamajima, N., Kuroishi, T., Kuzuya, K., Miura, S., and Tokudome, S. (1999) Comparative case-referent study of risk factors among hormone-related female cancers in Japan. *Jpn J Cancer Res* **90**, 255–261.

151. Lukanova, A., Toniolo, P., Lundin, E., Micheli, A., Akhmedkhanov, A., Muti, P., Zeleniuch-Jacquotte, A., Biessy, C., Lenner, P., Krogh, V., Berrino, F., Hallmans, G., Riboli, E., and Kaaks, R. (2002) Body mass index in relation to ovarian cancer: a multi-centre nested case-control study. *Int J Cancer* **99**, 603–608.

152. Schouten, L. J., Goldbohm, R. A., and van den Brandt, P. A. (2003) Height, weight, weight change, and ovarian cancer risk in the Netherlands cohort study on diet and cancer. *Am J Epidemiol* **157**, 424–433.

153. Beehler, G. P., Sekhon, M., Baker, J. A., Teter, B. E., McCann, S. E., Rodabaugh, K. J., and Moysich, K. B. (2006) Risk of ovarian cancer associated with BMI varies by menopausal status. *J Nutr* **136**, 2881–2886.

154. Olsen, C. M., Green, A. C., Whiteman, D. C., Sadeghi, S., Kolahdooz, F., and Webb, P.

M. (2007) Obesity and the risk of epithelial ovarian cancer: a systematic review and meta-analysis. *Eur J Cancer* **43**, 690–709.

155. Mink, P. J., Folsom, A. R., Sellers, T. A., and Kushi, L. H. (1996) Physical activity, waist-to-hip ratio, and other risk factors for ovarian cancer: a follow-up study of older women. *Epidemiology* **7**, 38–45.

156. Folsom, A. R., Kushi, L. H., Anderson, K. E., Mink, P. J., Olson, J. E., Hong, C. P., Sellers, T. A., Lazovich, D., and Prineas, R. J. (2000) Associations of general and abdominal obesity with multiple health outcomes in older women: the Iowa Women' Health Study. *Arch Intern Med* **160**, 2117–2128.

157. Schulz, M., Lahmann, P. H., Riboli, E., and Boeing, H. (2004) Dietary determinants of epithelial ovarian cancer: a review of the epidemiologic literature. *Nutr Cancer* **50**, 120–140.

158. Larsson, S. C., Giovannucci, E., and Wolk, A. (2004) Dietary folate intake and incidence of ovarian cancer: the Swedish Mammography Cohort. *J Natl Cancer Inst* **96**, 396–402.

159. Larsson, S. C. and Wolk, A. (2005) Coffee consumption is not associated with ovarian cancer incidence. *Cancer Epidemiol Biomarkers Prev* **14**, 2273–2274.

160. Riman, T., Dickman, P. W., Nilsson, S., Nordlinder, H., Magnusson, C. M., and Persson, I. R. (2004) Some life-style factors and the risk of invasive epithelial ovarian cancer in Swedish women. *Eur J Epidemiol* **19**, 1011–1019.

161. Baker, J. A., Boakye, K., McCann, S. E., Beehler, G. P., Rodabaugh, K. J., Villella, J. A., and Moysich, K. B. (2007) Consumption of black tea or coffee and risk of ovarian cancer. *Int J Gynecol Cancer* **17**, 50–54.

162. Whittemore, A. S., Wu, M. L., Paffenbarger, R. S., Jr., Sarles, D. L., Kampert, J. B., Grosser, S., Jung, D. L., Ballon, S., and Hendrickson, M. (1988) Personal and environmental characteristics related to epithelial ovarian cancer. II. Exposures to talcum powder, tobacco, alcohol, and coffee. *Am J Epidemiol* **128**, 1228–1240.

163. Cottreau, C. M., Ness, R. B., and Kriska, A. M. (2000) Physical activity and reduced risk of ovarian cancer. *Obstet Gynecol* **96**, 609–614.

164. Tavani, A., Gallus, S., La Vecchia, C., Dal Maso, L., Negri, E., Pelucchi, C., Montella, M., Conti, E., Carbone, A., and Franceschi, S. (2001) Physical activity and risk of ovarian cancer: an Italian case-control study. *Int J Cancer* **91**, 407–411.

165. Weiderpass, E., Margolis, K. L., Sandin, S., Braaten, T., Kumle, M., Adami, H. O., and Lund, E. (2006) Prospective study of physical activity in different periods of life and the risk of ovarian cancer. *Int J Cancer* **118**, 3153–3160.

166. Patel, A. V., Rodriguez, C., Pavluck, A. L., Thun, M. J., and Calle, E. E. (2006) Recreational physical activity and sedentary behavior in relation to ovarian cancer risk in a large cohort of US women. *Am J Epidemiol* **163**, 709–716.

167. Zhang, M., Xie, X., Lee, A. H., and Binns, C. W. (2004) Sedentary behaviours and epithelial ovarian cancer risk. *Cancer Causes Control* **15**, 83–89.

168. Franks, A. L., Lee, N. C., Kendrick, J. S., Rubin, G. L., and Layde, P. M. (1987) Cigarette smoking and the risk of epithelial ovarian cancer. *Am J Epidemiol* **126**, 112–117.

169. Smith, E. M., Sowers, M. F., and Burns, T. L. (1984) Effects of smoking on the development of female reproductive cancers. *J Natl Cancer Inst* **73**, 371–376.

170. Modugno, F., Ness, R. B., and Cottreau, C. M. (2002) Cigarette smoking and the risk of mucinous and nonmucinous epithelial ovarian cancer. *Epidemiology* **13**, 467–471.

171. Jordan, S. J., Whiteman, D. C., Purdie, D. M., Green, A. C., and Webb, P. M. (2006) Does smoking increase risk of ovarian cancer? A systematic review. *Gynecol Oncol* **103**, 1122–1129.

172. Singletary, K. W. and Gapstur, S. M. (2001) Alcohol and breast cancer: review of epidemiologic and experimental evidence and potential mechanisms. *JAMA* **286**, 2143–2151.

173. Gwinn, M. L., Webster, L. A., Lee, N. C., Layde, P. M., and Rubin, G. L. (1986) Alcohol consumption and ovarian cancer risk. *Am J Epidemiol* **123**, 759–766.

174. Adami, H. O., McLaughlin, J. K., Hsing, A. W., Wolk, A., Ekbom, A., Holmberg, L., and Persson, I. (1992) Alcoholism and cancer risk: a population-based cohort study. *Cancer Causes Control* **3**, 419–425.

175. Larsson, S. C. and Wolk, A. (2004) Wine consumption and epithelial ovarian cancer. *Cancer Epidemiol Biomarkers Prev* **13**, 1823; author reply 1823–1824.

176. Modugno, F., Ness, R. B., and Allen, G. O. (2003) Alcohol consumption and the risk of mucinous and nonmucinous epithelial ovarian cancer. *Obstet Gynecol* **102**, 1336–1343.

177. Goodman, M. T. and Tung, K. H. (2003) Alcohol consumption and the risk of borderline and invasive ovarian cancer. *Obstet Gynecol* **101**, 1221–1228.

178. Kelemen, L. E., Sellers, T. A., Vierkant, R. A., Harnack, L., and Cerhan, J. R. (2004) Association of folate and alcohol with risk of ovarian cancer in a prospective study of postmenopausal women. *Cancer Causes Control* **15**, 1085–1093.

179. Webb, P. M., Purdie, D. M., Bain, C. J., and Green, A. C. (2004) Alcohol, wine, and risk of epithelial ovarian cancer. *Cancer Epidemiol Biomarkers Prev* **13**, 592–599.

180. Peterson, N. B., Trentham-Dietz, A., Newcomb, P. A., Chen, Z., Hampton, J. M., Willett, W. C., and Egan, K. M. (2006) Alcohol consumption and ovarian cancer risk in a population-based case-control study. *Int J Cancer* **119**, 2423–2427.

181. Chang, E. T., Canchola, A. J., Lee, V. S., Clarke, C. A., Purdie, D. M., Reynolds, P., Bernstein, L., Stram, D. O., Anton-Culver, H., Deapen, D., Mohrenweiser, H., Peel, D., Pinder, R., Ross, R. K., West, D. W., Wright, W., Ziogas, A., and Horn-Ross, P. L. (2007) Wine and other alcohol consumption and risk of ovarian cancer in the California Teachers Study cohort. *Cancer Causes Control* **18**, 91–103.

182. Schouten, L. J., Zeegers, M. P., Goldbohm, R. A., and van den Brandt, P. A. (2004) Alcohol and ovarian cancer risk: results from the Netherlands Cohort Study. *Cancer Causes Control* **15**, 201–209.

183. Genkinger, J. M., Hunter, D. J., Spiegelman, D., Anderson, K. E., Buring, J. E., Freudenheim, J. L., Goldbohm, R. A., Harnack, L., Hankinson, S. E., Larsson, S. C., Leitzmann, M., McCullough, M. L., Marshall, J., Miller, A. B., Rodriguez, C., Rohan, T. E., Schatzkin, A., Schouten, L. J., Wolk, A., Zhang, S. M., and Smith-Warner, S. A. (2006) Alcohol intake and ovarian cancer risk: a pooled analysis of 10 cohort studies. *Br J Cancer* **94**, 757–762.

Chapter 21

Epidemiology, Pathology, and Genetics of Prostate Cancer Among African Americans Compared with Other Ethnicities

Heinric Williams and Isaac J. Powell

Abstract

Prostate cancer is the most common cancer affecting men in the Western world. In the United States, it is the second leading cause of cancer related deaths after lung and bronchus carcinoma. No definitive causes of prostate cancer (PCa) have been identified to date but, increasing age, a positive family history, and sub-Saharan African ancestry are strongly linked to its development. African American men (AAM) have the highest reported incidence rates in the United States and their mortality from the disease is markedly higher than that of European American men (EAM). Conversely, Asian American men and Pacific Islanders (API), American Indian and Alaskan Native (AI/AN) men, and Hispanic men all have lower incidence and mortality rates as compared with EAM. The reasons for these differences are unclear. However, it is clear that AAM have more advanced PCa when diagnosed. Several other reasons have been suggested and these include differences in treatments and health seeking behavior among the ethnic groups, cultural beliefs, environmental/lifestyle factors, dietary and genetic factors. In conclusion, there are multiple factors that impact prostate cancer outcome and that may be responsible for ethnic disparity. These factors are discussed in this chapter.

Key words: Epidemiology, prostate cancer outcome, racial differences, genetics.

1. Introduction

Prostate cancer (PCa) is the most common cancer affecting men in the Western world (1–4). In the United States, it is the second leading cause of cancer-related deaths after lung and bronchus carcinoma (1, 2). No definitive causes of PCa have been identified to date, but increasing age, a positive family history, and sub-Saharan

M. Verma (ed.), *Methods of Molecular Biology, Cancer Epidemiology, vol. 472*
© 2009 Humana Press, a part of Springer Science+Business Media, Totowa, NJ
Book doi: 10.1007/978-1-60327-492-0

African ancestry are strongly linked to its development (3, 5). African American men (AAM) have the highest reported incidence rates in the United States (1, 2, 6) and their mortality from the disease is markedly higher than that of European American men (EAM) (7). Conversely, Asian American men and Pacific Islanders (API), American Indian and Alaskan Native men (AI/AN), and Hispanic men all have a lower incidence and mortality rate as compared with EAM (1). The reasons for these differences have been the subject of much debate, but several explanations have been offered and these include variation in socioeconomic factors, nonfinancial barriers, cultural behaviors, and genetic susceptibility among the groups (2, 4, 8–12). The management of PCa (via measures ranging from primary prevention through screening to therapeutic intervention) imposes a substantial economic burden on individuals and society as a whole (13).

2. PCa Incidence and Mortality Rates

2.1. Incidence Rates

Data from the National Cancer Institute Surveillance Epidemiology and End Results (SEER) Program following PCa in both AAM and EAM from 1975–2002 and Hispanic, API, AI/AN from 1992–2002 showed that in the United States, the PCa incidence rates were highest for AAM (243/100,000 men) and lowest for AI/AN (70.7/100,000 men) (1). A closer review of the data demonstrated a steady and parallel rise in PCa incidence rates for both AAM and EAM from the 1970s to late 1980s. After the introduction of serum prostate-specific antigen (PSA) screening in the early 1990s, PCa incidence rates soared to their highest level in 1992 for EAM (237.6/100,000 men) and a year later for AAM (342.8/100,000 men). From those levels, the incidence declined sharply for both AAM and EAM until 1995. But, over the subsequent 7 years until 2002, AAM PCa incident rates marginally declined, while for EAM there was an increase. During the period 1992–2002, Hispanics (141/100,000 men) and API (104.2/100,000 men) had lower incidence rates as compared with EAM (156/100,000 men) (1).

The sharp rise in PCa incidence seem among AAM and EAM during the late 1980s and early 1990s probably reflect the improved detection of PCa by measuring serum PSA (7, 14). Since the introduction of PSA screening, the age at diagnosis and distribution of disease stage and grade has changed significantly (7, 14). In the 1980s, the median age at diagnosis for AAM and EAM was 70 and 72 years, respectively. However, during 1998–2002, men were being diagnosed at a younger age, 65 years for AAM and 68 years for EAM (1). In addition to the younger age at diagnosis seen during the PSA era, so too was there a shift in the type of disease being diagnosed. During the periods 1975–1978 and 1985–1989, 73% of PCa diagnoses were localized in comparison to the period 1995–2001, where 91% of the diagnoses were localized (1). During these same periods, the proportion of diagnoses with distant disease declined from 20% (1975–1978) to 16% (1985–1989) to 5% (1995–2001) (1).

Both PSA testing and improvements in transrectal ultrasonography have resulted in more cases being detected from a pool of men with previously unsuspected disease than was the case about 20 years ago, thus having a dramatic influence on local and national trends in PCa incidence in the United States (4). After the harvesting effect or clearing of the prevalence of PCa, there was a return to a new incidence level, which is higher than the pre-PSA screening levels but more consistent with the natural history of the disease and the slow increase of an aging population per 100,000 men.

The PCa incidence trends varied across the United States. The highest incidences of PCa were seen in District of Columbia, New Jersey, Michigan, and South Dakota and were lowest in Tennessee, Arizona, Hawaii, and Missouri (1). These differences may be related to relative prevalence of high-risk and low-risk men in these states as well as socioeconomic, environmental, and cultural factors.

Worldwide men of sub-Saharan African descent in countries such as Jamaica or Trinidad and Tobago have reported PCa incidence rates that exceed that of AAM (3, 15). For instance, in a 1998 analysis, Jamaican men of sub-Saharan descent were found to have a PCa incidence of 304/100,000 men. Interestingly, rates in African countries like Nigeria appear to be substantially lower, but recent evidence suggests that this may be secondary to underreporting and poor data collection (16). Nevertheless, these differing incidence rates within populations of African descent may represent environmental as well as genetic admixture differences (2, 17). A similar variation in PCa incidence rates was observed in men of Japanese descent based on their country of origin and migratory patterns (18). Japanese PCa incidence rates were lower for Japanese men in Japan as compared to men who migrated to Hawaii (18). The PCa incidence rates of Japanese men who migrated to Hawaii took one generation to approach that of EAM (18).

2.2. Mortality Rates

Deaths from PCa in the United States are more than twofold higher in AAM than in EAM (7, 19). The SEER data demonstrated that age-adjusted mortality rates from 1998 to 2002 were 68.9/100,000 men in AAM and 27.8/100,000 men in EAM (19). Although this increase did not mirror the sharp increase seen with the incidence rates for both groups, mortality rates still increased from 1975 to 2001 in both groups, and peaked in 1993 for AAM (81.9/100,000 men) and in 1991 for EAM (36.5/100,000 men) before decreasing to 66.4/100,000 men and 26.6/100,000 men, respectively, in 2001 (19). Reporting of mortality rate data for Hispanic men, API, and AI/AN began in 1992 and their age-adjusted mortality rates for 1998–2002 were 23, 18.3, and 12.1 per 100,000 men, respectively. Collectively, among the Hispanic men, API, and AI/AN, decreasing trends in mortality rates have also been noted. The most significant factors likely contributing to this decline include earlier diagnosis of PCa at a stage that is amenable to curative therapy, the relative decline in deaths from distant disease, and the earlier and more widespread use of andro-gen-deprivation therapy (20, 21).

Like PCa incidence rates, mortality rates vary across the United States. The highest mortality rates were seen in the District of Columbia, Mississippi, Alabama, and South Carolina, respec-tively, whereas the lowest rates were observed in Hawaii, Arizona, Nebraska, and California (1). It was interesting to note that states with high PCa incidence rates (1999–2003) did not covary with the states with high mortality rates (1999–2003) except for the District of Columbia (1).

A review of PCa mortality rates around the world showed that Western Europe, Australia, and North America had the high-est rates, whereas, the Far East and India experienced the lowest rates. Worldwide, the highest mortality rates were observed in men of sub-Saharan African descent, particularly in Trinidad and Tobago, Jamaica, and Brazil (2). In England, subgroup analy-sis showed the highest PCa mortality among men of Caribbean descent (22). Conversely, lower mortality rates of > 5.5/100,000 men were reported in China and Japan (2, 4). Within Europe, there is a dichotomy of PCa mortality rates between Northern Europe (Sweden, Norway, and Denmark) of 23–27/100,000 men and Southern Europe (Greece) with a mortality rate of 10.7/100,000 men. These international differences may be attributed to the prevalence of both environmental and genetic risk factors. Data from migration studies in men of Asian ancestry living in the United States showed that they had lower risks of PCa as compared with EAM, but had a higher risk of PCa when compared with men of similar ancestry living in Asia (18, 23).

3. Five-Year Relative Survival Rates

The reported 5-year survival rates have improved significantly for the two highest at-risk groups in the United States. For AAM and EAM with localized PCa diagnosed between 1996 and 2002 and followed through 2003, their 5-year survival rates were both 100%. Even for those men diagnosed with dis-tant disease, while their 5-year survival rates were significantly less as compared to those with localized disease, there was little difference in the rates for AAM and EAM, at 31% and 33% respectively (7).

4. Explanation of the Racial Differences

4.1. Genetics

An estimated 9% of PCa are due to an inherited predisposition (24). The risk of PCa increases with the number of relatives affected. In men with a first-degree relative, two relatives, and three relatives affected with PCa, there is a cumulative increased risk of developing PCa of 2.5, 5, and 11-fold, respectively (25). In the last 20 years, evidence that PCa may be caused by multiple genes, possibly interacting with endocrine and environmental factors, has continued to grow (3, 5, 11). Linkage studies have identified susceptibility loci for PCa on several chromosomes, including 1, 8, 10, 16, 17, 20, and X, with the strongest linked localized to chromosome 1 (5). The genes *HPC1* on chromosome 1q23–25, *PCAP* on chromosome 1q42–43, and *CAPB* on chromosome 1p36 are notable candidates (5).

Freedman et al. showed through admixture mapping that the 8q24 locus is associated with an increased risk of PCa in AAM with African ancestry at the 8q24 locus (26). It was also associated with an earlier age (<age 72 years) of PCa diagnosis in AAM with African ancestry as compared with European ancestry at the 8q24 locus (26). The microsatellite marker DG8S737 on 8q24 was also associated with PCa risk in Caucasian men from Iceland, Sweden, and Chicago men in the United States and AAM from Michigan, United States (27). Interestingly, this was found to be associated with only aggressive PCa.

Other genes of interest include *HPC2* on chromosome 17p, *HPC20* on chromosome 20q13, and *HPCX* on chromosome Xq27–28, linkage to chromosome 8p22–23, and several strong candidate genes have been mapped, including *RNASEL, ELAC2*, and *MSR1* (5). Kittles et al. recently reported that gene(ephB2) on chromosome 1p is associated with a family history of PCa in AAM but it is not found in EAM (28). The BRCA genes, especially BRCA2, may be involved in up to 2% of early-onset PCa. Studies show that altered expression of the *BCL-2* gene may be an important genetic factor underlying the greater aggressiveness of PCa in AAM (29).

4.2. Differences in Androgen Levels and Androgen Receptor Expression

PCa is a hormone-mediated cancer. There is significant evidence to show that the growth and maintenance of the prostate is dependent on androgens and that PCa regresses after androgen ablation or anti-androgen therapy (30). While testosterone is the principal androgen in circulation, it can passively diffuse in the prostate gland where it is converted to the more potent androgen, dihydrotestosterone (DHT), by the enzyme 5α reductase type 2 (SRD5A2). The action of DHT is mediated by the androgen receptor (AR), which binds DHT in the cytoplasm and enters the nucleus as a complex to mediate cell proliferation (31). In the absence of DHT, estradiol, insulin-like growth factors (IGFs), and vitamin D may also bind the AR and induce androgenic activity (32). Interestingly, increased testosterone and DHT have not been convincingly associated with an increased risk of PCa. Whereas some groups have reported that serum levels of these hormones are higher in patients with PCa than in age-matched control subjects, others were not able to detect such differences (33, 34). However, it was recently shown that a high level of serum testosterone is associated with an elevated risk of low-grade PCa and a reduced risk of high-grade PCa (35). Interestingly, a study in army veterans 31 to 50 years old also showed significantly higher mean serum testosterone in AAM than in EAM, a difference that may be relevant to the increased PCa risk in AAM (36).

Numerous studies have suggested that increased AR expression may have an important role in PCa (35–46). It is expressed in all stages of PCa. Numerous somatic mutations have been identified, and most of these have been detected in late-stage PCa (38). These mutations have been localized to exon 1 of the AR gene and include two trinucleotide repeat polymorphisms, namely (CAG)n and (GGN)n repeats (where N represents any nucleotide) (37–39). These trinucleotide repeats encode polyglutamine and polyglycine, respectively. In a recent meta-analysis, both (CAG)n and (GGN)n repeat lengths were found to have a small but significant role in PCa (37). In general, studies have shown that shorter (CAG)n repeats have been associated with more aggressive PCa, an earlier age of onset, and an increased time to recurrence, but this has not been consistently seen in all populations (38–41). For example, AAM were found to have a higher proportion of short (CAG)n repeats as compared with EAM and Asians, but this was not associated with an increased PCA risk (42, 43). Interestingly, the short (CAG)n repeats were associated with an increased PCa risk in Hispanic and Asian populations (44, 45). On the other hand, in a European study of French-German men, short (CAG)n repeats were not associated with an increased PCa risk (46).

4.3. Androgen-Related Genes

4.3.1. CYP17, CYP3A4, and SRD5A2

While few clinically meaningful associations of genetic polymorphisms with PCa risk have been demonstrated to date, the results of a recent meta-analysis suggested that *CYP17* polymorphisms may have a role in the susceptibility to PCa in men of sub-Saharan African but not of European descent (47).

In a study of the genetic variant *CYP3A4* and disease-free survival in a diverse population of men undergoing radical prostatectomy, EAM presented with an 8% variant G allele frequency, while AAM were observed to have an 81% variant G allele frequency. The variant G allele was associated with greater disease progression in men with pathologically locally advanced PCa than men diagnosed with the normal or wild-type (WT) A allele (11). In a case-control study, the variant G allele was strongly associated with aggressive PCa in AAM (48, 49).

SRD5A2 encodes the type2 steroid 5 alpha reductase enzyme, which is known to have numerous mutations (50). At least two of these mutations; A49T and V89L have been implicated in PCa risk. The T variant of the A49T mutation was shown to be associated with PCa in AAM and aggressive PCa. Interestingly, Asian men were found to have a high prevalence of the V89L LL genotype, which is associated with lower serum levels of 3 alpha-diol G and lower SRD5A2 activity (50).

4.4. IGF Axis

IGF-1 is a potent PCa growth factor that circulates bound to several IGF binding proteins (IGFBP) (51). Studies have shown that IGFBP-3, the most prominent IGFBP, is low in AAM as compared with EAM, resulting in higher serum levels of free IGF-1 (51). This combination of low IGFBP-3 and high IGF-1 is associated with development of advanced-stage PCa (51). IGFBP-3 is itself a proapoptotic agent with effect independent of IGF-1 (51). As a result, this may contribute to the increased risk of PCa in AAM.

4.5. Diet

Evidence supporting a role of dietary and/or environmental/lifestyle factors in the pathogenesis of PCa includes the strikingly different incidence and mortality rates evident in different geographic areas (2). Traditionally, PCa incidence and mortality rates in countries like Japan and China are reported lower than in the United States and Caribbean nations, and more interestingly, migrants from low- to high-incidence areas adopt a higher risk of the disease (2, 5, 8). A number of epidemiological studies have suggested a potential role for diet, specifically a high intake of saturated fat, red meat, and dairy products, in the pathogenesis of PCa (2, 3, 5, 32). Animal protein intake as a percent of protein intake is low in Asian countries and this could account for the > 20-fold decreased risk of PCa (52). Some have suggested that the mechanism may be related to the high androgen levels in the high-fat diets combined with the weak estrogenic activity of the soy components in the Asian diet (52, 53).

Obesity has been implicated in the development of PCa, but conclusive evidence is lacking. However, numerous studies suggest that obesity increases the risk of aggressive cancer while decreasing the risk of indolent disease (54). A retrospective study of 3,162 men in the United States showed that AAM had a significantly greater body mass index and significantly higher post-prostatectomy recurrence rates than EAM, possibly contributing to their outcome disparity (55).

In general, vegetable consumption has not been strongly associated with PCa risk with the exception of tomato-based products. Lycopene, a fat-soluble carotenoid principally found in tomatoes, is unusually concentrated in the prostate gland and is associated with a lower risk of PCa (56). This was shown in a Health Professionals Follow-up study in which 2,481 men with PCa were identified from a pool of 47,365 subjects, where high intake of tomato-based foods was associated with a relative risk of 0.84 (95% confidence interval [CI], 0.73–0.96; p = 0.003) (57). Interestingly, the Prostate, Lung, Colorectal and Ovarian cancer study analyzed the intake of lycopene and tomato products in 1,338 prostate cases and found that their intake was protective in individuals with a family history of PCa but that no overall protective effect of lycopene was observed (58).

A number of dietary supplements have been implicated in reduced PCa risk, but only selenium and vitamin E are currently the subject of a randomized controlled trial (Selenium and Vitamin E Cancer Prevention Trial) (59). A recent review has summarized the results of all ongoing and completed PCa chemoprevention trials (59).

5. Disease Presentation

Although SEER data for 1995 to 2000 indicate that the distribution of localized/regional, distant, and unstaged PCa is similar in AAM and EAM (60), some important differences in disease presentation, care patterns, and treatment outcomes have been reported. Moul et al. noted that AAM presenting with PCa have higher PSA values at initial diagnosis than EAM, and these higher PSA values were associated with larger tumor volumes within clinical (TNM) stage categories (60). While higher pretreatment PSA values could simply reflect later diagnosis in AAM due to decreased access to health care resources, there is evidence that the disease is more aggressive in AAM. Not only are they diagnosed at a younger age than EAM, they are also more frequently diagnosed with greater tumor volume, more advanced tumor stage, and higher Gleason grade, and they are more likely to experience bone pain and have poorer performance status (61–63). Even when studies were controlled for socioeconomic status, the greater likelihood of AAM to present with later-stage disease than EAM (64) and the differences in incidence and mortality were found to persist (4). However, a recent study of pretreatment PSA values, and stage and grade distributions in men in the United States in the 10-year period of 1988 through 1997 showed that there has been a more rapid decrease in pretreatment PSA values in AAM than in EAM (1.9% versus 0.6% yearly, respectively) and stage and grade distributions were indicative of a more favorable disease profile in AAM than was previously the case (14). The more rapid decrease in pretreatment PSA values in AAM may be a consequence of improved use of health care resources (14).

6. Patterns of Care and Treatment Outcomes

In addition to differences in the incidence and stage of the disease at presentation, another explanation for the disparity in mortality rates between the racial groups may lie in differences in treatment (65). Several studies show that AAM tend to receive aggressive therapy less often than EAM (66–68) or they go untreated more often (69). In a recent study, AAM were significantly more likely than non-Hispanic EAM to receive watchful waiting, which is an option appropriate in men diagnosed with early-stage disease and those with lower life expectancy. This racial difference in undergoing watchful waiting was not completely explained by differences in clinical characteristics, comorbidities, or life expectancy at diagnosis (70), suggesting that other factors may have had a greater influence. These factors may include differences in access to health care resources, the patient desire to avoid treatment side effects or have the cancer removed, nonfinancial barriers (fear of the diagnosis and distrust of the health system), religious beliefs, and differences in the recommendations or preferences of physicians and advice received from family and friends or from information sources such as the Internet (9, 70). In the United States military, where there is equal access to medical resources and these differences are less evident, it was reported that stage-specific treatments are similar in AAM and EAM with PCa (71) and the proportion of AAM electing radical prostatectomy for localized PCa increased in 1991 to 2000 from 14.0% in 1991 to 23.8% in 2000 (72). At a Veterans Administration Medical Center, where the distributions of race and annual income were similar, a significantly greater proportion of AAM presented with distant disease compared with EAM (25% versus 19%; $p = 0.045$). However, an interesting crossover effect in survival occurred. EAM younger than 70 years had better survival but there was a trend toward AAM older than 70 years to have better survival (73).

Higher disease recurrence rates and earlier failure following radical prostatectomy also point to a more aggressive variant of PCa in AAM (74, 75). Even when patients are stratified into risk categories based on clinical tumor stage, PSA values at diagnosis, and Gleason grade, African ancestry remained an independent predictor of disease recurrence following radical prostatectomy, suggesting that outcome differences following this intervention are not just a matter of more advanced disease at presentation (76, 77). In a study of men who underwent consecutive radical prostatectomy as monotherapy from 1990 to 1999, the influence of age, stage, and year of diagnosis, and the role of race/ethnicity on disease-free survival was examined (78). Results showed that when the majority of the cohort had pathologically organ-confined disease, which was the dominant stage in the late 1990s, and/or a mean age of 70 years or older, race/ethnicity was not an independent predictor of disease-free survival. However, if the cohort was diagnosed at a younger age and/or with more advanced PCa, which was the case in the early 1990s, race/ethnicity became an independent predictor. Thus, the influence of race/ethnicity as an independent predictor of PCa is conditional, and dependent on age, stage, and year of diagnosis. In general, studies in which the cohorts consist of subgroups of the entire spectrum of PCa are limited by these factors, especially by differences in stage at diagnosis and treatment. Although there is evidence that AAM have more aggressive disease biologically, if they are diagnosed and treated early enough (pathologically organ-confined disease), the role of race as a factor in outcome is significantly decreased (78).

7. Socioeconomic Factors

As discussed, differences in socioeconomic status, literacy, cultural beliefs, nonfinancial barriers, and environmental and lifestyle factors may also contribute to the differences in the PCa incidence and outcome between AAM and EAM. Although no clear environmental risk factors have been clearly delineated for AAM, negative health-seeking behavior and socioeconomic factors may influence access to health care and the type of care provided, contributing to the poor outcome (4), while low literacy, nonfinancial barriers, and cultural beliefs or concerns over the benefits versus risks of treatment may be a significant barrier to the diagnosis of early-stage disease.

8. Conclusions

If the lessons of other chronic diseases with a high prevalence in AAM, such as hypertension and diabetes mellitus, are to be heeded, studies targeting the testing of AAM for PCa along with focused education about the disease and its risks should be viewed as a priority health care initiative and scientific study in the United States to decrease the PCa outcome disparity as an end point. Although there is some evidence that racial differences in patterns of care are narrowing, particularly where there is equal access to health care resources, AAM still have a higher incidence of PCa, present at a younger age and with more advanced disease, and have a poorer prognosis than EAM. Whether this is a biological phenomenon or whether it reflects differences in socioeconomic factors, health-seeking behavior, literacy, cultural beliefs, or environmental/lifestyle factors has been debated, but a body of evidence indicates that PCa has a genetic basis.

Improving the outcome in AAM with PCa requires awareness of the epidemiological patterns of the disease as well as willingness on the part of physicians to implement targeted study initiatives with end points designed to detect the disease early in this population and begin appropriate management. In addition, there must be more education about PCa and its consequences in the African American community along with improved support initiatives for patients and their families. However, when doing so, it should be recognized that there may be significant barriers. In overcoming these barriers, the importance of tailored educational programs designed to help patients gain better understanding of the benefits and risks of treatment options, and increase their participation in the management decision-making process cannot be overemphasized. With this plan of action, a decrease in the racial/ethnic outcome disparity may be accomplished. We propose that a study should be performed to determine our ability to decrease racial outcome disparity by education, aggressive testing, and treatment.

References

1. American Cancer Society (2007) *Cancer facts and figures 2007*. Available at http://www.cancer.org/docroot/STT/stt_0.asp.
2. American Cancer Society (2003) *Cancer facts and figures 2003*. Available at http://www.cancer.org/docroot/STT/stt_0.asp.
3. Grönberg, H. (2003) Prostate cancer epidemiology. *Lancet* 361, 859–864.
4. Crawford, E. D. (2003) Epidemiology of prostate cancer. *Urology* 62 (6) (suppl 1), 3–12.
5. Schaid, D. J. (2004) The complex genetic epidemiology of prostate cancer. *Hum Mol Genet, suppl.* 13, R103–121.
6. Brawley, O. W. (1998) Prostate cancer and black men. *Semin Urol Oncol* 16,184–186.
7. American Cancer Society (2007) *Cancer facts and figures for AAMs 2007–2008*. Available at http://www.cancer.org/docroot/STT/stt_0.asp.
8. Liu, L., Cozen, W., Bernstein, L., Ross, R. K., Deapen, D. (2001) Changing relationship between socioeconomic status and prostate cancer incidence. *J Natl Cancer Inst* 93, 705–709.
9. Powell, I. J., Gelfand, D. E., Parzuchowski, J, Heilbrun, L., Franklin, A. (1995) A successful recruitment process of African American men for early detection of prostate cancer. *Cancer* 75, 1880–1884.
10. Robbins, A. S., Whittemore, A.S., Thom, D. H. (2000) Differences in socioeconomic status and survival among white and black

men with prostate cancer. *Am J Epidemiol*
151, 409–416.

11. Powell, I. J., Zhou, J., Sun, Y., Sakr, W. A,
Patel, N. P., Heilbrun, L. K., et al. (2004)
CYP3A4 genetic variant and disease-free survival among white and black men after radical
prostatectomy. *J Urol* **172**, 1848–1852.

12. Gaston, K. E., Kim, D., Singh, S., Ford 3rd,
O. H., Mohler, J.L. (2003) Racial differences in androgen receptor protein expression in men with clinically localized prostate
cancer. *J Urol* **170**, 990–993.

13. Mettlin, C. (1997) Recent developments in
the epidemiology of prostate cancer. *Eur J
Cancer* **33**, 340–347.

14. Jani, A. B., Vaida, F., Hanks, G., Asbell, S.,
Sartor O., Moul, J.W. et al. (2001) Changing face and different countenances of
prostate cancer: racial and geographic differences in prostate-specific antigen (PSA),
stage, and grade trends in the PSA era. *Int J
Cancer* **96**, 363–371.

15. Glover Jr, F. E., Coffey, D. S., Douglas, L.
L., Cadogan, M., Russell, H., Tulloch, T.,
et al. (1998) The epidemiology of prostate
cancer in Jamaica. *J Urol* **159**, 1984–1986.

16. Delongschamp, N. B., Singh A., Haas, G.
P. (2007) Epidemiology of prostate cancer
in Africa: Another step in the understanding of the disease? *Curr Prob Cancer* **31**,
226–236.

17. Ahluwalia, B., Jackson, M. A., Jones G.
W., Williams, A. O., Rao, M. S., Rajguru
S. (1981) Blood hormone profiles in prostate cancer patients in high-risk and low-risk
populations. *Cancer* **48**, 2267–2273.

18. Haenszel, W., Kurihara M. 1968 Study of
Japanese migrants. I. Mortality form cancer and other diseases among Japanese in
the United States. *J. Natl Cancer Inst* **40**,
43–68.

19. Ries, L. A. G., Eisner M.P., Kosary C.L.,
Hankey B.F., Miller B.A., Clegg L., et al.
(2002) SEER Cancer Statistics Review,
1975–2002, National Cancer Institute.
Bethesda, MD. Available at http://seer.
cancer.gov/csr/1975_2002/.

20. Chu, K. C., Tarone, R .E., Freeman, H. P.
(2003) Trends in prostate cancer mortality among black men and white men in the
United States. *Cancer* **97**, 1507–1516.

21. Lu-Yao, G., Albertsen P. C., Stanford J.L.,
Stukel T.A., Walker-Corkery, E. S., Barry
M. J. (2002) Natural experiment examining
impact of aggressive screening and treatment on prostate cancer mortality in two
fixed cohorts from Seattle area and Connecticut. *BMJ* **325**, 740.

22. Wild, S.H., Fischbacher, C. M., Brock, A.,
Griffiths, C., Bhopal, R. (2006) Mortality
from all cancers and lung, colorectal, breast
and prostate cancer by country of birth in
England and Wales, 2001–2003. *Br J Cancer* **94**, 1079–1085.

23. Yu, H., Jarris, R. E., Gao, Y. T., Gao, R.,
Wynder, E. L. (1991) Comparative epidemiology of cancer of colon, rectum, prostate
and breast in Shanghai, China versus the
United States. *Int J Epidemiol* **20**, 76–81.

24. Steinberg, G. D., Carter, B. S., Beaty, T. H.,
Childs, B., Walsh, P. C. (1990) Family history and the risk of prostate cancer. *Prostate*
17, 337–347.

25. Johns, L. E., Houlston, R. S. (2003) A systematic review and meta-analysis of familial
prostate cancer. *BJU Intl* **91**, 789–794.

26. Freedman, M. L., Haiman, C. A., Patterson,
N., McDonald, G. J., et al. (2006) Admixture mapping identifies 8q24 as a prostate
cancer risk locus in African-American men.
Proc Natl Acad Sci U S A **103**, 14068–
14073.

27. Suuriniemi, M., Agalliu, I., Schaid, D. J.,
Johanneson, B., McDonnell, S. K., et al.
(2007) Conformation of a positive association between prostate cancer risk and a locus
at chromosome 8q24. *Cancer Epidemiol
Biomarkers Prev* **16**, 809–814.

28. Kittles, R. A., Baffoe-Bonnie, A. B., Moses,
T. Y., Robbins, C. M., Ahaghotu, C., et al.
(2006) A common nonsense mutation in
EphB2 is associated with prostate cancer
risk in African American men with a positive
family history. *J Med Genet* **43**, 507–511.

29. DeVere White, R. W., Deitch, A. D., Jackson, A. G., Gandour-Edwards, R., Marshal-
leck, J., Soares, S.E., et al. (1998) Racial
differences in clinically localized prostate
cancers of black and white men. *J Urol* **159**,
1979–1982.

30. Richie, J. P. (1999) Anti-androgens and
other hormonal therapies for prostate cancer. *Urology* **54**, 15–18.

31. Kokontis, J. M., Liao, S. (1999) Molecular
action of androgen in the normal and neoplastic prostate *Vitam Horm* **55**, 219–307.

32. Culig, Z., Hobisch, A., Bartsch, G., Klocker,
H. (2000) Regulation of prostatic growth
by peptide growth factors. *Prostate* **28**,
392–405.

33. Parsons, J. K., Carter, H. B., Platz, E. A.,
Wright, E. J., Landis, P., Metter, E. J. (2005)
Serum testosterone and the risk of prostate
cancer: potential implications for testoster-
one therapy. *Cancer Epidemiol Biomarkers
Prev* **14**, 2257–2260.

34. Hsing, A. W., Comstock, G. W. (1993) Serological precursors of cancer: serum hormone and risk of subsequent prostate cancer. *Cancer Epidemiol Biomarkers Prev*, **2**, 27–32.

35. Platz, E. A., Leitzmann, M. F., Rifai, N., Kantoff, P. W., Chen, Y. C., Stampfer, M. J., Willet. W. C., Giovannucci, E. (2005) Sex steroid hormones and the androgen receptor gene CAG repeat and subsequent risk of prostate cancer in the prostate-specific antigen era. *Cancer Epidemiol Biomarkers Prev* **14**, 1262–1269.

36. Ellis, L., Nyborg, H. (1992) Racial/ethnic variations in male testosterone levels: a probable contributor to group differences in health. *Steroids* **57**, 72–75.

37. Zeegers, M. P., Kiemeney, L. A., Nieder, A. M., Ostrer, H. (2004) How strong is the association between CAG and GGN repeat length polymorphisms in the androgen receptor gene and prostate cancer risk? *Cancer Epidemiol Biomarkers Prev* **13**, 1765–1771.

38. Soronen, P., Laiti, M., Torn, S., Harkonen, P., Patrikainen, L., Li, Y., et al. (2004) Sex steroid hormone metabolism and prostate cancer. *Ster Biochem Mol Biol* **92**, 281–286.

39. Giovannucci E., Stampfer M. J., Krithivas K., Brown, M., Dahl, D., et al. (1997) The CAG repeat within the androgen receptor gene and its relationship to prostate cancer. *Proc Natl Acad Sci U S A* **94**, 3320–3323.

40. Bratt O., Borg A., Kristoffersson U., Lundgren, R., Zhang, Q. X., Olsson, H. (1999) CAG repeat length in the androgen receptor gene is related to age at diagnosis of prostate cancer and response to endocrine therapy, but not to prostate cancer risk. *Br J Cancer* **81**, 672–676.

41. Nam R. K., Elhaji, Y., Krahn, M. D., Lee, S. H., Kim, C. C., Hahn, S. H., et al. (2000) Significance of the CAG repeat polymorphism of the androgen receptor gene in prostate cancer progression. *J Urol* **164**, 567–572.

42. Gilligan, T., Manola, J., Sartor, O., Weinrich, S. P., Moul, J. W., Kantoff, P. W. (2004) Absence of a correlation of androgen receptor gene CAG repeat length and prostate cancer risk in an African-American population. *Clin Prostate Cancer* **3**, 98–103.

43. Powell, I. J., Land, S. J., Dey, J., Heilbrun, L.K., Hughes, M.R., Sakr, W., et al. (2005) Impact of CAG repeats in exon 1 of the androgen receptor on disease progression after prostatectomy. *Cancer* **103**, 528–537.

44. Balic, I., Graham, S. T., Troyer, D. A., Higgins, B. A., Pollock, B. H., Johnson-Pais, T. L., Thompson, I. M., Leach, R. J. (2002) Androgen receptor length polymorphism associated with prostate cancer risk in Hispanic men. *J Urol* **168**, 2245–2248.

45. Hsing A. W., Gao Y. T., Wu, G., Wang, X., Deng, J., Chen, Y. L., et al. (2000) Polymorphic CAG and GGN repeat lengths in the androgen receptor gene and prostate cancer risk: A population-based case-control study in China. *Cancer Res* **60**, 5111–5116.

46. Correa-Cerro L., Wohr G., Haussler J., Berthon, P., Drelon, E., Mangin, P., et al. (1999) (CAG)nCAA and GGN repeats in the human androgen receptor gene are not associated with prostate cancer in a French-German population. *Eur J Hum Genet* **7**, 357–362.

47. Ntais, C., Polycarpou, A., Ioannidis, J.P. (2003) Association of the CYP17 gene polymorphism with the risk of prostate cancer: a meta-analysis. *Cancer Epidemiol Biomarkers Prev* **12**, 120–126.

48. Rebbeck, T.R., Jaffe, J.M., Walker, A.H., Wein, A.J., Malkowicz, S.B. (1998) Modification of clinical presentation of prostate tumors by a novel genetic variant in CYP3A4. *J Natl Cancer Inst* **90**, 1225–1229.

49. Bangsi, D., Zhou, J.Y., Sun, Y., Patel, N. P., Darga, L. L., Heilbrun, L. K., et al. (2006) Impact of a genetic variant in CYP3A4 on risk and clinical presentation of prostate cancer among white and African-American men, *Urol Oncol* **24**, 21–27.

50. Makridakis, N, M., di Salle, E., Reichardt, J. K. (2000) Biochemical and pharmacogenetic dissection of human steroid 5 alpha-reductase type II. *Pharmacogenetics* **10**, 407–413.

51. Winters, D. L., Hanlon, A.L., Raysor, S. L., Watkins-Bruner, D., Pinover, W. H., et al. (2001) Plasma levels of IGF-1, IGF-2, and IGFBP-3 in white and African-American men at increased risk of prostate cancer. *Urology* **58**, 614–618.

52. Wang, C., Catlin, D. H., Starcevic, B., Heber, D., Ambler, C., Berman, N., et al. (2005) Low-fat high-fiber diet decreased serum and urine androgens in men. *J Clin Endocrinol Metab* **90**, 3550–3559.

53. Griffiths, K., Morton, M. S., Denis, L. (1999) Certain aspects of molecular endocrinology that relate to the influence of dietary factors on the pathogenesis of prostate cancer. *Eur Urol* **35**, 443–455.

54. Buschemeyer, W. C., Freedland, S. J. (2007) Obesity and prostate cancer, epidemiology and clinical implications. *Eur Urol* **52**, 1–13.

55. Amling, C. L., Riffenburgh, R.H., Sun, L., Moul, J.W., Lance, R.S., Kusuda, L., et al. (2004) Pathologic variables and recurrence rates as related to obesity and race in men with prostate cancer undergoing radical prostatectomy. *J Clin Oncol* **22**, 439–445.

56. Clinton, S. K., Emenhiser, C., Schwartz, S. J., et al. (1996) Cis-trans lycopene isomers, carotenoids, and retinol in human prostate cancer. *Cancer Epidemiol Biomarkers Prev* **5**, 823–833.

57. Giovannucci, E., Rimm, E. B., Liu Y., Stampfer, M. J., Willett, W. C. (2002) A prospective study of tomato products, lycopene, and prostate cancer risk. *J Natl Cancer Inst* **94**, 391–398.

58. Kirsh V. A., Mayne, S. T., Peters, U., Chatterjee, N., Leitzmann, M. F., Dixon, L. B., Urban, D. A., Crawford, E. D., Hayes, R. B. (2006) A prospective study of lycopene and tomato product intake and risk of prostate cancer. *Cancer Epidemiol Biomarkers Prev* **15**, 92–98.

59. Thorpe, J. F., Jain S., Marczylo, T. H., Gescher, A. J., Steward, W. P., Mellon, J. K. (2007) A review of phase III clinical trials of prostate cancer chemoprevention. *Ann R Coll Surg Engl* **89**, 207–211.

60. Moul, J. W., Sesterhenn, I. A., Connelly, R. R., Douglas, T., Srivastava, S., Mostofi, F. K., et al. (1995) Prostate-specific antigen values at the time of prostate cancer diagnosis in African-American men. *JAMA* **274**, 1277–1281.

61. Sakr, W. A., Grignon, D. J., Hass, G., Heilbrun, L. K., Pontes, J. E., Crissman, J. D. (1996) Age and racial distribution of prostate intraepithelial neoplasia. *Eur Urol* **30**, 138–144.

62. Hoffman, R. M., Gilliland, F. D., Eley, J. W., Harlan, L. C., Stephenson, R.A., Stanford, J. L., et al. (2001) Racial and ethnic differences in advanced-stage prostate cancer: the Prostate Cancer Outcomes Study. *J Natl Cancer Inst* **93**, 388–395.

63. Moul, J. W., Connelly, R. R., Mooneyhan, R. M., Zhang,W., Sesterhenn, I. A., Mostofi, F. K., et al. (1999) Racial differences in tumor volume and prostate specific antigen among radical prostatectomy patients. *J Urol* **162**, 394–397.

64. Ndubuisi, S.C., Kofie, V. Y., Andoh, J. Y., Schwartz, E. M. (1995) Black-white differences in the stage at presentation of prostate cancer in the District of Columbia. *Urology* **46**, 71–77.

65. Shavers, V. L., Brown, M. L. (2002) Racial and ethnic disparities in the receipt of cancer treatment. *J Natl Cancer Inst* **94**, 334–357.

66. Harlan, L. C., Potosky, A., Gilliland, F. D., Hoffman, R., Albertsen, P. C., Hamilton, A. S., et al. (2001) Factors associated with initial therapy for clinically localized prostate cancer: prostate cancer outcomes study. *J Natl Cancer Inst* **93**, 1864–1871.

67. Morris, C. R., Snipes, K. P., Schlag, R., Wright, W. E. (1999) Sociodemographic factors associated with prostatectomy utilization and concordance with the physician data query for prostate cancer (United States). *Cancer Causes Control* **10**, 503–511.

68. Klabunde, C. N., Potosky, A. L., Harlan, L. C., Kramer, B. S. (1998) Trends and black/white differences in treatment for nonmetastatic prostate cancer. *Med Care* **36**, 1337–1348.

69. Underwood, W., De Monner, S., Ubel, P., Fagerlin, A., Sanda, M. G., Wei, J. T. (2004) Racial/ethnic disparities in the treatment of localized/regional prostate cancer. *J Urol* **171**, 1504–1507.

70. Shavers, V. L., Brown, M. L., Potosky, A. L., Klabunde, C. N., Davis, W.W., Moul, J.W., et al. (2004) Race/ethnicity and the receipt of watchful waiting for the initial management of prostate cancer. *Gen Intern Med* **19**, 146–155.

71. Optenberg, S. A., Thompson, I. M., Friedrichs, P., Wojcik, B., Stein, C. R., Kramer, B. (1995) Race, treatment, and long-term survival from prostate cancer in an equal-access medical care delivery system. *JAMA* **274**, 1599–1605.

72. Moul, J. W., Wu, H., Sun, L., McLeod, D. G., Amling, C., Lance, R., et al. (2002) Epidemiology of radical prostatectomy for localized prostate cancer in the era of prostate-specific antigen: an overview of the Department of Defense Center for Prostate Disease Research national database. *Surgery* **132**, 213–219.

73. Powell, I.J., Schwartz, K., Hussain, M. (1995) Removal of the financial barrier to health care: does it impact on prostate cancer at presentation and survival? A comparative study between black and white men in a Veterans Affairs system. *Urology* **46**, 825–830.

74. Moul, J. W., Douglas, T. H., McCarthy, W. F., McLeod, D. G. (1996) Black race is an adverse prognostic factor for prostate cancer recurrence following radical prostatectomy in an equal access health care setting. *J Urol* **155**, 1667–1673.

75. Iselin, C. E., Box, J. W., Vollmer, R. T., Layfield, L. J., Robertson, J.E., Paulson, D.F. (1998) Surgical control of clinically localized prostate carcinoma is equivalent in African-American and white males. *Cancer* **83**, 2353–2360.

76. Powell, I.J., Dey, J., Dudley, A., Pontes, J.E., Cher, M.L., Sakr, W., et al., (2002) Disease-free survival difference between African-Americans and whites after radical prostatectomy for local prostate cancer: a multivariable analysis. *Urology* **59**, 907–912.

77. Grossfeld, G.D., Latini, D.M., Downs, T., Lubeck, D.P., Mehta, S.S., Carroll, P.R. (2002) Is ethnicity an independent pre-dictor of prostate cancer recurrence after radical prostatectomy? *J Urol* **168**, 2510–2515.

78. Powell, I.J., Banerjee, M., Bianco, F.J., Wood Jr, D.P., Dey, J., Lai, Z., et al. The effect of race/ethnicity on prostate cancer treatment outcome is conditional: a review of Wayne State University data. *J Urol* **171** (2004), 1508–1512.

Chapter 22

Racial Differences in Clinical Outcome After Prostate Cancer Treatment

Takashi Fukagai, Thomas Namiki, Robert G. Carlile, and Mikio Namiki

Abstract

Prostate cancer is the number one killer in the United States. A comparison of US and Japanese population is discussed in this chapter to identify risk factors for prostate cancer. Screening of prostate cancer is
common among Americans, but not among Japanese. A comparison of survival in different populations
is also presented; and prognosis after hormonal treatment in different populations is included.

Key words: Prostate cancer, clinical outcome, racial differences, prostate-specific antigen, PSA,
hormonal therapy.

1. Introduction

Prostate cancer is the most commonly diagnosed cancer in Western countries (*1*). It is increasing in incidence worldwide. However, the incidence of prostate cancer is still markedly different
among various races and countries. Asians, especially Japanese
and Chinese, have lower incidences than Caucasians (*2*). The
incidence in Japanese Americans (JA) is intermediate between
Japanese living in Japan and Caucasians in the USA (**Fig. 22.1**)
(*3*). The lower incidence among Japanese born in the USA compared with US whites may mean that Japanese immigrants retain
some genetic and/or lifestyle characteristics that make their risk
for prostate cancer less than that of US whites.

If the prostate cancer's behavior is due to any genetic differences related to race, this may result in different clinical responses
to treatment. Few publications have compared prostate cancer
treatment and patient survival among different ethnic groups.

M. Verma (ed.), *Methods of Molecular Biology, Cancer Epidemiology, vol. 472*
© 2009 Humana Press, a part of Springer Science + Business Media, Totowa, NJ
Book doi: 10.1007/978-1-60327-492-0

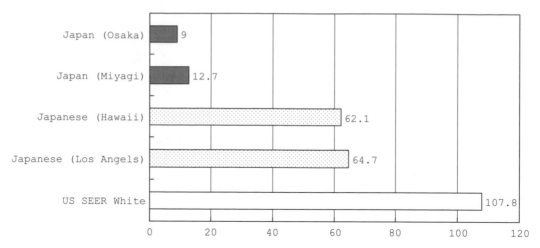

Fig. 22.1. Age-standardized incidence rates of prostate cancer (per 100,000): 1993–1997.

Several studies indicate that race is a prognostic factor for African American and white men. But the differences in survival between Asian and white men are unknown.

In this chapter, we show recent trends of prostate cancer incidence and mortality and discuss racial differences in clinical outcome after prostate cancer treatment, especially between Caucasians and Japanese.

2. Incidence and Mortality of Prostate Cancer in Caucasians and Japanese

Prostate cancer is the most common noncutaneous cancer in American men and the second most common cause of cancer death. In 2007, it is estimated that 218,890 new cases will be diagnosed and 27,050 men will die from the disease (1).

The incidence of prostate cancer in JA living in Hawaii is intermediate between Japanese living in Japan and Caucasians in the USA. But recently, the incidence of prostate cancer in JA has been getting higher and the difference between JA and Caucasians has been getting smaller (Fig. 22.2). This reason is not clear, but first-generation Japanese immigrants kept their Japanese lifestyle strictly after they immigrated to America, while subsequent generations changed their lifestyle and diet, which became more like the Caucasian lifestyle.

Regarding the incidence and mortality of prostate cancer in Japanese in Japan, in 2005, it is estimated that 37,060 new cases will be diagnosed and 10,045 men will die from the disease (4). It is the sixth most common cancer in incidence and the eighth

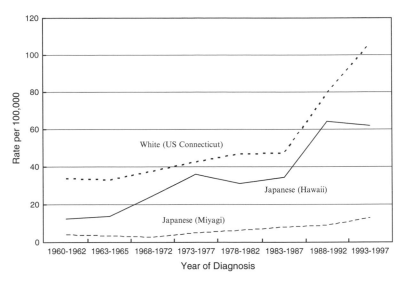

Fig. 22.2. Time trend in prostate cancer incidence.

most common cause of cancer death in Japanese men. The incidence and mortality of prostate cancer in North America has been reported to be declining since the early 1990s. But in Japan, although the incidence of prostate cancer is less than in the United States, the incidence of prostate cancer has been increasing steadily. The reported incidence of prostate cancer and the proportion of early stage cancer at diagnosis has increased in the USA following introduction of the prostate-specific antigen (PSA) test (*1*). Currently, about 50% of men in the United States have a PSA test annually, and about 75% of men have had a PSA test (*5*). On the other hand, although some Japanese prefectural and city government offices have conducted prostate cancer screening, nationwide, the percentage of municipalities conducting prostate cancer screening is still not large. Ito et al. reported that the cumulative exposure rate of PSA screening in Gunma prefecture, that has the most advanced PSA screening system in Japan, was estimated to be only 5.8% for 10 years (1992–2001) (*6*).

The increase in early-stage cancer detected in the US medical system has not yet appeared in the Japanese medical system; thus, the incidence of prostate cancer will be underestimated until the Japanese medical system achieves levels of screening for prostate cancer comparable to those in the USA. To accurately compare incidence of cancer between different countries, one must consider not only differences in ethnic origin, diet, and lifestyle, but also differences in case ascertainment reflecting the medical system in each country. The difference in incidence of prostate cancer in each country and ethnicity will probably decrease in next decade with the spread of PSA screening.

3. Clinical Outcomes After Prostate Cancer Treatment

3.1. Comparison Between Caucasians and African Americans

Most of the studies that investigated the ethnic differences in clinical outcomes after prostate cancer treatment compared the prognosis between African American and white men. Several studies showed the poor prognosis of African American men after prostatectomy. Earlier studies have shown that the black race is also associated with lower overall and disease specific survival after other prostate cancer treatments such as radiation therapy. But it is controversial as to whether this difference is a result of genetic and /or socioeconomic factors. A large recent study in Texas of over 60,000 men found that racial disparity in survival among men with local or regional prostate cancer can be largely explained by poverty and related factors. Eisenberger et al., in a review of the National Cancer Institute (NCI) Intergroup Study #0036 for prognostic factors in Stage D2 prostate cancer, concluded that African American race was an adverse prognostic factor in patients with stage D2 prostate cancer with hormonal therapy (7). Similar results have been found in other studies (8, 9). However, other authors did not find race to be an adverse prognostic factor in patients who had their prostate cancer treated with hormonal therapy (10, 11). McLeod et al. reported no difference in outcome of combined androgen blockade (CAB) for the treatment of prostate cancer between African American men and white men (10). These findings indicated that the clinical outcomes after treatments for prostate cancer were worse in African Americans regardless of treatment methods. But the cause of these difference is still controversial.

3.2. Comparison Between Caucasians and Japanese

Few publications have compared prostate cancer treatment and patient survival between Caucasian and Asian men. Young et al. reported with the SEER program data that Japanese had higher survival rates for prostate cancer (12). But the reason for this was not established and survival was not examined by the type of treatment received. Recently, we investigated the racial differences in clinical outcome after treatment for prostate cancer in Hawaii and reported part of our results (13). The findings of our research are as follows.

During 1992–2001, 2,074 prostate cancer patients were registered in the Tumor Oncology Registry of the Queen's Medical Center, Honolulu, Hawaii, USA. Of these prostate cancer patients, 642 Japanese men and 465 Caucasian men were included. We divided these patients according to race and treatment methods: prostatectomy, radiation therapy, hormonal therapy, or no treatments (watchful waiting), and compared the clinical outcomes between Caucasians and Japanese. Clinical information was also obtained from the hospital tumor registry. All living patients were followed to the end of 2001 and none were lost to follow-up. Age, stage, Gleason score, race, and pretreatment PSA values were abstracted. The Caucasian and Japanese patient groups were similar in terms of age, clinical stage, pretreatment PSA levels, and Gleason scores. Results indicated that the JA patients had significantly better outcomes after hormone treatment than their Caucasian counterparts (**Fig. 22.3**). We could not find any significant differences in clinical outcome after other treatments: prostatectomy, radiation therapy, and no treatment (**Figs. 22.4 and 22.5**).

3.3. Clinical Outcomes After Hormone Treatment

We investigated the prognosis of Caucasian and Japanese patients with hormone treatment in detail. The specific type of hormonal therapy each patient received (conventional surgical, medical castration alone, or CAB) was not available. Details of the patient's background of the two ethnic groups is given in **Table 22.1**. None of the patients received definitive surgical or radiation therapy. Differences in patient background between the two groups were estimated by using the t test and the χ^2 test. The clinical endpoint was survival. The Kaplan-Meier method was used for overall and cause-specific survival curves, which were compared using log-rank statistics. Age, stage, Gleason score, race, and pretreatment PSA values were assessed as to their interdependence and correlation with the clinical course using Cox's proportional hazards regression model. The hospital's Institutional Research Board approved the study. Median follow-up was 51 months (range, 2–126 months) for JA and 36 months (range, 2–88 months) for Caucasian men. There were no statistical differences in the

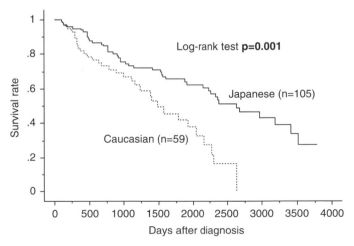

Fig. 22.3. Overall survival rate after hormone treatment according to race (© 2006, Blackwell Publishing).

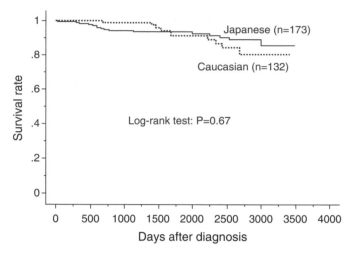

Fig. 22.4. Overall survival rate after prostatectomy according to race.

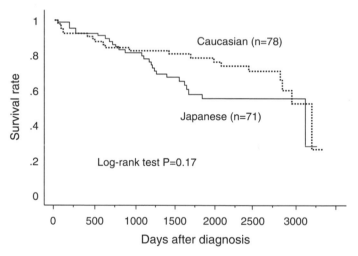

Fig. 22.5. Overall survival rate of the patients with watchful waiting according to race.

patients' backgrounds between the two groups (**Table 22.1**). Forty-five JA and 32 Caucasian men died during the follow-up period. At 60 months, the overall survival rate was 65.5% for JA and 41.7% for Caucasian men ($p = 0.01$). JA men who received hormonal treatment had a better overall and cause-specific survival rate compared with Caucasian men ($p = 0.001$ and 0.036, respectively) (**Figs. 22.3 and 22.6**). For patients with metastasis (Caucasian men, 15; JA men, 37) and without metastasis (Caucasian men, 44; JA men, 68), the overall survival rate was higher in JA men ($p = 0.032$ and 0.007, respectively). To clarify

Table 22.1
Baseline characteristics of ethnic groups

	Japanese (n = 105)	Caucasian (n = 59)	P value
Age			
Median (range)	77 (53–92)	77 (51–90)	
Mean ± SD	75.8 ± 8.1	76.5 ± 8.2	0.55
PSA			
Median (range)	46.1 (3.9–9,783)	16.2 (0.6–4,000)	
Mean ± SD	351.1 ± 1,437.4	152.3 ± 583.9	0.355
Clinical stage[a]			
I	0 (0%)	0 (0%)	
II	53 (50%)	37 (63%)	0.1[b]
III	10 (10%)	1 (2%)	
IV	42 (40%)	21 (36%)	
Gleason score			
2–6	14 (13%)	8 (14%)	
7	33 (31%)	18 (31%)	
8–10	52 (50%)	31 (53%)	
Unknown	6 (6%)	2 (3%)	
Median (range)	8	8	
Mean ± SD	7.7 ± 1.2	7.7 ± 1.4	0.883

SD, standard deviation [a]Clinical stage followed by 1997 International Union
Against Cancer (UICC)'s TNM classification.
[b]χ^2 test.

the relation between tumor progression and ethnic differences in
survival after hormone therapy in more detail, we compared the
survival curves between the two ethnic groups according to PSA
values. Among patients whose PSA value was over 100 ng/mL
(Caucasian men, 11; JA men, 26), there was no statistically significant difference in the survival curves between Caucasians and
Japanese (**Fig. 22.7**). We examined the simultaneous influence
of five covariables (age, clinical stage, race, Gleason score, and
pretreatment PSA value) on time to death. Race was a significant
prognostic factor on multivariate analysis ($p = 0.03$) along with
pretreatment PSA value ($p = 0.03$). The findings suggest a difference

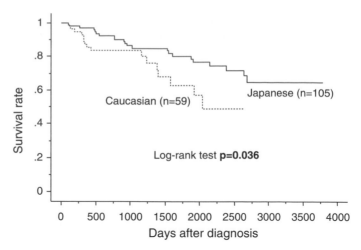

Fig. 22.6. Cause-specific survival rate after hormone treatment according to race (© 2006, Blackwell Publishing).

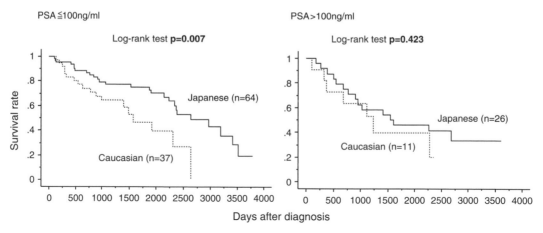

Fig. 22.7. Overall survival rate according to race by PSA value (© 2006, Blackwell Publishing).

in the effectiveness of hormonal therapy of prostate cancer in JA men living in Hawaii compared with Caucasian men living in Hawaii.

3.4. Comparison of Clinical Outcome After Hormone Treatment Among Other Races

After finding that Japanese patients showed better prognosis after hormone treatment, we investigated the clinical outcome after hormone treatment in other races. This research is ongoing. We found 126 Filipino and 36 Chinese the same tumor registry

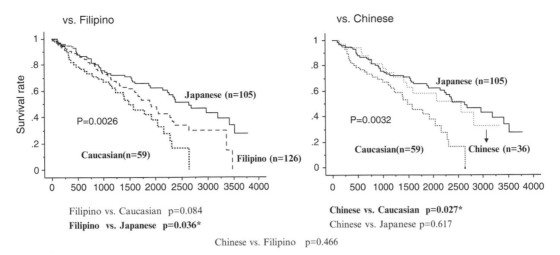

Fig. 22.8. Overall survival rate after hormone treatment according to race: comparison among Japanese, Caucasian, Chinese, and Filipino in Hawaii.

in Hawaii who had hormone treatment. We compared these patients' clinical outcome with that of Caucasians and Japanese. Interestingly, Chinese men show almost the same prognosis as Japanese and better prognosis than Caucasian men. Filipinos show a worse prognosis after hormonal therapy than Japanese, but a better prognosis than Caucasian men (**Fig. 22.8**).

4. Discussion

As we mentioned already, few publications have compared prostate cancer treatment and patient survival between Caucasian and Asian men. To our knowledge, this is the first study to compare the prognosis, especially after hormonal therapy, between Caucasians and Japanese in the USA. Our study consisted of a relatively small number of patients and the information on progression-free survival rate was not available. All patients were treated by the same group of urologists in a single institution, with follow-up management in cases of relapses. It is also unlikely that only one ethnic group, the Japanese, had a large proportion of CAB treatment, because both ethnic groups had almost the same clinical background and were treated by the same urologists. Therefore, we believe that our study is significant even though we did not have the information on progression-free survival. This study showed a better overall and disease-specific survival for JA men with hormone treatment for prostate cancer. In contrast, no racial differences in overall survival were found in the group of patients who received no treatment for prostate cancer during the same period. But our analysis showed that for patients' whose PSA value was over 100 ng/mL, a more advanced stage, there was no statistically significant difference in survival between Caucasians and Japanese. PSA is a strong prognostic factor that correlates with the extension of prostate cancer. It is well known that prostate cancer shows various genetic changes associated with progression (*14*). Genetic changes in the more advanced stage cancer may reduce the effects of ethnic differences in prognosis after hormone treatment as noted in this study. One of the putative reasons for the difference may be fewer side effects, especially cardiovascular disease, associated with hormonal therapy in Japanese patients. Although our outcome data did not include the cause of death except cancer death, we found that Japanese patients showed better prognosis in cause-specific survival rates as well as in overall survival rates. Also, recent hormonal treatment methods, luteinizing hormone-releasing hormone (LHRH) agonist treatment, anti-androgen agent treatment, and orchiectomy do not have the cardiovascular side effects associated with previously used estrogen administration. The findings may indicate different sensitivities for hormonal therapy in Japanese patients.

Several studies have shown racial differences in CAG repeat alleles (*15*, *16*). Irvine et al. found that the prevalence of short CAG alleles was highest in African American men with the highest risk for prostate cancer, intermediate in intermediate risk non-Hispanic whites, and lowest in Asians at very low risk for prostate cancer (*15*). Bratt et al. found an association between long CAG repeat length and a good response to hormonal therapy (*16*). These findings may explain our results showing better prognosis in Japanese after hormonal therapy, corresponding to the low prevalence of short CAG repeats and the high prevalence of long CAG repeats in Asians. However, other studies report conflicting results. Suzuki et al. found that shorter CAG repeat length was correlated with better response to hormonal therapy and prognosis in Japanese prostate cancer patients (*17*). Others also note a higher frequency of short CAG repeat length in African American men compared with whites and Asians, but no difference in CAG repeat length between whites and Asians (*18–20*). Another racial difference in association with androgen levels is 5α-reductase activity. Ross et al. measured serum testosterone, dihydrotestosterone (DHT), and metabolites of DHT among young American blacks and whites and native Japanese (*21*). In this study, both black and white men had significantly higher serum levels of DHT metabolites than did native Japanese men. The influence of the different serum levels of DHT metabolites on the effectiveness of hormone treatment is unclear, but may potentially have an influence on the different effectiveness of hormone treatment between Japanese and Caucasian men. Further studies are needed to clarify the relation between CAG repeat alleles, 5α-reductase activity, and response to hormonal therapy.

As we showed already, an ongoing study of other ethnic groups in Hawaii has also shown different prognosis after hormonal therapy. Chinese men show almost the same prognosis as Japanese and better prognosis than Caucasian men. Filipinos show a worse prognosis after hormonal therapy than Japanese but better than Caucasian men. Interestingly, the prognosis after hormonal therapy is inversely correlated with the prostate cancer incidence of the ethnic group. As previously noted, the incidence of prostate cancer within ethnic groups may relate to the exogenous or endogenous hormonal environment, which in turn may also relate to the different effectiveness of hormonal therapy.

5. Conclusions

Some recent studies have indicated that the real incidence of prostate cancer in Japan is higher than expected, and actually closer to that of the United States.

A marked racial difference in clinical outcome after hormonal therapy was observed in our study between Japanese and Caucasians. A prospective study with a larger number of patients may be necessary to elucidate the differential effectiveness of hormonal therapy of prostate cancer in different races, especially between Japanese and Caucasians.

References

1. Jemal, A., Siegel, R., Ward, E., Murray, T., Xu, J., and Thun, M.J. (2007) Cancer statistics, 2007. *CA Cancer J Clin.* **57**, 43–66.

2. Wynder, E.L., Fujita, Y., Harris, R.E., Hirayama, T., and Hiyama, T. (1991) Comparative epidemiology of cancer between the United States and Japan. *Cancer.* **67**, 746–763.

3. Zaridze, D.G., Boyle, P., and Smans, M. (1984) International trends in prostatic cancer. *Int J Cancer.* **33**, 223–230.

4. Oshima, A., Kuroishi, T., Tajima, K., (eds) (2004) Cancer Statistics in Japan 2004-Mortality, Incidence and Survival (In Japanese). Shinohara Publishers, Tokyo, Japan.

5. Thompson, I.M., Canby-Hagino, E., and Lucia, M.S. (2005) Stage migration and grade inflation in prostate cancer: Will Rogers meets Garrison Keillor. *J Natl Cancer Inst.* **97**, 1236–1237.

6. Ito, K., Yamamoto, T., Ohi, M., Takechi, H., Kurokawa, K., and Suzuki, K.(2006) Impact of exposure rate of PSA-screening on clinical stage of prostate cancer in Japan. *J Urol.* **175**, S477–478.

7. Eisenberger, M.A., Crawford, E.D., Wolf, M., Blumenstein, B., McLeod, D.G., Benson, R., Dorr, F.A., Benson, M., and Spaulding, J.T. (1994) Prognostic factors in stage D2 prostate cancer; important implications for future trials: results of a cooperative intergroup study (INT.0036). The National Cancer Institute Intergroup Study #0036. *Semin Oncol.* **21**, 613–619.

8. Thompson, I., Tangen, C., Tolcher, A., Crawford, E., Eisenberger, M., and Moinpour, C. (2001) Association of African-American ethnic background with survival in men with metastatic prostate cancer. *J Natl Cancer Inst.* **93**, 219–225.

9. Pienta, K.J., Demers, R., Hoff, M., Kau, T.Y., Montie, J.E., and Severson, R.K. (1995) Effect of age and race on the survival of men with prostate cancer in the Metropolitan Detroit tricounty area, 1973 to 1987. *Urology.* **45**, 93–101.

10. McLeod, D.G., Schellhammer, P.F., Vogelzang, N.J. Soloway, M.S., Sharifi, R., Block, N.L., Venner, P.M., Patterson, A.L., Sarosdy, M.F., Kelley, R.P., and Kolvenbag, G.J. (1999) Exploratory analysis on the effect of race on clinical outcome in patients with advanced prostate cancer receiving bicalutamide or flutamide, each in combination with LHRH analogues. The Casodex Combination Study Group. *Prostate.* **40**, 218–224.

11. Koff, S.G., Connelly, R.R., Bauer, J.J., McLeod, D.G., and Moul, J.W. (2002) Primary hormonal therapy for prostate cancer: experience with 135 consecutive PSA-ERA patients from a tertiary care military medical center. *Prostate Cancer Prostatic Dis.* **5**, 152–158.

12. Young, J.L. Jr., Ries, L.G., and Pollack, E.S. (1984) Cancer patient survival among ethnic groups in the United States. *J Natl Cancer Inst.* **73**, 341–352.

13. Fukagai, T., Namiki, S.T., Carlile, R., Yoshida, H., and Namiki, M. (2006) Comparison of the clinical outcome after hormonal therapy for prostate cancer between Japanese and Caucasian men. *BJU Int.* **97**, 1190–1193.

14. Bostwick, D.G., Pacelli, A., and Lopez-Beltran, A. (1996) Molecular biology of prostatic intraepithelial neoplasia. *Prostate.* **29**, 117–134.

15. Irvine, R.A., Yu, M.C., Ross, R.K., and Coetzee, G.A. (1995) The CAG and GGC microsatellites of the androgen receptor gene

in linkage disequilibrium in men with prostate cancer. *Cancer Res.* **55**, 1937–1940.

16. Bratt, O., Borg, A., Kristoffersson, U., Lundgren, R., Zhang, Q.X., and Olsson H. (1999) CAG repeat length in the androgen receptor gene is related to age at diagnosis of prostate cancer and response to endocrine therapy, but not to prostate cancer risk. *Br J Cancer.* **81**, 672–676.

17. Suzuki, H., Akakura, K., Komiya, A., Ueda, T., Imamoto, T., Furuya, Y., Ichikawa, T., Watanabe, M., Shiraishi, T., and Ito, H. (2002) CAG polymorphic repeat lengths in androgen receptor gene among Japanese prostate cancer patients: potential predictor of prognosis after endocrine therapy. *Prostate.* **51**, 219–224.

18. Sartor, O., Zheng, Q., and Eastham, J.A. (1999) Androgen receptor gene CAG repeat length varies in a race-specific fashion in men without prostate cancer. *Urology.* **53**, 378–380.

19. Jin, B., Beilin, J., Zajac, J., and Handelsman, D.J. (2000) Androgen receptor gene polymorphism and zonal volumes in Australian and Chinese men. *J Androl.* **21**, 91–98.

20. Hsing, A.W., Gao, Y.T., Wu, G., Wang, X., Deng, J., Chen, Y.L., Sesterhenn, I.A., Mostofi, F.K., Benichou, J., and Chang, C. (2000) Polymorphic CAG and GGN repeat lengths in the androgen receptor gene and prostate cancer risk: a population-based case-control study in China. *Cancer Res.* **60**, 5111–5116.

21. Ross, R.K., Bernstein, L., Lobo, R.A., Shimizu, H., Stanczyk, F.Z., Pike, M.C., and Henderson, B.E. (1992) 5-alpha-reductase activity and risk of prostate cancer among Japanese and US white and black males. *Lancet.* **339**, 887–889.

Chapter 23

Epidemiology of Stomach Cancer

Hermann Brenner, Dietrich Rothenbacher, and Volker Arndt

Abstract

Despite a major decline in incidence and mortality over several decades, stomach cancer is still the fourth most common cancer and the second most common cause of cancer death in the world. There is a 10-fold variation in incidence between populations at the highest and lowest risk. The incidence is particularly high in East Asia, Eastern Europe, and parts of Central and South America, and it is about twice as high among men than among women. Prognosis is generally rather poor, with 5-year relative survival below 30% in most countries. The best established risk factors for stomach cancer are *Helicobacter pylori* infection, the by far strongest established risk factor for distal stomach cancer, and male sex, a family history of stomach cancer, and smoking. While some factors related to diet and food preservation, such as high intake of salt-preserved foods and dietary nitrite or low intake of fruit and vegetables, are likely to increase the risk of stomach cancer, the quantitative impact of many dietary factors remains uncertain, partly due to limitations of exposure assessment and control for confounding factors. Future epidemiologic research should pay particular attention to differentiation of stomach cancer epidemiology by sub-site, and to exploration of potential interactions between *H. pylori* infection, genetic, and environmental factors.

Key words: Gastric cancer, *Helicobacter pylori*, incidence, mortality, smoking, stomach cancer.

1. Introduction

Stomach cancer (gastric cancer) emerges from gastric tissue. More than 90% of stomach cancers are adenocarcinomas, and the remaining gastric malignancies are lymphomas or originate from gastrointestinal stromal tissue (sarcomas). Still, stomach cancer is

M. Verma (ed.), *Methods of Molecular Biology, Cancer Epidemiology, vol. 472*
© 2009 Humana Press, a part of Springer Science + Business Media, Totowa, NJ
Book doi: 10.1007/978-1-60327-492-0

one of the leading causes of cancer related deaths in the world, although a permanent decrease in incidence has been recorded within the past decades. Furthermore, on a global scale, large geographic differences exist (1). The underlying reasons for these differences are still not very well understood.

In addition, the reasons for the overall observed declining incidence are not clear yet. Notably, this decline is especially related to gastric carcinoma located in the distal stomach. The relatively small proportion of gastric cancers related to the proximal stomach and to the gastroesophageal junction seems to be on a constant rise. As proximal and distal stomach cancer seem to have different pathogenesis, a change of precursor conditions or related environmental risk factors may most likely explain these changes. What is good for one entity may not be good for the other.

Nutritional factors had long been under suspect as main risk factors of stomach cancer. However, studies investigating the role of preserved foods, low intake of fruits, and other nutritional factors often showed inconsistent results, and dietary factors may only explain a small part of the variation in stomach cancer risk. Since the year 1994, infection with the gastric bacterium *Helicobacter pylori* has been classified as a definite carcinogen for stomach cancer (2). Recent evidence suggests the role of this agent to be even more important than initially suspected. However, only distal cancers are related to *H. pylori* infection, cancers located proximally are not. Furthermore, some large populations with high prevalence of *H. pylori* infection have low gastric cancer rates (3), indicating that other factors may be of importance, too.

Undoubtedly, during the last 20 years, important contributions have been made to shed light on the risk factors of stomach cancers, but there is still an urgent need for a better understanding of the underlying causes of this important cancer in order to define successful means of cancer prevention. This is of especial urgency, as the prognosis of the affected patients is still rather poor (4).

2. Descriptive Epidemiology

2.1. Global Burden

Until recently, gastric cancer was the second most common cancer worldwide. But now with an estimated number of 900,000–950,000 new cases per year at the beginning of the 21st century, it is in forth place behind cancers of the lung, breast, colon, and rectum (5). Due to its poor prognosis, gastric cancer is the second most common cause of death from cancer and accounts for

700,000 deaths annually. As with most other solid tumors, the incidence rate of gastric cancer increases with age and the cancer is relatively rare in male or female patients younger than 45 years. Most patients are between 60 and 80 years old at diagnosis. In general, incidence and mortality rates in men are approximately double to those in women.

Almost two thirds of the cases of gastric cancer occur in developing countries and 42% in China alone. However, gastric cancer cannot readily be categorized as being associated with less developed economies (6). As can be seen from **Table 23.1**, overall age-standardized incidence rates are comparable between so-called "more developed" and "less developed" countries.

2.2. Geographic Variation

As with most of the common forms of cancer, there is considerable geographic variation in incidence of gastric cancer around the world. High-risk areas (age-standardized rates in men >20 per 100,000) include East Asia, Eastern Europe, and parts of Central and South America (5). Incidence rates are low in Southern Asia, North and East Africa, North America, Australia, and New Zealand (**Fig. 23.1**). Patterns in women are broadly similar to those in men.

Table 23.1
Global gastric cancer incidence and mortality estimates (rates per 100,000) for 2002

Region	Men			Women		
	Cases	Crude rate	ASR(W)[a]	Cases	Crude rate	ASR(W) [a]
Incidence						
World	603,419	19.3	22.0	330,518	10.7	10.4
More developed regions	195,782	33.7	22.4	115,372	18.8	10.0
Less developed regions	405,211	15.9	21.5	214,024	8.7	10.4
Mortality						
World	446,052	14.3	16.3	254,297	8.3	7.9
More developed regions	128,721	22.2	14.5	83,515	13.6	6.9
Less developed regions	315,603	12.4	17.0	169,972	6.9	8.3

[a]ASR(W), age-standardized rate according to world standard population From ref. (1)

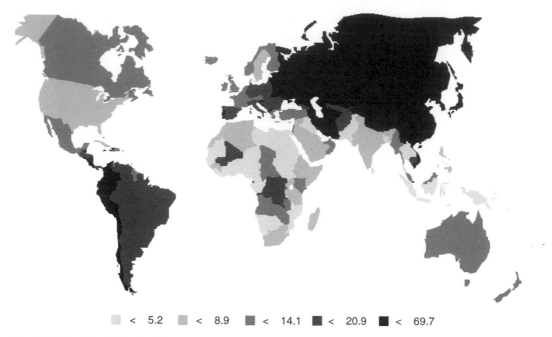

Fig. 23.1. Age-standardized incidence rates (per 100,000) of gastric cancer in men in 2002 (1).

The distribution of gastric cancer does not, however, follow a clear geographical pattern. Thus although some of the world's highest risk populations are in Asian countries, such as Japan, Korea, and China, other Asian countries have relatively low rates (e.g. India). There are also some very high-risk groups within low-risk populations (e.g. Koreans living in the USA) (6, 7).

2.3. Survival

In contrast to many other cancer sites, for which impressive improvements in prognosis have been reported (4), survival rates for patients with gastric cancer are poor, in general (5). The EUROCARE study estimated European survival for cases diagnosed in the period 1990–1994 to be around 24% at 5 years after diagnosis (8). Similar survival rates have been observed for most other industrialized countries outside of Europe (9, 10). Prognosis for gastric cancer is moderately good only in Japan (52%), where mass screening by photofluoroscopy has been practiced since the 1960s (5).

2.4. Time Trends

In the 1930s, gastric cancer was the most common cause of cancer death in the USA and Europe (11). Incidence as well as mortality rates have substantially declined over the past decades in many countries (**Fig. 23.2**). The most recent worldwide estimates of age adjusted incidence (22.0 per 100,000 in men and 10.3 per 100,000 in women) are about 15% lower than the values estimated in 1985

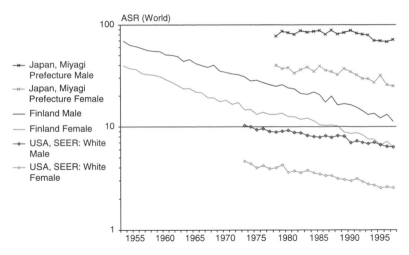

Fig. 23.2. Age-standardized incidence rate (ASR) (world standard population) of gastric cancer in Finland, USA, and Japan by time period (7).

(5). This decline may be related to improvements in preservation and storage of foods; it may also represent changes in the prevalence of *H. pylori* by birth cohort, perhaps as a result of reduced transmission in childhood, following a trend to improved hygiene and reduction of crowding (12, 13). As, in case of gastric cancer, mortality is closely associated with incidence, the trend in mortality rates has shown a very similar pattern.

Despite this notable decline in incidence rates, gastric cancer will remain an important component of the global cancer burden in absolute terms. Even if the current decline in incidence will continue in the future, the predicted growth in world population combined with increased longevity will most likely result in a net increase in the overall number of gastric cancers being diagnosed for several decades to come (6).

3. Risk Factors and Preventive Factors

3.1. Helicobacter pylori *Infection*

H. pylori, a Gram-negative bacterium has been redetected as a common inhabitant of the human stomach in 1984 (14). Numerous ecological, case–control and cohort studies conducted since then have consistently found *H. pylori* infection to be related to an increased risk of stomach cancer. In 1994, *H. pylori* was classified as a definite carcinogen for stomach cancer by the International Agency for Research on Cancer (2). In 2001, a pooled analysis from 12 prospective cohort studies demonstrated a sixfold increased risk of stomach cancer after 10 years of follow-up (15). *H. pylori* infection specifically increases the risk of cancer in the distal part of the stomach, where the vast majority of stomach cancers have been located in the past, whereas there is no increase in risk of proximal (cardia) cancer. Failure to distinguish proximal cancer from distal gastric cancer in previous studies may thus have led to dilution of effects of *H. pylori* infection and other risk factors. Furthermore, more recent evidence suggests that the role of *H. pylori* infection for the risk of distal stomach cancer may have been strongly underestimated in epidemiological studies due to additional methodological pitfalls, such as the secondary clearance of the infection in the process of stomach cancer development from atrophic gastric epithelium. Estimates of relative risk of distal stomach cancer associated with *H. pylori* infection increased to about 20 in studies from Sweden and Germany, when potential misclassification of infection status from this source was minimized (16, 17), and it was even suggested that *H. pylori* infection may be a (close to) necessary risk factor for distal stomach cancer development.

Given that about half of the adult world population has been infected with *H. pylori* in the past (18), this infection is likely to account for a very large share of the global burden of stomach cancer cases and deaths. On the other hand, the high prevalence of the infection also implies that only a small proportion of infected subjects will eventually develop stomach cancer, and identification of factors associated with increased risk among infected individuals and of interactions between the infection and other risk factors are therefore crucial for a better understanding of disease etiology and approaches for prevention. On the side of the infectious agent, a number of virulence factors being associated with increased risk have been identified, the best established being carriage of the cytotoxin-associated gene A (*cagA*) (19). On the host side, genetic predisposition likely plays a major role. For example, the risk of distal stomach cancer has been found to strongly increase with the number of proinflammatory polymorphisms (20). In addition, the combination of *H. pylori* infection with other risk factors, such as smoking or a positive family history, may lead to strongly elevated risks of distal stomach cancer and may point to approaches for targeted prevention and early detection (21, 22).

Regarding potential approaches to targeted prevention and early detection, a number of additional issues have to be addressed. Prevention of the *H. pylori* infection would have to take place among infants, given that most infections are acquired within the first few years of life (23). Preventive vaccination might have a large impact, but, despite major research efforts, is not available so far. Fortunately, rates of acquisition of persistent

H. pylori infection in childhood seem to decline rapidly in younger birth cohorts, at least in developed countries, possibly as a side effect of antibiotic therapy for other indications (24), which may accelerate the decline in incidence of distal stomach cancer in future generations of older adults. Given that the mother appears to be the main source for transmission of the infection, at least in developed countries (25), testing for and eradication of *H. pylori* infection among young women might be another approach for decreasing infection rates of future generations. To what extent eradication of *H. pylori* infection among adults may reduce their own cancer risk has yet to be established. A randomized trial from China could not show an overall beneficial effect of *H. pylori* eradication on stomach cancer occurrence, but suggested that prevention might be possible if eradication occurs before the onset of premalignant changes in the gastric mucosa (26). If confirmed in future studies, potential preventive eradication strategies might be considered. To extend preventive eradication strategies beyond established high-risk groups, while keeping them as cost-effective as possible, further enhanced risk stratification would be highly desirable (27).

3.2. Other Factors

In addition to *H. pylori* infection, further environmental factors have long been recognized as potential factors related to risk of stomach cancer. Immigrants coming from high-prevalence countries to low-prevalence countries have still a similar risk to the population of the country from which they origin. Their offspring, however, have a risk that is more or less already similar to the risk of the population of the country to which they immigrated, pointing to environmental influences that may already act at early life (28).

Dietary factors may partly explain these patterns. Certain foods containing large amounts of salt and nitrites for conservational purposes have been suggested to be important contributors to cancer risk. Although most epidemiological studies support these associations, evidence from large, prospective studies is still inconclusive (29). A diet rich in fruit and vegetables was found to be beneficial as a result of a meta-analysis summarizing the results of observational studies up to the year 2003. However, the results were no more statistically significant if only prospective studies were considered (30), and were not confirmed by the large-scale European Prospective Investigation Into Cancer and Nutrition (EPIC) study (31), pointing to potential sources of error in earlier retrospective studies.

The intake of meat and processed meat was both associated with an increased cancer risk in the EPIC study. This increase was related to distal (non-cardia) cancer and affected especially *H. pylori*-seropositive subjects (32). Whereas the intake of antioxidants, vitamins, and dietary supplementations may play a role in high-risk population such as in China, a prospective study in a US population found no influence on stomach cancer mortality associated with the self-reported intake of such substances (33). In this area, future studies might profit from the use of biological markers to define the exposure status and overcome some of the limitations of the studies based on self-report.

In contrast, smoking is an established causal risk factor for stomach cancer. An analysis in the EPIC study attributed about every sixth case of gastric cancer to cigarette smoking (34).

Other comorbid conditions such as pernicious anemia are long known risk factors associated with gastric cancer and the risk in presence of this condition is increased about threefold (35). Intake of non-steroidal anti-inflammatory drugs (NSAIDs), including aspirin, shows a preventive effect on stomach cancer in a dose–dependent manner. However, the gastrointestinal complications and the associated risk of the long-term use demand a thorough risk–benefit analysis, which may nevertheless result in a useful strategy in a high-risk population (36).

A positive family history is also associated with an increased risk for stomach cancer. Beside sharing some genetic commonalities, it may also express the familial exposure to other risk factors, such as infection with *H. pylori* (37).

Obesity is a further associated risk factor of gastric cancer as well as of other cancers (38). Notably, in a prospective study including over 900,000 US adults, a clear increase in risk was only seen in men in the highest body mass category. It was almost double in the category 35–40 kg/m² when compared with men of normal weight (18.5–24.9 kg/m²).

Several occupational factors such as dusts, exposure to nitrogen oxides, *N*-nitroso compounds, and ionizing radiation have been described as related to stomach cancer in certain occupational groups such as carpenters, steel workers and tin miners, and workers of the chemical and coal mining industry (39). However, their contribution to overall risk on a population-based level seems to be small.

4. Conclusions

Discovery of *H. pylori* and disclosure of its key role in the development of distal stomach cancer within the past 25 years has revolutionized the understanding of stomach cancer, which can now be considered, to a large extent, as a disease of infectious origin. However, many of the co-factors leading from infection to development of stomach cancer among a minority of infected individuals remain poorly understood and need to be focused on in future epidemiological research. The strong reduction in stomach cancer incidence and mortality in the past decades was achieved without specific, targeted measures of prevention. On the basis of identification of mechanisms and factors leading from *H. pylori* infection to stomach cancer, specific prevention measures, such as targeted eradication of the infection, especially among high-risk groups, may become a promising strategy for further reduction of the burden of the disease in the future.

References

1. Ferlay, J., Bray, F., Pisani, P., and Parkin, D. M. (2004) GLOBOCAN 2002: Cancer incidence, mortality and prevalence worldwide. IARC CancerBase No. 5. Version 2.0, IARC Press, Lyon, France [online available from http://www-dep.iarc.fr].

2. International Agency for Research on Cancer, World Health Organization (1994) Infection with *Helicobacter pylori*, in *Schistosomes, liver flukes and Helicobacter pylori*, IARC Monogr. Eval. Carcinog. Risks Hum. Vol. 60, Lyon, France, pp. 177–240.

3. Campbell, D. I., Warren, B. F., Thomas, J. E., Figura, N., Telford, J. L., and Sullivan, P. B. (2001) The African enigma: low prevalence of gastric atrophy, high prevalence of chronic inflammation in West African adults and children. *Helicobacter.* **6**, 263–267.

4. Brenner, H. (2002) Long-term survival rates of cancer patients achieved by the end of the 20th century: a period analysis. *Lancet* **360**, 1131–1135.

5. Parkin, D. M., Bray, F., Ferlay, J., and Pisani, P. (2005) Global cancer statistics, 2002. *CA Cancer J. Clin.* **55**, 74–108.

6. Forman, D. and Burley, V. J. (2006) Gastric cancer: global pattern of the disease and an overview of environmental risk factors. *Best Pract. Res. Clin. Gastroenterol.* **20**, 633–649.

7. Parkin, D. M., Whelan, S. L., Ferlay, J., and Storm, H. (2005) Cancer incidence in five continents, Vol I to VIII, IARC CancerBase No. 7, IARC Press, Lyon, France [online available from http://www-dep.iarc.fr].

8. Berrino, F. (2003) The EUROCARE Study: strengths, limitations and perspectives of population-based, comparative survival studies. *Ann. Oncol.* **14** Suppl 5, v9–13.

9. Gatta, G., Capocaccia, R., Coleman, M. P., Gloeckler Ries, L. A., Hakulinen, T., Micheli, A., Sant, M., Verdecchia, A., and Berrino, F. (2000) Toward a comparison of survival in American and European cancer patients. *Cancer* **89**, 893–900.

10. Verdecchia, A., Mariotto, A., Gatta, G., Bustamante-Teixeira, M. T., and Ajiki, W. (2003) Comparison of stomach cancer incidence and survival in four continents. *Eur. J. Cancer* **39**, 1603–1609.

11. Crew, K. D. and Neugut, A. I. (2006) Epidemiology of gastric cancer. *World J. Gastroenterol.* **12**, 354–362.

12. Banatvala, N., Mayo, K., Megraud, F., Jennings, R., Deeks, J. J., and Feldman, R. A. (1993) The cohort effect and *Helicobacter pylori*. *J. Infect. Dis.* **168**, 219–221.

13. Roosendaal, R., Kuipers, E. J., Buitenwerf, J., van Uffelen, C., Meuwissen, S. G., van Kamp, G. J., and Vandenbroucke-Grauls, C. M. (1997) *Helicobacter pylori* and the birth cohort effect: evidence of a continuous decrease of infection rates in childhood. *Am. J. Gastroenterol.* **92**, 1480–1482.

14. Marshall, B. J. and Warren, J. R. (1984) Unidentified curved bacilli in the stomach of patients with gastritis and peptic ulceration. *Lancet* **1**, 1311–1315.

15. Helicobacter pylori and Cancer Collaborative Group (2001) Gastric cancer and *Helicobacter pylori*: a combined analysis of 12 case control studies nested within prospective cohorts. *Gut* **49**, 347–353.

16. Ekström, A. M., Held, M., Hansson, L. E., Engstrand, L., and Nyren, O. (2001) *Helicobacter pylori* in gastric cancer established by CagA immunoblot as a marker of past infection. *Gastroenterology* **121**, 784–791.

17. Brenner, H., Arndt, V., Stegmaier, C., Ziegler, H., and Rothenbacher, D. (2004) Is *Helicobacter pylori* infection a necessary condition for noncardia gastric cancer? *Am. J. Epidemiol.* **159**, 252–258.

18. Rothenbacher, D. and Brenner, H. (2003) Burden of *Helicobacter pylori* and *H. pylori*-related diseases in developed countries:

recent developments and future implications. *Microbes Infect.* **5**, 693–703.

19. Huang, J. Q., Zheng, G. F., Sumanac, K., Irvine, E. J., and Hunt, R. H. (2003) Meta-analysis of the relationship between cagA seropositivity and gastric cancer. *Gastroenterology* **125**, 1636–1644.

20. El-Omar, E. M., Rabkin, C. S., Gammon, M. D., Vaughan, T. L., Risch, H. A., Schoenberg, J. B., Stanford, J. L., Mayne, S. T., Goedert, J., Blot, W. J., Fraumeni, J. F., Jr., and Chow, W. H. (2003) Increased risk of noncardia gastric cancer associated with proinflammatory cytokine gene polymorphisms. *Gastroenterology* **124**, 1193–1201.

21. Brenner, H., Arndt, V., Bode, G., Stegmaier, C., Ziegler, H., and Stumer, T. (2002) Risk of gastric cancer among smokers infected with *Helicobacter pylori. Int. J. Cancer* **98**, 446–449.

22. Brenner, H., Arndt, V., Stürmer, T., Stegmaier, C., Ziegler, H., and Dhom, G. (2000) Individual and joint contribution of family history and *Helicobacter pylori* infection to the risk of gastric carcinoma. *Cancer* **88**, 274–279.

23. Rothenbacher, D., Inceoglu, J., Bode, G., and Brenner, H. (2000) Acquisition of *Helicobacter pylori* infection in a high-risk population occurs within the first 2 years of life. *J. Pediatr.* **136**, 744–748.

24. Rothenbacher, D., Bode, G., and Brenner, H. (2002) Dynamics of *Helicobacter pylori* infection in early childhood in a high-risk group living in Germany: loss of infection higher than acquisition. *Aliment. Pharmacol. Ther.* **16**, 1663–1668.

25. Weyermann, M., Adler, G., Brenner, H., and Rothenbacher, D. (2006) The mother as source of *Helicobacter pylori* infection. *Epidemiology* **17**, 332–334.

26. Wong, B. C., Lam, S. K., Wong, W. M., Chen, J. S., Zheng, T. T., Feng, R. E., Lai, K. C., Hu, W. H., Yuen, S. T., Leung, S. Y., Fong, D. Y., Ho, J., Ching, C. K., and Chen, J. S. (2004) *Helicobacter pylori* eradication to prevent gastric cancer in a high-risk region of China: a randomized controlled trial. *JAMA* **291**, 187–194.

27. Fuccio, L., Zagari, R. M., Minardi, M. E., and Bazzoli, F. (2007) Systematic review: *Helicobacter pylori* eradication for the prevention of gastric cancer. *Aliment. Pharmacol. Ther.* **25**, 133–141.

28. Kamineni, A., Williams, M. A., Schwartz, S. M., Cook, L. S., and Weiss, N. S. (1999) The incidence of gastric carcinoma in Asian migrants to the United States and their descendants. *Cancer Causes Control* **10**, 77–83.

29. Jakszyn, P. and Gonzalez, C. A. (2006) Nitrosamine and related food intake and gastric and oesophageal cancer risk: a systematic review of the epidemiological evidence. *World J. Gastroenterol.* **12**, 4296–4303.

30. Riboli, E. and Norat, T. (2003) Epidemiologic evidence of the protective effect of fruit and vegetables on cancer risk. *Am. J. Clin. Nutr.* **78**, 559S–569S.

31. Gonzalez, C. A., Pera, G., Agudo, A., Bueno-de-Mesquita, H. B., Ceroti, M., Boeing, H., Schulz, M., Del Giudice, G., Plebani, M., Carneiro, F., Berrino, F., Sacerdote, C., Tumino, R., Panico, S., Berglund, G., Siman, H., Hallmans, G., Stenling, R., Martinez, C., Dorronsoro, M., Barricarte, A., Navarro, C., Quiros, J. R., Allen, N., Key, T. J., Bingham, S., Day, N. E., Linseisen, J., Nagel, G., Overvad, K., Jensen, M. K., Olsen, A., Tjonneland, A., Buchner, F. L., Peeters, P. H., Numans, M. E., Clavel-Chapelon, F., Boutron-Ruault, M. C., Roukos, D., Trichopoulou, A., Psaltopoulou, T., Lund, E., Casagrande, C., Slimani, N., Jenab, M., and Riboli, E. (2006) Fruit and vegetable intake and the risk of stomach and oesophagus adenocarcinoma in the European Prospective Investigation into Cancer and Nutrition (EPIC-EURGAST). *Int. J. Cancer* **118**, 2559–2566.

32. Gonzalez, C. A., Jakszyn, P., Pera, G., Agudo, A., Bingham, S., Palli, D., Ferrari, P., Boeing, H., del Giudice, G., Plebani, M., Carneiro, F., Nesi, G., Berrino, F., Sacerdote, C., Tumino, R., Panico, S., Berglund, G., Siman, H., Nyren, O., Hallmans, G., Martinez, C., Dorronsoro, M., Barricarte, A., Navarro, C., Quiros, J. R., Allen, N., Key, T. J., Day, N. E., Linseisen, J., Nagel, G., Bergmann, M. M., Overvad, K., Jensen, M. K., Tjonneland, A., Olsen, A., Bueno-de-Mesquita, H. B., Ocke, M., Peeters, P. H., Numans, M. E., Clavel-Chapelon, F., Boutron-Ruault, M. C., Trichopoulou, A., Psaltopoulou, T., Roukos, D., Lund, E., Hemon, B., Kaaks, R., Norat, T., and Riboli, E. (2006) Meat intake and risk of stomach and esophageal adenocarcinoma within the European Prospective Investigation Into Cancer and Nutrition (EPIC). *J. Natl. Cancer Inst.* **98**, 345–354.

33. Jacobs, E. J., Connell, C. J., McCullough, M. L., Chao, A., Jonas, C. R., Rodriguez, C., Calle, E. E., and Thun, M. J. (2002) Vitamin C, vitamin E, and multivitamin supplement use and stomach cancer mortality in the Cancer Prevention Study II

cohort. *Cancer Epidemiol. Biomarkers Prev.*
11, 35–41.

34. Gonzalez, C. A., Pera, G., Agudo, A., Palli, D., Krogh, V., Vineis, P., Tumino, R., Panico, S., Berglund, G., Siman, H., Nyren, O., Agren, A., Martinez, C., Dorronsoro, M., Barricarte, A., Tormo, M. J., Quiros, J. R., Allen, N., Bingham, S., Day, N., Miller, A., Nagel, G., Boeing, H., Overvad, K., Tjonneland, A., Bueno-De-Mesquita, H. B., Boshuizen, H. C., Peeters, P., Numans, M., Clavel-Chapelon, F., Helen, I., Agapitos, E., Lund, E., Fahey, M., Saracci, R., Kaaks, R., and Riboli, E. (2003) Smoking and the risk of gastric cancer in the European Prospective Investigation Into Cancer and Nutrition (EPIC). *Int. J. Cancer* **107**, 629–634.

35. Brinton, L. A., Gridley, G., Hrubec, Z., Hoover, R., and Fraumeni, J. F., Jr. (1989) Cancer risk following pernicious anaemia. *Br. J. Cancer* **59**, 810–813.

36. Wang, W. H., Huang, J. Q., Zheng, G. F., Lam, S. K., Karlberg, J., and Wong, B. C. (2003) Non-steroidal anti-inflammatory drug use and the risk of gastric cancer: a systematic review and meta-analysis. *J. Natl. Cancer Inst.* **95**, 1784–1791.

37. Brenner, H., Bode, G., and Boeing, H. (2000) *Helicobacter pylori* infection among offspring of patients with stomach cancer. *Gastroenterology* **118**, 31–35.

38. Calle, E. E., Rodriguez, C., Walker-Thurmond, K., and Thun, M. J. (2003) Overweight, obesity, and mortality from cancer in a prospectively studied cohort of U.S. adults. *N. Engl. J. Med.* **348**, 1625–1638.

39. Raj, A., Mayberry, J. F., and Podas, T. (2003) Occupation and gastric cancer. *Postgrad. Med. J.* **79**, 252–258.

INDEX